PSYCHIATRY LEARNING SYSTEM

(Revised Edition)

Patricia M. Randels, M.D.
Lorenz Villeponteaux, Ph.D.
Luis A. Marco, M.D.
Darlene L. Shaw, Ph.D.
Layton McCurdy, M.D.

Health Sciences Consortium
200 Eastowne Drive
Chapel Hill, North Carolina 27514

ISBN 0-938938-03-7

Cover: Josephine A. Killeffer & Bogara

Printed in the United States of America

DEDICATION

INGA TAYLOR, M.D.
December 28, 1943 - July 14, 1980

Dr. Inga Taylor was Associate Professor of Psychiatry at the Medical University of South Carolina and staff psychiatrist at the Charleston Veterans Administration Hospital. Energetic, purposeful, dedicated, enthusiastic, and devoted are words which have been used to describe her. To the editors and many of the contributors to the Psychiatry Learning System she was a friend and colleague.

It is with affection and sadness that we dedicate this edition of the Psychiatry Learning System to the memory of Inga who, while only thirty-six years old at her death, taught us all.

PREFACE

This text has been written specifically for the medical student who is doing a clerkship in psychiatry. Since 1972, previous editions of the *Psychiatry Learning System* (PLS) have been used at the Medical University of South Carolina to replace didactic lectures during the psychiatry clerkship. The PLS has not been used as a substitute for ward experience or for faculty supervision. On the contrary, we view this material as a means of enhancing the experiential aspects of the clerkship.

While this edition, like the previous editions, is written in a programmed format, we now have gone to a somewhat different style which presents the material in longer sections rather than in very short "frames." The feedback questions, or, as we call them, the "Quiz Questions," are grouped at the end of sections rather than being interspersed throughout the chapter. This has been done on the assumption that medical students do not need feedback at intervals as frequent as the intervals in previous editions. Furthermore, we think that this new format makes "working" the text a much more smooth and coherent process. Additionally, the pre- and post-tests are included in the text rather than in a separate workbook. We think that this will facilitate the use of the program. The PLS consists of a text interdigitated with videotaped clinical examples. The text has nineteen chapters which are divided into three sections. In Section I there are four chapters on the assessment of patients with mental disorders. There are eleven chapters in Section II which describe the mental disorders and provide the diagnostic criteria for these disorders. Section III is composed of four chapters all dealing with treatment modalities.

While the text and the videotaped examples were designed to be used together, this edition of the text has been written in such a way that it can stand alone, i.e., without the videotapes. Our experience, however, has been that the videotapes, used with the text, greatly enhance and reinforce the learning process.

Nearly all of the tapes for this revised edition have been made from new patient material. In a few instances, actors were used instead of "real" patients. These actors are listed in the Acknowledgments. The vast majority of the videotapes, however, are from interviews with actual patients. While we have gone to great lengths to obtain informed consent from the patients and, in some instances, from the patients' families, this material is still considered CONFIDENTIAL. We expect that users will treat the videotapes as such. The tapes are distributed for professional education only.

We have made extensive efforts to adhere to the third edition of the *Diagnostic and Statistical Manual of Mental Disorders* (DSM-III, 1980), and we have attempted to find case examples which fit the diagnostic categories of that manual. Whenever diagnostic criteria for mental disorders appear in the text they come directly from the DSM-III.

Here is one final note of caution. There are many instances in the text where appropriate pharmacological interventions of mental disorders are noted. Knowledge about drugs accumulates rapidly. Therefore, before prescribing drugs for any disorder, one should go to the current literature to verify dosage, side effects, precautions, and new insights on mechanisms of action.

PREFACE

HOW TO USE THE PLS

First, it is important to use the materials only as long as you are alert because fatigue interferes with efficient learning. We advise you to take frequent short breaks, preferrably at 20- to 30-minute intervals.

Begin with the written text. Read the chapter outline and the learning objectives. Answer the pre-test questions, and then check your answers. This will tell you how much you already know about the material in the chapter, as well as how much you do not know. Now read the text. You will come to groups of "Quiz Questions" which are designed to give you feedback about whether or not you have learned the material. We suggest that you actually write your responses (or circle the appropriate response) to the "Quiz Questions." This is another aid to learning.

Continue with the written material until you come to an instruction which directs you to:

****

GO TO VIDEOTAPE

****

At this point you should insert the appropriate videotape in the playback machine and view the designated segment. At the end of the taped segment you will hear a series of "beeps" and will see a written instruction on the television screen to:

STOP TAPE
*****
RETURN TO TEXT

Continue to work through the text and the videotapes until you complete the chapter. You should then take the post-test at the end of the chapter. This is for self-assessment and will tell you how well you have learned the material.

You may start with almost any chapter, especially in the section on specific disorders. This will allow you to integrate your course of study with your clinical work with patients.

ACKNOWLEDGMENTS

A great many people have contributed large amounts of time and energy to the production of this edition of the *Psychiatry Learning System*. In a general way, the Medical University of South Carolina and the Department of Psychiatry and Behavioral Sciences provided both financial and moral support, as well as encouragement for the project.

Grateful appreciation is extended to Maria Brown, Lynn McBride, and Audrey DeLong, who as research technicians, did much of the library work, and proofing, the organizational details, and hundreds of other editorial chores in connection with the text and the videotapes.

Much of the typing on the text, including the several drafts of each chapter, as well as the final copy, was done by Hannah Dimmock and Vicki Brumbelow. We are especially grateful to Pam Thompson, who both typed and edited the final manuscript, and to Jane Britt, who always made time to help. We also very much appreciate the work of Mary Villeponteaux in proofreading the entire text.

We wish to thank Pat Clute and his staff at the Medical University of South Carolina Print Shop who performed so many tasks for us and who were quite tolerant of our errors. We also admire and appreciate the work of the Audiovisual Services of the Medical University, especially the Art Section. Florence E. Goodwin and Kevin J. McPhillips did all of our figures and tables and made our lead-in board for all of the videotapes.

The Television Section of the Division of Continuing Education of the Medical University of South Carolina spent enormous amounts of time, both in Charleston, South Carolina, and in Coatesville, Pennsylvania, taping interviews and editing hundreds of hours of videotape to produce the final product. We are indebted to Daniel J. Mallard, Director of Television Production Operations, Norman E. Cooper, Jr., Kenneth L. Repsher, and Charles L. Riecke, III, Jack R. Petit, Jr., and William Edmund Bates, III. We also greatly appreciate the work of the two narrators for the videotapes, Gerald Donovan M.D., and Mrs. Mariett R. Wicks.

The sources of patient material were primarily the Medical University of South Carolina Psychiatry Inpatient Service and the Veterans Administration Medical Centers at Charleston, South Carolina, and at Coatesville, Pennsylvania. To the administrators and staff of those clinical facilities we are greatly indebted.

ACKNOWLEDGMENTS

In a few instances, we used actors to portray patients. We wish to acknowledge their skill and express our appreciation for their willingness to perform. The actors are:

John Diamond, M.D.	Cognitive Therapy tape
Lynn McBride	Biofeedback tape
Julia C. S. Keefe	Sexual Dysfunctions tape
Shelia D. Johnston	Sexual Dysfunctions tape
Ronald D. Holmes	Sexual Dysfunctions tape
William Bender	Sexual Dysfunctions tape

We are also enormously grateful to all who conducted interviews with patients and were willing to have those interviews videotaped:

Jeffry J. Andresen, M.D.
Michael R. Bartos, M.D.
Oliver J. W. Bjorksten, M.D.
Miriam DeAntonio, M.D.
Gerald M. Donovan, M.D.
Donald W. Fennell, M.D.
Leo C. Freeman, M.D.
David L. Goldberg, M.D.
John H. Heiligenstein, M.D.
Valerie L. Holmstrom, Ph.D.
James B. Hoyme, M.D.
J. Eric Jones, M.D.
Charles S. Jordan, Ph.D.
Ada Kirkman, M.D.
E. Michael Lampkin, M.D.
Kenneth T. Lennington, M.D.
Layton McCurdy, M.D.
J. Bryce McLaulin, M.D.

Donald E. Manning, M.D.
Luis A. Marco, M.D.
Joseph H. Marshall, M.D.
Patrick M. O'Neil, Ph.D.
Victor Prockow
Patricia M. Randels, M.D.
Elizabeth E. Read, M.D.
Eric L. Ressner, M.D.
Rob Richardson, M.D.
John M. Roberts, M.D.
John C. Roitzsch, Ph.D.
Alberto B. Santos, M.D.
Bahman Sholevar, M.D.
Robert H. Sinnott, M.D.
Thomas E. Steele, M.D.
Margery S. Sved, M.D.
Lorenz Villeponteaux, Ph.D.
Brian L. West, Ph.D.

The preparation of the PLS was greatly enhanced by the work of the Health Sciences Consortium, Chapel Hill, North Carolina. Frank Penta, Ed.D., and his staff provided invaluable assistance by obtaining peer review of the text. Uldarico P. Dátiles, Ed.D., spent many hours tediously proofing the manuscript and offering excellent instructional design suggestions.

For the provision of support for typing, videotaping, organizing, and getting the work done we are very grateful to Hal S. Currey, Business Manager of the Department of Psychiatry and Behavioral Sciences.

Finally, we owe a great deal of thanks to the many patients who were willing to appear on videotape in order to help teach mental health professionals.

TABLE OF CONTENTS

VIDEOTAPES
AND
VIDEOTAPE EDITORS

Psychiatric Evaluation	C1-1	Patricia M. Randels, M.D. Layton McCurdy, M.D.
Psychodynamic Considerations and Defense Mechanisms	C2-1	Layton McCurdy, M.D. Miriam DeAntonio, M.D. Lorenz Villeponteaux, Ph.D.
Psychological Evaluation	C3-1	Darlene L. Shaw, Ph.D. Valerie L. Holmstrom, Ph.D.
Psychosocial Factors in Physical Illness	C4-1	Robert Malcolm, M.D. Brian L. West, Ph.D.
Organic Mental Disorders	C5-1	Luis A. Marco, M.D. Patricia M. Randels, M.D.
Schizophrenic Disorders, Psychoses Not Elsewhere Classified, and Paranoid Disorders	C7-1 C7-2	Patricia M. Randels, M.D.
Affective Disorders	C8-1 C8-2	Thomas E. Steele, M.D. Lorenz Villeponteaux, Ph.D.
Anxiety Disorders	C9-1	Lorenz Villeponteaux, Ph.D. Miriam DeAntonio, M.D.
Somatoform and Dissociative Disorders	C10-1 C10-2	Donald E. Manning, M.D. Lorenz Villeponteaux, Ph.D.
Psychosexual Disorders	C11-1 C11-2	Lorenz Villeponteaux, Ph.D. Darlene L. Shaw, Ph.D.
Impulse Control Disorders	C12-1	Lorenz Villeponteaux, Ph.D.
Personality Disorders	C13-1 C13-2	Donald E. Manning, M.D. Lorenz Villeponteaux, Ph.D.
Disorders of Infancy, Childhood, and Adolescence	C15-1 C15-2	Lorenz Villeponteaux, Ph.D.
Behavioral Treatment	C18-1 C18-2	Alberto B. Santos, M.D. Lorenz Villeponteaux, Ph.D.
Other Treatment Modalities	C19-1	Alberto B. Santos, M.D. Lorenz Villeponteaux, Ph.D.

Section I

Assessments

This section consists of four chapters all dealing with the assessment of mental disorders. The assumption is made that you have previously studied normal human behavior in a behavioral sciences or life cycle course.

Chapter 1, Psychiatric Evaluation, provides one approach to the interview, that of Norman Kagan. There are others, of course, but our goal is not to provide an exhaustive survey of interviewing techniques and styles. Rather, we hope to give you a clear, cogent view of a usable approach. In this chapter you also will learn about the basic assessment tool of the psychiatrist, the "mental status examination."

Chapter 2, Psychodynamic Considerations and Ego Defense Mechanisms, deals with theories of the unconscious and with some of the ways the unconscious is manifested verbally and behaviorally. Any assessment of human behavior must take into consideration ways in which human beings alter reality in a self-protective way.

Chapter 3, Psychological Evaluation, reviews the use of various psychological tests in the assessment of patients. Issues of reliability and validity of tests, of what can and cannot be expected from testing, and of when to seek psychological consultation are addressed.

Chapter 4, Psychosocial Factors in Physical Illness, contains material on the relationship between the mind and the body. This is a subject of more than passing interest to the primary care physician who sees a significant number of patients in whom there is a prominent interaction between physical illness and mental functioning.

To reiterate from the Preface, you will not learn all there is to know about the assessment of mental disorders merely by studying this section. You will need clinical experience and supervision to be able to effectively collect data about a patient and then organize those data to formulate an evaluation.

CHAPTER 1

Psychiatric Evaluation
Patricia M. Randels, M.D.
Layton McCurdy, M.D.
Pamela J. Saunders, M.S.W.

CHAPTER OUTLINE

LEARNING OBJECTIVES

After completing this chapter you will be able to:

1. Describe appropriate techniques for beginning, conducting, and terminating the interview.

2. Describe the process of conducting a psychiatric evaluation, including taking a history and doing a mental status examination.

3. Formulate a multiaxial diagnosis including the concepts of psychosocial stressors and predisposing factors.

4. Define the following terms:

    Rapport
    Empathy
    Mood
    Affect
    Circumstantiality
    Tangentiality
    Delusion
    Hypochondriasis
    Phobia
    Hallucination
    Judgement
    Reality testing

PRE-TEST

For each of the following questions, <u>one</u> or <u>more than one</u> answer may be correct. Circle the correct answer(s).

1. Which of the following is/are true concerning the psychiatric evaluation?

   a. Establishing rapport makes it more likely that the physician will obtain pertinent information from the patient.
   b. A complete psychiatric diagnosis can usually be made once you have completed the psychiatric history and mental status examination.
   c. The mental status examination provides information about the patient's functioning at the time of the exam, while the psychiatric history gives a more longitudinal view.
   d. When rating the severity of a stress, it is important to take into account the individual's vulnerability to a particular stress, rather than how an average person might experience the stress.

2. In obtaining a psychiatric history,

   a. it is necessary to elicit the existence of delusions, hallucinations, or ideas of reference in order to make a diagnosis of an Affective Disorder.
   b. loss of recent memory for important information is indicative of a neurotic reaction.
   c. suicidal tendencies in the patient are likely to be aggravated by the physician's inquiring about them.
   d. psychological or emotional processes in the physician can influence the type of information he obtains.

3. Note-taking during the psychiatric evaluation

   a. may be considered by the patient as a sign of the physician's interest.
   b. should be discontinued if the patient objects.
   c. is permissible with reassurance to the patient that all notes are confidential.
   d. will <u>not</u> be necessary if the physician has a well-trained memory.

4. Open-ended questions should be used in which of the following interviewing situations?

   a. during the opening phase
   b. when the patient is hesitant in talking about himself
   c. when questioning the patient about his feelings
   d. when the patient tends to be very circumstantial

5. When terminating an interview, which of the following steps is/are useful?

    a. Summarize for the patient what you have learned.
    b. Define your role beyond this encounter.
    c. Ask the patient if he has any questions for you.
    d. End the interview on a positive note.

For each of the following questions, circle the letter corresponding to the one correct response.

6. The term rapport is defined as

    a. the development of a fondness between the patient and physician.
    b. the displacement of affect from one object to another.
    c. the process of helping the patient to speak freely and describe his problems fully.
    d. the arousal of the physician's repressed feelings by the interview situation.
    e. a harmonious and unconstrained relationship between the patient and physician.

7. "Transference" is a term used to designate the

    a. physician's reaction to the patient.
    b. referral of the patient to another physician.
    c. carry-over of feelings and attitudes from previous relationships.
    d. establishment of positive feelings toward the doctor.
    e. need for terminating the treatment.

The statements or questions that follow are posed by patients in evaluative and therapeutic interviews. In each instance, select the most appropriate response for the physician.

8. Early in her first interview with a male physician a female patient says, "I think all men are jerks."
   Physician:

    a. "Your experience with men must certainly have been disagreeable for you to have this feeling."
    b. "What makes you feel this way?"
    c. "I understand why you feel this way now."
    d. "With an attitude like this, you'll get nowhere."
    e. "Perhaps you would like me to refer you to another physician."

9. A 33-year-old bachelor presents as his initial complaint: "I feel cold and detached in the presence of women."
Physician:

   a. "That's because you are afraid of women."
   b. "Tell me about your experience."
   c. "You must want to destroy women, and thus you have to protect yourself from them."
   d. "Don't worry. That feeling is very common."
   e. "It is probable that this reflects your feeling toward your mother."

10. During an initial interview, a woman, after mentioning that she has been married three times previously, reviews her current husband's frequent angry outbursts toward her in some detail. Of the following, the best immediate response from the physician would be:

   a. "What do you do to arouse his anger?"
   b. "Have you always chosen ill-tempered men?"
   c. "Were there similar problems with your previous husbands?"
   d. "Perhaps you make men angry."
   e. "Perhaps you just don't like men."

11. A 42-year-old man comes to your office and states, "I've had a problem with drinking, and my wife says she'll leave if I don't get help. I'm not an alcoholic. I haven't drunk anything for a week, and I've made up my mind to stop, so I don't believe I need a doctor."
You would now respond:

   a. "As long as you're here, we might as well talk about how you're getting along."
   b. "Would you give me a dollar for every time you've made up your mind to stop?"
   c. "Most alcoholics act just as you do."
   d. "Your wife seems to think you do."
   e. "Have you ever had hallucinations while coming off alcohol?"

12. The patient goes on to state that if he has a problem it is only because his wife has been refusing to participate in sexual intercourse which makes him tense and angry.
You would now respond:

   a. "Have you tried getting someone else?"
   b. "How do you feel about that?"
   c. "Have you talked with her about it?"
   d. "Have you had sexual troubles in the past?"
   e. "Sometimes women act that way, but why do you handle it by drinking?"

13. A married woman in psychotherapy for anxiety attacks, initially evasive about why she is anxious when alone at home, admits that she is afraid a man might break into the house. She then says, "I don't see anything abnormal about that. None of the women I know like to be alone at night." The most appropriate intervention might be:

    a. "From what you've told me, I really don't think that you have anything to worry about."
    b. "I agree, that's not abnormal."
    c. "Let's try to understand your feelings about this particular situation."
    d. "Perhaps you could get a friend to stay with you."
    e. "Don't you think it would be best not to limit your life just because you're afraid?"

14. A 26-year-old woman appeared in the emergency room requesting help. She spoke in a very soft manner, resembling that of a small child. Although her narrative was somewhat disorganized and rambling, she did relate that her father had just called her to tell her that her mother had died that day from a heart attack. She reported that shortly after this she felt "dazed" and began to feel that she had, in some way, been responsible for causing her mother's death. Then she began to cry and was unable to continue speaking for several minutes.
    At this point in the interview, the best technique would be to say:

    a. "That's all right, dear. Don't cry. I'm certain that everything will work out all right."
    b. "These feelings are very interesting. We must talk more about them."
    c. Nothing, and wait for the patient to regain her composure.
    d. "I can appreciate how you feel after hearing such upsetting news."
    e. "It must be difficult for you if you have guilt feelings about your mother."

15. You are in family practice. A 28-year-old woman comes into your office and complains about having pain while having intercourse. She states that she has been having problems with her husband who drinks. She states that she has not enjoyed intercourse with him ever, but the pain is new and worries her. You would now respond:

    a. "When did you last have a gynecological exam?"
    b. "What do you mean by 'with him'?"
    c. "Tell me more about things."
    d. "Have you spoken to a marriage counselor?"
    e. "How bad is your husband's problem with alcohol?"

16. Later in the interview she states, with hesitation, that she does feel guilty about the fact that she did get so angry with her husband that she had an affair, just before the pain started.
Your response would be:

   a. "Do you think your pain might represent unconscious guilt over the affair?"
   b. "Did he find out?"
   c. "Have you had pain after the affair?"
   d. "Tell me more about your pathological guilt feelings."
   e. Silence to find out if the patient will continue.

Match each concept with the appropriate description. Lettered items may be used once, more than once, or not at all.

___17. open-ended question
___18. facilitation
___19. empathy
___20. respect
___21. genuineness
___22. mental status
___23. insight
___24. reality testing

   a. specifies topic in general terms
   b. a response that indicates you are listening, interested, and want the patient to continue talking
   c. the ability to understand another person and to communicate that understanding
   d. ability of patient to comprehend his current situation correctly
   e. evaluation of current psychological functioning
   f. positive regard
   g. authenticity
   h. the ability to distinguish between productions of one's own mind and the real world

Match the following axes of a multiaxial diagnosis with the appropriate definitions.

___25. Axis I
___26. Axis II
___27. Axis III
___28. Axis IV
___29. Axis V

   a. physical disorders
   b. personality disorders
   c. highest level of adaptive functioning during past year
   d. clinical psychiatric syndromes
   e. psychosocial stressors

I. INTRODUCTION

The psychiatric evaluation of a patient may involve a variety of procedures, including a physical and neurological examination. By far, the most frequently used procedure is what is called the mental status examination (MSE). This chapter focuses on the MSE and the means of conducting the examination, the psychiatric interview.

A. PURPOSES OF THE INTERVIEW

The interview is a basic tool of the physician. It is a systematic attempt to gain knowledge of the patient and the nature of the illness. It is through the interview that a history of the patient's present illness and past life is elicited, and the same principles apply in the interview of patients, whether they are seen in a psychiatric or medical setting. It is also through the interview that a mental status examination, an essential part of the physical examination, is performed.

A complete physical examination is necessary, but here we will focus on mental and psychological evaluation. A physical examination including a neurological examination should be performed, because some types of psychopathology may be precipitated or perpetuated by physical illness, and because a patient with somatic complaints may need to have these investigated before he can accept that his complaints may have a psychological cause and thus respond to psychiatric treatment.

The psychiatric history attempts to answer the question, "How did this person happen to become the way he is now?" and thus gives a longitudinal view of the patient. The psychiatric history encompasses chief complaints and history of the present illness, as well as a personal and family history and other features included in a general medical history. It should focus on relationships between occurrence of symptoms and life events and feelings.

See page 26 for an Outline for a Psychiatric History.

The Mental Status Examination (see page 29 for an outline) is an evaluation of the patient's current behavior and mental functioning, providing a cross-sectional perspective. Repetition of the patient's mental status is a reliable way of determining the patient's progress.

Both physical and psychiatric illnesses occur when the individual cannot adapt to external and/or internal events. Therefore, it is always important to examine the patient's environmental circumstances, as well as his internal make-up, when trying to determine the cause of the illness. With regard to the notion of causality in psychiatric illness, we are generally trying to examine the "psychodynamic cause," only because other specific etiological agents are not known for most psychiatric disorders. A dynamic formulation should include:

1) Psychosocial stressors (or precipitating events)
2) Predisposing factors
3) Areas of conflict about instinctual drives
4) Defense mechanisms used

We shall define each of these in turn.

1) <u>Psychosocial stressors</u>.
These stressors are environmental events or changes involving the individual's interpersonal relations, work, and living circumstances. Developmental phases such as puberty and the menopause are also considered to be psychosocial stressors. Physical illness can also be a psychosocial stressor. As described in DSM-III, the severity of the stress is based on how an average person with similar sociocultural values would experience the same stress. Thus the rating of the severity of the stress is not based on the individual's predisposition or vulnerability. According to recommendations in DSM-III, the judgement of severity should take into account: a) the amount of change in the individual's life caused by the stress; b) the degree to which the event is desired and under the individual's control, such as accepting a promotion or getting married; and c) the number of stressors.

2) <u>Predisposing factors</u>.
When psychosocial stressors, i.e., external precipitants, cannot be discovered, one may assume that the internal make-up of the individual strongly predisposes him to the psychiatric disorder. He is especially vulnerable and may experience as stressful something the average person would not. Predisposing factors may be due to genetic contributions or to the occurrence of psychosocial stresses during critical developmental periods. For example, the loss of a parent during childhood may predispose the individual to depression in later years.

3) <u>Conflict about instinctual drives</u>.
A special area of psychiatric evaluation pertaining to predisposing factors is the patient's conflict about instinctual drives, i.e., sex, aggression, and dependency. Conflict about instinctual drives is discussed more fully in Chapters 2 and 8. A psychiatric illness is often precipitated by stress relating to conflicts about instinctual drives; the conflict generally derives from past events, such as the familial and cultural norms in which the patient grew up.

4) <u>Defense mechanisms</u>.
The manner in which a person tends to cope with conflict about sex, aggression, and dependency may in itself be of etiological importance in the development of psychiatric symptoms. Sometimes a person may develop defense mechanisms (synonyms: coping mechanisms, mental mechanisms) to disguise from himself and others

the nature of his conflict. These mechanisms are sometimes pathological; that is, they are symptoms or produce symptoms. Defense mechanisms are presented in detail in Chapter 2.

QUIZ, Section I.A.

Match the numbered items with the lettered choices. Lettered items may be used once, more than once, or not at all.

___1.   history of present illness
___2.   mental status examination
___3.   assessment of conflict about instinctual drives

a.   necessary for evaluation of physical disorder
b.   necessary for evaluation of psychiatric disorder
c.   necessary for both

TRUE or FALSE: Indicate whether the following question is true (T) or false (F) by circling the appropriate letter.

T   F   4.   The mental status examination provides information about the patient's functioning at the time of the exam, while the psychiatric history gives a more longitudinal view.

Circle the letter corresponding to the one correct answer.

Use the following case study to answer questions 5-6.

This 35-year-old woman states that she has been hospitalized for treatment of her "basic problem...alcoholism." She describes feelings of "deep emptiness," an inability to give to her children, and a wish to escape from these feelings. She tries to escape by drinking. These feelings are accentuated when her husband, who travels in his work, is away. Her feelings of loneliness date from childhood. Her father was in the Army and the family moved frequently, so it was difficult for her to form close or lasting friendships. Her father died when she was 13, and she has sustained numerous other personal losses, saying, "Life is a series of goodbyes."

5.   Identify the likely psychosocial stressor(s).

a.   husband's traveling
b.   death of father
c.   a and b

6.   Identify the likely predisposing event(s).

a.   death of father
b.   frequent moving
c.   a and b

B. MULTIAXIAL DIAGNOSIS

A psychiatric evaluation should provide sufficient information to permit a complete or multiaxial diagnosis. DSM-III suggests five dimensions or "axes" to consider when making a psychiatric diagnosis:

Axis I	lists the specific clinical psychiatric syndrome(s)
Axis II	includes personality disorders and specific developmental disorders
Axis III	current physical disorders that may affect the psychiatric problems are listed here
Axis IV	psychosocial stressors and their severity are listed here
Axis V	describes the highest level of adaptive functioning during the past year

All the psychiatric diagnoses are listed on the first two axes, Axis I being psychiatric syndromes and Axis II being personality disorders. The DSM-III specifies criteria for each disorder. This text has included these criteria in the chapters describing the various disorders.

Recall that psychosocial stressors are events or changes involving the individual's interpersonal relationships, work, and living circumstances. The specific event or change should be listed on Axis IV, and the severity of the stress should be rated. The terms for grading the severity of psychosocial stressors include: 1, none; 2, minimal; 3, mild; 4, moderate; 5, severe; 6, extreme; 7, catastrophic. Examples of these ratings will be given in cases presented throughout the text.

Axis V is an assessment of the individual's adaptive functioning during the past year and takes into account interpersonal relations, work, and use of leisure time. The ratings range from superior to grossly impaired. Examples of the use of these ratings will be given throughout the text as case studies are presented. The level of adaptive functioning has prognostic implications in that usually an individual can be expected to return to a level of functioning that he has previously attained once the illness or problem has subsided.

QUIZ, Section I.B.

TRUE OR FALSE: Circle the correct letter.

T   F   1.   A complete psychiatric diagnosis can usually be made once you have completed the psychiatric history and mental status examination.

T   F   2.   When rating the severity of a stress, it is important to take into account the individual's vulnerability to a particular stress, rather than how an average person might experience the stress.

3.   Complete the following table by supplying the Axis numbers.

   a. Axis _____   psychiatric disorders
   b. Axis _____   personality disorders
   c. Axis _____   physical disorders
   d. Axis _____   psychological stressors
   e. Axis _____   highest level of adaptive functioning during past
                          year

4.   Using the DSM-III Axis IV rating scale, how would you rate the severity
     of stress in the following case?_____

     You are called to the emergency room to see a fireman who, that
     afternoon, narrowly escaped death in the collapse of a building
     roof when his team was fighting a fire. Two of the crew mem-
     bers were killed at that time. The patient is a 30-year-old
     married man who is cooperative and verbal. For the past eight
     years he has worked with the same fire-fighting team, and the
     two men who were killed were his best friends. As he describes
     the events he is physically shaking and periodically stops talking
     because of tears. He says he can still see in his mind his two
     friends falling under the crashing roof and hear their screams as
     they died. He repeatedly describes how "awful" it was.

II.   CONDUCTING AN INTERVIEW

A.   SETTING

Effective interviewing is undertaken in an atmosphere of attentiveness and
emotional objectivity. Not only is there freedom from interruption, but also
the assurance of privacy. There is no possibility of being overheard, no
possibility that confidential material will unwittingly be disclosed to persons
other than whom the patient designates.

The physical setting of the interview should be chosen for relative comfort
and unquestionable privacy for the benefit of both interviewer and patient.
It is generally helpful to arrange the seating so that the patient has a
clear path to the exit. This formality serves as an indication that the
patient is present by his own choice and has the option of leaving the
interview at any time; also, it is unlikely that you will want to serve as an
obstruction should the patient decide to terminate the interview.

What to do about permitting smoking in the office is a subtle issue. On
the one hand, there are pressures against smoking, and physicians should
not advocate smoking because of health reasons. On the other hand, your
patient comes to you, perhaps filled with anxieties and feeling that he
needs the crutch of smoking in order to relax and open up about his
problems. Psychiatrists appear more tolerant of smoking and usually
provide an ash tray in the office for the patient.

ANSWERS, Section I.A. _____

1.   c
2.   c
3.   c
4.   T
5.   a
6.   c

A convenient box of tissues is an item that should always be provided.

It is in this comfortable and private setting that, with the encouragement of the attentive and emotionally objective physician, the patient is free to address his concerns. It is this atmosphere which is conducive to the establishment of rapport, that quality of a relationship characterized by mutuality - mutual honesty, mutual participation, mutual responsibility, mutual trust, mutual respect. Encouraging the patient to be a responsible, sincere participant in matters concerning his well-being is the principal objective of establishing rapport. Rapport is important for at least two reasons:

1) It is essential that the doctor attain the patient's trust and cooperation in obtaining the information needed to make a diagnosis and develop a treatment plan.

2) Any treatment process or subsequent contact with the patient will be greatly influenced by the quality of initial encounters.

QUIZ, Section II.A.

Circle the correct answer(s). One or more than one answer may be correct.

1.   An appropriate setting in which to conduct an interview provides

a.   an atmosphere of attentiveness and emotional objectivity.
b.   physical comfort for patient and doctor.
c.   privacy.
d.   all of the above.

2.   The term "rapport" is defined as

a.   the development of a fondness between the patient and physician.
b.   the displacement of affect from one object to another.
c.   the process of helping the patient to speak freely and describe his problems fully.
d.   the arousal of the physician's repressed feelings by the interview situation.
e.   a harmonious and unconstrained relationship between the patient and physician.

TRUE or FALSE: Circle the correct letter.

T   F   3.   Establishing rapport makes it more likely that the physician will obtain pertinent information from the patient.

B. QUALITIES OF THE INTERVIEWER

It is of interest to consider the nature of the doctor-patient relationship in the context of the medical interview. The so-called "good patient," from the standpoint of the examiner, is one who is cooperative, objective, and not excessively demanding or dependent. The "good doctor," from the patient's standpoint, is one who possesses the qualities of empathy, respect, and genuineness.

Empathy is the ability to identify and understand the emotions and behavior of the patient and accurately communicate this understanding to the patient.

Respect or positive regard for the patient is communicated by the interviewer's efforts to understand the patient and by his real concern for the patient.

Genuineness is the quality of being authentic, real, and spontaneous; the degree to which interviewer's responses appear to reflect his true feelings.

It is for the sake of this latter quality - genuineness - that interviewing technique must necessarily be integrated by each individual student to suit his own personality.

There are attitudinal considerations important to the doctor-patient relationship in the context of the interview. For example, there may be personal qualities of your patient that discourage or prevent you from becoming truly empathic with them. Which patient is it that leaves you feeling angry, depressed, or ineffective? What sensitivity in yourself can you identify that allows this to happen? Are you able to manage your own sensitivity for the benefit of your patient and the professional relationship you have with him?

Similarly, the interviewer needs to be aware of shortcomings or defects of his personality that weaken his credibility and thereby his effectiveness as an interviewer.

Are there certain topics that are difficult or uncomfortable for you to discuss (e.g., sexuality, aggression, dependency)? Are there problems that you cannot or will not take seriously (e.g., your patient may consider his problem to be more problematical than you do)?

Do you tend to initially demonstrate concern and positive regard, only to withdraw these supportive gestures when your patient becomes dependent upon them? If so, what about this patient's dependency frightens you?

ANSWERS, Section I. B. _____

1. F
2. F
3. a. I
    b. II
    c. III
    d. IV
    e. V
4. 6

Is it realistic? Are there other patterns that seem to fit your relationships with patients? Considering these self-inquiry questions can be valuable to each physician.

Ask your patients and colleagues for the invaluable gift of feedback and let them know if you have learned something from the experience of working with them.

There are three ways to assess our effectiveness as interviewers:

1) Patient feedback
2) Colleague feedback
3) Self-inquiry (i.e., your personal assessment of your effectiveness)

Transference is defined as a reaction based on a distortion of past experience rather than a realistic response to the current situation. The physician's responses based on his own past experience are referred to as countertransference.

QUIZ, Section II.B.

Match the following terms with the appropriate definitions.

___1. empathy
___2. respect
___3. genuineness

a. positive regard
b. the ability to understand another person and to communicate understanding
c. authenticity

Circle the letter corresponding to the one correct response.

4. In obtaining a psychiatric history,

    a. it is necessary to elicit the existence of delusions, hallucinations, or ideas of reference in order to make a diagnosis of an Affective Disorder.

    b. loss of recent memory for important information is indicative of a neurotic reaction.

    c. suicidal tendencies in the patient are likely to be aggravated by the physician's inquiring about them.

    d. psychological or emotional processes in the physician can influence the type of information he obtains.

5. Transference is a term used to designate the

    a. physician's reaction to the patient.

    b. referral of the patient to another physician.

    c. carry-over of feelings and attitudes from previous relationships.

    d. establishment of positive feelings toward the doctor.

    e. need for terminating the treatment.

C. TECHNIQUES FOR INTERVIEW CONDUCT

The important steps in initiating an interview with a new patient include:

    1) Introducing yourself (shaking hands)

    2) Greeting the patient by name

    3) Defining your role or status

    4) Making explicit the purpose of the interview

    5) Telling the patient how much time is available for the task

    6) Asking the patient if he is at ease prior to the task

    7) If you plan to take notes or use an audiotape during the interview, asking the patient if he has any objections

During the course of several interviews you will want to obtain the data outlined under the Psychiatric History, obtaining information pertinent to chief complaint, present illness, and so forth. During the interview you will note the mental status of the patient and subsequently may ask specific questions relating to the mental status examination. All patients cannot adjust to the physician's frame of reference so you must adjust your information gathering to what the patient is willing and able to describe. In general, the interviewer should follow the patient's leads and postpone discussion of topics for which the patient seems unprepared. Indications that the patient is not prepared to discuss a topic suggested by the interviewer include vagueness, avoidance, long hesitations, and difficulty in organizing the response. Thus, you must permit the patient to structure the interview to some extent. The patient structures the interview by way of information he spontaneously reports and by avoiding topics he is not prepared to discuss.

Important interviewing techniques that promote communication and rapport include avoiding jargon, clarifying what the patient says, following the

ANSWERS, Section II.A. _____

1.   d
2.   e
3.   T

_____

leads the patient gives, the use of open-ended questions and brief questions, avoiding repetition, and the use of facilitating responses. The interviewer also needs to be able to deal with emotionally loaded material.

1.   Open-ended Question.
     A useful way to get at what is troubling the patient and yet al-
     low him latitude in what he wishes to say is to ask an open-ended
     question.   An open-ended question asks for information, specifying
     the topic in general terms.   For example, "What sort of problems
     are you having?"   "What brought you to the hospital?"   "Tell me
     what other things were going on at that time?"

     Exception: If the patient is confused or if thinking is disorganized,
     open-ended questions should be avoided.

2.   Clarifying and Following Leads.
     The patient supplies you with clues of which he may not recognize
     the full import.   The interviewer needs to be responsive to state-
     ments by the patient that may indicate unexplored problems.   The
     interviewer needs to clarify the situation.   You should question in
     depth to elicit full information, resolve ambiguities and inconsis-
     tencies.

     Suppose, in response to your open-ended question, you learn that
     your patient is fearful of closed spaces.   You don't just drop the
     subject there; you need to learn more about that symptom.   Just
     as you would follow up on a physical complaint, you ask "Under
     what circumstances?   When did it start?"   and so forth.

3.   Avoiding Jargon.
     You should avoid using technical or ambiguous words and request
     definitions of technical or ambiguous words used by your patient.
     Terms such as "nervous," "depression," and "paranoid" are exam-
     ples of those to be avoided because the meanings are often idiosyn-
     cratic.   You must get your patient to describe what he means by
     these words.   There are many slang words for drugs among sub-
     stance abusers; be sure you find out just what drugs your patient
     has been on.

     On the other hand, if you use jargon such as telling your patient
     he is employing "defense mechanisms" or is suffering from "Schizo-
     phrenia" or an "oedipus complex," then communication will be hin-
     dered.   Communication will be facilitated if doctor and patient use
     the same language, as simple, yet as precise as possible.

4. Brief Questions.
    The interviewer should avoid lengthy, complex questions, because not only will these serve to confuse the patient, but may also indicate what you expect to hear.

    Often a lengthy question can be answered by a yes or no from the patient, generally from which very little is learned. The interviewer should avoid qualifying what he wants the patient to tell him. For example, if you ask, "Did you come from a happy home?," it may make it more difficult for the patient to describe his unhappy home life. Or if you say, "Now let me ask you to do some simple math problems," the patient may feel belittled if he is unable to do those problems. Thus, it would be better to say: "What sort of home did you have?," "Now let me ask you to do some math problems."

    Sometimes it may be necessary to prompt reticent patients with choices such as "Was that because you were tired? or sick? or sad?" But most often you should allow the patient to supply you with the information.

5. Facilitating responses.
    This means that the interviewer encourages the patient to begin talking, or continue talking about a subject. Open-ended questions are one means of facilitation.

    Other facilitating responses the interviewer can use include:

    a) Facilitation: This is just a word such as "uh-huh," "yes," that indicates that you are listening, interested and that you want the patient to continue talking.
    b) Silence: The occasional use of silence, if the nonverbal behavior of the interviewer indicates interest, is useful in encouraging the patient to continue talking.
    c) Reflection: This is a response that repeats a word or phrase the patient just said. Examples: "You could not sleep?" "Nervous?" "Problem?" "Frightened?" The patient is prompted to go on with what he was talking about.

6. Handling of Emotionally Loaded Material.
    Emotionally loaded material means information about which the patient has intense emotions. In general, the subject areas that generate strong feelings are sex, aggression, and dependency. In psychoanalytic terminology these are the areas of instinctual drives, and psychoanalysts tend to think that learning to cope with these drives and the emotions generated by them in socially acceptable methods is the ideal of maturity. An attentive and empathic attitude on the part of the physician better enables the patient to discuss disturbing topics.

ANSWERS, Section II.B. _____

1. b
2. a
3. c
4. d
5. c

_____

Enelow and Wexler (1966) define empathy as "Putting oneself into the psychological frame of another, so that the other person's thinking, feeling and acting are understood" (p. 59). This understanding may be communicated to the patient by labeling the emotion (Kagan, 1971) he is experiencing. There are two important reasons for labeling of emotion: Attention is focused on the emotional communication, so the patient may if he wishes, recognize and delve deeper into what he is feeling; and the patient's feeling that he is understood will generally improve the doctor-patient relationship.

D. TERMINATING THE INTERVIEW

Before terminating the interview, it is generally helpful to let the patient know that there are only a few minutes left to talk. This provides some closure for the interview and allows the patient to complete any unfinished business, ask questions, and prepare himself emotionally to leave.

Additionally, the following steps should be included in the termination.

1) Summarize for the patient what you have learned.
2) Use reassurance and support in giving the patient encouragement in coming to terms with himself.
3) Define your role beyond this encounter.
4) Ask the patient if he has any questions for you, particularly if your questions have dominated the interview.
5) If possible, end the interview on a positive note; it is important for the patient and interviewer to part company with the feeling that each has been effective and constructive.

****

GO TO VIDEOTAPE

****

Quiz, Section II.C.

Circle the correct answer(s). <u>One</u> or <u>more</u> <u>than</u> <u>one</u> answer may be correct.

1.   Open-ended questions should be used in which of the following inter-
      viewing situations?

      a.   during the opening phase
      b.   when the patient is hesitant in talking about himself
      c.   when questioning the patient about his feelings
      d.   when the patient tends to be very circumstantial

Circle the letter corresponding to the <u>one</u> correct response.

2.   Which of the following statements concerning note-taking during an
      evaluation - interview is <u>not</u> correct?

      a.   may be considered by the patient as a sign of the physician's
           interest
      b.   should be discontinued if the patient objects
      c.   is permissible with reassurance to the patient that all notes are
           confidential
      d.   will not be necessary if the physician has a well-trained memory

The statements or questions that follow are posed by patients in evaluative
and therapeutic interviews. In each instance, circle the most appropriate
response for the physician.

3.   Early in her first interview with a male physician a female patient says,
      "I think all men are jerks."
      Physician:

      a.   "Your experience with men must certainly have been disagreeable
           for you to have this feeling."
      b.   "What makes you feel this way?"
      c.   "I understand why you feel this way now."
      d.   "With an attitude like this, you'll get nowhere."
      e.   "Perhaps you would like me to refer you to another physician."

4.   A 33-year-old bachelor presents as his initial complaint: "I feel cold
      and detached in the presence of women."
      Physician:

      a.   "That's because you are afraid of women."
      b.   "Tell me about your experience."
      c.   "You must want to destroy women, and thus you have to protect
           yourself from them."
      d.   "Don't worry. That feeling is very common."
      e.   "It is probable that this reflects your feeling toward your mother."

5. During an initial interview, a woman, after mentioning that she has been married three times previously, reviews her current husband's frequent angry outbursts toward her in some detail. Of the following, the best immediate response from the physician would be:

   a. "What do you do to arouse his anger?"
   b. "Have you always chosen ill-tempered men?"
   c. "Were there similar problems with your previous husbands?"
   d. "Perhaps you make men angry."
   e. "Perhaps you just don't like men."

6. A 42-year-old man comes to your office and states, "I've had a problem with drinking, and my wife says she'll leave if I don't get help. I'm not an alcoholic. I haven't drunk anything for a week, and I've made up my mind to stop, so I don't believe I need a doctor."
   You would now respond:

   a. "As long as you're here, we might as well talk about how you're getting along."
   b. "Would you give me a dollar for every time you've made up your mind to stop?"
   c. "Most alcoholics act just as you do."
   d. "Your wife seems to think you do."
   e. "Have you ever had hallucinations while coming off alcohol?"

7. The patient goes on to state that if he has a problem it is only because his wife has been refusing to participate in sexual intercourse which makes him tense and angry.
   You would now respond:

   a. "Have you tried getting someone else?"
   b. "How do you feel about that?"
   c. "Have you talked with her about it?"
   d. "Have you had sexual troubles in the past?"
   e. "Sometimes women act that way, but why do you handle it by drinking?"

8. A married woman in psychotherapy for anxiety attacks, initially evasive about why she is anxious when alone at home, admits that she is afraid a man might break into the house. She then says, "I don't see anything abnormal about that. None of the women I know like to be alone at night." The most appropriate intervention might be:

   a. "From what you've told me, I really don't think that you have anything to worry about."
   b. "I agree, that's not abnormal."
   c. "Let's try to understand your feelings about this particular situation."
   d. "Perhaps you could get a friend to stay with you."
   e. "Don't you think it would be best not to limit your life just because you're afraid?"

9. A 26-year-old woman appeared in the emergency room requesting help. She spoke in a very soft manner, resembling that of a small child. Although her narrative was somewhat disorganized and rambling, she did relate that her father had just called her to tell her that her mother had died that day from a heart attack. She reported that shortly after this she felt "dazed" and began to feel that she had, in some way, been responsible for causing her mother's death. Then she began to cry and was unable to continue speaking for several minutes. At this point in the interview, the best technique would be to say:

    a. "That's all right, dear. Don't cry. I'm certain that everything will work out all right."
    b. "These feelings are very interesting. We must talk more about them."
    c. Nothing, and wait for the patient to regain her composure.
    d. "I can appreciate how you feel after hearing such upsetting news."
    e. "It must be difficult for you if you have guilt feelings about your mother."

10. You are in family practice. A 28-year-old woman comes into your office and complains about having pain while having intercourse. She states that she has been having problems with her husband who drinks. She states that she has not enjoyed intercourse with him ever, but the pain is new and worries her.
    You would now inquire:

    a. "When did you last have a gynecological exam?"
    b. "What do you mean by 'with him'?"
    c. "Tell me more about things."
    d. "Have you spoken to a marriage counselor?"

11. Later in the interview she states, with hesitation, that she does feel guilty about the fact that she did get so angry with her husband she had an affair just before the pain started.
    Your response would be:

    a. "Do you think your pain might represent unconscious guilt over the affair?"
    b. "Did he find out?"
    c. "Have you had pain after the affair?"
    d. "Tell me more about your pathological guilt feelings."
    e. Silence to find out if patient will continue.

For each of the following pairs of interviewer responses, circle the one which illustrates the better technique.

12. a. Now, I want to give you an easy proverb.
    b. Tell me what this proverb means.

13. a. I know this may be an unpleasant subject to discuss, but studies show that the more you can talk about your feelings, the greater likelihood you can get relief. In fact, most patients with manic depressive illness should be allowed to ventilate as much as possible, provided they don't act on their feelings.
    b. Tell me more.

14. a. Do you have a loving mother?
    b. What kind of person is your mother?

15. In the following transcript, identify the points at which the interviewer facilitates (encourages) the patient to continue talking.

    Pt: I would say that I am better now, but I seem to lack a sense of direction. I don't know what to expect.

    a. Dr.: Expect?

    Pt: Yes, what to expect out of life. I used to enjoy painting, but now I think it was mainly because of the impression it made on other people. You know, being an artist.

    b. Dr.: Oh?

    Pt: Now I'm not so much interested in impressing other people. I used to be very particular about the way I dressed. Every little thing had to be just right. But now I don't care.

    c. Dr.: Tell me more about it.

    Pt: Now I come home late and rush to get dressed to go out and I don't care as much that my shoes ought to be brown, and I only have black. But the way I dressed before, something seemed to be lacking.

    d. Dr.: Something seemed to be lacking?

Match the following statements with the appropriate descriptions.

___16. I need to conduct this interview in order to be evaluated on interviewing technique.

___17. I need to find out as much as possible about you in order to determine how I will be able to be of help to you.

___18. I am a student doctor.

___19. I will be your physician while you are in the hospital.

___20. I am Dr. Smith.

a. defining of role
b. making explicit purpose of interview
c. neither

Match the following definitions with the appropriate terms.

___21. specifies topic in general terms   a. open-ended
___22. a response that indicates you are   question
        listening, interested, and want   b. facilitation
        the patient to continue talking   c. empathy
___23. the ability to understand another person
        and to communicate that understanding

===

III.   OUTLINE FOR PSYCHIATRIC HISTORY

A.   PATIENT IDENTIFICATION

1.   Name, age, sex, marital status, cultural background, occupation.

2.   Source of referral.

3.   History of hospitalizations.

4.   Estimated reliability of information.

B.   CHIEF COMPLAINT/PRESENTING COMPLAINT

The chief complaint should be recorded <u>verbatim</u>. The patient's perception of why he is undergoing psychiatric examination is of critical value to the examiner. If the psychiatric patient is unable for some reason to describe the current problem, the informant should be identified and the problem stated in the informant's exact words.

C.   PRESENT ILLNESS

This is a chronological story of the difficulties which prompted the patient to see the psychiatrist (or the difficulties which prompted others to refer him to a psychiatrist). The report of the present illness should contain precise descriptions of symptoms of the first occurrence of symptoms. Attention should be given to possible <u>relationships between symptoms and life events</u>, especially feelings, fantasies, and thoughts associated with these life events.

Permit the patient to tell the story spontaneously as much as possible. Observations of his associations, digressions, repetitions, emotional responses, etc., will provide information for the mental status examination.

D.   SYSTEMIC REVIEW

Follow the general medical outline. Under "Central Nervous System" expand as follows: Investigate thoroughly any history of seizures, tremors, disturbances of gait or coordination, paralysis, head trauma, or alterations of consciousness.

E. PERSONAL HISTORY

A longitudinal view of the patient's personality development and origin of his psychopathology.

1. FAMILY HISTORY

    a. Economic and social status of parents, personality of parents, quality of patient's relationship with parents, compatibility of parents.

    b. Personality of siblings, relationship of patient to siblings, birth order of patient.

    c. Remarkable family history, medical history, particularly family history of psychiatric illness, suicide, eccentric relatives.

2. INFANCY AND EARLY CHILDHOOD

The patient can report only what he has been told. Sometimes an interview with the patient's parents is indicated.

3. CHILDHOOD

    a. School: Special likes and dislikes in school subjects; relationships with peers, teachers; sports and extracurricular activities; interference with schooling by illness, accidents, trouble at home.

    b. Health: Illness, accidents, surgery, and reactions to them.

    c. Childhood personality: Passivity/aggressiveness, independence/dependence, rebelliousness/conformity, attitudes toward responsibility, competition, frustration, pleasure, reactions to family events such as births, deaths, illnesses, separations, etc.

4. ADOLESCENCE

    a. School, special relationships with teachers, issues of achievement, sports.

    b. Religious upbringing.

    c. Relationship to family, examples of rebelliousness.

    d. Special interests.

    e. Health and physical development, reactions to onset of puberty.

    f. Personality: changes in disposition and temperament.

    g. Psychosexual development: attitudes toward peers of same and opposite sexes, how information about sexuality was acquired;

interest in sex literature, homosexual information, interests, experiences, heterosexual contact (dating, intercourse, parties, dancing).

5. ADULT ADJUSTMENT PRIOR TO ILLNESS

    a. Education: chronologic educational events.

    b. Occupation: employment history and ambitions, gains.

    c. Psychosexual: marital history and current status, sexual adjustment; parenting history and attitudes toward child rearing, relationship with children prior to onset of present illness.

    d. Family: nature of relationship to family of origin.

    e. Military record: date of service, type of discharge, combat experience, hospitalizations, rank in service.

    f. Social adjustment: organizations, community activities, friends, political activities, antisocial activities, criminal record.

    g. Habits: smoking and a careful history of drug and alcohol use.

    h. Interests: hobbies, sports, recreation, etc.

6. FURTHER EXAMINATION OF PREMORBID PERSONALITY AND ONSET OF PRESENT ILLNESS

    a. Elicit patient's perception of his personality as reflected by: typical mood, dominant interests, interpersonal relationships, and attitudes toward work, religion, sexuality, material possessions, self.

    b. Recent or past personality changes should be noted by the above, but will also be reflected by changes in: personal appearance, personal habits, mental alertness, ability to concentrate, memory, subjective awareness of periods of anxiety, suspiciousness or increased dependence on others.

IV.   THE MENTAL STATUS EXAMINATION

The mental status examination is a part of the interview having the purpose of evaluating the present status of intellectual and psychological functioning of an individual. The information gathered during the mental status examination is of diagnostic, therapeutic and prognostic significance and also serves as a baseline against which future mental status examinations can be compared. The mental status examination is sometimes viewed as a long and arduous task better left to neurologists and psychiatrists, but a thorough working knowledge of the mental status exam is crucial to every physician. It is learned easily and with practice becomes as readily incorporated in the physician's armamentarium as the examination of the heart and lungs.

OUTLINE OF THE MENTAL STATUS EXAMINATION

Under each heading examples are given. These are not all of the possible descriptors for each heading, but rather a limited list.

A. GENERAL OBSERVATIONS

These observations are made in the normal course of the interview and generally do not require special test procedures.

1. The setting of the examination.

2. Any special circumstances affecting the examination.

3. General appearance and behavior of the patient.

   a. Physical characteristics: attractiveness, normality of weight and height, any apparent physical deformity, congruence between apparent and stated age, personal hygiene (nails, hair, etc.).

   b. Dress: cleanliness of clothing, fastidious dress.

   c. Posture: slumped, relaxed, tense, erect, rigid, unusual, etc.

   d. Facial expression: eye contact, facial mobility, predominant grimacing; expressions: fixed, bland, angry, suspicious, sad, perplexed, anxious, cheerful, euphoric.

   e. Motor activity: stuporous, hypoactive, normal, hyperactive, agitation, mannerisms, stereotypes, tics, repetitive gestures, ataxias, etc.

   f. Behavior toward examiner: cooperativeness, accessibility, indifference, flirtatiousness, ingratiation, fearfulness, evasiveness, anger, suspiciousness, helplessness, easily distracted, etc.

B.   EMOTIONAL STATE, MOOD, AND AFFECT

Mood refers to the prevailing emotional feeling during the examination. Is the mood sustained or variable? While mood refers to a more overall sustained emotional state, affect is the feeling tone which the patient is feeling at the moment and is normally related to the current content of one's thoughts and verbal expressions. Mood and affect are inferred from direct behavioral observation and from what the patient reports. Asking "How have your spirits been?" will often serve to get the patient to discuss his mood. The issues that are important include:

1) What is the prevailing mood? Sadness, elation, apathy, anger, etc.
2) Does mood fluctuate?
3) What is the range of mood?
4) Is there a flatness of affect--a constant, apathetic mood without variation?
5) Is there an apparent dissociation of affect from the content of the patient's speech--inappropriate affect--i.e., smiling while discussing a misfortune?

C.   CHARACTERISTICS OF SPEECH AND THOUGHT

Thought processes and thought content are deduced from the patient's speech.

1. Form of Speech.
   The tone, the pitch, the rate--slowed speech is often seen in depressed persons and very rapid speech is often seen in manics.

   Mutism is an extreme speech disorder which may derive from an organic brain lesion or may be simple uncooperativeness.

2. Thought Process.
   Generally abnormalities in this area are observed during the course of the interview without requiring specific questions. If the examiner observes verbal productions that seem to reflect an abnormality of thought process, follow-up inquiry is often helpful. Some abnormalities are listed below:

   a) Circumstantiality is an abnormality evidenced by the patient's digressing into unnecessary detail while communicating the central idea. It is often seen with schizophrenic patients, obsessional conditions, and in organic mental disorders.
   b) Tangentiality is seen when the patient follows a target leading further and further from the central idea.
   c) Flight of Ideas is a rapid succession of thoughts without apparent connection, often seen in manic patients.
   d) Word Salad is an incoherent stream of words and phrases.
   e) Clang Association is a rhyming of words without apparent meaning.

f) Thought Retardation is an abnormal slowing of thoughts.

g) Blocking is an obstruction of thought process. It appears as a sudden stop of thought process as if the person's speech had been momentarily turned off.

h) Perseveration is the pathological repetition of the same response to different questions.

i) Derailment (Loose Associations), a frequently seen sign in Schizophrenia, wherein the patient's thoughts do not seem logically connected. Do thoughts logically follow another or do they seem loosely connected?

j) Neologisms are new words or condensations of words idiosyncratic to the patient's own thinking. They are often used to express complex ideas or schemes.

3. Thought Content.

The content of the patient's thought can be discerned generally while obtaining the history; the person's preoccupations, concerns, daydreams, etc. Often probing questions are necessary to explore verbal cues indicating possible abnormalities in this area, particularly with regard to delusions.

a. Delusions.

A fixed, false belief inconsistent with the person's educational and cultural background. The patient will adhere to his delusion in the face of evidence to the contrary. Logic and reason do not seem to influence the firmly held belief system.

Types include:

1) Delusions of grandeur - an exaggerated sense of one's powers or importance.

2) Delusions of persecution - the thought that one is being harmed or harrassed.

3) Ideas of reference - the belief that others are discussing one.

4) Nihilistic delusions - the belief that the person or all persons are doomed.

5) Delusions of control - the belief that one's mind or other functions are under external control.

6) Delusions of infidelity - pathological jealousy for one's spouse or mate.

7) Delusions of worthlessness - the belief that one is of no value.

8) Somatic delusions - a belief that some bodily function is operating abnormally. This belief must be distinguished from Hypochondriasis (see page 32).

b. Obsessions.

The persistence of a thought, feeling, or impulse that one can not exclude from one's conscious mind. The obsession is generally perceived by the patient as being pathological and is unwanted. Often obsessive thoughts are coupled with compulsive acts - a powerful pressure to repetitively perform simple or complex motor tasks - e.g., a handwashing ritual. Obsessions must be differentiated from delusions.

c. Phobia.
An unrealistic fear or dread of an object or a situation and avoidance of that object or situation. The patient usually recognizes the phobia as pathological. Many common phobias have been assigned special names. A few examples of phobia are:

1) Claustrophobia - fear of close spaces.
2) Agoraphobia - fear of open places.
3) Acrophobia - fear of high places.
4) Xenophobia - fear of strangers.

d. Hypochondriasis.
An exaggerated concern for one's own health and bodily function. The patient feels ill, although there are generally no physical findings to support the patient's belief. On other occasions, the person will elaborate and enlarge on a genuine physical problem. Hypochondriasis must be differentiated from somatic delusions--the latter involves a belief system which has bizarre qualities, e.g., the patient may feel that something is wrong with his bowel function. When questioned about the nature of the problem, the hypochondriacal patient might complain of not having a bowel movement each day, while the delusional patient might say that his large intestine has died and is obstructed with maggots.

D. PERCEPTIONS

Distortions in the perception of a reality include illusions and hallucinations.

1. Illusions are the misinterpretation of some real sensory experience. The patient who has a toxic lesion condition will often be frightened by shadows in his room.

2. Hallucinations are false sensory perceptions in the absence of external stimuli. Some types of hallucinations are:

a) Auditory - hearing
b) Visual - sight
c) Olfactory - smell
d) Tactile - touch
e) Gustatory - taste

Many healthy people will experience hallucinations during that phase between being awake and falling asleep (hypnagogic hallucinations) and upon awakening (hypnopompic hallucinations).

There are other kinds of hallucinations seen under certain circumstances. The "phantom limb syndrome" seen after an amputation in which the person falsely perceives movement or sensation in the missing limb is a kinesthetic hallucination.

E.   HIGHER CORTICAL FUNCTIONS

In many instances, dysfunction will indicate some organic brain damage (Chapter 5).

The examiner must exercise special judgement and skill in determining the intactness of these functions. Often specific testing of some area is not indicated. But the examiner must be confident that the functions are intact. In relating the history, the patient may have presented clear evidence of a full orientation. It might be awkward under these circumstances to ask, "Do you know where you are?" Nevertheless, the examiner must be confident that each function is intact. If there is a question, then specific testing must be done.

    1.   Orientation.

        a.   Time (time of day, date, month, year; season, if severely impaired).

        b.   Place (location of examination, street address, city, state).

        c.   Person (the patient's perception of the role of the examiner, other staff, other patients, who he is).

    2.   Attention and Concentration.
The patient's level of attention and his ability to concentrate within normal limits can generally be judged from his behavior in the interview. When there is some doubt, this can be formally tested by the use of serial subtraction: asking the patient to subtract 7 from 100 and continue subtracting 7 until he can go no further. If educational level does not permit this test, have him count backwards from 38 to 27.

An alternative assessment can be made by way of the digit span exercise: the examiner gives the patient a series of digits to repeat. The examiner must be careful not to group the numbers as he says them, or his assessment will be inaccurate. The digits should be spoken at one-second intervals. First 2 digits, then 3 digits, then 4 digits, etc. After finding the patient's limitation with digit retention forward, ask the person to repeat the digits in reverse order. The average norms for the digit span are 6-7 numbers forward and 4-5 numbers backward. Digit retention also tests recent memory.

    3.   Memory.

        a.   Recall of remote past experiences can be tested formally by obtaining such information as time and place of birth, past occupations, schooling, date of marriage, birth of children, etc. Be alert to the possibility that the patient may be making up the answers (confabulating). Information can be confirmed by medical records or family members.

b. Recall of recent past experience can be tested formally by asking questions regarding events in the patient's experience which have occurred during the past 24 hours. This information can be validated by the nursing staff or other staff members who were likely to have witnessed these events.

c. Immediate memory can be tested formally by giving the patient the task of remembering three nonrelated words or phrases (e.g., chair, blue, a piece of cake) and having him repeat them in approximately five minutes. Also the use of digit retention (see above) tests immediate memory.

4. Intellect and Fund of Information.
A general intellectual evaluation can be inferred from the patient's vocabulary, his use of language, his educational achievements, vocational success, and social adjustment. Questions regarding general information may be employed if a deficit is suspected, e.g., name the last four presidents, why do people have lungs, the distance from New York to Los Angeles, events of current interest in the newspapers, etc.

5. Symbolization and Abstract Reasoning.
This can be tested formally by asking for differences in meaning between words such as idleness and laziness, poverty and misery, character and reputation. An alternative method is proverb interpretation: "What is the meaning of the saying, 'People who live in glass houses shouldn't throw stones,' 'Rome wasn't built in a day,' " etc. Note the extent to which the patient personalizes the interpretation of the proverb and the degree of concreteness or appropriate abstraction involved. Asking familiar proverbs often tests memory to a greater degree than abstraction. Use of a proverb unfamiliar to the patient is often more indicative of abstract reasoning ability. Remember that the educational and cultural background of the patient must be taken into account when proverb interpretation is assessed. Some proverbs many patients may not have heard are:

"Man has the gun, but God carries the bullets."

"The golden key opens the iron door."

"The minnows laugh when the whale gets into shallow water."

6. Insight into Illness, Judgement, and Reality Testing.

a. Insight into illness represents the patient's ability to comprehend his current situation correctly: To what extent does the patient realize that he suffers from illness or from personal difficulties? Does the patient recognize areas of stress in his life situation or certain internal conflicts?

b. Judgement. The range of judgement is considerable. Much can be inferred from the patient's sensitivity to the social setting. Often a person will make statements that are socially awkward; they are "out of context" for the situation. Judgement can be formally tested by asking what behavior would be appropriate in a given social situation, such as "What would you do if you were the first to discover a fire in a crowded movie theater?" However, look particularly at the patient's current behavior for evidence of the extent to which his judgement is impaired.

c. Reality testing is the ability to evaluate the external world objectively and to differentiate between self and nonself. Adequate reality testing is reflected both in the patient's judgement and his insight into his illness. Can the patient differentiate the real world and what is the creation of his own mind?

After the evaluation is complete, a diagnostic statement should be made. In psychiatry, the diagnosis initially may be unclear. Continued observation and examination may provide additional needed information.

****

GO TO VIDEOTAPE

****

F.   MULTIAXIAL DIAGNOSIS

The Diagnostic and Statistical Manual III of the American Psychiatric Association (1980) provides a classification of psychiatric disorders. Directions are provided for evaluating a person on five (5) different axes. Wherever possible, all five (5) axes should be used.

Use any factual data that you have obtained from the psychiatric history and mental status examination, along with your impressions about the patient which would account for psychopathology, in order to formulate the diagnosis. Use a narrative style. Include under the formulation:

1) Predisposing factors: Factors from the patient's personal or family history which are likely to account for the present psychopathology.
2) Precipitating events: Stresses or events which may have precipitated the present illness.
3) Areas of conflict: (e.g., sex, aggression, dependency).
4) Defense mechanisms: See Chapter 2.
5) Differential diagnosis.

READING NOTE: For more information about Dynamic Formulations see: Levine, M. Principles of psychiatric treatment. In F. Alexander & H. Ross (Eds.), Dynamic psychiatry. Chicago: The University of Chicago Press, 1952, 307-368.

G.   MANAGEMENT

Often a treatment plan evolves over several contacts with the patient. As far as possible, outline a proposed therapeutic program under the following headings:

1) Hospitalization versus outpatient treatment.
2) If hospitalized, what sort of milieu?
3) Further investigative procedures (list).
4) Chemotherapy (antipsychotics, antianxiety agents, antidepressants, lithium).
5) Other somatic therapies (e.g., ECT).
6) Psychotherapy (individual, insight; individual, supportive; family; marital; group).
7) Behavior modification (systematic desensitization, aversive conditioning, operant conditioning, relaxation training, assertiveness training, biofeedback).
8) Other recommendations (be specific and include long-range goals such as modification of patient's future environment, vocational counseling, further education, etc.)

QUIZ, Section IV.

Match the following terms with their appropriate definitions.

___1.   mental status
___2.   insight
___3.   reality testing

a.   ability of patient to comprehend his current situation correctly
b.   evaluation of current psychological functioning
c.   ability to evaluate external world objectively and to differentiate adequately between self and nonself

V.   INTERVIEW RATING SCALE

Following are a series of items which make up an interviewer rating scale. These items can be used to evaluate the quality of the psychiatric examination as described in this chapter.

Psychiatric Evaluation

Score "1" if behavior is observed or not applicable; "0" if absent.

		Yes	No
A.	**INITIAL APPROACH**		
1.	Greeted patient by name	1	0
2.	Introduced self	1	0
3.	Defined role or status	1	0
4.	Made explicit purpose of interview	1	0
5.	Mentioned time available for interview	1	0
6.	Asked if patient at ease prior to task	1	0

B. AREAS OF INFORMATION COVERED

1. Details of chief complaints	Yes	No
a. Elicited the chief complaints	1	0
b. Established onset of problems within one month	1	0
c. Elicited precipitating factors	1	0
d. Elicited main events in course of problems	1	0
e. Covered treatment of current episode including:		
1. Type of treatment	1	0
2. Duration	1	0
3. Medication - types, doses, wanted effects, side effects	1	0

2. Effect of illness on patient and family Determined extent of disruption of normal functioning due to current problems in relation to:	Yes	No
a. Work or school	1	0
b. Interpersonal relationships	1	0
c. Sex	1	0
d. Social activities	1	0
e. Leisure activities	1	0

3. Insight	Yes	No
Elicited patient's attitude to problems	1	0

4. Factors predisposing to the development of similar problems	Yes	No
a. Obtained description of previous personality	1	0

b. Obtained relevant information about previous episodes of mental illness:	Yes/NA	No
(1) Type	1	0
(2) Similarity to present problems	1	0
(3) Treatment	1	0
(4) Effect and outcome	1	0

		Yes	No
c.	Checked if family history of mental illness	1	0
	(1) Type	1	0
	(2) Similarity to patient's problems	1	0
	(3) Treatment	1	0
	(4) Effect and outcome	1	0

		Yes	No
d.	Obtained relevant information about episodes of physical illness	1	0

		Yes/NA	No
	(1) Type	1	0
	(2) Similarity to present problem	1	0
	(3) Treatment	1	0
	(4) Effect and outcome	1	0

		Yes	No
5.	Asked screening questions	Yes	No
a.	For substance use/abuse		
	(1) Alcohol	1	0
	(2) Drugs	1	0
	(3) Tobacco	1	0
b.	For symptoms of depression		
	(1) Depressive mood	1	0
	(2) Appetite	1	0
	(3) Weight	1	0
	(4) Energy	1	0
	(5) Sleep patterns	1	0
	(6) Diurnal variation	1	0
	(7) Feelings about the future	1	0
c.	For suicide risk Elicited if any suicidal ideas or attempts	1	0
d.	For symptoms of anxiety		
	(1) Palpitation	1	0
	(2) Sweating	1	0
	(3) Headaches	1	0
	(4) Nausea	1	0
	(5) Tremor	1	0
	(6) Diarrhea	1	0
	(7) Shortness of breath	1	0
	(8) Feelings of nervousness	1	0
e.	For psychosis		
	(1) Hallucinations	1	0
	(2) Delusions	1	0
	(3) Change in thinking	1	0

ANSWERS, Section IV. _____

1. b
2. a
3. c

_____

		Yes	No
f.	For organic impairment		
	(1) Orientation	1	0
	(2) Memory	1	0
	(3) Abstraction	1	0
g.	For physical illness		
	(1) Cardiovascular	1	0
	(2) Central nervous system	1	0
	(3) Respiratory system	1	0
	(4) Gastrointestinal	1	0
	(5) Locomotor	1	0
	(6) Urogenital	1	0

	Yes	No
C. TERMINATION OF INTERVIEW		
Interviewer ended the interview appropriately	1	0

D. CONDUCT OF INTERVIEW
Score interviewer's use of each technique as follows:

Poor use of technique, total omission	Score 0
Fairly poor use of technique, many omissions	Score 1
Fairly good use of technique, some omissions	Score 2
Good use of technique, few omissions	Score 3
Excellent use of technique, no omissions	Score 4

1. Clarifying
Interviewer questions in depth to elicit
full information, resolve ambiguities
and inconsistencies

No   Yes
0 1 2 3 4

2. Avoiding jargon
Interviewer avoids using technical
or ambiguous wording

0 1 2 3 4

3. Rejecting jargon
Interviewer asks for definition of
technical or ambiguous words used
by patient

0 1 2 3 4

4. Handling of emotionally loaded
material. Interviewer does not avoid,
and handles sensitively, topics which
may be disturbing or embarrassing
to the patient

No   Yes
0 1 2 3 4

5. Avoiding repetition
    Interviewer does not request, or
    allow the patient to persist in giving,
    information which has already been
    elicited in the interview   0   1   2   3   4

6. Following leads of patient   No   Yes
    Interviewer is responsive to statements
    by the patient which may indicate unex-
    plored problems   0   1   2   3   4

7. Facilitating
    Interviewer encourages the patient's
    responses   0   1   2   3   4

8. Open-ended questions
    Interviewer asks questions which
    do not direct the patient's answers   0   1   2   3   4

9. Use of brief questions
    Interviewer asks single, brief
    questions; does not ask long,
    complex questions   0   1   2   3   4

E. GLOBAL RATINGS
    Scoring for each item:

    Very poor   Score 0
    Poor   Score 1
    Moderate   Score 2
    Good   Score 3
    Excellent   Score 4

    1. Self-assurance
        The interviewer seems confident,
        open, and relaxed; does not show
        confusion, hesitancy, shyness,
        or embarrassment   0   1   2   3   4

    2. Empathy
        The interviewer shows empathy by ask-
        ing appropriate questions and making
        appropriate responses that he understands
        the nature of the patient's illness, the
        effect the illness has on his life, and
        the way in which the patient himself
        perceives the problem   0   1   2   3   4

	No				Yes

3. Warmth
    The interviewer shows that he
    has regard and concern for the
    patient   0 1 2 3 4

4. Competence (over-all)
    The interviewer uses appropriate
    interview skills to elicit key
    information from the patient
    while maintaining a relaxed and
    mutually responsive relationship 0 1 2 3 4

POST-TEST

Circle the letter corresponding to the <u>one</u> correct response.

1.   Transference is a term used to designate the

   a.   physician's reaction to the patient.
   b.   referral of the patient to another physician.
   c.   carry-over of feelings and attitudes from previous relationships.
   d.   establishment of positive feelings toward the doctor.
   e.   need for terminating the treatment.

2.   The term "rapport" is defined as

   a.   the development of a fondness between the patient and physician.
   b.   the displacement of affect from one object to another.
   c.   the process of helping the patient to speak freely and describe his problems fully.
   d.   the arousal of the physician's repressed feelings by the interview situation.
   e.   a harmonious and unconstrained relationship between the patient and physician.

The statements or questions that follow are posed by patients in evaluative and therapeutic interviews. In each instance, select the most appropriate response for the physician.

3.   During an initial interview, a woman, after mentioning that she has been married three times previously, reviews her current husband's frequent angry outbursts toward her in some detail. Of the following, the best immediate response from the physician would be:

   a.   "What do you do to arouse his anger?"
   b.   "Have you always chosen ill-tempered men?"
   c.   "Were there similar problems with your previous husbands?"
   d.   "Perhaps you make men angry."
   e.   "Perhaps you just don't like men."

4.   A married woman in psychotherapy for anxiety attacks, initially evasive about why she is anxious when alone at home, admits that she is afraid a man might break into the house. She then says, "I don't see anything abnormal about that. None of the women I know like to be alone at night." The most appropriate intervention might be:

   a.   "From what you've told me, I really don't think that you have anything to worry about."
   b.   "I agree, that's not abnormal."
   c.   "Let's try to understand <u>your</u> feelings about this particular situation."
   d.   "Perhaps you could get a friend to stay with you."
   e.   "Don't you think it would be best not to limit your life just because you're afraid?"

5. A 33-year-old bachelor presents as his initial complaint: "I feel cold and detached in the presence of women."
    Physician:

    a. "That's because you are afraid of women."
    b. "Tell me about your experience."
    c. "You must want to destroy women, and thus you have to protect yourself from them."
    d. "Don't worry. That feeling is very common."
    e. "It is probable that this reflects your feeling toward your mother."

6. Early in her first interview with a male physician, a female patient says, "I think all men are jerks."
    Physician:

    a. "Your experience with men must certainly have been disagreeable for you to have this feeling."
    b. "What makes you feel this way?"
    c. "I understand why you feel this way now."
    d. "With an attitude like this, you'll get nowhere."
    e. "Perhaps you would like me to refer you to another physician."

7. A 42-year-old man comes to your office and states, "I've had a problem with drinking and my wife says she'll leave if I don't get help. I'm not an alcoholic. I haven't drunk anything for a week, and I've made up my mind to stop, so I don't believe I need a doctor."
    You would now respond:

    a. "As long as you're here, we might as well talk about how you're getting along."
    b. "Would you give me a dollar for every time you've made up your mind to stop?"
    c. "Most alcoholics act just as you do."
    d. "Your wife seems to think you do."
    e. "Have you ever had hallucinations while coming off alcohol?"

8. The patient goes on to state that if he has a problem, it is only because his wife has been refusing to participate in sexual intercourse which makes him tense and angry.
    You would now respond:

    a. "Have you tried getting someone else?"
    b. "How do you feel about that?"
    c. "Have you talked with her about it?"
    d. "Have you had sexual troubles in the past?"
    e. "Sometimes women act that way, but why do you handle it by drinking?"

9. A 26-year-old woman appeared in the emergency room requesting help. She spoke in a very soft manner, resembling that of a small child. Although her narrative was somewhat disorganized and rambling, she did relate that her father had just called her to tell her that her mother had died that day from a heart attack. She reported that shortly after this she felt "dazed" and began to feel that she had, in some way, been responsible for causing her mother's death. Then she began to cry and was unable to continue speaking for several minutes.
    At this point in the interview, the best technique would be to say:

    a. "That's all right, dear. Don't cry. I'm certain that everything will work out all right."
    b. "These feelings are very interesting. We must talk more about them."
    c. Nothing, and wait for the patient to regain her composure.
    d. "I can appreciate how you feel after hearing such upsetting news."
    e. "It must be difficult for you if you have guilt feelings about your mother."

10. You are in family practice. A 28-year-old woman comes into your office and complains about having pain while having intercourse. She states that she has been having problems with her husband who drinks. She states that she has not enjoyed intercourse with him ever, but the pain is new and worries her.
    You would now respond:

    a. "When did you last have a gynecological exam?"
    b. "What do you mean by 'with him'?"
    c. "Tell me more about things."
    d. "Have you spoken to a marriage counselor?"
    e. "How bad is your husband's problem with alcohol?"

11. Later in the interview she states, with hesitation, that she does feel guilty about the fact that she did get so angry with her husband that she had an affair, just before the pain started.
    Your response would be:

    a. "Do you think your pain might represent unconscious guilt over the affair?"
    b. "Did he find out?"
    c. "Have you had pain after the affair?"
    d. "Tell me more about your pathological guilt feelings."
    e. Silence to find out if patient will continue.

Circle the correct answer(s). <u>One</u> or <u>more</u> <u>than</u> <u>one</u> answer may be correct.

12. Which of the following is/are true concerning the psychiatric evaluation?

    a. Establishing rapport makes it more likely that the physician will obtain pertinent information from the patient.
    b. A complete psychiatric diagnosis can usually be made once you have completed the psychiatric history and mental status examination.
    c. The mental status examination provides information about the patient's functioning at the time of the exam, while the psychiatric history gives a more longitudinal view.
    d. When rating the severity of a stress it is important to take into account the individual's vulnerability to a particular stress, rather than how an average person might experience the stress.

13. In obtaining a psychiatric history,

    a. it is necessary to elicit the existence of delusions, hallucination, or ideas of reference in order to make a diagnosis of an Affective Disorder.
    b. loss of recent memory for important information is indicative of a neurotic reaction.
    c. suicidal tendencies in the patient are likely to be aggravated by the physician's inquiring about them.
    d. psychological or emotional processes in the physician can influence the type of information he obtains.

14. Note-taking during the psychiatric evaluation

    a. may be considered by the patient as a sign of the physician's interest.
    b. should be discontinued if the patient objects.
    c. is permissible with reassurance to the patient that all notes are confidential.
    d. will <u>not</u> be necessary if the physician has a well-trained memory.

15. When terminating an interview which of the following steps is/are useful?

    a. Summarize for the patient what you have learned.
    b. Define your role beyond this encounter.
    c. Ask the patient if he has any questions for you.
    d. End the interview on a positive note.

16. Open-ended questions should be used in which of the following interviewing situations?

    a. during the opening phase
    b. when the patient is hesitant in talking about himself
    c. when questioning the patient about his feelings
    d. when the patient tends to be very circumstantial

Match each concept with the appropriate description. Lettered items may be used more than once.

___17. facilitation
___18. open-ended question
___19. mental status
___20. reality testing
___21. empathy
___22. respect
___23. genuineness
___24. insight

a. the ability to understand another person and to communicate that understanding
b. evaluation of current psychological functioning
c. a response that indicates you are listening, interested, and want the patient to continue talking
d. positive regard
e. authenticity
f. ability of patient to comprehend his current situation correctly
g. specifies topic in general terms
h. the ability to distinguish between productions of one's own mind and the real world

Match the following axes of a multiaxial diagnosis with the appropriate definitions.

___25. Axis IV
___26. Axis V
___27. Axis III
___28. Axis II
___29. Axis I

a. personality disorders
b. clinical psychiatric syndromes
c. psychosocial stressors
d. physical disorders
e. highest level of adaptive functioning during past year

PRE-TEST ANSWERS

1.	a,c	11.	a	21.	g
2.	d	12.	c or b	22.	e
3.	a,b,c	13.	c	23.	d
4.	a,b,c	14.	d	24.	h
5.	a,b,c,d	15.	c	25.	d
6.	e	16.	e	26.	b
7.	c	17.	a	27.	a
8.	b	18.	b	28.	e
9.	b	19.	c	29.	c
10.	c	20.	f		

POST-TEST ANSWERS

1.	c	11.	e	21.	a
2.	e	12.	a,c	22.	d
3.	c	13.	d	23.	e
4.	c	14.	a,b,c	24.	f
5.	b	15.	a,b,c,d	25.	c
6.	b	16.	a,b,c	26.	e
7.	a	17.	c	27.	d
8.	c or b	18.	g	28.	a
9.	d	19.	b	29.	b
10.	c	20.	h		

REFERENCES

Bernstein, L., Bernstein, R. S., & Dana, R. H. Interviewing: A guide for health professionals. New York: Appleton-Century-Crofts, 1974.

Davis, J. C., & Foreyt, J. P. Mental examiner's source book. Springfield, Illinois: Charles C. Thomas, 1975.

Enelow, A. J., & Wexler, M. Psychiatry in the practice of medicine. New York: Oxford University Press, 1966.

Freedman, A. M., Kaplan, H. I., & Sadock, B. J. Comprehensive textbook of psychiatry II. Baltimore: The William & Wilkins Company, 1975.

Froelich, R. E., & Bishop, F. M. Clinical interviewing skills. St. Louis: The C.V. Mosby Company, 1977.

Kagan, N. Influencing human interaction. East Lansing, Michigan: Instructional Media Center, Michigan State University, 1971.

MacKinnon, R. A., & Michels, R. The psychiatric interview in clinical practice. Philadelphia, Pa.: W.B. Saunders Company, 1971.

Masserman, J. H., & Schwab, J. J. The psychiatric examination. New York: Intercontinental Medical Book Corporation, 1974.

CHAPTER 2

Psychodynamic Considerations and Defense Mechanisms
Miriam DeAntonio, M.D.
Bryce McLaulin, M.D.
Layton McCurdy, M.D.

CHAPTER OUTLINE

LEARNING OBJECTIVES

After completing this chapter you will be able to:

1. List basic assumptions necessary to understanding psychodynamic theory (psychoanalytic theory).

2. List and describe the three conceptual components of the psychic apparatus--id, ego, and superego.

3. Describe the adaptive functions of the ego.

4. Describe the interrelationships of the three components of the psychic apparatus.

5. Define and describe conscious mind, nonconscious mind, instinctual drives, affect, ego-syntonic, ego-dystonic (ego-alien).

6. Understand and be able to recognize the use of the following ego defense mechanisms:

    Identification (including incorporation and introjection)
    Repression
    Regression
    Rationalization
    Sublimation
    Displacement
    Intellectualization
    Reaction formation
    Denial
    Projection

7. Relate the concept of personality characteristics to the individual's use or repertoire of defense mechanisms and coping style.

PRE-TEST

For the following questions, circle the letter corresponding to the <u>one</u> correct answer.

1. The groundwork for psychoanalysis was laid by

    a. Alfred Adler.
    b. Karen Horney.
    c. Sigmund Freud.
    d. Carl Jung.

2. One of the basic assumptions of the psychoanalytic model is that

    a. a portion of the mind is unconscious, but most of the mind is conscious.
    b. a portion of the mind is unconscious, but this portion has little or no effect on behavior.
    c. a portion of the mind is unconscious, and none of this unconscious material can be made conscious.
    d. a portion of the mind is unconscious, and some of this material can be made conscious by certain techniques.

3. Having the patient freely report passing thought activity without censorship or reservation is known as

    a. thought broadcasting.
    b. free association.
    c. projection.
    d. thought dissociation.
    e. affect analysis.

4. Freud described three functional components of the mind. Which of the following is <u>not</u> part of his schema?

    a. id
    b. archetype
    c. superego
    d. ego

5. Instinctual components of the id are most easily seen in the

    a. 2-year-old.
    b. newborn.
    c. college student.
    d. 6-year-old.

6. Which of the following statements concerning the ego is _not_ true?

    a. The ego is the integrative adaptive portion of the mind.
    b. The ego houses moral and ethical standards.
    c. Ego functions include intelligence, memory, motivation, and sensory perception.
    d. Some ego functions are conscious, others are not.
    e. The capacity to do creative and purposeful work is an ego function.

7. Ego defense mechanisms

    a. were just introduced by Charcot in 1873.
    b. are used to bring areas of conflict into consciousness to relieve anxiety.
    c. generally determine all personality characteristics.
    d. are used normally and/or pathologically to cope with dysphoric emotions.
    e. are used to the same degree, regardless of the stress.

8. Which of the following statements concerning identification is _not_ true?

    a. Identification does not occur in adult life.
    b. Identification is crucial in normal healthy development.
    c. Adolescents tend to identify with their peer group.
    d. Young children usually tend to identify with the same sex parent.

9. A 30-year-old woman married for seven years has been unsuccessful in becoming pregnant. A fertility work-up reveals bilateral stenosis of the Fallopian tubes. Upon hearing the results from her physician she states, "I don't believe it. I'll find another doctor!" This woman is using

    a. projection.
    b. denial.
    c. both.

10. A 40-year-old male has devoted his life to his domineering, obnoxious, invalid father. He is extremely solicitous and protective to his unappreciative parent. This man is using the defense mechanism known as

    a. denial.
    b. displacement.
    c. reaction formation.
    d. projection.
    e. rationalization.

11. A young pediatrics intern cares for an extremely ill six-year-old. While he is on call, the child dies. The following morning he calmly discusses the case with his attending. Upon arriving home, he kicks his dog and accuses his wife of being incompetent in managing household affairs. In the order of appearance in this vignette, select the defense mechanisms evident.

    a. denial, rationalization, projection
    b. repression, sublimation, intellectualization
    c. isolation of affect, displacement, projection
    d. regression, denial, undoing

12. In the months following the child's death, the intern decides that rather than remain frustrated and angry over the child's death, he will actively study the disease which killed the child. The intern may be using the defense mechanism known as

    a. intellectualization.
    b. displacement.
    c. sublimation.
    d. undoing.
    e. rationalization.

For the following questions, one or more than one answer may be correct. Circle the correct answer(s).

13. The ego seeks to achieve and maintain a homeostatic state by

    a. mediating between external reality and internal demands.
    b. mediating between id demands and superego standards.
    c. using defense mechanisms.
    d. none of above.

14. Which of the following describe(s) the id?

    a. seat of instinctual drives
    b. present at birth
    c. operates on the pleasure principle
    d. has been definitively demonstrated anatomically

15. Which of the following describe(s) the ego?

    a. compromises between internal demands and external reality
    b. like the id, follows the pleasure principle
    c. functions include intelligence, memory, and sensory perception
    d. all ego functions are conscious

16. The superego

    a. is derived from the id in early infancy.
    b. is influenced during its development by cultural values and standards.
    c. usually has no relationship to the ethical teaching of parents.
    d. can vary in degree from very permissive to very punitive.

17. Ego-dystonic demands

    a. can produce conflict leading to unpleasant emotional experiences.
    b. virtually never occur in daily life.
    c. may arise from the id, superego, or environment.
    d. are generally in keeping with the ego's principles and functions.

18. Repression

    a. is a primitive basic defense mechanism that should be considered pathological if seen past age 5 years.
    b. operates exclusively in awareness.
    c. refers to using earlier modes of adaptation.
    d. is represented by the inability of individuals to remember physical pain and post-hypnotic suggestions.

19. Projection

    a. is a primitive mechanism, seen normally in infancy.
    b. is attributing one's unacceptable feelings, wishes or attributes to others.
    c. is evident in paranoid behavior.
    d. can be observed in "normal" individuals.

20. Regression

    a. is a common defense mechanism seen in schizophrenics and physically ill individuals, among others.
    b. causes irreparable damage to personality development.
    c. is characterized by a return to an earlier, more primitive mode of functioning.
    d. is virtually unknown past the teenage years.

21. Rationalization

    a. involves use of socially acceptable explanations for questionable behavior.
    b. could be seen as a means to appease the superego.
    c. may be used by the ego to keep selfish motives out of awareness.
    d. usually occurs in consciousness, thus may be thought of as lying.

22.   Intellectualization and displacement

   a.   are alike in that both are defense mechanisms that deal with un-
        pleasant affects.
   b.   are alike in that both use substitute objects to relieve anxiety.
   c.   are commonly used unconscious mechanisms.
   d.   are primitive defense mechanisms like projection.

Match the following drives with the corresponding characteristics.

_____23. hunger drive
_____24. sexual drive
_____25. aggressive drive

a.   hostility
b.   social needs
c.   dependency needs

I. INTRODUCTION

The psychodynamic model of mental function is derived largely from the work of Sigmund Freud whose first published work appeared in 1895. Over a period of years he elaborated a complex theory of human behavior, as well as a treatment method for emotional disorders, both of which have been incorporated under the general heading of "psychoanalysis." Freud's impact on psychiatry and psychology cannot be overestimated. Some of Freud's students later modified and extended Freud's work. This chapter will present one model of the extension of psychoanalytic theory which is called the psychodynamic model.

In order to develop the psychodynamic model two fundamental assumptions which are basic to understanding this model must be granted.

Assumption 1: Our conscious awareness forms only a small portion of the brain's activity. There are portions of each person's experience, memory, feelings, wishes, etc., which are outside of one's consciousness. Called the unconscious, this portion of the individual's mind contains memories, feelings, and drives. Some of this unconscious material at times emerges into conscious awareness; other material may remain buried in the unconscious mind at all times. Often an individual will experience some event in a dream which had not been thought of in years. That material was in the unconscious mind.

We often infer the content of the unconscious mind from the individual's behavioral expression. The material in this chapter will examine various inferences that can be made concerning the connection between the individual's outward behavioral activity and the forces in the unconscious mind which generate that behavior. Freud's psychoanalytic approach involved bringing material from the unconscious into the patient's awareness. The first technique he utilized was hypnosis. He later abandoned the notion of hypnosis for the technique of free association and dream content analysis. Free association is that psychoanalytic technique in which the patient attempts to verbalize without reservation or censorship the passing thought activity in his mind. The trained analyst then notices the connections between these thought fragments. Through this activity various unconscious memories, emotions, and drives are inferred and subsequently made conscious.

Assumption 2: Instinctual drives are present in all human beings, largely in the unconscious mind. These instinctual drives include:

(1) The drive to maintain homeostasis, that state of physical and emotional well-being free of physical and emotional discomfort or pain. Stated another way, this is the drive for the preservation of the self.

(2) The drive for the preservation of the species. This drive is linked to the individual's sexual urges.

These drives are related to each other in complex ways. For example, the drive for intimacy with another person involves the urge to procreate, as well as to meet the need for emotional comfort.

QUIZ, Section I.

Complete the following:

1. A basic assumption of the psychodynamic model is the existence of the _____, a part of the mind out of awareness. Sigmund Freud first used _____ to bring unconscious material into consciousness; later he developed the techniques of _____ _____ and _____ to achieve the same goal.

2. Another assumption of the psychodynamic model is the ubiquitous presence of instinctual drives. Maintaining a state of physical and emotional well being is the drive to maintain _____, in essence, the drive for _____ of the self. Another drive, preservation of the species, is linked to _____ urges.

II. STRUCTURAL THEORY OF PERSONALITY

Freud suggested that the mental functions could be best understood if the mind was viewed as having three functional components--the id, the ego, and the superego. These represent functional concepts and are not related to specific areas of the brain, although newer neural anatomic research is beginning to identify various brain locations related to specific emotional drives.

Reading Note: The student interested in reading further concerning relationships of various parts of the brain to emotional drive is referred to the following article: Sherwin & Geschwind, Neural substrates of behavior. In Nicholi, The Harvard guide to modern psychiatry, Harvard University Press, 1978.

The id is a functional portion of the psychic apparatus present at birth and the repository of instinctual drives. The id operates on the pleasure principle; that is to say, it seeks to immediately discharge instinctual drives. These instinctual drives can be organized around three fundamental types.

(1) The drive for hunger -- this instinctual drive becomes elaborated into dependency needs.
(2) The sexual drive -- this becomes elaborated into the individual's social needs, i.e., the need for interaction with other persons.
(3) The aggressive drive -- this is related to hostility and anger.

These instinctual components of id are most easily seen in the newborn infant. The infant experiences the physiologic feelings of hunger and responds to these feelings with anger and crying. If the mother does not provide feeding immediately, the infant escalates its expression of anger and frustration. This drive for hunger is expressed through anger and is the signal to the mother to provide feeding which may be viewed as a social interaction (the involvement with another person).

While the id does not have an absolute representation in brain anatomy, portions of the mesencephalic brain seem to be related to various drives such as hunger and sexual drives. Remember that translating from animal experiments to the human is a very difficult matter. The interested student is referred to the reference cited on the preceding page which explains in greater detail current research work in this area.

In order to adapt to the social environment in which one lives, one must learn to modify and adapt the id to the environment around the individual. Adaptation is accomplished by that portion of the psychic apparatus known as the ego. The ego follows the reality principle. Using specific adjustment techniques, the ego is the executive aspect of the mind and stands, as it were, between the id and the environment. It compromises internal demands with external reality.

This executive, integrative, and adaptive portion of the mind - the ego - has a host of functions critical to personality development and to adaptive capacity. Functions of the ego include intelligence, memory, motivation, and sensory perception. Other more complex functions of the ego involve defense mechanisms which will be described later. Our capacity to relate with other people and our capacity to do creative and purposeful work are also functions of the ego. Some ego functions are conscious, others are not. For example, the use of ego defense mechanisms is generally an unconscious process.

The superego derives from the ego during the early phases of infant development. Roughly comparable to a person's conscience, the superego develops from the ego as the individual incorporates or takes in the moral standards, first of his parents or parent substitutes and then of the family. Subsequently, the values and moral structures of the individual's culture are involved in superego development. The superego in some individuals may be permissive and in others punitive. Much of this superego function is related to the standards first learned from parents and then from society.

The ego's function is to stand between the superego and the id and the environment. Consequently, we regard the ego as the adaptive portion of the psychic apparatus. Just as the id makes demands on the ego via instinctual drives seeking gratification, so, too, the superego makes demands on the ego concerning moral and ethical standards and prohibitions. Clearly one of the most important functions of the ego is to mediate between the internal demands of the id and of the superego and the external demands of reality. The ego strives to compromise between these demands, i.e., to achieve and maintain a homeostatic state.

1.   unconscious
     hypnosis
     free association
     dream content analysis
2.   homeostasis
     preservation
     sexual

Figure 2 - 1

SCHEMATIC REPRESENTATION OF THE PSYCHIC APPARATUS

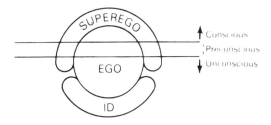

Reading Note: Those interested in learning more about ego development should read: Hartman, H., Kris, E., & Lowenstein, R. _Psychoanalytic studies of the child_, volume 2, 1946, 11-38.

These three persons further developed Freudian theory and are known as the originators of a field of study called ego psychology.

Now consider what kinds of unpleasant events may occur when conflict arises between the ego, the id, the superego, and/or environment. Conflict can produce fear, anxiety, sadness, guilt and emotional pain.   If the ego receives demands in keeping with its functions and principles, those demands are ego-syntonic.   Demands upon the ego not in keeping with its principles and functions are ego-dystonic.   The chart below gives a simple representation of these kinds of interactions:

Environmental Stress	→	Ego	→	Fear
Id Threat	→	Ego	→	Anxiety
Superego Disturbance	→	Ego	→	Sadness
Body Trauma	→	Ego	→	Guilt

This illustration is adapted from Hofling, 1968, p. 73.

As we can see from the above illustration, events in the environment or within our own psyche can produce unpleasant emotions.   Loss of a loved one can cause sadness.   Unacceptable impulses from the id can produce conflict leading to anxiety.   Stress from the environment can produce fear or anxiety within our own awareness or can escalate a conflict area in our nonconscious mind.   The function of the ego through all of these events is to maintain psychological homeostasis and facilitate adaptation.

Adaptation is the goal of our efforts to maintain psychological homeostasis. Our body is endowed with many adaptive mechanisms. The hierarchy of mechanisms used in maintaining internal body temperature is a useful analogy for understanding some aspects of psychological adaptation. The number of body temperature regulatory systems called into service is determined by the size of the task, namely the difference between ambient temperature and 98.6° Fahrenheit. Increasing the temperature difference brings more regulatory systems into play. Similarly, our capacity to adapt to emotional stress from the environment or emotional discomfort created by intrapsychic conflict will be based on the repertoire of our adaptive mechanisms. This chapter offers a consideration of ego defense mechanisms and a useful adaptive system. Sigmund Freud first introduced the notion of ego defense mechanisms as a part of a dynamic balance within our psychic apparatus. Freud postulated that we utilize varying mechanisms normally and pathologically to cope with dysphoric emotions or affects. Freud also postulated that defense mechanisms are used to keep certain areas of conflict out of our awareness, thus the anxiety associated with these conflicts is effectively bound up (inactivated).

The development of personality characteristics in an individual is often viewed as the manifestation of the most frequently used mechanisms of defense, although certainly all personality characteristics are not derivations of the standard list of ego mechanisms of defense. Competitiveness is an example of a personality characteristic determined by many factors. Sometimes competitiveness is used to compensate for a self-perceived deficiency. Other factors contributing to the development of competitiveness might include family norms and cultural norms. The individual's unique experiences during childhood and early adult life also might play a role.

QUIZ, Section II.

Complete the following.

1. Name the three functional components of the mind.

    _____

2. The id seeks immediate discharge of instinctual drives, thus operating on the _____ principle. The three fundamental drives of the id are: _____ _____ _____.

3. Portions of the _____ brain seem to be related to the hunger and sexual drives.

4. The _____ mediates between the id and the environment following the _____ principle.

5. The prohibition against stealing is a function of the _____.

6. Having overslept and missed breakfast, the junior medical student arrives on the ward. Midway through attending rounds, he is famished and feels he must have something to eat immediately (_____ function). He dares not leave attending rounds though (_____ function). He then remembers a vending machine nearby and plans a quick stop immediately after attending rounds (_____ function).

7. Environmental stress is mediated through the _____ to maintain homeostasis.

8. In attempting to deal with unpleasant emotions, the ego employs _____ to bind _____.

Match the following descriptions with the lettered items. Lettered items may be used once, more than once, or not at all.

____ 9. present at birth	a. id
____10. pleasure principle	b. ego
____11. reality principle	c. both
____12. completely unconscious	d. neither
____13. capacity to relate to others	
____14. moral standards	

Match the following descriptions with their corresponding lettered items.

____15. conflict free ego state	a. ego-dystonic
____16. unacceptable id impulses	b. ego-syntonic
____17. punitive superego	c. both
____18. sensory perception	d. neither

===

III. EGO DEFENSES

The development and use of ego defense mechanisms are normal adaptive processes. Specific ego defense mechanisms can be adaptive or maladaptive. The extent and the circumstances under which the mechanism is used are basic in determining when the use is adaptive and when it is maladaptive. Further, the individual's flexibility and the range of defense mechanisms available for use are also determinants of adaptive success. Moreover, often the degree of stress will determine the nature of the defense mechanism used. Consider the use of denial (see page 64). Many psychologically healthy, obese persons will deny the health hazard of being overweight. A psychologically healthy, young mother will refuse to accept the news of the accidental death of her child. Both of these are examples of the ego mechanism of denial. Both are normal, adaptive responses; differing only in degree of stress.

A. REPRESSION

Repression is said to be the basic defense mechanism, taking the form of forgetting. Repression involves putting into the unconscious things like wishes, impulses, feelings, or dysphoric affects. An example of the normal use of repression is the inability of a person to retain the memory of the quality and intensity of pain. If the memory of these aspects of physical pain were not repressed, people would be unlikely to undergo multiple surgical procedures, and many women would bear only one child. When a person uses repression, that person retains the repressed material in the nonconscious mind. The most common use of repression is seen in everyday forgetting. Consider a young physician just starting in practice and with limited financial means who receives a request to give money to his alumni association. He wants to give the money but feels the pinch. He finally decides to give, writes the check, and puts it in an envelope. One week later he finds the envelope in his coat pocket. He did not forget to mail the envelope with the payment for his electric bill. This is an example of repression. Other external manifestations of repression seen in medicine, particularly psychiatry, include slips of the tongue (Freudian slips).

Example: An intern on a medical service has considerable difficulty in his work with an overbearing, complaining, argumentative, obese lady who constantly demands pain medication for complaints he believes are non-organic. He withholds pain medication and avoids her. When X-rays reveal evidence of considerable spinal arthritis the attending physician suggests that he order aspirin prn. Respecting the attending, he agrees to do so. Three days later, while reviewing the charts, the attending points out that the intern "forgot" to order aspirin for the unpleasant woman who has since angrily signed out of the hospital. The intern later realizes how much the patient reminded him of his mother with whom he had spent many unhappy years. Forgetting to order the aspirin is an example of repression.

Example: A man comes home from a particularly hard day at work. He finds that his two small children are especially noisy, active, and argumentative. Finally his wife asks him to tell the children to get ready for dinner. He steps into the next room where the children are playing and says, "Children, it's time for you to get ready for bed." Substituting the word "bed" for "dinner" is a slip of the tongue reflecting a wish which may be nonconscious.

Repression can also be seen operating in hypnosis. For example, the subject is given a post-hypnotic suggestion and is instructed to forget that he has been given the suggestion. After recovery from the hypnotic trance, the subject performs the act which he was instructed to do. When questioned about his behavior, he tries to offer some rational explanation. His inability to remember the instructions given him during hypnosis is another example of repression.

B.   IDENTIFICATION (including incorporation and introjection)

Incorporation, introjection, and identification are defense mechanisms essential for normal psychological development. This chapter will not differentiate the three. In definition, these mechanisms are very similar

ANSWERS, Section II. _____

1. id, ego, superego
2. pleasure; hunger, sexual, aggressive
3. mesencephalic
4. ego, reality
5. superego
6. id, superego, ego
7. ego
8. defense mechanisms, anxiety
9. a

10. a
11. b
12. a
13. b
14. d
15. b
16. a
17. a
18. d

---

and, in the interest of simplicity, will be grouped under the broad heading of identification.

Identification is a process of taking into our development those character-istics which we admire in other people. Identification is an important developmental phenomenon. As children and adolescents, we all found that we could identify with other people in order to get some notion of what kind of person we wanted to be. Parents, movie stars, athletes, and various famous people serve as models for imitation and identification. Young children reach a point when they want to be like father or mother. Generally, they identify with the parent of the same sex. Little boys pretend to shave; little girls play with makeup. In adolescence, the use of identification is extremely important for normal healthy development. Adolescents choose a variety of persons with whom to identify, but very importantly they also tend to identify with their peer group. They and their friends tend to dress alike, talk alike, and adopt the same value systems.

While identification is an important developmental concept, the identification may be maladaptive. A person may deal with an unacceptable impulse to be aggressive by identifying with a very aggressive person. If the process of identification continues long enough, the person may take on the aggressive behavior and find the impulse to act aggressively acceptable.

A concern in choosing faculty members in a college of medicine is their suitability as role models for students, another example of identification occurring in adult life.

C. PROJECTION

Projection, a primitive mechanism, is seen in normal development during infancy. Projection can be seen during the first year of life. Exclusive use of projection in adults implies a seriously compromised adaptation. Projection is the mechanism whereby unacceptable feelings, wishes, or attributes originating within one's self are attributed to other persons.

Example: A tired and irritable child is taken to bed by his mother and told that he must take a nap. His instantaneous inner feeling is anger with his mother. He cries out, "You're mean, Mommy, you hate me." The child is projecting his unacceptable angry feelings onto his mother.

Example: A married man in his early 50's begins to experience strong sexual impulses for women in his office.   His fundamental religious upbringing has provided him a superego that would not permit consciousness of these sexual thoughts.   As the intensity of his feelings increases, he begins to suspect his wife of going to bed with the postman during the day.   He begins to search for evidence and assigns unrealistic importance to everyday events such as a comment from his wife that she is eager to receive a certain letter.   This is an example of maladaptive or pathological projection, resulting in a behavioral style which we call paranoia.

****

GO TO VIDEOTAPE

****

D.   DENIAL

Denial is the refusal to believe or allow awareness of some unpleasant or threatening aspect of external reality.   Denial is another primitive mechanism developing in early life.   The standard mechanism used in learning about the unexpected death of a loved one is the initial feeling of "It can't be true." Denial is often called into force when gross abrupt stress is experienced. The example above of the young mother learning of the death of her child is such an instance.   That mother may go on denying the death of the child for several hours.   Another example is the mother who receives the telegram from the War Department concerning the death of a child in combat.   She may go on for several weeks preparing for the child's return, denying the death.

Much research has been done with people who have recently experienced acute myocardial infarctions.   Interestingly, the survival rate of individuals who are acutely post-MI and hospitalized in coronary care units is greater if they manifest denial during the acute episode.   The form of this denial varies from person to person but can be characterized by the individual who says, "Yes, I've had a heart attack, but then a lot of people do. Most people think that it actually makes you take better care of yourself and so could be a good thing."   If one examines that statement carefully, it becomes difficult to explain how a myocardial infarction could possibly be a good thing.

****

GO TO VIDEOTAPE

****

E.   REGRESSION

Regression, a very common mechanism of defense, is manifest when an individual returns to an earlier, more primitive level of functioning.   When regression occurs, personality development and maturation suffer some degree of loss, at least temporarily.   Most families are familiar with regression in their young children with the arrival of a new baby in the home. Frequently encountered is a more demanding youngster, who reverts to baby talk, asks for a bottle again, or soils his or her pants. Such regressive behavior occurs when the youngster feels threatened about losing the parents' love and care.

Regression is commonly seen when someone is physically sick. Illnesses may require bed rest, physical limitations, restricted diets, numerous tests, and, in general, a certain dependency on others. This kind of threat will cause many people to regress, feeling the wish and need for someone to take care of them.

Schizophrenia is a major psychiatric disorder that includes regression as a significant component of the illness. The schizophrenic patient returns to an earlier mode of thinking and functioning.

QUIZ, Section III. A-E.

Circle the correct answer(s). <u>One</u> or <u>more than one</u> answer may be correct.

1. Which of the following is (are) true of ego defense mechanisms?

    a. generally maladaptive
    b. independent of degree of stress
    c. absent in psychologically healthy people
    d. keep certain conflicts out of awareness, binding anxiety
    e. are derivatives of cultural values

2. Projection

    a. is a primitive defense mechanism.
    b. when used to excess in adults may result in paranoid thinking.
    c. occurs normally in infancy.
    d. is never seen in healthy adults.

TRUE or FALSE: Circle the correct letter.

T   F   3. Repression is operative with the technique of hypnosis, but rarely occurs in daily life.

Complete the following:

4. A 10-year-old boy develops a consuming interest in baseball, telling everyone he wants to grow up to be just like Reggie Jackson. This example illustrates a normal process of _____ .

5. An inexperienced intern admires his Chief Resident's diagnostic skills and hopes to be as skillful one day. This is an example of _____ occurring in adult life.

6. Faced with an abrupt, unpleasant stress many individuals use _____ initially to deal with the stress.

7. A 21-year-old schizophrenic requires constant reminding to maintain personal hygiene. Such behavior might represent _____ .

F. RATIONALIZATION

Rationalization involves the use of socially acceptable explanations for behavior that may be interpreted as questionable. Behavior is usually prompted by a combination of inner motives, some of which may be moralistic and altruistic, and some of which may be selfish and instinctual. Unable to tolerate behavior based on other than noble motives, individuals verbally attempt to justify their actions in virtuous tones. Ethical incentives are selected out for conscious reasoning, while unacceptable motives are kept hidden in the nonconscious. (This differs from an untruth, wherein the falsehood is in the conscious mind.)

Example: Asked to dictate a patient's discharge summary before leaving the ward, the third year medical student states that the patient's chart could not be located. The fact that the student thus had time to attend an afternoon intramural soccer game is not considered by him to have influenced his not dictating the summary.

Example: Having done poorly on an important exam, the student attempts to maintain self-respect by stating that the professor asked unfair questions and "has never liked me anyway." The student refuses to remember that his preparation for the exam was done at the last minute, and that the course was one he did not enjoy.

Example: Not having been selected to represent the residents at a conference in San Francisco, the individual reasons that the trip would have been too time consuming and expensive anyway.

While rationalization generally includes an element of truth, the "whole truth" remains in the unconscious.

****

GO TO VIDEOTAPE

****

G. INTELLECTUALIZATION

Closely related to rationalization, intellectualization is the overuse of logic, reasoning, or intellectual concepts to avoid confrontation with an unacceptable affect or expression of feeling.

ANSWERS, SECTION III. A-E._____

1. d
2. a,b,c
3. F
4. identification
5. identification
6. denial
7. regression

_____

H. DISPLACEMENT

Transferring emotions or affects from one idea or object to a more acceptable substitute idea or object to relieve anxiety is displacement. Then
the affects, which were previously threatening or unacceptable, may
surface into consciousness and be displaced onto the safer idea or object
to which the person is ordinarily indifferent. The individual is thus
spared the pain of dealing with the original source of the conflict.

Example: A 36-year-old successful physician is discovered to have
inoperable bronchogenic carcinoma of the lung. He is hospitalized for
palliative treatment, and his condition rapidly deteriorates. The intense
emotions he feels in this most difficult situation are displaced onto those
treating and caring for him. He angrily yells, "These residents and
interns don't know what they're doing!...These nurses are incompetent!...
This food is terrible!"

I. REACTION FORMATION

Reaction formation occurs when a person develops attitudes and behaviors
that are in direct opposition to underlying unconscious impulses. This
defense mechanism thus hides the real urge or instinct by providing an
opposing acceptable position. A person who harbors unconscious, hostile
feelings toward his mother may behave toward her in an overprotective,
oversolicitous manner. An intensely insecure individual may adopt a
stance that is quite aggressive. Doubtful of his masculinity, a young
man may display a "Don Juan" behavior. The reformed alcoholic preaches
that to take a drink dooms one to a life of degradation. The behaviors
adopted are formed in reaction to underlying unacceptable and threatening impulses.

J. ISOLATION OF AFFECT

This defense mechanism relieves anxiety by separating emotions or affects
from ideas, objects, or memories originally associated with them. The
emotionally charged affect is repressed, and the idea, object, or memory
can then be discussed or reported "safely." The person who recalls the
details surrounding the death of a loved one without showing any signs
of affect or emotional feeling tone exhibits isolation of affect. The individual who speaks of his pending execution without any display of feeling or

emotion exemplifies isolation of affect. The medical student may call on this mechanism of defense at the time of his first autopsy, isolating his emotional response associated with the autopsy and devoting his energies to studying the pathology. The lack of feeling tone seen in patients diagnosed as obsessive-compulsive personality type is a clinical example of this mechanism.

****

GO TO VIDEOTAPE

****

K.   SUBLIMATION

Unlike other defense mechanisms, sublimation does not involve opposition between the ego and the id, but rather is a cooperative effort, whereby the ego helps the id gain external expression in a socially acceptable way. The anxiety, coupled with basic needs and impulses, is channeled by means of sublimation into development of lifestyles, vocations, and interests that provide gratification and reward for the individual and society. Aggressive tendencies may lead to a professional football career; intense curiosity may lead to a highly successful scientific career.

L.   UNDOING

Undoing is another method of coping with the anxiety associated with unacceptable thoughts or impulses by performing repetitive acts. Usually these acts are symbolically associated with the unacceptable thought or impulse. This mechanism of defense is often seen in the obsessive compulsive patient. We frequently see undoing as a compulsive act in response to an obsessive thought.

Handwashing and counting compulsions are among the more frequently encountered examples of undoing. Other examples include such things as checking time after time to make sure a door is locked or having to return to the kitchen as soon as one leaves to ensure the stove is turned off.

****

GO TO VIDEOTAPE

****

QUIZ, Section III. F-L.

Match the following descriptions with the most appropriate ego defense.

___ 1.	revealed by slips of the tongue forgetfulness	a. projection
___ 2.	logical explanation for behavior and feelings	b. regression
___ 3.	blaming others for despised tendencies in ourselves	c. denial
___ 4.	actively taking in qualities by imitation	d. repression
___ 5.	disowning of unacceptable thoughts, behavior, or reality factors	e. identification
___ 6.	stressing the opposite of true feelings	f. rationalization
___ 7.	return to earlier patterns of behavior	g. reaction formation

Match the following descriptions with the most appropriate ego defenses.

___ 8.	"the basic defense mechanism"	a. identification
___ 9.	obsessive compulsive, rituals	b. repression
___ 10.	Schizophrenia	c. isolation of affect
___ 11.	sports, creativity, vocation	d. projection
___ 12.	obsessive compulsive, aloof	e. reaction formation
___ 13.	adolescence	f. displacement
___ 14.	paranoia	g. undoing
		h. sublimation
		i. regression

ANSWERS, Section III, F-L. _____

1.	d		8.	b
2.	f		9.	g
3.	a		10.	i
4.	e		11.	h
5.	c		12.	c
6.	g		13.	a
7.	b		14.	d

POST-TEST

For the following questions, <u>one</u> or <u>more</u> <u>than</u> <u>one</u> answer may be correct. Circle the correct answer(s).

1.   The superego

    a.   is derived from the id in early infancy.
    b.   is influenced during its development by cultural values and standards.
    c.   usually has no relationship to the ethical teaching of parents.
    d.   can vary in degree from very permissive to very punitive.

2.   Which of the following describe(s) the ego?

    a.   compromises between internal demands and external reality
    b.   like the id, follows the pleasure principle
    c.   functions include intelligence, memory, and sensory perception
    d.   all ego functions are conscious

3.   Ego-dystonic demands

    a.   can produce conflict leading to unpleasant emotional experiences.
    b.   virtually never occur in daily life.
    c.   may arise from the id, superego, or environment.
    d.   are generally in keeping with the ego's principles and functions.

4.   Which of the following describe(s) the id?

    a.   seat of instinctual drives
    b.   present at birth
    c.   operates on the pleasure principle
    d.   has been definitively demonstrated anatomically

5.   Projection

    a.   is a primitive mechanism, seen normally in infancy.
    b.   is attributing one's unacceptable feelings, wishes, or attributes to others.
    c.   is evident in paranoid behavior.
    d.   can be observed in "normal" individuals.

6.   Rationalization

    a.   involves use of socially acceptable explanations for questionable behavior.
    b.   could be seen as a means to appease the superego.
    c.   may be used by the ego to keep selfish motives out of awareness.
    d.   usually occurs in consciousness, thus may be thought of as lying.

7. Regression

    a. is a common defense mechanism seen in schizophrenics and physically ill individuals, among others.
    b. causes irreparable damage to personality development.
    c. is characterized by a return to an earlier, more primitive mode of functioning.
    d. is virtually unknown past the teenage years.

8. Repression

    a. is a primitive basic defense mechanism that should be considered pathological if seen past age 5 years.
    b. operates exclusively in awareness.
    c. refers to using earlier modes of adaptation.
    d. is represented by the inability of individuals to remember physical pain and post-hypnotic suggestions.

9. Intellectualization and displacement

    a. are alike in that both are defense mechanisms that deal with unpleasant affects.
    b. are alike in that both use substitute objects to relieve anxiety.
    c. are commonly used unconscious mechanisms.
    d. are primitive defense mechanisms like projection.

10. In the months following a child patient's death, an intern decides that rather than remain frustrated and angry over the child's death, he will actively study the disease which killed the child. The intern may be using the defense mechanism known as

    a. intellectualization.
    b. displacement.
    c. sublimation.
    d. undoing.
    e. rationalization.

11. A 30-year-old woman married for seven years has been unsuccessful in becoming pregnant. A fertility work-up reveals bilateral stenosis of the Fallopian tubes. Upon hearing the results from her physician she states, "I don't believe it. I'll find another doctor!" This woman is using

    a. projection.
    b. denial.
    c. both.

12. Ego defense mechanisms

    a. were just introduced by Charcot in 1873.
    b. are used to bring areas of conflict into consciousness to relieve anxiety.
    c. generally determine all personality characteristics.
    d. are used normally and/or pathologically to cope with dysphoric emotions.
    e. are used to the same degree, regardless of the stress.

13. A 40-year-old male has devoted his life to his domineering, obnoxious, invalid father. He is extremely solicitous, and protective to his unappreciative parent. This man is using the defense mechanism known as

    a. denial.
    b. displacement.
    c. reaction formation.
    d. projection.
    e. rationalization.

14. Which of the following statements concerning identification is not true?

    a. Identification does not occur in adult life.
    b. Identification is crucial in normal healthy development.
    c. Adolescents tend to identify with their peer group.
    d. Young children usually tend to identify with the same sex parent.

15. A young pediatrics intern cares for an extremely ill six-year-old. While he is on call, the child dies. The following morning he calmly discusses the case with his attending. Upon arriving home, he kicks his dog and accuses his wife of being incompetent in managing household affairs. In the order of appearance in this vignette, select the defense mechanisms evident.

    a. denial, rationalization, projection
    b. repression, sublimation, intellectualization
    c. isolation of affect, displacement, projection
    d. regression, denial, undoing

16. Having the patient freely report passing thought activity without censorship or reservation is known as

    a. thought broadcasting.
    b. free association.
    c. projection.
    d. thought dissociation.
    e. affect analysis.

17. Which of the following statements concerning the ego is not true?

    a. The ego is the integrative adaptive portion of the mind.
    b. The ego houses moral and ethical standards.
    c. Ego functions include intelligence, memory, motivation, and sensory perception.
    d. Some ego functions are conscious, others are not.
    e. The capacity to do creative and purposeful work is an ego function.

18. The ego seeks to achieve and maintain a homeostatic state by

    a. mediating between external reality and internal demands.
    b. mediating between id demands and superego standards.
    c. using defense mechanisms.
    d. none of the above.

For the following questions, circle the letter corresponding to the one correct answer.

19. The groundwork for psychoanalysis was laid by

    a. Alfred Adler.
    b. Karen Horney.
    c. Sigmund Freud.
    d. Carl Jung.

20. One of the basic assumptions of the psychoanalytic model is that

    a. a portion of the mind is unconscious, but most of the mind is conscious.
    b. a portion of the mind is unconscious, but this portion has little or no effect on behavior.
    c. a portion of the mind is unconscious, and none of this unconscious material can be made conscious.
    d. a portion of the mind is unconscious, and some of this material can be made conscious by certain techniques.

21. Instinctual components of the id are most easily seen in the

    a. 2-year-old.
    b. newborn.
    c. college student.
    d. 6-year-old.

22. Freud described three functional components of the mind. Which of the following is not part of his schema?

    a. id
    b. archetype
    c. superego
    d. ego

Match the following drives with the corresponding characteristics.

_____23. sexual drive

_____24. hunger drive

_____25. aggressive drive

a.   dependency needs

b.   social needs

c.   hostility

PRE-TEST ANSWERS

1.	c	10.	c	18.	d
2.	d	11.	c	19.	a,b,c,d
3.	b	12.	c	20.	a,c
4.	b	13.	a,b,c	21.	a,b,c
5.	b	14.	a,b,c	22.	a,c
6.	b	15.	a,c	23.	c
7.	d	16.	b,d	24.	b
8.	a	17.	a,c	25.	a
9.	b				

POST-TEST ANSWERS

1.	b,d	10.	c	18.	a,b,c
2.	a,c	11.	b	19.	c
3.	a,c	12.	d	20.	d
4.	a,b,c	13.	c	21.	b
5.	a,b,c,d	14.	a	22.	b
6.	a,b,c	15.	c	23.	b
7.	a,c	16.	b	24.	a
8.	d	17.	b	25.	c
9.	a,c				

REFERENCES

Hirsia, L. E., & Campbell, R. J. <u>Psychiatric dictionary</u> (4th ed.). New York: Oxford University Press, 1970.

Kaplan, H. I., Freedman, A. M., & Sudock, B. J. <u>Comprehensive text-book of psychiatry III</u>. Baltimore: William & Wilkins, 1980.

McCurdy, L., & Villeponteaux, L. Personality and ego defenses. In L. Villeponteaux & D. Kilpatrick (Eds.), <u>The correctional learning system</u>. Charleston, SC: Deligamus, 1978.

CHAPTER 3

Psychological Evaluation

Darlene L. Shaw, Ph.D.
Valerie L. Holmstrom, Ph.D.

CHAPTER OUTLINE

LEARNING OBJECTIVES

After completing this chapter you should be able to:

1. List four uses of psychological tests in clinical settings.

2. Define the characteristics of a "good" psychological test: objectivity, reliability, validity, and standardization.

3. Define: frequency distribution, normal distribution curve, arithmetic mean, and standard deviation.

4. Define intelligence.

5. Describe five factors which affect measured intelligence.

6. Describe the WAIS-R, WISC-R, WPPSI, and Stanford-Binet, including the age groups with which they are commonly used.

7. Describe the general purposes of objective and projective personality assessment and describe the following personality tests: Rorschach, MMPI, and TAT.

8. Describe the two principal purposes for making psychological assessments for organicity.

9. Describe the following tests which are commonly used to evaluate patients for organicity: Wechsler Intelligence Scales, Wechsler Memory Scale, Graham-Kendall Memory-for-Designs Test, Bender-Gestalt Visual Motor Test, and the Halstead-Reitan battery of tests.

10. List the five components of behavioral assessment.

11. List the three elements to include in a request for psychological consultation and list the reasons for including these elements.

PRE-TEST

For the following questions, <u>one</u> or <u>more</u> <u>than</u> <u>one</u> answer may be correct. Circle the correct answer(s).

1. Psychological tests are used in clinical settings to

    a. assign the proper diagnostic label to psychiatric disorders.
    b. identify symptomatic behaviors.
    c. determine the etiology of pathological behaviors.
    d. establish baseline levels and monitor change in behavior.

2. Common characteristics among the WAIS, WISC, WPPSI, and Stanford-Binet include that they

    a. are measures of intelligence.
    b. provide information regarding impairment of higher cortical functioning indicative of organic brain dysfunction.
    c. measure performance in a variety of functional areas.
    d. are self-administered tests taken in a group.

3. Factors which have been found to affect measured intelligence include

    a. academic experiences.
    b. cultural influences.
    c. heredity.
    d. certain psychiatric disorders.

4. Which of the following are characteristics of a good psychological test which also apply to the MMPI?

    a. objectivity
    b. standardization
    c. validity
    d. projectivity

5. Validity of a psychological test is best defined as

    a. uniformity of procedures in administering and scoring a test.
    b. consistency of the scores received by the same person on each administration of the test.
    c. the extent to which a test measures an individual's perceptual organization of ambiguous stimuli.
    d. the extent to which a test measures what it purports to measure.

6. Which of the following is/are a purpose(s) for making a psychological assessment for organicity in a patient?

    a. to establish the etiology of organic dysfunction
    b. to determine the nature and extent of functional loss in order to plan the patient's rehabilitation program
    c. to determine the relationship between social adjustment and maturation level
    d. to provide information to assist in making a diagnosis

7.   A behavioral assessment entails

    a.   identification of adaptive behaviors in the individual's repertoire.
    b.   quantification of the problematic behavior.
    c.   identification of environmental events which trigger and maintain the problematic behavior.
    d.   identification of stimuli which the individual finds reinforcing and those which are aversive for him.

Use the following case study to answer questions 8-9.

Mr. J. is a 62-year-old, retired, white, male patient who has been hospitalized three times in the past for depression. His last hospitalization was 15 years ago. Since that time he has required no outpatient psychiatric treatment. He has now been admitted to an inpatient psychiatric service at the encouragement of his wife who reports that her husband is agitated and irritable at home, that he does not sleep through the night, is not going out to socialize with friends, and seems forgetful.

On mental status examination, Mr. J. appears somewhat disheveled and unkempt. He is moderately dysphoric in mood and becomes agitated when asked how he feels about his wife bringing him to the hospital. His attention and concentration are poor, and while remote memory is intact, recent memory and immediate recall are poor.

8.   Which of the following statements is/are true?

    a.   A request for psychological consultation may be useful to evaluate Mr. J.'s personality and the severity of his depression.
    b.   In order to establish a clinical diagnosis of Mr. J., more information is needed.
    c.   A systematic behavioral assessment may be useful in evaluating Mr. J., either for depression or organicity.
    d.   Neuropsychological assessment of Mr. J.'s memory could be used to establish the nature and extent of functional loss.

9.   Which of the following statements is/are true?

    a.   Given the long period of time since Mr. J.'s last psychiatric hospitalization, information about previous psychiatric problems is not relevant to evaluating him at this time.
    b.   Mr. J.'s poor recent memory may be a function of emotional factors.
    c.   Neuropsychological testing would be of no use with this patient because he also has symptoms of depression.
    d.   Mr. J.'s poor recent memory may be a function of organic factors.

Use the figure below to answer questions 10-13.

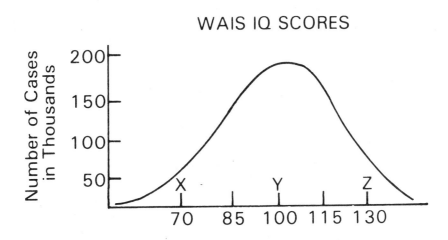

WAIS IQ SCORES

Circle the letter corresponding to the <u>one</u> correct response.

10. The graph in the figure above represents

    a. reliability distribution.
    b. baseline distribution.
    c. normal distribution.
    d. incremental validity distribution.

11. The arithmetic mean of the distribution in the figure above is at

    a. Point X.
    b. Point Y.
    c. Point Z.

12. The point in the distribution which is two standard deviations above the mean is

    a. X.
    b. Y.
    c. Z.

13. Eighty-four percent of the population represented in the preceding figure falls below an IQ score of

   a. 70.
   b. 85.
   c. 100.
   d. 115.
   e. 130.

Match the following descriptions with the corresponding psychological tests.

___14. standardized objective, self-administered personality test

___15. individually administered, projective personality test using standardized inkblots

___16. individually administered, projective personality test in which the individual creates a story about the pictures he is presented

___17. a self-administered projective personality test in which the individual interprets ambiguous stimuli

___18. individually administered intelligence test

a. TAT
b. Rorschach
c. Stanford-Binet
d. MMPI
e. none of the above

Match the following descriptions with the corresponding psychological tests.

___19. an intelligence test which yields a Verbal, Performance, and Full Scale IQ Score

___20. a standardized perceptual motor memory test

___21. a battery of several tests to evaluate functional losses secondary to organic brain dysfunction

___22. a test of six areas of short- and long-term memory functions

___23. a perceptual motor test which is effective for screening for organic brain dysfunction

a. Halstead-Reitan
b. Bender-Gestalt
c. WAIS
d. Wechsler Memory Scale
e. Graham-Kendall Memory-for-Designs

I. FUNDAMENTALS OF PSYCHOLOGICAL TESTING

A. PURPOSES AND USES OF TESTS

The fundamental purposes of psychological tests are to measure differences among individuals and differences among responses of the same individual on different occasions. People differ from one another in numerous ways. These differences include variations in abilities, attitudes, aptitudes, behaviors, achievements, interests, and personality characteristics. In addition to being different from one another, individuals show variability over time and situation. Psychological tests measure individual variability related to time and situation and permit comparison of individuals.

The historical roots of testing lie in the ancient Chinese empire where examinations were used in the civil service system. Testing became a part of the educational system in ancient Greece. Tests were first used in clinical settings in the nineteenth century. During that period, the movement toward humane treatment of the mentally retarded and insane made it necessary to differentiate between these two diagnostic groups. The historical uses of tests are not dissimilar from the current uses of tests.

In clinical settings tests are used to measure acquisition and retention of information and skills, as well as to identify specific symptomatic behaviors. Psychological tests are also used to classify individuals along a particular dimension (e.g., intellectual ability) and to aid in diagnosis. Prediction of behavior such as suicide or response to psychotherapy is another application of psychological testing. Tests are also used to establish baseline levels of a behavior or characteristic, in order that changes in that behavior or characteristic may be monitored. For example, a clinician might collect psychological and behavioral measures before and after prescribing a tricyclic drug, in order to determine whether the drug effected a change in depressive symptomatology. Finally, tests serve an important function in clinical research involving identification and quantification of individual differences and monitoring change. In summary, psychological tests aid in identifying, classifying, predicting, and monitoring change in behavior.

B. CHARACTERISTICS OF A GOOD TEST

We said earlier that the purpose of psychological tests is to measure differences between individuals or between the responses of the same individual on different occasions. We all make informal evaluations of one another on a daily basis. Informal ratings, however, have several flaws. They are often based on a limited, possibly nonrepresentative sample of behavior; they are subjectively rendered; and they may be biased by preconceived notions regarding the person. Psychological tests attempt to minimize the faults of informal evaluations by providing standard samples of behavior and objective ways of rating behavior. Thus, a psychological test is defined as "an objective and standardized measure of a sample of behavior" (Anastasi, 1978). In order to be a good test - that is, one that can be confidently and accurately used to evaluate people - a psychological test must have several characteristics: primarily objectivity, reliability, validity, and standardization. Some tests possess these desirable attributes to a greater extent than others. Although the characteristics of reliability, objectivity, validity, and standardization are interrelated, we will define them separately.

Objectivity refers to uniformity of procedures in the administration, scoring, or interpretation of a test. Testing conditions and scoring procedures must be the same for all persons if the performance by different persons is to be comparable.

Reliability means consistency - consistency of the scores or rank received by the same person on each administration of the test or an equivalent form of the test. If chance or random error largely determines the score an individual obtains on a test, the test is unreliable. The usefulness of an I.Q. test, for example, would be very limited if a student obtained an I.Q. of 105 one day and an I.Q. of 135 the next day. Thus, reliability is essential for a good psychological measure. A test may be highly reliable, however, and still not measure what it intends to measure. Reliability, in other words, is necessary, but not sufficient for validity.

Validity refers to the extent to which a test measures what it purports to measure. In other words, validity is the extent to which a measuring device accomplishes its intended purpose. Therefore, validity is never abstract, but always specific to a particular purpose. For example, a yard stick is a highly reliable and valid measure of a person's height, but it is not a valid measure of his intelligence. Typically, the validity of a measuring instrument is determined by comparing the results of the measure with a standard or criterion. The results of a personality test, for example, might suggest a diagnosis. On the other hand, agreement by a panel of expert clinicians is a widely accepted method of diagnosis. Therefore, the validity of the personality test might be measured by comparing the diagnosis obtained using the test with the criterion diagnosis assigned by the experts. The ability of a measuring device to predict a future criterion is called predictive validity. If, for example, scores on an admission test are found to be highly correlated with the criterion of grades subsequently received in medical school, the test would have predictive validity.

The usefulness or validity of a measuring instrument is affected by the extent to which it provides information beyond that which can be obtained by chance. The increase in predictive ability attributable to a test is called incremental validity. For example, if chance assignment of a diagnostic category is correct 25% of the time, and a psychological test leads to correct diagnostic assignment 40% of the time, the rise from 25 to 40 represents the incremental validity.

It is very unlikely, however, that decisions regarding classification, selection, or evaluation of individuals are made on the basis of chance. Usually other information such as history, interview data, and the like is considered in the decision process. Thus, the contribution of a test should be judged by the extent to which the test improves the predictive ability of existing decision-making methods.

When considering the contribution of psychological measures to the decision process, the base rate of the phenomenon under consideration must also be taken into account. The base rate is the frequency of a given phenomenon in the population under consideration. For example, if 95% of all residents in a particular nursing home have organic brain dysfunction, the base rate of that condition is 95%. Although the use of a valid psychological measure will always improve decision accuracy, in cases of extreme base rates, either high (near 100%) or low (near 0%), a test provides little improvement in the decision (predictive) process. The improvement in prediction is greatest when the base rate is near 50%. Given a 95% base rate of organic brain dysfunction in a nursing home population, a clinician who diagnosed all patients in such a setting as organic would be correct 95% of the time, and any improvement in prediction provided by a psychological test would likely be negligible.

Standardization involves administering a test under standard conditions to a large, well-defined group of individuals representative of the group for whom the test was devised. The purpose of standardization is to provide a frame of reference or norm to which a particular person's or group of persons' scores can be compared. Many tests have more than one set of norms for different sexes, age groups, etc. so that comparisons can be made with whatever group(s) is (are) appropriate. In order for comparison of an individual's score with the test norm to be fair, the test norms must have been gathered on a group having similar characteristics to that individual. For example, if a test in basic science knowledge is being used to select medical school applicants, the standardization group could be the general population; however, a more appropriate normative group would be medical school freshmen.

In summary, in order to be helpful in prediction or decision making, a psychological test must not only be valid, but must also have incremental validity - that is, it must measure what it was intended to measure and increase prediction beyond the level attainable by chance, base rates, and customary decision-making methods. A prerequisite for validity is reliability. That is, the test must give consistent results on repeated administrations. To be reliable, it must be objective in that a uniform procedure for administration and scoring is provided. Finally, in order for an individual's score to convey meaningful information, the test must be standardized which permits comparison to the scores of similar persons. The psychological measures described in this chapter have these characteristics; however, some of the measures fulfill the criteria of a good test better than others. Information regarding the fundamentals of testing will permit the student to judge the relative strengths and weaknesses of the various tests described.

C. INTERPRETATION OF TEST SCORES

It was noted earlier that in psychological assessment, we are almost always interested in comparing people. A psychological characteristic is not like years or inches; it is a relative measure. Carrying this point to absurdity, if 95% of all individuals in our society reported on a psychological test that they regularly hallucinated pink snakes on the wall, this behavior would be the "norm," would no longer be defined as deviant, and consequently, would be of little interest psychologically.

Since the presence of psychological traits is relative, a raw numerical score on a test is meaningless in itself. You may score 50 on a scale measuring depression and 75 on a scale measuring anxiety, and we still can say nothing meaningful about your psychological adjustment. Statistical procedures are used to organize, summarize, and compare testing data. Therefore, an understanding of rudimentary statistical concepts is necessary for interpreting and understanding the results of psychological testing.

A convenient and frequently used way to organize data is in the form of a graph where the horizontal axis represents the number values of whatever is being measured, and the vertical axis depicts the number of persons who obtained each number value (Figure 3-1). A graph constructed in this way is called a frequency distribution.

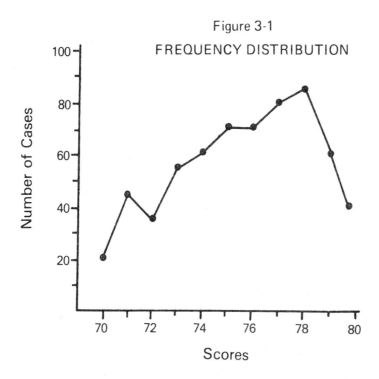

Figure 3-1

FREQUENCY DISTRIBUTION

When psychological and biological characteristics such as intelligence and height are measured in a very large, unselected population, the frequency distribution usually approaches a symmetrical, "bell-shaped" curve. A frequency distribution with this shape of a curve is called a normal distribution or the normal curve.

As can be seen in Figure 3-2, in a normal distribution most individuals fall near the middle of the distribution, and fewer and fewer individuals are found toward the extremes of the distribution.

Figure 3-2

THE NORMAL CURVE

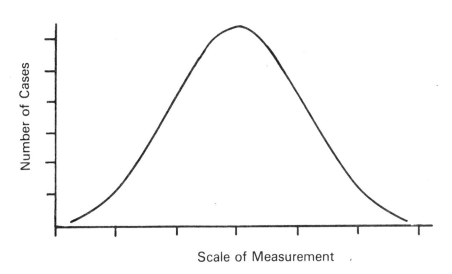

Two kinds of statistics are used to summarize a distribution of data: (1) measures of central tendency and (2) measures of variability. Measures of central tendency define the center of the distribution and, in this way, provide a single representative score which characterizes the performance of the whole group (Anastasi, 1978). The most frequently used measure of central tendency is the well known "average," technically called the arithmetic mean ($\bar{x}$). To obtain the mean, simply add all the scores in a distribution and divide by the total number of scores. For example, in the distribution of scores shown in Table 3-1, the mean equals 6 ($\bar{x}= 6$).

TABLE 3-1
COMPUTATION OF THE MEAN OF
A GROUP OF SCORES

SCORES	
2	
4	
4	Mean = $\bar{X}$ = 42/7 = 6
5	Range = 11-2 = 9
7	Standard Deviation = SD = 3.2
9	
11	
TOTAL = 42	

In addition to knowing the central value (mean) of a set of scores, you must also measure the spread or variability of the scores in order to describe the distribution. The variability of a distribution reflects the degree to which the individuals in the group differ from one another. A group of secretaries, for example, might have the same mean ($\bar{x}$) intelligence as the general population; however, the secretaries would likely cluster around the mean, having relatively little variability, while the general population would have much greater variability, since both extremely intelligent and retarded individuals would be included in the distribution.

The simplest measure of variability is called the range. The range is the difference between the highest and lowest score in a distribution. For example, the range for the group of scores in Table 3-1 is 9.

The most frequently used measure of variability is the standard deviation (SD). While you need not know how the standard deviation is calculated, you should know what it means. The standard deviation tells how closely the scores are clustered around the mean. Figure 3-3 demonstrates how the degree of variability around the mean is reflected by the standard deviation; the two distributions have equal means but different standard deviations.

Figure 3-3

THE STANDARD DEVIATION
INDICATES THE SPREAD OF A
DISTRIBUTION

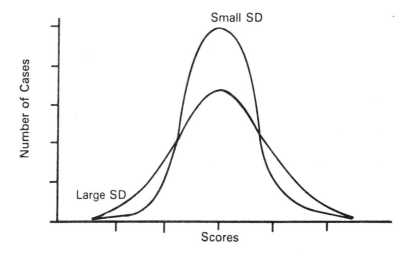

In any normal or approximately normal distribution, there is an exact relationship between the standard deviation and the proportion of cases falling below or above a specific point or between two points on the scale. The relationship between standard deviation and percentages of a normal distribution is summarized in Figure 3-4. It can be seen that 68.3 (34.13 + 34.13 = 68.26) percent of the cases in a normal distribution fall between 1 SD above and 1 SD below the mean. Approximately 95 percent lie between 2 SD's above and 2 SD's below the mean, and 99.7 percent of the cases fall between ± 3 SD's. Because there is an exact relationship between the standard deviation and the proportion of scores falling below a given score in a normal distribution, the standard deviation provides the basis for comparing a person's performance on two different tests or on the same test on two different occasions, relative to the normative sample. For example, if the mean on an intelligence test is 100 ($\bar{x}$ = 100) and the standard deviation is 15 (SD = 15), then an individual obtaining a raw score of 115 falls one standard deviation unit above the mean, with 84 percent of the population scoring below him (see Fig. 3-4 for Percentiles). If the same individual scored 200 on a test of manual dexterity for which the mean score was 225 and the standard deviation was 25, his performance would place him one standard deviation below the mean or at the 16th percentile on that test. It could then be said that the individual scored relatively better on the test of general intelligence than he did on the test of manual dexterity.

Figure 3-4

RELATIONSHIPS AMONG STANDARD DEVIATION,
PERCENTAGES, PERCENTILES AND DIFFERENT
TEST SCORES IN A NORMAL DISTRIBUTION

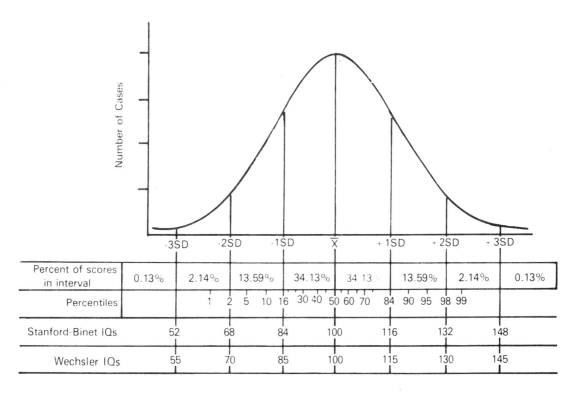

	-3SD		-2SD		-1SD		$\bar{x}$		+1SD		+2SD		+3SD
Percent of scores in interval	0.13%		2.14%		13.59%		34.13%		34 13		13.59%		2.14%		0.13%
Percentiles			1	2	5	10 16	30 40	50 60 70	84	90 95	98 99		
Stanford-Binet IQs		52		68		84		100		116		132		148
Wechsler IQs		55		70		85		100		115		130		145

QUIZ, Section I.

Circle the correct answer(s). <u>One</u> or <u>more</u> <u>than</u> <u>one</u> answer may be correct.

1. Psychological tests measure

    a. differences between persons.
    b. differences among responses of the same person at different times.

2. Psychological tests permit measurement of change in an individual's behavior by establishing

    a. classifications of behavior.
    b. predictors of behavior.
    c. baseline levels of behavior.

3. Test administration and scoring procedures must be the same for all persons if a test is to meet the criterion of

    a. objectivity.
    b. standardization.
    c. validity.

4. Standardization

    a. involves administering a test to a large group of people.
    b. provides a measure of a test's validity.
    c. permits comparison of an individual's score with the performance of a representative group.

5. A good psychological test has

    a. objectivity.
    b. reliability.
    c. validity.
    d. standardization.

6. The arithmetic mean

    a. measures the reliability of a test.
    b. is denoted by "$\bar{x}$."
    c. is commonly called the "average."

7. In normal distributions, the standard deviation

    a. provides information regarding the reliability of the test.
    b. provides information regarding the proportion of cases lying below, above, or between two points in the distribution.
    c. provides the basis for comparing scores.

8. When psychological and biological traits are measured for a large group of the general population,

    a. most individuals fall near the middle of the distribution of possible scores.
    b. the frequency distribution formed by the scores is a symmetrical "bell-shaped" curve.
    c. a normal curve is formed.

Circle the letter corresponding to the <u>one</u> correct response.

9. Psychological tests differ from informal evaluations of behavior in that psychological tests provide _____ ways of measuring _____samples of behavior.

    a. classical, baseline
    b. objective, standard
    c. subjective, predictor
    d. none of the above

10. As the influence of chance or random error on a test score decreases, the consistency of the score increases, and the reliability of the score

    a. decreases.
    b. increases.
    c. stays the same.
    d. may increase or decrease depending on the objectivity of the test.

11. If clinical interviews of patients in a particular population result in accurate diagnosis of Schizophrenia 50% of the time, and a psychological test results in correct diagnosis of Schizophrenia 60% of the time, the improvement in diagnostic accuracy provided by the test represents

    a. the base rate of Schizophrenia.
    b. an improvement in the base rate of Schizophrenia.
    c. the incremental validity of the test.
    d. the predictive validity of the test.

12. In a normal distribution approximately _____% of the cases fall between 2SD's above and 2SD's below the mean.

    a. 95
    b. 68
    c. 100
    d. 50

TRUE or FALSE: Indicate whether the following questions are true (T) or false (F) by circling the appropriate letter.

T   F   13. Reliability is a necessary, but not sufficient, condition for a test to be valid.

T   F   14. All psychological tests are equally objective, reliable, and valid.

T   F   15. Since psychological characteristics are relative, a raw score on a psychological test is meaningless by itself.

T   F   16. Statistical procedures, applied to scores on psychological measures, make these scores meaningful and permit comparison of individuals.

T   F   17. The range and standard deviation provide information regarding the degree to which individuals in a group differ from one another.

T   F   18. The smaller the numerical value of a standard deviation, the larger the variability of scores around the mean of a distribution.

Match the following descriptions with the corresponding lettered items.

___19.   the ability of a test to measure   a.   validity
          what it is supposed to measure   b.   predictive validity
___20.   the extent to which a test improves   c.   predictive criterion
          the predictive ability of existing   d.   incremental validity
          decision-making methods   e.   base rate
___21.   the ability of a test to predict   f.   criterion population
          a criterion measure
___22.   the frequency of a phenomenon
          in a population

Match the following descriptions with the corresponding lettered items.

___23.   consistency of test scores   a.   reliability
          on different administrations   b.   objectivity
___24.   uniformity of test administration   c.   validity
          and scoring procedures   d.   standardization
___25.   test administration to a large
          group with resulting group norms
___26.   the ability of a test to measure the
          variable it is intended to measure

II.   INTELLIGENCE TESTING

A.   THE NATURE OF INTELLIGENCE

Intelligence is a construct used to describe a collection of complex mental abilities, such as the ability to recall general information, the ability to reason abstractly, or the ability to reproduce a geometric design. Development of intellectual ability is dependent on both genetic potential and environmental encounters that promote learning of information or skills.

There are several popular misconceptions regarding the nature of intelligence. For example, intelligence is frequently thought of as a unitary measure of ability rather than as a measure of varied abilities. That is, laymen might label an individual as "bright" or "dumb" while actually the individual is skilled at mechanical tasks and deficient on verbal tasks. Other erroneous beliefs portray intelligence as an innate fixed quality, which explains a person's behavior--"Joe does not have enough intelligence to do well in therapy." Another myth is that intelligence represents a universally agreed upon concept which spans socioeconomic and cultural barriers and is measured the same by all intelligence tests.

Let us examine each of these misconceptions. First, intelligence is not a unitary quality. Rather, multiple abilities constitute intelligence. Individuals obtaining the same score on an intelligence test may have completely different patterns of specific abilities and deficiencies. While one individual might excel on items measuring manual skills, another might do best on verbal tasks. Secondly, intelligence is better regarded as a descriptive rather than an explanatory concept. That is, a score on an intelligence test (IQ score) is a shorthand description of an individual's performance on a specific set of tasks at a given time. A given score does not explain the reasons for a particular performance.

Thirdly, measured intelligence is neither fixed, nor is it solely determined by heredity. Performance on any test of ability is determined by four factors: (1) innate ability, (2) environmental/experiential influences, (3) motivation, and (4) the content of the test items. Furthermore, a change in one of these factors will affect the test score, and the test provides no means for untangling these components. Finally, the component abilities constituting intelligence are not universal, but at least in part, culture specific. Moreover, even within a given culture a particular intelligence test may emphasize measurement of a sub-class of the multiple abilities constituting intelligence to the relative exclusion of other types of abilities. Therefore, a particular intelligence test will predict some abilities better than others, and the item content of the test will influence an individual's IQ score.

B. INTELLIGENCE TESTS

The first intelligence test was devised by a French psychologist, Alfred Binet, in 1905. It was used in the Paris school system to identify children of low intelligence who were not expected to benefit from attending school. A revision of Binet's original test was published for American school children in 1916 and came to be known as the Stanford-Binet Scale.

The Stanford-Binet (since revised) is administered individually and remains a popular scale for testing the intelligence of children. The test consists of a series of subscales arranged according to age levels. Measurement of intelligence was predicated on the assumption that mental ability progressively increases with chronological age. An individual's mental age (MA) is equal to the chronological age at which the "average" person performs as well as the individual. For an "average" child, mental age should be consistent with chronological age. For example, a normal five-year-old child should have a mental age of five. Similarly, a "slower" five-year-old who performs at the level of an average four-year-old would have a mental age of four. Based on this assumption, intelligence or the intelligence quotient (IQ) was originally expressed as a ratio of mental age (MA) to chronological age (CA), multiplied by 100.

$$\text{Example:} \quad IQ = MA/CA \times 100$$
$$MA = 6.0$$
$$CA = 5.7$$
$$IQ = 6.0/5.7 \times 100 = 105$$

Since this way of computing the IQ proved problematic, the ratio IQ is no longer used. The Stanford-Binet IQ is now derived from the standard deviation and is expressed as a standard score. As Figure 3-4 denotes, for each age group the mean IQ is 100, and the standard deviation is 16. Thus, a given IQ score provides information about the individual's performance relative to his age group. For example, a Stanford-Binet IQ score of 116 always indicates that an individual has scored at or above the performance level of 84 percent of individuals his age.

There remains, however, another important limitation of the Stanford-Binet Scale. Although it measures other skills to some extent, it is predominantly a test of verbal ability. This limitation is less important when testing children but more problematic for an adult population in which the user wishes to predict a wider range of skills. Therefore, while there are Stanford-Binet norms for the adult population, the test is used more frequently with children.

The most widely used intelligence test for adults was devised by David Wechsler and is called the Wechsler Adult Intelligence Scale (WAIS). In 1980 a revised edition of this test (WAIS-R) was developed. Both the WAIS and the WAIS-R are commonly used for the intellectual assessment of persons 16 years of age and older. The WAIS and the WAIS-R, like the Stanford-Binet, are individually administered and composed of several subtests. The subtests, however, are not scaled according to age as in the Stanford-Binet, but according to increasing difficulty for the type of ability measured by each subtest. Although the subtests are grouped into two categories, the Verbal Scale and the Performance Scale, the subtests are scored separately so that an individual's performance in each ability area may be compared. In addition, the Verbal and Performance Scales are scored separately, yielding a Verbal Scale IQ and a Performance Scale IQ as well as a Full Scale IQ.

In addition to the WAIS, Wechsler devised two additional intelligence scales - the Wechsler Intelligence Scale for Children (WISC) for ages 5 through 15 years, and the Wechsler Preschool and Primary Scale of Intelligence (WPPSI) for ages 4 through 6½ years. Both the WISC and WPPSI are individually administered, have separately scored subtests similar to those of the WAIS, and are divided into a Verbal and Performance Scale, yielding a Verbal Scale IQ, a Performance Scale IQ, and a Full Scale IQ.

As with the Stanford-Binet, IQ's obtained from the Wechsler scales (WAIS, WISC, and WPPSI) are expressed in the form of standard scores. The

ANSWERS, Section I.

1. a,b	10. b	19. a
2. c	11. c	20. d
3. a	12. a	21. b
4. a,c	13. T	22. e
5. a,b,c,d	14. F	23. a
6. b,c	15. T	24. b
7. b,c	16. T	25. d
8. a,b,c	17. T	26. c
9. b	18. F	

mean IQ for each age is 100 and the standard deviation for each age is 15. Therefore, for example, an individual obtaining a raw score one standard deviation below the mean for his age group has an IQ score of 85, and an individual scoring one standard deviation above the mean for his age group would obtain an IQ of 115. In this way, IQ scores are comparable across age groups, and the percentage of individuals having IQ's above, below, or between particular IQ values is predictable from the normal curve (see Figure 3-4).

In addition to providing information regarding intelligence, the Wechsler Scales, Stanford-Binet, and other individual intelligence tests potentially provide information concerning: (1) motivation; (2) concentration; (3) impairment of higher cortical functioning indicative of organic brain dysfunction; and (4) behaviors reflective of personality characteristics and/or symptoms such as anxiety, psychomotor retardation, and impulsivity suggestive of functional disorders. Therefore, in clinical settings, individual intelligence scales are most frequently used. Potential drawbacks of individual intelligence tests, however, include the expense in terms of professional time and training needed to administer and interpret the scales.

Group administered intelligence tests such as the Otis SA, the Armed Forces Qualification Test, or the Shipley Institute of Living Scales, are sometimes used in clinical settings when inexpensive, rapid assessment of a large number of individuals is needed or when a trained professional is unavailable. Although less information is provided by group intelligence tests and some reliability is sacrificed, group tests are particularly useful for "routine" or "screening" assessment when a rougher estimate of intelligence is adequate.

Regardless of whether an individual or group intelligence test is used, it is important to choose a test which measures the criterion the examiner is attempting to predict. Particular tests predict some criteria better than others. For example, the Stanford-Binet, along with several other IQ tests, is heavily weighted on verbal skills. Hence, it predicts performance on tasks requiring verbal skills better than tasks requiring motor skills.

Considerations such as these are important when selecting a test from the myriad of tests on the market--a job which is best left to a qualified psychologist.

C. DETERMINANTS OF INTELLIGENCE

Some people are of average intelligence, while others are intellectually re-tarded, and still others are exceptionally bright. Similarly, particular groups of individuals are popularly viewed as having greater intellectual ability than other groups. Foreigners, Blacks, and women have been viewed stereotypically as intellectually inferior to American-born, White males. Research indicates that differences among groups do exist, but often these differences are neither as great as the layman thinks, nor are the determi-nants of these differences what the layman imagines.

We said earlier that intelligence is determined by an interaction of four components: heredity, motivation, test content, and environmental or ex-periential factors. The relative contributions of these components have been studied by research conducted on groups of people. A brief summary of research findings will be provided in order to give a better understanding of intelligence and the factors influencing it.

A great deal of interest has centered on whether heredity or environment is the primary determinant of intelligence. Studies have typically held either heredity or environment constant, while varying the other. Identical twins reared together have been found to have very similar IQ's (average differ-ence less than 8 IQ points); moreover, IQ scores of identical twins reared apart are almost as similar as those for identical twins reared together (Shields, 1958). When identical and fraternal twins reared together were compared, the correlations between the scores of identical twins were much higher than between those of fraternal twins (Blewett, 1954). Another find-ing which supports the importance of heredity is that children reared in foster homes have IQ's much more closely related to those of their biological parents than those of their foster parents (Skodak & Skeels, 1949).

Other studies have pointed to environmental factors as important determinants of intelligence. It has been found, for example, that children placed in superior foster homes have IQ's as much as 15 points higher than would be predicted from their biological parents' IQ's (Morgan & King, 1971). More-over, psychological environment may be more important than physical environ-ment. Children moved from an orphanage to an equally drab institution for the mentally retarded where they were "adopted" by a retarded, though attentive and loving foster mother, showed dramatic gains in intelligence and significantly better adult-life adjustment as compared to a control group left behind in the orphanage (Skeels, 1966). Taken as a whole, research on the environment versus heredity issue points to the importance of the interaction between the two factors. A stimulating environment may increase measured intelligence, but no amount of favorable environmental influence can create potentials that do not exist genetically.

Just as home environment influences measured intelligence, different cultural environments foster development of different patterns of ability.

This conclusion is supported by studies comparing rural versus urban children (Morgan & King, 1971), Ceylonese versus American college entrants (Straus, 1951), and children from different ethnic and socioeconomic groups (Stodolsky & Lesser, 1967). Findings such as these and attempts to compare individuals from different socioeconomic groups have raised the problem of finding test materials which do not favor or penalize one group or the other. Since most intelligence tests were devised by well-educated members of the middle and upper socioeconomic classes, there has been a danger that current intelligence tests penalize less advantaged groups. Since it is nearly impossible to devise test items which do not utilize some past experience, a test can never be entirely culture free. There is a push toward developing culture-fair tests which sample a wider range of mental abilities than traditional tests and have items equally common and equally motivating to all socioeconomic and ethnic groups. To date, however, no widely accepted culture-fair test has been developed.

Along with cultural differences in ability patterns, there appear to be sex differences in patterns of abilities. Although overall IQ's of males and females of any age are virtually the same, boys exceed girls in performance on spatial relations and mechanical tasks, whereas girls surpass boys on memory tests, verbal tasks, and problems requiring quick and accurate perception of details. Whether these differences are due to genetics or to different roles assigned and reinforced from infancy remains unanswered.

Age is another factor which contributes to measured intelligence. Intelligence scores obtained during preschool years, and particularly below the age of two, are not very reliable and may measure general development and factors such as attention rather than specific mental ability. Scores obtained after age six correlate more highly with adult intelligence than scores obtained at earlier ages, and it is generally accepted that when conditions such as physical and emotional health, social environment, and home situation remain the same, measured intelligence does not change markedly (more than 10-20 points) after age seven or eight.

Different types of abilities show different patterns of change with regard to age. The peak of perceptual-motor ability occurs earlier, in the mid-twenties, while the peak of verbal ability occurs in the early thirties. After these peaks, performance skills tend to decline more rapidly than verbal skills. Elderly individuals perform as well as younger persons on vocabulary and general information tasks, but tend to do worse on tasks requiring adaptation to novel problems, new learning, or speed.

In summary, the factors influencing measured intelligence are multiple--including heredity, home environment, cultural environment, sex, motivation, and age. Certainly additional research is needed to clarify the interactions among these variables, and it seems unlikely that any simple cause and effect relationships will be found. From our discussion, however, it can be seen that intelligence should be viewed as a complex adaptive behavior involving multiple component skills whose development requires both hereditary potential and optimal environmental stimulation.

QUIZ, Section II.

Circle the correct answer(s). <u>One</u> or <u>more</u> <u>than</u> <u>one</u> answer may be correct.

1. The ratio IQ

   a. is computed by the formula IQ = MA/CA + 100.
   b. is no longer used.
   c. is based on the assumption that mental age increases with chronological age, hence the IQ of an "average" child is always 100 regardless of his age.

2. Because all Stanford-Binet IQ scores are expressed in the form of a standard score,

   a. mental age does not affect the computation of an individual's IQ.
   b. the mean IQ and standard deviation of the IQ scores are the same for all age groups.
   c. each IQ score indicates how well an individual performed relative to his age group.

3. The revised Wechsler Adult Intelligence Scale

   a. is individually administered.
   b. has several subtests which measure different abilities.
   c. yields a Verbal, Performance, and Full Scale IQ.
   d. is commonly called the WAIS-R.

4. IQ scores obtained from the Wechsler scales

   a. have different means and standard deviations, depending on the scale.
   b. are expressed as ratios in which IQ = MA/CA × 100.
   c. provide information about an individual's standing relative to the normal population of his age.

5. Group intelligence tests as compared to individual intelligence tests

   a. provide more information, since an individual's score can be compared to the rest of the group.
   b. are more reliable.
   c. are less dependent on an individual's motivation.
   d. are a less expensive way of testing a number of people.

6. The Stanford-Binet Intelligence Test

   a. is used most frequently with adults.
   b. consists of several subscales arranged according to age level.
   c. is administered individually.

7. All of the Wechsler Intelligence Scales

    a. are administered individually.
    b. have several subtests which measure different abilities.
    c. yield a Verbal, Performance, and Full Scale IQ score.

TRUE or FALSE: Circle the correct letter.

T   F   8. Intelligence is a fixed, unitary quality.

T   F   9. Heredity and environmental influence are the sole determinants of performance on intelligence tests.

T   F   10. An IQ score is a description of an individual's performance on a specific test.

T   F   11. Test content and motivation affect IQ scores.

T   F   12. Intelligence represents a collection of abilities, and a given IQ score can result from different ability patterns.

T   F   13. Twin studies have generally supported the notion that heredity is an important determinant of intelligence.

T   F   14. It is likely that hereditary factors determine the range of intellectual potential, and environmental conditions affect the degree to which this potential is realized.

T   F   15. Several studies have found that different ethnic and socio-economic environments lead to development of different patterns of ability.

T   F   16. Culture-free tests are heavily dependent on prior experiences.

T   F   17. Ideally, the items on a culture-fair test would be equally interesting and equally familiar to individuals from all cultural environments.

T   F   18. Research has shown that boys and girls have different ability patterns which are genetically determined.

T   F   19. After the age of eight, IQ scores remain fairly stable.

T   F   20. Verbal skills peak at an earlier age but decline more slowly than performance skills.

Match each of the Wechsler Scales with the population which it tests.

___21. WISC   a. pre-schoolers
___22. WAIS   b. children and early adolescents
___23. WPPSI   c. late adolescents and adults

III. PERSONALITY ASSESSMENT

A. PURPOSE OF PERSONALITY ASSESSMENT

Personality assessment is concerned with systematically evaluating the ways an individual perceives, organizes, and responds to both internal and external stimuli. Such assessment is generally pursued in order to understand the internal process or functions which underlie behavioral patterns, particularly when the individual's behavior deviates from the cultural norm.

When the clinician is evaluating a patient manifesting symptoms of emotional pathology, he organizes the available information and makes decisions about what additional information is needed to formulate the case, make a diagnosis, and select an appropriate treatment approach. The early steps in this evaluation process generally include conducting a mental status examination, making behavioral observations, and taking a history of present illness and pertinent developmental factors. Following these steps, the clinician may have a clear picture of the patient's personality structure or style of coping in the world. If he does not, a consultation for personality assessment is indicated.

The clinical psychologist is trained to evaluate personality by using both objective and projective personality tests, systematic behavioral assessment, and interview assessment. Often, more than one kind of assessment approach is used in order to formulate a response to questions about personality structure.

B. OBJECTIVE PERSONALITY ASSESSMENT

Objective personality assessment is based on two major assumptions: (1) that personality abnormality is defined by the degree of difference between the individual's pattern of test response and the pattern of the cultural norm; and (2) that individuals of similar personality type will respond in the same way to questions about their feelings, mood, energy, thinking process, etc. An objective personality test is a standardized instrument which the psychologist can use to compare any specific patient's pattern of response to a normative sample. Objective personality tests are generally paper-and-pencil tests which can be administered to a group of individuals at the same time. They offer limited options for response which can be objectively scored. Therefore, results can generally be obtained quickly and at relatively low cost.

The Minnesota Multiphasic Personality Inventory (MMPI) is the most popular and widely used objective personality test. The MMPI has ten clinical scales which are: Hypochondriasis (Hs), Depression (D), Hysteria (Hy), Psychopathic Deviation (Pd), Masculinity/Femininity (Mf), Paranoia (Pa), Psychasthenia (Pt) (measuring obsessive compulsive defenses), Schizophrenia (Sc), Mania (Ma), and Social Introversion (Si). The test also has four validity scales: unanswered items (?), Lie (L), Validity (F), and Correction (K), which provide information about test-taking attitudes, including identifying patients who are either extremely defensive about acknowledging problems or are attempting to exaggerate their pathology.

ANSWERS, Section II.

1.	b,c	9.	F	17.	T
2.	a,b,c	10.	T	18.	F
3.	a,b,c,d	11.	T	19.	T
4.	c	12.	T	20.	F
5.	d	13.	T	21.	b
6.	b,c	14.	T	22.	c
7.	a,b,c	15.	T	23.	a
8.	F	16.	F		

Scores for each of the MMPI scales can be plotted to make a profile, which when compared to norms for the general population or specific clinical populations provides inferential information about the patient's personality style, defense mechanisms, moods, and expected benefits from different kinds of treatment. (See Figure 3-5 below.)

Figure 3-5

SAMPLE MMPI PROFILE

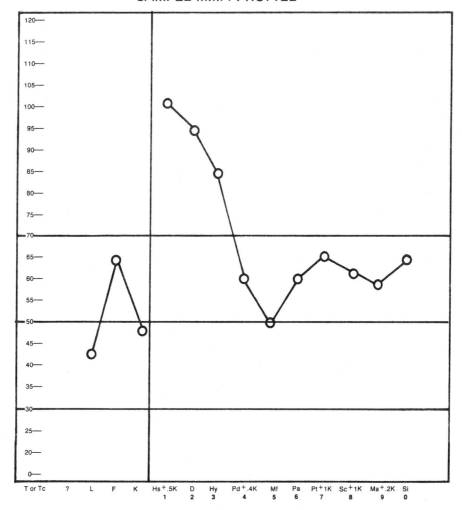

Each scale is standardized such that the mean is a standard score (T or Tc) of 50, and the SD is equal to 10. Therefore, on each scale a standard score of 30 is 2 SD's below the mean, and a standard score of 70 is 2 SD's above the mean. Generally, scores on any scale which are above a standard score of 70 or below a standard score of 30 are considered to be in the "clinical range," indicating evidence of psychopathology. Profiles are interpreted both on the basis of significantly high or low scales and also on the basis of profile configuration, or the relationship among scales. Both elevation and configuration contribute to the evaluation of severity of symptoms or pathology and to the evaluation of personality style, character structure, and differential diagnosis. The profile in Figure 3-5 has significant elevations on the Hypochondriasis, Depression, and Hysteria scales. One may infer from this profile that the patient's symptomatology includes many somatic complaints, signs of depression, and a tendency towards psychological denial of emotions, particularly anger. Furthermore, persons with profiles of this configuration tend to be passive, dependent, whining, and complain about physical discomfort. These inferences are based on what is known clinically about other persons who have similar profiles to the one in the example.

The MMPI is only one of many objective measures which assess emotional pathology. There are other general objective personality tests (e.g., California Personality Inventory, Adjective Checklist, and the Symptom Checklist 90). There are also many measures of specific dimensions of personality functions. Some of those most commonly used include: Beck's Depression Scale, the Profile of Mood States, the State-Trait Anxiety Index, and the Zung Depression Scale. Limitations of objective personality tests include their use with individuals who cannot read, who are too disturbed to attend well to an independent task, or who are culturally dissimilar from the standardization sample.

C. PROJECTIVE PERSONALITY ASSESSMENT

Projective personality assessment is based on the assumption that an individual's personality will determine his perceptual organization of ambiguous stimuli. For example, if several people look at the same cloud formation and report what the clouds look like, one might infer that the personality differences among the participants account for their different responses. Projective personality tests are constructed to provide a task requiring the patient to structure a set of ambiguous stimuli. The clinician assumes the projective test results reveal the principles by which the patient organizes reality and operates in the world. Uses of this information include: the inference of psychological defense mechanisms and personality traits, the development of working hypotheses about responses to life stress and therapeutic interventions, and the labeling or diagnosis of psychopathology. Many attempts have been made to establish scoring systems and norms to aid in clinical interpretation of projective test results. However, most clinicians rely heavily on subjective norms based on clinical experience. Two of the most widely used projective tests for adults are the Rorschach and the Thematic Apperception Test (TAT). These will be described in further detail. Other adult projective tests include: The Draw-a-Person Test (DAP), the Rotter Incomplete Sentence Blank and word association tests.

The <u>Rorschach</u> test consists of ten standardized inkblots which the psychologist uses as unstructured visual stimuli for the patient to structure. The patient's task is to first describe to the examiner what he sees; then, after responding to all 10 cards, the patient provides information about the determinants of his responses. Clinical interpretations are principally based on: content or theme of responses; level of visual integration of form; response to color, shading, and texture; and use of movement in determining responses. Personality structure, areas of conflict, and reality testing are primary foci which are assessed with this particular projective test.

The <u>Thematic Apperception Test</u> (TAT) consists of 20 cards with pictures of scenes which are somewhat ambiguous in their meaning. The task for the patient taking this test is to make up a story from beginning to end, in which a given picture is a scene from the middle of the story. The story is also expected to include thoughts and feelings of the characters. The TAT is frequently used to test hypotheses about patients' feelings about parent figures and peers, self-concept, motivation, and expectations about self and others. The test is individually constructed by the clinician in that he selects several cards from the set of 31. The clinician selects those cards which he expects will elicit the information needed to test the clinical hypotheses. While the TAT is not particularly useful in helping with differential diagnosis, it can be especially useful in obtaining access to thoughts and feelings of withdrawn patients who are initially reticent to discuss their emotions or life problems.

In making an appropriate selection of personality tests to answer clinical questions, the psychologist selects the test or combination of tests which will best provide the desired information. If more than one test could provide the necessary information, he generally uses whichever test is the most economical. As mentioned earlier, objective personality tests such as the MMPI have two potential advantages. First, since they are generally self-administered or can be administered to a group of patients at the same time, they are relatively inexpensive in that a psychologist is needed only to interpret the test results. A second advantage of objective tests is their empirical basis. In contrast, projective personality tests such as the Rorschach and TAT are costly in administration time, requiring a skilled clinician to individually administer and interpret them. These tests also produce such individual protocols that clinical norms are less available and are considered less valid. Nevertheless, results from projective personality assessment often do afford more specific clinical data about a patient which may be useful in planning therapeutic intervention.

QUIZ, Section III.

Circle the correct answer(s). <u>One</u> or <u>more</u> <u>than</u> <u>one</u> answer may be correct.

1. Personality assessment is concerned with systematically evaluating the ways an individual

    a. perceives internal and external stimuli.
    b. organizes internal and external stimuli.
    c. responds to internal and external stimuli.

2. Which of the following is/are underlying assumptions of objective personality tests?

    a. The difference between the normative test response pattern of an individual's culture and that individual's test pattern defines the degree of personality abnormality.
    b. The individual will project his feelings and attitudes into test questions in such a manner that the examiner can reliably identify personality structure on the basis of quality of test responses.
    c. Individuals of similar personality type will respond to test questions in a similar way.

3. Which of the following is/are general objective personality tests?

    a. Profile of Mood States
    b. MMPI
    c. Beck's Depression Scale
    d. California Personality Inventory

4. In contrast to objective personality tests, projective personality tests are generally

    a. more costly to administer.
    b. less likely to have available clinical norms.
    c. generally considered less valid.

TRUE or FALSE: Circle the correct letter.

T   F   5. The MMPI is made up of six (6) clinical scales and four (4) validity scales.

T   F   6. An advantage of the MMPI is that it measures test-taking defensiveness and attempts to exaggerate pathology.

T   F   7. The "clinical range" for all of the MMPI scales is the range of scores greater than two (2) standard deviations above or below the mean score for that scale.

T   F   8. In projective personality tests, the patient's way of structuring ambiguous stimuli is used as the basis for inferring his personality structure.

T   F   9. The Rorschach is an <u>objective</u> test of personality structure and reality testing.

T   F   10. The TAT is a projective test eliciting information about the patient's thoughts and feelings.

IV. ASSESSMENT OF ORGANICITY

A. INTRODUCTION

When evaluating the patient with psychiatric symptoms it is important to consider the range of possible explanations accounting for the presenting deviant behavior or symptom pattern. The mental status exam and history may raise questions about possible neurologic or organic bases of functional limitations. When such questions arise, a consult for <u>neuropsychological assessment</u> to obtain further information about the nature and extent of functional loss may be a necessary step in making a diagnosis and formulating a treatment plan. Depending on the nature of the diagnostic question and the information already available, neuropsychological assessment may range from establishing the current level of functioning in a particular area to a comprehensive assessment of functioning in many areas.

B. ASSESSMENT FOR DIAGNOSTIC PURPOSES

A common question asked of psychologists is "Is the patient organic?" or "Does he have an Organic Brain Syndrome?". Such questions are so broad and unspecific that they are relatively meaningless to a psychologist who is asked to assess a patient's functioning. Furthermore, it is important to remember that psychological tests measure functional behaviors, not etiologic factors or pathogenetic mechanisms, so that an organic basis underlying functional deficits can only be inferred from neuropsychological test results.

Neuropsychological tests can provide systematic information about a patient's functioning in a wide variety of areas. When significant differences are found between different areas of performance at a given time, or when performance in one or more areas changes over a period of time, the clinical hypotheses of functional losses which occur secondary to organic changes can be tested. For example, if a patient who has functioned successfully as an automotive mechanic for many years presents with symptoms which include marked difficulty in performing adequately at his job, it is reasonable to question whether or not there is an organic basis to the problem. Neuropsychological tests may be useful in answering the following questions in such a case:

(1) Does the patient currently demonstrate intellectual functioning sufficient to perform as a mechanic?
(2) If not, what are his specific functional limitations?
(3) If he has specific functional limitations, is there evidence of progressive deterioration?

In order to answer the third question, the psychologist may first establish current performance on tests and then repeat the same measures at later intervals to determine whether there is progressive deterioration. The answers to the questions above may be useful to establish the presence of a brain lesion or to diagnose an acute or chronic brain syndrome (see Chapter 5). The clinical history, neurological studies, and observation of the patient's behavior provide other important sources of information essential in establishing the diagnosis.

C.　ASSESSMENT FOR TREATMENT PURPOSES

In cases in which a diagnosis has already been established, neuropsychological tests may be useful to determine the nature and extent of functional loss for the purpose of planning the patient's rehabilitation program. For example, children who are deficient in their ability to process information presented through the visual, auditory, or tactile modality may require individually constructed special education programs which maximize their opportunity to learn. For adults who have organic deficits secondary to head trauma or a cardiovascular accident (CVA), retraining for a vocation which utilizes their functional strengths and helps them compensate for deficits is often possible.

D.　SPECIFIC NEUROPSYCHOLOGICAL TESTS

The selection of tests administered in any evaluation of organic impairment depends upon both the nature of the clinical question and the extent of the existing data base. It is the psychologist's role to select specific tests which can best answer the question of the referring clinician. However, it is important to be familiar with the nature and purpose of some of the most commonly administered tests for organicity. These include the Wechsler Intelligence Scales (WAIS, WAIS-R, WISC, WISC-R, and WPPSI), the Wechsler Memory Scale (WMS), the Graham-Kendall Memory-for-Designs (MFD), the Benton Visual Retention Test, the Wisconsin Card Sorting Test, the Bender-Gestalt, and the tests which make up the Halstead-Reitan Battery.

The Wechsler Intelligence Scales, which have been previously discussed (pp. 96-97), provide an overall assessment of intellectual functioning, with a breakdown into two basic categories of intellectual functions: those which are controlled primarily by the left cerebral hemisphere (Verbal Scale) and those which are controlled primarily by the right cerebral hemisphere (Performance Scale). Within each Scale, subdivisions of functions by the several subtests provide descriptive information regarding abilities to recall past learning and abilities to acquire and process new information. An additional advantage of the scoring systems of the Wechsler Intelligence Scales is that an individual's score on any subtest may be compared to norms for his specific age group.

Tests which are most often used to explore memory functions for adults are the Wechsler Memory Scale (WMS) and the Graham-Kendall Memory-for-Designs (MFD). The WMS is made up of subtests for various kinds of memory functions, including immediate recall and short-term and remote memory. The WMS has been standardized on the WAIS so that an individual's overall score for memory functioning can be easily compared with overall intellectual functioning on the WAIS. This way, the clinician can evaluate impairment of memory functions relative to general intelligence. Within the WMS, however, subtests have not been scaled to provide easy comparison of strengths and weaknesses of the seven areas of memory functions tested.

The Graham-Kendall Memory-for-Designs Test (MFD) consists of a series of 15 standardized designs. Each design is visually presented to the patient, then removed from view, and the patient's task is to draw the design from

ANSWERS, Section III. _____

1.	a,b,c	6.	T
2.	a,c	7.	T
3.	b,d	8.	T
4.	a,b,c	9.	F
5.	F	10.	T

memory. Scoring criteria and norms have been established for both normal and diagnosed brain damaged populations.

The Bender-Gestalt Test is another measure of perceptual motor functioning used as a part of an evaluation for organicity. Unlike the MFD, the Bender requires the patient to copy designs, not to reproduce them from memory. In other words, the Bender has a visual perception and motor component, but no standardized memory component. In spite of the limited area of performance measured by the Bender, this test has been found to be quite effective as a screening test for organic brain dysfunction (Lezak, 1976).

The Halstead-Reitan test battery is a collection of several different tests covering a wide range of abilities. The WAIS and MMPI, which have been previously described, are two tests in this battery. The other tests include: the Aphasia Screening Test, the Category Test, the Critical Flicker Fusion Test (CFF), the Tactual Performance Test, the Seashore Rhythm Test, the Speech Sounds Perception Test, the Finger Tapping Test, the Time Sense Test, and the Trail Making Test. The primary purpose of the Halstead-Reitan battery is to assess performance in such a specific manner as to help locate the specific area or areas of the brain where organic damage may be present. Since the battery requires specialized equipment and special training to administer and interpret, it is most often used in cases in which there is suspicion of a growing neurological lesion.

One of the problems with all of the tests which are used to evaluate patients for organic impairment is the general absence of norms for psychiatric populations. Since there is some overlap between clinical symptoms for psychiatric disorders and clinical symptoms for neurologic disorders, including decrements in performance on psychological tests for intellectual functioning, it is especially difficult to interpret findings from neuropsychological testing for individuals having a concomitant psychiatric disorder.

QUIZ, Section IV.

Circle the correct answer(s). One or more than one answer may be correct.

1.   To test hypotheses regarding functional changes which occur secondary
     to organic changes, neuropsychologists may look for

     a. decreases in performance over time in one or more areas of intel-
         lectual functioning.
     b. significant differences between different areas of performance at the
         same time.

2.   Treatment or training programs for individuals with neuropsychological
     deficits can often be more effectively designed if an assessment has
     been made of the nature and extent of the

     a. functional loss.
     b. systemic loss.
     c. patient's subjectivity.

3.   The Wechsler Memory Scale measures

     a. immediate recall.
     b. long-term memory.
     c. short-term memory.

Circle the letter corresponding to the one correct response.

4.   Tests are selected for neuropsychological assessments on the basis of
     both the question to be answered and the extent of the _____ base.

     a. organic
     b. functional
     c. data
     d. etiologic

5.   The Verbal Scale of the Wechsler Intelligence Scales measures those
     functions primarily controlled by the _____ cerebral hemisphere.

     a. right
     b. left

6.   The Performance Scale of the Wechsler Intelligence Scales measures
     functions primarily controlled by the _____ cerebral hemisphere.

     a. right
     b. left

7. A test standardized for adults with the components of visual perception, motor functioning, and memory is

    a. the Bender-Gestalt.
    b. the Graham-Kendall Memory-for-Designs.

TRUE or FALSE: Circle the correct letter.

T   F   8. One advantage of obtaining neuropsychological testing when there is a question of organicity is that such tests are constructed to measure the <u>etiologic</u> basis of impairment.

T   F   9. The Halstead-Reitan battery has generally been used to help localize lesions in the brain.

T   F   10. The absence of norms for neuropsychological tests for psychiatric populations contributes to the difficulty in interpretation of results from such tests for psychiatric patients.

V. BEHAVIORAL ASSESSMENT

The behavioral model views problematic behavior as the result of the same learning processes that govern and affect all behavior--i.e., behavior is shaped, maintained, or extinguished by reinforcement contingencies naturally occurring in the environment. The focus of the behavioral model is on behaviors or "symptoms," not on psychodynamic processes such as ego defenses. Therefore, unlike traditional psychological assessment, behavioral assessment is aimed neither at personality description, diagnosis, identification of underlying defense mechanisms, nor toward using this type of information to make inferences about etiology, prognosis, or treatment.

The focus of behavioral assessment is on identifying problematic behaviors and the events occurring in the environment which maintain the undesirable behaviors. More specifically, behavioral assessment involves: (1) identification and quantification of problematic or "target" behaviors, (2) identification of environmental and internal contingencies which trigger and maintain the target behavior, (3) determination of adaptive behaviors or skills in the individual's repertoire for use in the therapeutic program, (4) identification of particular persons, events, or objects which serve as reinforcers and those which because of their aversiveness prompt avoidance responses, and (5) construction of a treatment plan (including behavior modification techniques) aimed at changing the undesirable behavior from its baseline level.

<u>Identification</u> of the problematic or target behavior includes defining the behavior operationally and ideally, in terms of observable events. Most target behaviors, such as crying and headbanging, are easily defined, and some behaviorally oriented clinicians limit the range of target behaviors to such observable events. Other behaviorally oriented clinicians extend the range of potential target behaviors to include internal events such as hallucinatory and cognitive behaviors which are difficult to define in terms of observables.

Quantification of the target involves measuring and recording the frequency, intensity, and duration of the behavior. While several methods are used to collect these measures, the simplest method is self-report logs or records of the problematic behavior. In most logs the behavior is recorded each time it occurs. Weight management programs, for example, often require that patients record the kind and amount of food consumed, and the duration of the eating occasions. In cases where the behavior is less easily directly observed, a record may be kept of some observable manifestation of the target behavior. With visual hallucinations, for example, self-reports of hallucinatory experiences or occasions on which the patient stares for a prolonged period of time might be recorded. When recording each occurrence of a target behavior is not feasible, as with behaviors which occur very frequently or almost continually, a time-sampling technique may be used. In time-sampling the behavior is monitored and recorded for brief, randomly selected periods of time. The particular time interval used for the sample is largely determined by the nature of the target behavior. For example, thumbsucking might be monitored for one minute of each 10 minutes while depressed mood would be monitored once during a 4-hour period using a self-rating scale.

Identification of internal and environmental contingencies which trigger and maintain a target behavior involves answering several questions including: where the behavior occurs, when (time of day, etc.) the behavior occurs, and what happens before and after the behavior is emitted (e.g., how the patient feels and how others respond). In weight control programs, for example, the patient might record for each eating occasion, where, when, and how (e.g., alone, standing, watching TV) the food was consumed, as well as completing a brief rating scale describing their feeling state (e.g., anxious, depressed, degree of hunger, etc.) before and after eating. Identification of the events maintaining a particular behavior permits, in turn, manipulation of these events with a consequent change in the target behavior. If, for example, a behavioral log revealed an individual often overate in response to feelings of anxiety, a competing response such as relaxation exercises could be taught as an adaptive way of coping with anxiety.

Identification of an individual's adaptive behaviors or skills is important in behavioral assessment because these behaviors can often be used in the therapeutic program. If, for example, a particular psychotic patient does not hallucinate when engaged in interpersonal activity, a program could be devised to, in part, increase the amount of interpersonal behaviors such as engaging in cooperative games.

Identification of persons, events, or objects which an individual finds rewarding or aversive is an important part of a behavioral analysis, since rewarding and aversive events are idiosyncratic. The purpose of obtaining this information is so that reinforcers and aversive events can be manipulated in the therapeutic program to increase adaptive behaviors and decrease maladaptive responses.

In summary, behavioral analysis involves empirical measurement of behavior and the environmental contingencies maintaining that response. Adaptive

ANSWERS, Section IV.

1. a,b	6. a
2. a	7. b
3. a,b,c	8. F
4. c	9. T
5. b	10. T

---

skills, reinforcers, and punishers are identified in order that they may be utilized in a behavior change program. Although behavioral assessment is used primarily by psychologists, it has wide applicability in a variety of medical specialty areas. A behavioral assessment of many physical symptoms such as headache, dizziness, or chronic pain is important for making a differential diagnosis and devising a treatment plan. Behavioral analysis techniques such as self-report logs of symptomatic behaviors, collection of baseline data, and simple behavior change programs could serve as important adjuncts in the treatment repertoires of most medical practitioners.

QUIZ, Section V.

Circle the correct answer(s). One or more than one answer may be correct.

1. In order to identify the contingencies which trigger and maintain a target behavior one must determine

   a. where and when the behavior occurs.
   b. what defense mechanisms underlie the behavior.
   c. what are the consequences of the behavior.

2. Identification of an individual's adaptive behaviors and stimuli which he finds reinforcing and punishing

   a. is not important in behavioral assessment.
   b. is an important part of neuropsychological assessment.
   c. is a prerequisite for developing a behavior change program.

TRUE or FALSE: Circle the correct letter.

T F 3. The behavioral model views problematic behaviors as resulting from the same type of environmental processes which effect nonproblematic behaviors.

T F 4. Both behavioral assessment and traditional assessment focus on identifying feelings and defenses which affect personality.

T F 5. Behavioral assessment involves identifying problem behaviors.

T F 6. Behavioral assessment does not involve identifying adaptive behaviors.

T F 7. Behavioral assessment involves identifying environmental events which trigger problem behavior.

T　　F　　8. Behavioral assessment involves identifying events and stimuli which an individual finds reinforcing or rewarding.

T　　F　　9. Since behavioral assessment requires that each target behavior be carefully defined, no internal events can be the subject of this type of assessment.

T　　F　　10. Quantification of a target behavior involves recording the frequency, intensity, and duration of the behavior.

T　　F　　11. Self-kept logs are an easy way of measuring the frequency of a target behavior.

T　　F　　12. In time-sampling techniques the individual is monitored constantly, and each occurrence of the target behavior is recorded.

T　　F　　13. Behavioral assessment techniques are useful only to psychologists who treat psychiatric patients.

VI.　PSYCHOLOGICAL CONSULTATION

Patient assessment and treatment consists of an ongoing process of formulating and testing clinical hypotheses. Generally this process is divided into four phases: (1) assessment, (2) treatment planning, (3) implementation of treatment plan, and (4) outcome evaluation. This division is somewhat deceptive, however, as treatment begins to some extent with the initial contact with the patient. Also, throughout the treatment process new data are incorporated with previously obtained data to clarify the formulation of the clinical problem and sometimes to change the direction of therapeutic interventions. At any point along the path from initial assessment through completion of treatment, clinical questions may arise which might be answered by consultation with a psychologist for further psychological assessment.

As noted earlier, clinical psychologists use a variety of assessment tools to obtain information to assist in: (1) describing pathology, (2) understanding the functional basis of deficits, (3) formulating treatment plans, and (4) evaluating treatment outcome. In order to maximize the effectiveness of the consultation process, several principles should be observed when requesting a psychological consult. The consultation request should include:

(1) Problem definition or the clinical question the psychologist is to answer.
(2) Relevant data for defining the problem or answering the question.
(3) Reason for referral (e.g., to establish baseline data, make a diagnosis, assess prognosis, or formulate treatment plan).

A.　PROBLEM DEFINITION

In order to obtain the desired information from a psychological consultation, it is important to define as clearly as possible the clinical question or hypothesis to be tested. For example, some clear statements of questions which might be answered by a psychological assessment would include:

(1) Does this patient have sufficient intellectual ability to participate in a home renal dialysis program?

(2) Does this patient have sufficient intellectual ability to complete a trade school program?

(3) Would this patient be a candidate for behavioral training in relaxation techniques?

(4) Are this patient's "memory lapses" likely to be based on psychogenic or organic processes?

(5) Does this patient show evidence of psychosis?

(6) Is this patient a candidate for insight oriented psychotherapy?

(7) What is the patient's current level of memory functioning?

B. RELEVANT DATA

Providing the consulting psychologist with relevant information from the existing data base will minimize duplication of effort and increase the effectiveness of the consultation process. Relevant data include those specific pieces of information from the history, clinical assessment, and observations of the patient's behavior which provide possible clues in solving the clinical puzzle.

Generally, when the consultation question is about intellectual functioning, existing data of the following kinds are useful:

(1) Patient's educational level (highest grade completed and degrees or certificates obtained).

(2) Known problems in school.

(3) Vocational level (jobs held).

(4) Mental status exam findings of intellectual and memory functions.

(5) Previous findings from intellectual assessments.

Consultation requests for personality assessment and/or psychological treatment recommendations should include:

(1) Past psychiatric diagnosis.

(2) Brief psychiatric treatment history, including outcome (e.g., fifth psychiatric hospitalization successfully treated with ECT, unresponsive to tricyclics).

(3) Positive mental status exam findings (e.g., hallucinations, recent memory impairment).

(4) Significant aspects of social/interpersonal behavior (e.g., patient brought alcohol onto ward and lost temper with nurse).

(5) Recent or current life stresses (e.g., loss of job or significant other, marital discord, etc.).

Consultation requests for neuropsychological assessment should include:

(1) Highest known level of intellectual and vocational adjustment.

(2) History of head trauma, high fever, CVA, cardiac arrests, substance abuse, and any other possible etiologic factors.

(3) Positive findings from neurologic studies.

(4) Positive findings from mental status exam.

(5) History of behavioral and personality changes.

C. REASON FOR REFERRAL

When requesting psychological consultation, a statement of the reason for referral or the purpose for which the information will be used gives direction to the psychologist. This facilitates his selection of assessment instruments and helps him provide the appropriate information when responding to the consult request. For example, a neuropsychological consultation on a patient with a recent CVA may be requested to establish a baseline of functional deficits prior to some retraining program. This way, the same measures can be taken later to evaluate treatment programs. Another purpose of the initial evaluation with such a patient may simply be to document the nature and extent of functional impairment. A third possible purpose for the neuropsychological assessment of this patient may be to obtain suggestions for designing a treatment plan to help the patient compensate for his organic deficit.

In summary, requests for psychological consultation should include three principal elements. These are the definition of the problem or question to be answered, known data relevant to the problem or question, and the reason for referral or purpose for obtaining the information. Consultation requests which include these elements maximize the possibility of obtaining information which is useful in understanding and treating the patient. The statement of problem definition or clinical hypotheses, relevant data, and the reason for referral can often be conveyed in one or two statements. An example of this would be:

> This 32-year-old white male with prior diagnosis of Paranoid Schizophrenia, admitted for his second psychiatric hospitalization, displays symptoms of acute paranoia. Personality assessment of this patient is requested to help differentiate between a possible Affective Disorder and Schizophrenia in order to select an appropriate plan for psychotropic medication.

QUIZ, Section VI.

Circle the correct answer(s). One or more than one answer may be correct.

1. Which of the following is/are <u>not</u> essential elements to include in a request for psychological consultation?

    a. relevant data
    b. reason for referral
    c. developmental history
    d. problem definition

2. Which of the following consultation requests lack(s) clear problem definition?

    a. Please give patient MMPI.
    b. Is patient organic?
    c. Is patient's pain psychogenic?

3. Which of the following would generally <u>not</u> be relevant data to include on a consultation request <u>for neuropsychological evaluation</u>?

    a. work adjustment
    b. hallucinations
    c. number of siblings
    d. history of excessively high fever

4. Which of the following would generally be relevant data to include on a consultation request <u>for intellectual functioning</u>?

    a. achievement level in school
    b. activities in which a person excels
    c. activities in which a person fails
    d. past performance on IQ tests

5. Consultation requests for <u>psychological treatment recommendations</u> should include mention of previous forms of psychiatric interventions, including the

    a. prognosis.
    b. etiology.
    c. motor functioning.
    d. treatment outcomes.

6. A statement in the consult request about the purpose for which the information will be used guides the psychologist in his _____ of tests and reporting of the information obtained.

    a. administration
    b. selection
    c. evaluation
    d. all of the above

ANSWERS, Section VI._____

1.   c
2.   a,b,c
3.   c
4.   a,b,c,d
5.   d
6.   b

_____

POST-TEST

Circle the letter corresponding to the <u>one</u> correct answer.

Use the figure below to answer questions 1-4.

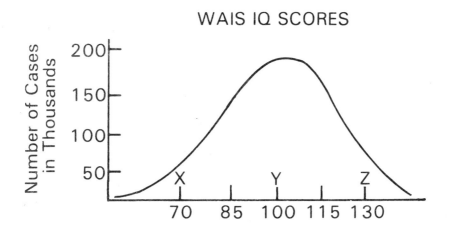

1. The point in the distribution which is two standard deviations above the mean is

    a. X.
    b. Y.
    c. Z.

2. The arithmetic mean of the distribution in the figure above is at

    a. Point X.
    b. Point Y.
    c. Point Z.

3. Eighty-four percent of the population represented in the figure above falls below an IQ score of

    a. 70.
    b. 85.
    c. 100.
    d. 115.
    e. 130.

4. The graph in the figure above represents

    a. reliability distribution.
    b. baseline distribution.
    c. normal distribution.
    d. incremental validity distribution.

For the following questions, <u>one</u> or <u>more</u> <u>than</u> <u>one</u> answer may be correct. Circle the correct answer(s).

5. Factors which have been found to affect measured intelligence include

    a. academic experiences.
    b. cultural influences.
    c. heredity.
    d. certain psychiatric disorders.

6. Which of the following is a purpose for making a psychological assessment for organicity in a patient?

    a. to establish the etiology of organic dysfunction
    b. to determine the nature and extent of functional loss in order to plan the patient's rehabilitation program
    c. to determine the relationship between social adjustment and maturation level
    d. to provide information to assist in making a diagnosis

7. Psychological tests are used in clinical settings to

    a. assign the proper diagnostic label to psychiatric disorders.
    b. identify symptomatic behaviors.
    c. determine the etiology of pathological behaviors.
    d. establish baseline levels and monitor change in behavior.

8. Validity of a psychological test is best defined as

    a. uniformity of procedures in administering and scoring a test.
    b. consistency of the scores received by the same person on each administration of the test.
    c. the extent to which a test measures an individual's perceptual organization of ambiguous stimuli.
    d. the extent to which a test measures what it purports to measure.

9. Which of the following are characteristics of a good psychological test which also apply to the MMPI?

    a. objectivity
    b. standardization
    c. validity
    d. projectivity

10. Common characteristics among the WAIS, WISC, WPPSI, and Stanford-Binet include that they

   a. are measures of intelligence.
   b. provide information regarding impairment of higher cortical functioning indicative of organic brain dysfunction.
   c. measure performance in a variety of functional areas.
   d. are self-administered tests taken in a group.

11. A behavioral assessment entails

   a. identification of adaptive behaviors in the individual's repertoire.
   b. quantification of the problematic behavior.
   c. identification of environmental events which trigger and maintain the problematic behavior.
   d. identification of stimuli which the individual finds reinforcing and those which are aversive for him.

Use the following case study to answer questions 12-13.

Mr. J. is a 62-year-old, retired, white, male patient who has been hospitalized three times in the past for depression. His last hospitalization was 15 years ago. Since that time he has required no outpatient psychiatric treatment. He has now been admitted to an inpatient psychiatric service at the encouragement of his wife who reports that her husband is agitated and irritable at home, that he does not sleep through the night, is not going out to socialize with friends, and seems forgetful.

On mental status examination, Mr. J. appears somewhat disheveled and unkempt. He is moderately dysphoric in mood and becomes agitated when asked how he feels about his wife bringing him to the hospital. His attention and concentration are poor, and while remote memory is intact, recent memory and immediate recall are poor.

12. Which of the following statements is/are true?

   a. Given the long period of time since Mr. J.'s last psychiatric hospitalization, information about previous psychiatric problems is not relevant to evaluating him at this time.
   b. Mr. J.'s poor recent memory may be a function of emotional factors.
   c. Neuropsychological testing would be of no use with this patient because he also has symptoms of depression.
   d. Mr. J.'s poor recent memory may be a function of organic factors.

13. Which of the following statements is/are true?

   a. A request for psychological consultation may be useful to evaluate Mr. J.'s personality and the severity of his depression.
   b. In order to establish a clinical diagnosis of Mr. J., more information is needed.

c. A systematic behavioral assessment may be useful in evaluating Mr. J., either for depression or organicity.

d. Neuropsychological assessment of Mr. J.'s memory could be used to establish the nature and extent of functional loss.

Match the following descriptions with the corresponding psychological tests.

_____ 14. individually administered intelligence test

_____ 15. individually administered, projective personality test in which the individual creates a story about the pictures he is presented

_____ 16. individually administered, projective personality test using standardized inkblots

_____ 17. a self-administered projective personality test in which the individual interprets ambiguous stimuli

_____ 18. standardized objective, self-administered personality test

a. MMPI
b. Rorschach
c. Stanford-Binet
d. TAT
e. none of the above

Match the descriptions with the corresponding psychological tests.

_____ 19. a test of six areas of short- and long-term memory functions

_____ 20. a perceptual motor test with no standardized memory component

_____ 21. a standardized perceptual motor memory test

_____ 22. a battery of several tests to evaluate functional losses secondary to organic brain dysfunction

_____ 23. an intelligence test which yields a Verbal, Performance, and Full Scale IQ Score

a. Halstead-Reitan
b. Bender-Gestalt
c. WAIS
d. Wechsler Memory Scale
e. Graham-Kendall Memory-for-Designs

PRE-TEST ANSWERS

1.	b,d	13.	d
2.	a,b,c	14.	d
3.	a,b,c,d	15.	b
4.	a,b,c	16.	a
5.	d	17.	e
6.	b,d	18.	c
7.	a,b,c,d	19.	c
8.	a,b,c,d	20.	e
9.	b,d	21.	a
10.	c	22.	d
11.	c	23.	b
12.	d		

POST-TEST ANSWERS

1.	d	13.	a,b,c,d
2.	c	14.	c
3.	d	15.	d
4.	c	16.	b
5.	a,b,c,d	17.	e
6.	b,d	18.	a
7.	b,d	19.	d
8.	d	20.	b
9.	a,b,c	21.	e
10.	a,b,c	22.	a
11.	a,b,c,d	23.	c
12.	b,d		

REFERENCES

Anastasi, A. Psychological testing (3rd. ed.). New York: MacMillan, 1978.

Blewett, D. B. An experimental study of the inheritance of intelligence. Journal of Mental Science, 1954, 100, 922-933.

Lezak, M. D. Neuropsychological assessment. New York: Oxford University Press, 1976.

Morgan, C. T., & King, R. A. Introduction to psychology (4th ed.). New York: McGraw Hill Book Company, 1971.

Shields, F. Twins brought up apart. Eugenics review, 1958, 50, 115-123.

Shodak, M., & Skeels, H. M. A final followup of one hundred adopted children. Journal of Genetic Psychology, 1949, 25, 3-19.

Skeels, H. M. Adult status of children with contrasting early life experiences. Monographs of the Society for Research in Child Development, 1966, 31(3), 1-63.

Stodolsky, S., & Lesser, G. S. Learning patterns in the disadvantaged. Harvard Educational Review, 1967, 37(4), 546-593.

Straus, M. A. Mental ability and cultural needs: A psychocultural interpretation of the intelligence test performance of Ceylon University entrants. American Sociological Review, 1951, 16, 371-375.

SUGGESTIONS FOR FURTHER READING

Anastasi, A. Psychological testing (3rd ed.). New York: MacMillan, 1968.

Lezak, M. D. Neuropsychological assessment. New York: Oxford University Press, 1976.

CHAPTER 4

Psychosocial Factors in Physical Illness

Robert Malcolm, M.D.
Brian L. West, Ph.D.

CHAPTER OUTLINE

LEARNING OBJECTIVES

After reading this chapter you will be able to:

1.   List major reasons why the interactions between biological and psycho-social factors are important in understanding health and disease.

2.   Define psychosomatics.

3.   Compare and contrast disease and illness.

4.   List the major contributions of Charcot, Freud, Pavlov, Alexander, and Dunbar in the development of psychosomatics.

5.   Cite four ways in which psychosocial and biological factors interact in clinical practice.

6.   Define behavioral medicine.

PRE-TEST

For each of the following questions, one or more than one answer may be correct. Circle the correct answer(s).

1. An understanding of psychosocial and biological factors that contribute to disease is important because

   a. individuals are affected by social, biological, and psychological factors spontaneously.
   b. many medical patients have psychological disorders.
   c. missing the identification of a psychological disorder is costly.
   d. psychological factors may contribute to the initiation or exacerbation of a physical disorder.

2. Psychosomatic medicine is

   a. a scientific discipline.
   b. holistic medicine.
   c. a body of clinical knowledge.
   d. an interdisciplinary branch of medicine.

3. Psychosocial disturbances may contribute to disease

   a. as a complication of a disease.
   b. by contributing to pathophysiologic mechanisms.
   c. by acting as a risk factor.
   d. by determining illness behavior.

4. Behavioral medicine is

   a. equivalent to psychosomatic medicine.
   b. biofeedback.
   c. the application of behavioral principles and techniques to medical treatment.
   d. the study of psychopathology in medical patients.

5. Operant conditioning is

   a. a means for learning a reflexive response.
   b. a method used for learning in behavioral psychology.
   c. employed in biofeedback treatment.

TRUE or FALSE: Indicate which of the following statements are true (T) and which are false (F) by circling the appropriate letter.

T   F   6.   Illness and disease are synonymous.

T   F   7.   Separation of psychosocial and biomedical issues in health care began in the early twentieth century.

T   F   8.   Extreme forms of illness behaviors are only seen in mentally ill individuals.

T   F   9.   Behavioral analysis of smoking behavior in a patient should include knowledge of the antecedents and consequences of smoking.

T   F   10. Stress management is a grouping of different techniques primarily intended to reduce tension in a patient and replace that response with one of relaxation in the presence of a formerly stress-inducing stimulus.

I. INTRODUCTION AND DEFINITIONS

This chapter is concerned with the interaction between psychosocial and biological factors that contribute to health and disease. This interaction is important to the holistic treatment of patients since most complex health disorders are determined by multiple factors occurring simultaneously at social, psychological, and biological levels. Between 30% and 60% of medical inpatients and between 50% and 80% of medical outpatients suffer from psychosocial difficulties, either in conjunction with, or in addition to their presenting medical complaints. There is also the widespread tendency among patients to define their psychosocial distresses and problems of living in terms of medical complaints and, therefore, seek help from health systems. The failure to understand and manage the psychosocial problems that accompany patients leads to their greater suffering and debilitation, interference with medical regimens, greater costs by leading to excessive medical evaluations and hospitalizations, and ultimately greater aggravation and concern, both on the part of the patient and the health care provider.

The DSM-III category of psychological factors affecting physical disorders does not, alone, constitute a diagnosis. Instead it documents the judgment that psychological factors are contributing to the initiation or exacerbation of a physical disorder. A diagnosis of physical disorder (Axis III) must first be made. Then the judgment that psychological factors are affecting the physical disorder may be made on one of two levels of certainty. Psychological factors probably affecting physical disorders should be used when a causal or correlated relationship is suspected but evidence of certainty is lacking. Psychological factors definitely affecting physical disorders is to be used when there is great evidence of such a relationship. The DSM-III refers to psychological (intrapsychic) rather than psychosocial factors affecting physical disorders. Social factors (interpersonal) are major determinants of health and disease. Therefore, "psychosocial" will be used in this chapter.

Diagnostic criteria for Psychological Factors
Affecting Physical Disorder include:

A. The presence of a physical disorder coded on Axis III.

B. There is a temporal relationship between psychologically meaningful environmental stimuli and the initiation or exacerbation of the physical disorder.

C. The psychologically meaningful environmental stimuli are judged to be contributory, in this particular individual, to the initiation or exacerbation of the physical disorder.

Subtypes of psychological factors affecting physical disorder are:
316.10--Psychological Factor Probably Affecting Physical Disorder
316.20--Psychological Factor Definitely Affecting Physical Disorder

Psychosomatic medicine is the interdisciplinary branch of medicine which is interested in the clinical relationships between psychosocial and biological events that promote health or disease. "Psychosomatic" is derived from the Greek words, psyche, "spirit, soul," and soma meaning "body." The term was actually first used in the early 19th century to describe the two indivisible aspects of the self. A contemporary definition of psychosomatic medicine includes:

(1) The scientific discipline that is concerned with the understanding, prediction, and control of the relationships of biological, psychological, and social determinants of health and disease.

(2) It is a set of philosophical guidelines embodying a holistic approach to the practice of medicine.

(3) It is a major portion of the clinical knowledge that comprises the specialty of consultation/liaison psychiatry.

Most of the common and complex health disorders of Western civilization are determined by multiple risk factors from biological, social, and psychological areas. All of these factors act in concert in that many of them together are necessary, but no one of them alone is sufficient to produce a particular disorder. Common examples of physical disorders in which psychological and/or social factors play a role include: obesity, muscle contraction and migraine headaches, angina pectoris, painful menstruation, low back pain, acne, rheumatoid arthritis, asthma, tachycardia, arrhythmias, gastric ulcer, duodenal ulcer, regional enteritis, ulcerative colitis, frequency of micturition, hyperthyroidism, and diabetes mellitus. Psychophysiologic disorders are conditions that were formerly believed to be primarily caused or very strongly influenced by psychological factors. Asthma, ulcerative colitis, and peptic ulcer disease are examples of psychophysiologic disorders. It is now recognized that multiple biological, social, and psychological factors come together to contribute to the incidence and manifestations of these conditions. For example, it is incorrect to assume that adult onset diabetes mellitus is purely caused by genetic factors. Likewise, there is no evidence to support the assumption that maternal deprivation per se causes asthma in childhood.

Another useful distinction in psychosomatics is illness versus disease. Illness is the experience of not being well. The illness is the summation of the patient's subjective symptoms of pain, discomfort, and disability. It is what the patient believes he has. Disease refers to structural or functional disorders of cells, tissues, or organs which lead to signs of pathology and altered physiology or biochemistry. The following table summarizes the distinction between illness and disease:

TABLE 4-1

DISTINCTIONS BETWEEN ILLNESS AND DISEASE

Disease	Illness
Seen by physician	Felt by patient
Signs	Symptoms
Objective	Subjective
Altered structure and/or function of cells, tissue, or organs	Alterations in the functions of the whole person
Life threatening	Life-style threatening

Illness and disease may coexist or they may exist independently of one another. The prudent health providers attend to and treat both conditions.

The <u>biomedical</u> model of disease is a set of <u>postulates</u> and assumptions that states that defects in health are produced by an interaction between an environmental agent and a susceptible host, leading to a predictable pathogenesis, pathophysiology, tissue pathology, clinical course, and prognosis. This model is essentially binary in that either you have it or you don't. This is the implicit model of medical practice in most of Western society at the present time. This model is most applicable to infectious disease and some surgical conditions.

The <u>biopsychosocial</u> model of illness and disease, in addition to incorporating the factors from the biomedical model, takes into account the patient with his or her behaviors, attitudes, emotions, the social context of his or her life, the role of the health provider, and the type of health delivery system. This model recognizes that the boundaries between health and disease and well and sick are far from clear and fall on a continuum that is ever in change. Figure 4-1 illustrates the dimensions of the biopsychosocial model. This figure is useful in demonstrating the interaction of the three dimensions for the purpose of clinical formulations.

READING NOTE: The interested student is referred to Engel, 1977, for an elaboration of the biopsychosocial model.

QUIZ, Section I.

For the following questions, <u>one</u> or <u>more than one</u> answer may be correct. Circle the correct answer(s).

1. Psychosomatic medicine is

    a. a scientific discipline.
    b. holistic medicine.
    c. a body of clinical knowledge.
    d. an interdisciplinary branch of medicine.

TRUE or FALSE: Circle the correct letter.

T   F   2.   Illness and disease may coexist or operate alone in an individual.

II. HISTORY

In primitive cultures no distinctions were made between disorders of mind or body with the possible exception of those produced by trauma. Treatment rituals were, therefore, holistic and aimed at returning the afflicted individual to a useful position within his community. The cause of most disorders in primitive communities was usually seen as magical and produced by forces external from the patient (spirits and spells). As cultures developed, treatment rituals initially remained holistic, but causes of disease were seen

Figure 4-1
BIOPSYCHOSOCIAL MODEL

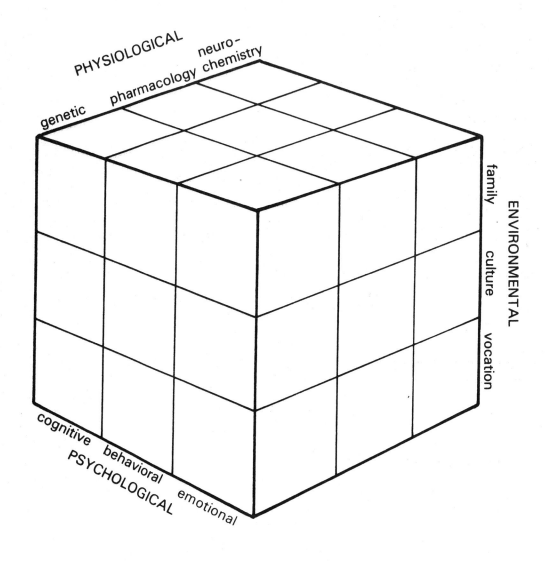

ANSWERS, Section I.

1. a
   b
   c
   d
2. T

---

as religious and illness was punishment for sin. In Babylonian and Egyptian cultures, diseases were seen as productions of the body for improprieties of conduct. Remnants of such thinking remain with us today. Greek culture stressed both external and internal influences in health and sickness and began identifying psychological disorders which were felt to emanate from the mind. During the Renaissance, Descartes furthered the notion of separation of mind from body. Religious thinking of the day had made distinctions between the soul, mind, and body. Morgagni and other anatomists during the Renaissance increased the mind-body distinction by recognizing that a disturbance in organs often leads to death or disease. In the 19th century, the cell became the focus of the soma and thus the location for health or disease. The lag in the development of the social sciences also enhanced the mind-body dichotomy. Despite the overwhelming force of the thinking which separated psyche from soma, isolated individuals in the 19th century attempted to link the two. Heinroth coined the term "psychosomatic" in 1818. Mesmer, and later Charcot and Freud, found that they could dramatically modify physical complaints through hypnosis. In the early 1900's, Sherrington demonstrated that even simple reflex arcs were subject to modification by central cognitive influences. Pavlov demonstrated visceral learning and showed that animals presented with ambiguous stimuli which they could not discriminate developed agitation, aggression, weight loss, and alopecia. Cannon pioneered the early work on the relationship between behavior, emotions, and hormonal status. He used the term "homeostasis" to denote total body equilibrium. Hans Selye in the 1940's clarified many of the physiologic phenomena that occur in reaction to environmental stresses. Wolff observed that emotional states greatly influenced gastric secretory activities and led to symptomatic behaviors. Flanders Dunbar, aware of the preceding work, speculated that psychosomatic disorders were a result of autonomic and endocrine overactivity. Franz Alexander developed the hypothesis that stresses evoke unconscious conflicts which result in disturbances of specific organ physiology. Alexander and others studied several illnesses (asthma, peptic ulcer disease, migraine, ulcerative colitis, hypertension, thyrotoxicosis, rheumatoid arthritis, and neurodermatitis) which they believed were primarily psychologically determined. They, therefore, felt that psychoanalytic treatment was the therapy of choice for these conditions. Although Dunbar's and Alexander's original hypotheses have not been supported by more recent psychosomatic research, they laid the foundations for the modern field of psychosomatic medicine.

Contemporary psychosomatic theory and research are diverse and include work in the areas of psychosocial stresses, neuroendocrine arousal mechanisms, the role of family structure in illness, sociocultural determinations of illness behaviors, the role of personality as a risk factor in disease, the psychosocial adaptation to disease, and the use of techniques derived from experimental analysis of behavior (Behavioral Medicine; see section V).

Consider how man has used the institutions of magic, science, and religion to explain health and disease. Consider how thinking from all three areas is interwoven in our own conduct when we become sick.

III. MODES OF INTERACTION BETWEEN BIOLOGICAL AND PSYCHOSOCIAL EVENTS

In clinical practice, biological, social, and psychological variables are always acting on the patient, the health provider, and the health care delivery system. The types of interactions may be arbitrarily grouped into four categories. Several of these factors are operating simultaneously, and there is considerable overlap as well.

A. PSYCHOSOCIAL SYNDROMES AS A RESPONSE TO DISEASE

This area is often referred to as somatopsychics. During or after a disease an individual may develop a specific psychiatric disorder. Although many of the syndromes discussed in this book may be seen, the most common reactions to disease are anxiety and depression. Delirium following surgical procedures or during severe medical illnesses is also frequent in susceptible individuals. Any of these syndromes may be mistaken for another manifestation of the original disease or merely overlooked. Frequently, these secondary psychiatric conditions produce the greater disability for patients and family. It is estimated that 40% to 80% of patients on chronic renal dialysis develop psychological adjustment disorders that are clinically significant (Armstrong, 1978). Prompt identification and treatment of these secondary psychiatric syndromes are essential.

Examples:
1) Generalized anxiety syndrome following myocardial infarction.
2) Depression following chronic infections, i.e., mononucleosis, influenza, or hepatitis.
3) Phobic behaviors following treatment for neoplastic disease.

B. PSYCHOSOCIAL FACTORS AS PART OF A PATHOPHYSIOLOGIC MECHANISM OF ILLNESS

Anxiety is a good example of a psychological disorder which may ultimately produce symptoms of physical illness. Anxiety is directly involved in the pathophysiology that leads to the condition known as the hyperventilation syndrome. Signs and symptoms of the hyperventilation syndrome occur in many organ systems and can be best understood as manifestations of anxiety plus the pathophysiologic changes induced by overbreathing. Overbreathing leads to excessive amounts of CO_2 being exhaled. This leads to a decrease in pCO_2 in the blood and a corresponding shift in blood pH toward alkalosis. Alkalosis decreases ionized calcium and possibly other ions leading to increased neuromuscular irritability and to alterations of consciousness (the exact mechanism of the latter is not understood). Increased neuromuscular irritability leads to variable difficulties including headaches, muscular pains and cramps, tremor, and paresthesias. For the signs and symptoms directly produced by anxiety, please review Chapter 9. Figure 4-2 summarizes the hyperventilation syndrome.

Acute hyperventilation is easy to recognize since many of the signs and symptoms are present to a florid degree. Acute anxiety and the hyperventilation syndrome frequently follow acute traumatic events in a person's life. Patients with chronic hyperventilation tend to have only marginally increased respiration, may only report one or two complaints, and may be difficult to diagnose. In addition, two so-called "pseudophobias," avoidance of auto driving and avoidance of church attendance, have been associated with the chronic hyperventilation syndrome. These are called "pseudophobias" since they do not have the symbolic meanings of true phobias (Chapter 9). They are forms of avoidance behaviors generally generated by concerns that he or she will have a hyperventilation attack in the feared setting.

Treatment of the acute hyperventilation syndrome consists of having the patient hold his breath intermittently or breathe into a paper bag or rebreathing mask. Occasionally, the patient requires an anxiolytic drug to reduce the anxiety. After the patient is calmed, identification of the anxiety-promoting conditions is important. Treating the chronic hyperventilation syndrome is more difficult and may involve elements of patient education, psychotherapy, and psychopharmacology.

Case Study: Mrs. G. T., a 43-year-old white female, wife of a minister, was admitted to the hospital for evaluation of possible hyperthyroidism. For six weeks she had suffered from fatigue, tachycardia, tremor, and weight loss. Her husband sought her hospitalization after she began refusing to go to church. Thyroid function studies proved negative, and when the endocrinologist suspected a psychiatric problem, a psychiatric consultation was requested. The cause of Mrs. T.'s difficulties remained obscure until she reluctantly admitted to the consultant that seven weeks ago she had learned that her 19-year-old daughter was involved with a college faculty member.

The patient was evaluated for the hyperventilation syndrome by having her breathe rapidly for one minute. At 30 seconds, she had reproduced most of her symptomatology. Her condition was explained in detail and she was instructed how to time and slow her breathing when having difficulties. Brief family therapy was undertaken involving mother, father, and daughter. Mrs. T. was placed on an anxiolytic agent (lorazepam), but only required it for the first four weeks after discharge.

C. PSYCHOSOCIAL VARIABLES AS ASSOCIATED RISK FACTORS IN DISEASE[1]

There are individual behaviors, attitudes, and major life events that contribute to the onset or exacerbation of multifactorially determined diseases. Major life events represent psychosocial stressors that correlate temporally with the onset of physical or mental disorders. Examples of psychosocial stressors include change in marital status, death of a close friend or relative, financial difficulties, legal problems.

---

[1] The authors wish to thank Dr. Donald Riopel for his contributions to this section.

Figure 4 - 2

Summary of Hyperventilation Syndrome

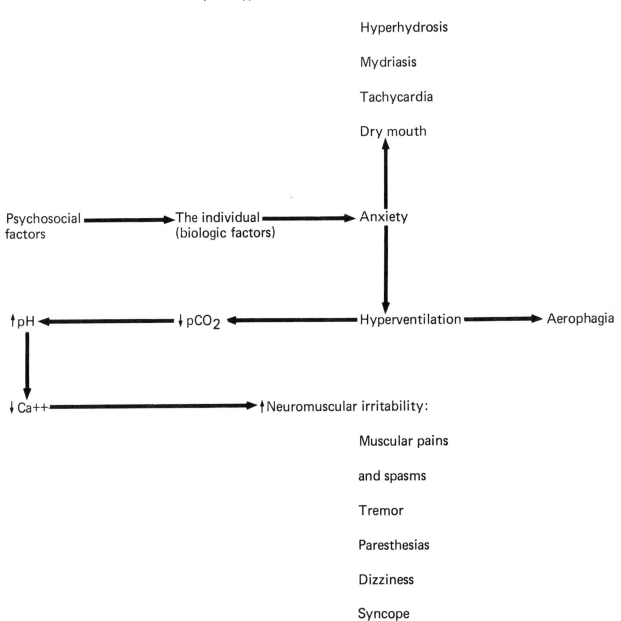

Atherosclerotic-related diseases are the greatest causes of mortality among adult citizens of the U.S. Behavior and attitudes concerning smoking, sedentary life style, maladaptive eating patterns leading to obesity, and substance abuse appear to be major risk factors in the development or worsening of these diseases (AHA, 1980). The best scientific support for the association between psychological factors and heart disease related to the Type A/B behavior pattern was first described by Friedman and Rosenman (Friedman & Rosenman, 1959). This type of pattern has often been mislabeled a "personality type." The response or behavior pattern can be observed and catalogued, and this approach forms a basis for categorization of Type A/B behavior pattern. Type A behavior pattern is primarily characterized by intense ambition, competitive "drive," constant preoccupation with occupational "deadlines," and a sense of time urgency. Type B pattern is the converse.

The relationship between Type A behavior pattern and coronary disease is independent of other important risk factors: serum cholesterol, blood pressure, and cigarette smoking (Harlan et al., 1981). Friedman and Rosenman have dealt with a fairly homogeneous group of white, middle-aged, middle-class individuals. However, available reports do not provide data for a variety of ethnic groups or persons with diverse backgrounds, socio-economic status, and work situations. Furthermore, there is little information of changes in personality with age and with changing social status. Behavioral patterns may vary in different societies. Cohen (Cohen et al., 1975) found that Japanese-Americans have a lower prevalence of Type A characteristics originally described in American males, but men of this group who displayed what was interpreted as an Eastern manifestation of Type A pattern had 2-3 times the risk of developing coronary heart disease. With respect to environmental influences, little data are available that indicate what effect differing environments might have on behavior patterns in their relationship to coronary heart disease. More recently (Rosenman & Friedman, 1977), modifications of the behavior patterns have been attempted by changing situations, age, or training.

****

GO TO VIDEOTAPE

****

D.   PSYCHOSOCIAL FACTORS DETERMINING THE PHENOTYPIC RESPONSE
     TO DISEASE

Most individuals begin to conduct themselves differently when they define themselves as being ill. This altered conduct is referred to as <u>illness behavior</u>. Illness behaviors are complex and are derived from cultural, familial, and individual sources. Sometimes the cultural differences in illness behavior are particularly striking. Irish people complain less of pain than do Italians. European, Arab, and Asian females react quite differently to the onset of the menopause. In Western society "being ill" often means taking off from work, changing one's diet, and consulting a physician. In other societies illness is associated with ritual dancing, isolation in a special hut, or a pilgrimage to a shrine. Since many diseases are self-limited, a plethora of personal "cures" develops. For example, alcohol may be offered as an excellent remedy for nonpoisonous snake bite because it relieves the anxiety of being bitten.

Physicians are often mystified as to why a patient seeks medical aid at a particular time. McWhinney (1972) proposed a five part classification of medical help-seeking behaviors which is useful in categorizing the precipitating causes of a medical visit:

1. Limit of Tolerance; The patient initiates physician contact because the pain, discomfort, or a loss of function becomes intolerable.

2. Limit of Anxiety; The patient initiates contact because a symptom provokes anxiety. A young woman who finds a breast mass is an example of this.

3. Problems of living presenting as a medical symptom (Heterothetic presentation); Heterothetic means "putting forward other things." The patient initiates physician contact for a symptom that is neither intolerable nor anxiety producing, but occurs in the context of great emotional stress. An example is a man who sees a physician for low back pain of fifteen years' duration following separation from his wife. The individual is attempting to find relief from emotional distress in a manner that is socially acceptable, both to him and to a medically oriented health provider.

4. Administrative; The patient initiates physician contact to have a form filled out, etc.

5. No Illness; The patient (or physician) initiates contact for preventive care only. This includes annual checkups and prenatal visits.

Medical help-seeking behavior is only one type of help-seeking strategy. Prior to seeing a physician, many patients obtain advice from a family member, friend, clergyman, chiropractor, or faith healer. Questioning patients about these help-seeking patterns will reveal much about the patients' health beliefs and perceptions of their health problem.

One serious error made by health providers (especially physicians) is to assume that ill people use illness behavior all of the time. This erroneous assumption often leads to the labeling of people with extreme forms of illness behaviors as "crocks" or "hateful patients" (Groves, 1978). "Crocks" are patients with numerous medical complaints, but who have no biomedical disorder. (They frequently have multiple psychological problems.) "Hateful" patients are demanding, often hostile patients who evoke anger in health care providers. Illness behaviors are usually role specific and are usually terminated when the patient perceives himself as no longer ill.

Listed below are common forms of illness behaviors that have been frequently recorded by observers.

Complaining
Demanding
Passivity
Helplessness
Increased self-observation
Moodiness
Nervousness

Suspiciousness
Withdrawal
Daydreaming
Sympathy seeking
Food cravings
Reassurance seeking
Expression of guilt

EXERCISE: Pick out the above terms that describe your own illness behaviors.

Some people react to perceived illness in themselves as a grave physical threat. The reasons for their extreme forms of illness behavior are often idiosyncratic and in part based on psychological features such as personality structure, previous diseases, or serious disease in another family member or friend. These individuals react dramatically to disorders that might be seen as minor by others, especially by health care providers. Patients with extreme forms of illness behaviors are seen by physicians as very dependent, demanding, manipulating, and frustrating. These circumstances usually lead to expectations on the part of the patient that cannot be met, "doctor hopping," and early referral to a specialist (the dumping syndrome).

The key to the management of these patients is the understanding of the personal meaning of their illness. The case below illustrates this.

Case Study: Mrs. J., a 31-year-old female, was admitted to a medicine service for evaluation and treatment of a hemorrhagic cystitis and possible pyelonephritis. The family history disclosed a brother who was under treatment for carcinoma of the bladder. Her resident physician became concerned that she was psychotic. She had repeatedly mentioned her great fear of having carcinoma of the bladder. Attempts at reassurance were unsatisfactory. Her exaggerated complaints appeared to be a blatant attempt to convince nurses and physicians of the seriousness of her condition. A psychiatric consultation was requested because of her demanding and manipulative style. This consultation revealed that she was afraid of the pain, suffering, and a return to dependency on her estranged husband. A check with family sources revealed a very poor social, vocational, and personal adjustment since her separation. The psychiatric consultant suggested to the patient that perhaps unknowingly she wished to return to her husband. She became furious at this, but immediately ceased her demanding and manipulative tactics.

Remember, "problem patients" with extreme forms of illness behaviors often function very well when not ill.

"There are many good people who are not what I call good patients."

Dr. Oliver Wendell Holmes, Sr.

QUIZ, Section III.

Circle the letter corresponding to the <u>one</u> correct response.

1. Which one of the following is usually <u>not</u> seen in the hyperventilation syndrome?

    a. muscular pain
    b. tremor
    c. syncope
    d. globus hystericus
    e. aerophagia

2. Which one of the following is usually <u>not</u> increased when a person is ill?

    a. dependency
    b. passivity
    c. moodiness
    d. self-reliance

****

GO TO VIDEOTAPE

****

IV.   CONSULTATION/LIAISON PSYCHIATRY

This is the branch of psychiatry which contributes to the evaluation and management of psychosocial difficulties arising in medical and surgical patients in both inpatient and outpatient settings. This specialty uses a multidisciplinary team approach and a biopsychosocial model of health care delivery. Liaison is maintained with individuals, medical units, or agencies that have a high proportion of psychosocial problems among their patients. Consultation/liaison teams are often comprised of psychologists, psychiatrists, social workers, and psychiatric nurses, all working with primary care practitioners.

For an example of how one can use a biopsychosocial approach in gathering a health assessment data base, please see Fisher, 1979.

V.   BEHAVIORAL MEDICINE

As discussed above, interest in the relationship of behavior and illness has a long history in the practice of medicine. Health practitioners, from the past "country doctor" to the contemporary family physician, have recognized the importance of a patient's attitude and environment in the process of recovery from illnesses. Frequently, however, the psychological intervention methods for rectifying poor personal habits, negative attitudes, and disruptive affectual responses (to disease) have not been equal to the challenge. With the application of behavioral techniques to these medical patient problems, the new and promising field of behavioral medicine has emerged.

Although many times confusing labels are used to describe the study of interaction between the medical and psychological bodies of knowledge, behavioral medicine refers to a more precise process. Blanchard (1977) has defined behavioral medicine as "the systematic application of the principles and technology of behavioral psychology to the field of medicine, health, and illness" (p. 2). Additionally Pomerleau and Brady (1979) have offered that behavioral medicine is "(a) the clinical use of techniques derived from experimental analysis of behavior - behavior therapy and behavior modification (see chapter 18) - for the evaluation, prevention, management, or treatment of physical disease or physiological dysfunction; and (b) the conduct of research contributing to the functional analysis and understanding of behavior associated with medical disorders and problems in health care" (p.xii).

Behavioral medicine can be conceptualized as an extension of the application of learning principles and behavioral analysis beyond the traditional mental health field. Because of this emphasis on behavioral constructs and technologies, a limited review of these topics is warranted.

READING NOTE: For more detailed description, the reader is referred to Joseph Brady's chapter on Learning and Conditioning in Pomerleau & Brady's book, Behavioral medicine: Theory and practice (1979).

The basic components in the behavioral sciences are stimuli and response. These are segregated into various classifications. Stimuli may be placed in one of these categories: eliciting stimuli, which are those events which precede and induce a reflexive response (i.e., rubber hammer hitting patella tendon elicits a knee jerk); discriminating stimuli, which are events that provide information about a situation and therefore promote responses, particularly responses which have been reinforced (rewarded) in that situation previously (i.e., stopping automobile for red light and driving with green light); or reinforcing stimuli, those events which follow a response and increase the frequency of that response occurring in the future (i.e., a 98 on an anatomy examination). Responses are similarly divided into either respondents, involuntary reaction to a previously experienced stimulus (i.e., knee jerk); or instrumental (operant) responses which are those emitted to a stimulus because of a previous reinforcing experience with that response. With these basic components, behavioral scientists have been able to observe and describe three basic paradigms for learning: classical conditioning, operant conditioning, and modeling.

All behavioral techniques have been derived from one or a combination of these paradigms. Classical conditioning is the process whereby a formerly neutral event (e.g., ringing a bell) comes to elicit a response (e.g., salivation) after having been temporally paired with an unconditioned stimulus (e.g., food). The conditioned stimulus (ringing bell) can thus recreate the response (salivation) without the presence of the unconditioned stimulus (food). This type of learning is differentiated from operant conditioning, since in the latter case an instrumental response is not reflexively given to the emitting stimuli. Instead, a stimulus (e.g., light) emits the operant response (e.g., bar press) from the organism because previous responses (of a bar press) in the presence of the stimulus (light) have accrued the consequence of a reinforcing stimulus (e.g., food pellet). Thus the organism has learned a way to achieve something needed or desired. It is this latter type of conditioning that can be observed most often in higher order behaviors (e.g., working for money). Modeling, sometimes called vicarious learning, is the process of observing a stimulus-response sequence and mimicking that response when presented with the stimuli (e.g., patterning one's own illness behavior from a hypochondriacal parent).

There are many other principles which influence the acquisition process, maintenance, and modification of a stimulus-response contingency; unfortunately the explanation of these is beyond the intended scope of this chapter. Nonetheless, the full appreciation of the concept that behavioral responses are under the control of external and internal environmental stimuli (including physiological events) is imperative in the understanding of the techniques employed in behavioral medicine. In addition, the student of behavioral analysis should understand that changing the contingencies (the connection between a behavior and reinforcement of that act) in a behavioral sequence will alter the frequency of the behavior under study.

A. BEHAVIORAL ANALYSIS AND TREATMENT TECHNIQUES

Behavioral analysis is the common denominator initiating all behavioral techniques. Primarily, the analysis process is the study of problem behaviors including the antecedent stimuli that preceded and elicited the behavior, as well as the consequences of that behavior(s). As discussed above, all behaviors, whether they be mopping one's brow, lighting a cigarette, or drinking a cup of coffee, are responses to a stimulus which has previously been followed by some reinforcing consequence(s). As is the case with most cigarette smokers, the antecedents may be a break from work, or after a meal, in an interpersonal situation, or with a cup of coffee. The behaviors of lighting the cigarette and inhaling are then followed by reinforcing consequences. Smokers describe these in different ways - "tastes good," "relaxing," "stimulating" - but in general, pleasant experiences. In addition, the pleasant event may represent the reduction of tensions which, behaviorally defined, is a process of negative reinforcement where an aversive condition is removed and thus reinforces the preceding responses. For instance, the junior executive may light up after a demanding meeting with his boss and through the ingestion of nicotine reduces tension or "calms down." In time he may become conditioned to having a cigarette after meeting with his boss, regardless of whether their discussion was anxiety producing or not. Furthermore, this smoking may occur in his office, in the corridor, or at lunch in the local diner. Subsequently then, these become conditioned stimuli (formerly neutral stimuli which have preceded a reinforced response) and may begin to elicit the response of lighting a cigarette. In this way, the behavior of smoking (or any operant behavior) is generalized to many different settings and situations. The smoking of course will be maintained as a response in these settings as long as the

ANSWERS, Section III. _____

1.   d
2.   d

_____

behavior is reinforced, either by the effects of the nicotine, social approval, tension reduction, and as long as the act is not punished, such as through social disapproval or excessive throat irritation.

As one might expect, smoking cessation programs attempt to change the contingencies in this pattern by following smoking behavior with an aversive stimuli (electrical shock, warm, smokey air, etc.) and through reinforcing nonsmoking behavior (i.e., praise for putting cigarettes down before lighting, or extinguishing the cigarette before inhaling).

B. STRESS MANAGEMENT

A major area of interest in behavioral medicine has been stress management. Although there is no consensus among practitioners as to an exact procedure for the management of stress, the basic concept of reducing anxiety and tension as a response to daily occurrences and replacing these with a more "relaxed" physical and mental state seems widely accepted. Two facts significant to this type of therapy should be emphasized here. First, as we have discussed, operant technology provides a method for modifying an individual's behavior, including internal responses. Second, humans are capable of implementing their own self-control by initiating the necessary stimuli to elicit a desired response and maintain that response through self-reinforcement. Most programs developed for reducing stress have, therefore, included both an operant procedure for developing a relaxed state and then, through self-control procedures, attempted to generalize and maintain that relaxation response across situations. We will now turn to a discussion of some examples of the specific methods employed in this therapy and the medical disorders indicated for this type of treatment.

The basic premise of behavioral psychology is that all responses (thus all behaviors) are under the control of stimuli and can, therefore, be modified by new and different stimuli. Applying this same approach to an individual's internal state has led to the development of biofeedback. Biofeedback can be defined as the "application of operant conditioning methods to the control of visceral, somatomotor and central nervous system activities" (Shapiro & Surwit, 1979; p. 45). For instance, objective reports of a patient's electromygraphic (EMG) activity (muscle tonus or tension) over a period of time can enable the individual to learn when he is tense and how to relax those muscles being monitored. Subsequently, the patient elicits his own relaxation, not only when given EMG recordings in the clinic, but in situations which are stressful and anxiety producing in his everyday environments.

Another method for minimizing physiological signs of tension while maximizing a relaxed state is Progressive Relaxation Training (PRT). In this approach, the patient learns to discriminate between tension and relaxation of the major muscle groups in the body. This is accomplished by having the patient first tense up the muscle, followed immediately by relaxing that same muscle group. In PRT, emphasis is placed initially on making sure the patient can appreciate the differences in the proprioceptive (internal) cues from these two states. Subsequently, the individual is instructed to induce the relaxed state when involved in his daily activities. This might include relaxing the face, shoulder, and chest regions while working at his desk at work or while waiting in line at the bank, even though late for his next appointment. The object in this phase of treatment is to generalize the ability of self-induced relaxation into those situations that previously elicited tension.

Of course, other methods for relaxing have also been employed (i.e., hypnosis, warm baths, meditation, etc.), but the underlying objective of recalling through self-elicitation this relaxed state in formerly stressful situations remains the same.

****

GO TO VIDEOTAPE

****

It should be obvious to the reader that an important component in successful stress management is the individual's ability to modify his own behaviors through operant procedures, commonly called <u>self-management</u>. The behavioral principles, of course, remain the same in self-management, including the fact that a given stimulus will elicit a response and that the frequency of that response will increase if rewarded. In addition, it should be recognized that cognitions (thoughts, mental imagery) represent "behaviors" and are believed to be under the same control as observable behaviors. Therefore, a patient who learns to identify his behavior of picking up a cigarette (<u>discriminative stimulus</u>) as a step towards smoking will also be able to use that cognitive state of awareness (which incidentally is serving as a <u>conditioned response</u> and a <u>conditioned stimulus</u> for the next step) to begin a new chain of events that includes thoughts of not smoking (<u>conditioned response(s)</u> followed by self-reinforcement (<u>reinforcement stimulus</u>) statements (i.e., "I don't smell like smoke" or "no emphysema for me") or behaviors (i.e., a break from work, placing money in a "crazy money" jar for a larger reward later). Some other behavioral techniques which have been employed for medically related problems include <u>assertiveness</u> and <u>social skills training</u> (for migraine headaches), <u>contingency management</u> (for improving adherence to medical procedures), <u>systematic desensitization</u> (for reducing anxiety responses to medical procedures), and <u>contingency contracting</u> (for compliance problems, among others).

C. DISORDERS TREATED THROUGH BEHAVIORAL MEDICINE TECHNIQUES

Behavioral medicine, in its relatively short history, has developed several subdomains of emphasis. Blanchard (1977) has distinguished these as: 1) behavioral treatment for more traditional medical concerns such as obesity, hypertension, headache, epilepsy, Raynaud's phenomenon, insomnia, etc.; 2) the use of behavioral techniques to facilitate psychophysiological changes via biofeedback or relaxation training (the promotion of change in the patient's physiological occurrences by teaching the patient to gain more effective self-control over these events); 3) the enhancement of medical care through improvement in compliance to medical procedures; and 4) the development and maintenance of health-promoting behaviors that are believed to reduce disease risks (i.e., smoking cessation, increasing the occurrence of annual medical checkups, or breast self-examinations, etc., in clinics and mass media).

It is important for the reader to understand that these divisions have been made based on the intent or goal of the behavioral intervention factor (treating a specific disorder versus removing a disease risk factor, etc.), and not along treatment lines. For instance, the same PRT or biofeedback procedures may be used for 1) reducing frontalis muscle tension in a headache patient; 2) decreasing feelings of anxiety in cardiac catheter candidates; and, 3) enabling a post-myocardial infarction patient to remove risk factors from his life (i.e., time urgency, tension, smoking, etc.). Blanchard's subdomains illustrate the many different areas of health care that behavioral medicine is currently involved in.

As was discussed in the previous section, stress management methods have recently had a prominent place in applied behavioral medicine. In part, this is because those procedures are effective in treating a number of different disorders. Promising results with stress management procedures have been reported for reducing blood pressure in hypertensives, decreasing the frequency and intensity of headache episodes in muscle contraction headache patients, reducing the occurrences of pain in tempromandibular joint syndrome and bruxism and other chronic pain syndromes, decreasing the frequency of epileptic seizures, and decreasing insomniac episodes. Although the stress-management approach as described above is relatively new, the initial results are quite promising.

D. FACTITIOUS DISORDERS

Factitious Disorders are medical or psychiatric syndromes which are fabricated by an individual and, it is assumed, are under the voluntary control of the patient. There is quite frequently a compulsive quality to the behavior of the patient, i.e., the patient will continue to commit acts which produce signs of diseases which have serious consequences to health. The alternative, of course, is being "caught." The diagnosis of Factitious Disorder is usually made by excluding other etiologic phenomena and/or catching the person in the act of fabrication. For example, Factitious Disorder was diagnosed in a young female who had recurrent episodes of joint infections. The infecting agents were found to be similar to bacteria found in feces. Ultimately, the diagnosis was made after a nurse discovered the patient injecting feces into her knee.

Factitious Disorders are distinguished from malingering by the goal of the fabrication of the illness. In the case of the malingerer the goal is usually to manipulate the environment for some recognizable end. For example, avoiding being drafted into the military, altering vocational circumstances, or improving one's conditions in prison might lead to malingering. Individuals with Factitious Disorder, on the other hand, appear to produce their illness in order to be treated as a patient, that is, to receive the benefit of diagnostic and therapeutic procedures, hospitalization, and nursing care. These persons usually have profound psychological disturbances, frequently Personality Disorders.

The DSM-III distinguishes among three Factitious Disorders. The first is Factitious Disorder with Psychological Symptoms (Ganser syndrome, and pseudocyesis, for example). The second is Factitious Disorder with Physical Symptoms (for example, Münchausen syndrome). The third is Atypical Factitious Disorder with Physical Symptoms (for example, dermatitis artifacta).

There is no good epidemiological information on the incidence and prevalence of Factitious Disorders. Finding definite causative factors for most individuals is illusive since many, when found out, will flee the medical facility in which they are discovered, only to duplicate their illness elsewhere. Some individuals have a history of severe childhood or adolescent illnesses in themselves or in the parents. Often underlying dependent masochistic or sociopathic personality features are present. The treatment of these disorders   is   extremely   difficult.

QUIZ, Section V.

Circle the correct answer(s). <u>One</u> or <u>more</u> <u>than</u> <u>one</u> answer may be correct.

1.   Behavioral Medicine is

    a.   the study of psychosocial issues in medical patients.
    b.   the application of behavioral psychology to medical treatment.
    c.   another name for Health Psychology.
    d.   the utilization of the behavioral analysis process to study behaviors associated with health and illness.

(See answer to this question below.)

ANSWERS, Section V.

1.   b,d

POST-TEST

Circle the correct answer(s). <u>One</u> or <u>more</u> <u>than</u> <u>one</u> answer may be correct.

1. Psychosocial disturbances may contribute to disease in which of the following ways?

    a. as a complication of a disease
    b. contribute to pathophysiologic mechanisms
    c. act as a risk factor
    d. determine illness behavior

2. An understanding of psychosocial and biological factors that contribute to disease is important because

    a. individuals are affected by social, biological, and psychological factors spontaneously.
    b. many medical patients have psychological disorders.
    c. missing the identification of a psychological disorder is costly.
    d. psychological factors may contribute to the initiation or exacerbation of a physical disorder.

3. Psychosomatic medicine is

    a. a scientific discipline.
    b. holistic medicine.
    c. a body of clinical knowledge.
    d. an interdisciplinary branch of medicine.

4. Behavioral medicine is

    a. equivalent to psychosomatic medicine.
    b. biofeedback.
    c. the application of behavioral principles and techniques to medical treatment.
    d. the study of psychopathology in medical patients.

5. Operant conditioning is

    a. a means for learning a reflexive response.
    b. a method used for learning in behavioral psychology.
    c. employed in biofeedback treatment.

TRUE or FALSE: Circle the correct letter.

T   F   6.   Extreme forms of illness behaviors are only seen in mentally ill individuals.

T   F   7.   Behavioral analysis of smoking behavior in a patient should include knowledge of the antecedents and consequences of smoking.

T   F   8.   Stress management is a grouping of different techniques primarily intended to reduce tension in a patient and replace that response with one of relaxation in the presence of a formerly stress inducing stimulus.

T   F   9.   Illness and disease are synonymous.

T   F   10.   Separation of psychosocial and biomedical issues in health care began in the early twentieth century.

PRE-TEST ANSWERS

1. a,b,c,d   6.   F

2. a,b,c,d   7.   F

3. a,b,c,d   8.   F

4. c   9.   T

5. b,c   10. T

POST-TEST ANSWERS

1. a,b,c,d   6.   F

2. a,b,c,d   7.   T

3. a,b,c,d   8.   T

4. c   9.   F

5. b,c   10. F

REFERENCES

American Heart Association Committee Report: Risk Factors and Coronary Disease. Circulation, 1980, 62, 449A.

Armstrong, S. H. Psychological maladjustment in renal dialysis patients. Psychosomatics, 1978, 19, 169.

Blanchard, E. B. Behavioral medicine: A perspective. In R. B. Williams, Jr. & W. D. Gentry (Eds.), Behavioral approaches to medical treatment. Cambridge, Mass.: Ballinger, 1977.

Cohen, B., Syone, S. L., & Jenkins, C. D. The cultural context of a type A behavior and the risk of congenital heart disease. American Journal of Epidemiology, 1975, 102, 434.

Engel, J. L. The need for a new medical model: A challenge for biomedicine. Science, 1977, 196, 129.

Fisher, J. V. Diagnosis by inclusion. Psychosomatics, 1979, 20, 90.

Friedman, M., & Rosenman, R. H. Association of specific overt behavior pattern with blood and cardiovascular findings. Journal of American Medical Association, 1959, 169, 1286.

Friedman, M., & Rosenman, R. H. Type A behavior and your heart. New York: Knopf, 1974.

Garrety, T. F., Marx, M. B., & Somes, G. W. The relationship of recent life change to seriousness of later illness. Journal of Psychosomatic Research, 1978, 22, 7.

Greer, S. Psychological inquiry: A contribution to cancer research. Psychological Medicine, 1979, 9, 81.

Groves, J. E. Taking care of the hateful patient. New England Journal of Medicine, 1978, 298, 883.

Hackett, T. P., & Cassem, N. H. (Eds.). Handbook of general hospital psychiatry. St. Louis: C. V. Mosby, 1978.

Harlan, W. R., Sharrett, A. R., Weill, H., Turino, G. M., Borhani, N. O., & Resnekov, L. Impact of environment on cardiovascular disease; report of the American Heart Association Task Force on Cardiovascular Disease. Circulation, 1981, 63, 242A-271A.

Lipowski, Z. A. Psychosomatic medicine in the 70's: An overview. American Journal of Psychiatry, 1977, 134, 233.

McWhinney, I. R. Beyond diagnosis. New England Journal of Medicine, 1972, 287, 384-387.

Malcolm, R., Foster, H. K., & Smith, C. The problem patient as perceived by family physicians. Journal of Family Practice, 1977, 5, 361.

Pomerleau, O. F., & Brady, J. P. Behavioral medicine: Theory and practice. Baltimore: Williams and Wilkins, 1979.

Rosenman, R. H., & Friedman, M. Modifying type A behavior pattern. Journal of Psychosomatic Research, 1977, 21, 323-332.

Shapiro, D., & Surwit, R. S. Biofeedback. In O. F. Pomerleau & J. P. Brady (Eds.), Behavioral medicine: Theory and practice. Baltimore: Williams and Wilkins, 1979.

Section II
Disorders

The eleven chapters in this section follow the Third Edition of the *Diagnostic and Statistical Manual of Mental Disorders* (DSM-III), both in the overall organization of the section and in the diagnostic criteria for the specific disorders.

You may notice that the criteria for the disorders are phenomenologically based on behavior which is observable and reportable by the patient. This also means that the diagnostic criteria do not necessarily imply causation. Our view is that this system of classifying mental disorders is an important step forward in psychiatry. At the same time we recognize that etiology is important too for the planning and implementation of treatment. Therefore, you will find that the chapters in this section deal with questions of etiology.

There is some overlap between two chapters in this section, Organic Mental Disorders and Substance Use Disorders. The Organic Mental Disorders include a number of disorders which are "substance induced." These same substances (alcohol, barbiturates, opioids, amphetamines, etc.) are also viewed from the standpoint of abuse and/or dependence.

We have omitted two groups of diagnostic categories found in the DSM-III. The first is a group of eight "Adjustment Disorders" which are responses to an "identifiable psychosocial stressor" (DSM-III, p. 299). The assumption is that the disturbance (anxiety, depression, inhibition, etc.) is transient and directly related to the stressor. These disorders may occur at any age, but obviously if all the criteria of one of the mental disorders are met, Adjustment Disorder is not used.

The second group of categories which has been omitted is made up of the "V" codes based on the *International Classification of Diseases*, Ninth Revision (ICD-9). They have to do with conditions which do not meet the criteria for any of the mental disorders, but conditions for which individuals seek treatment. For example, malingering, borderline intellectual functioning, marital problems, and academic problems, are all conditions which may bring an individual to his primary care physician, a psychiatrist, or a clinic.

Both of these groups are listed, with code numbers, in the DSM-III, but are only referred to in the *Psychiatry Learning System* in relation to diagnosable mental disorders, specifically as differential diagnoses in instances when the diagnostic criteria for certain disorders are not met. Appendices A and B provide lists of these two groups of disorders.

CHAPTER 5

ORGANIC MENTAL DISORDERS
Luis A. Marco, M.D.

CHAPTER OUTLINE

Learning Objectives

Pre-Test

Q. Amphetamine Withdrawal
R. Hallucinogen Mental Disorders
S. Cannabis Mental Disorders
T. Tobacco Withdrawal
U. Caffeine Intoxication or Caffeinism
V. Other or Unspecified Substance

Post-Test

Pre-Test Answers

Post-Test Answers

References

LEARNING OBJECTIVES

After completing this chapter you will be able to:

1. Define the following terms: pathogenesis, etiology, functional, and Organic Mental Disorders.

2. Describe and diagnose approximately 30 Organic Brain Syndromes listed in DSM-III.

3. Select treatment for these syndromes.

PRE-TEST

For the following questions, circle the letter corresponding to the <u>one</u> correct response.

1. Dementia characteristically includes all the following features <u>except</u>

    a. memory impairment.
    b. impairment of abstract thinking.
    c. impairment in judgement.
    d. personality change.
    e. autonomic arousal.

2. Differential diagnosis of Dementia includes all the following <u>except</u>

    a. Schizophrenia.
    b. depression with cognitive deficit.
    c. normal process of aging.
    d. Somatization Disorder.
    e. Delirium.

3. Usual features of the Alcohol Amnestic Syndrome include all of the following <u>except</u>

    a. attention is intact.
    b. short-term memory is intact.
    c. confabulation.
    d. apathy and emotional blandness.
    e. some disorientation as to time.

4. A 24-year-old man comes to the emergency room in a state of agitation and restlessness. He complains of loss of appetite and insomnia. Examination shows an elevated blood pressure, tachycardia, a clear sensorium, and paranoid delusions. Of the following, the most likely cause is

    a. Anxiety Disorder.
    b. cocaine withdrawal.
    c. Barbiturate Intoxication.
    d. Delirium Tremens.
    e. Amphetamine Intoxication.

5. Among the following, visual hallucinations are most common in

    a. Schizophreniform Disorder.
    b. Bipolar Affective Disorder.
    c. Delirium.
    d. Catatonic Schizophrenia.
    e. Amnestic Syndrome.

6. The most fundamental feature of Delirium is

    a. disorder of attention.
    b. anxiety.
    c. fine tremor of hands.
    d. auditory hallucinations.
    e. pressure of speech.

7. The usual course of Delirium may best be described as

    a. slow onset with rapid recovery.
    b. rapid onset and progressively deteriorating.
    c. chronic and unremitting.
    d. rapid onset and brief duration.
    e. gradual onset with periodic recurrence at biweekly intervals.

8. The management of Delirium includes all the following EXCEPT

    a. provide light in the room.
    b. Valium, 10 mg qid.
    c. haloperidol, 1 mg q 4-6 hrs.
    d. provide environmental orientation.
    e. ask family members to remain in room with patient.

9. A 28-year-old man is hospitalized for pneumonia. He states that he is addicted to heroin and is going into withdrawal. This can be verified by

    a. presence of needle tracks.
    b. detection of hepatitis.
    c. detection of opiates in urine during the first hospital day.
    d. presence of rhinorrhea, restlessness, and muscle twitches.
    e. intravenous injection of naloxone.

10. Which of the following is not characteristic of a patient with Dementia?

    a. neologisms
    b. emotional lability
    c. impairment of social judgement
    d. neglect of personal appearance
    e. disorientation to time

11. Delirium is characterized by all the following except

    a. memory impairment.
    b. emotional lability.
    c. normal sleep patterns.
    d. perceptual disturbances.
    e. autonomic arousal.

12. Any patient sufficiently recovered from an intentionally suicidal overdose of barbiturates or related drugs

a. should be left alone unless he tries again.
b. can be discharged since most overdose patients are hysterical and inconsequential.
c. should have a thorough psychiatric evaluation since many are depressed, very angry, or frustrated.
d. should receive pharmacological education because most overdose patients are only confused and can be conceptualized as involuntary suicides.
e. should be discouraged from discussing the idea of suicide.

13. A known male heroin addict has just been admitted to your licensed inpatient facility, and he begins to develop signs of abstinence (i.e., tachypnea, sweating, lacrimation, rhinorrhea, yawning, piloerection). You know for a fact that his last IV "fix" of heroin was about 16 hours earlier, but you do not know the amount he injected. You choose to give him 20 mg of methadone orally. Following that, he becomes somnolent. The next dose that evening should be

a. less than 20 mg.
b. 20 mg again.
c. more than 20 mg.
d. withheld indefinitely; allow patient to go "cold turkey."
e. based on the amount the patient usually takes.

14. You examine a 23-year-old male college graduate with skull depression on left frontal region, enophthalmos and total blindness of the eye on the same side, poor vision in the right eye, and great difficulty reading optotype paragraphs of large size. History reveals severe craniofacial injury two years earlier resulting from a fight with an individual who was trying to rape the patient's fiancee. He has been unable to return to school to get his Master's Degree, to find a job, or to retain his fiancee's interest in him. He appears severely depressed and seriously considering suicide. There are no major cognitive deficits, delusions, or hallucinations. The most likely diagnosis in this case is

a. Traumatic Dementia.
b. Affective Syndrome.
c. Delirium.
d. Organic Personality Syndrome.
e. Organic Hallucinosis of auditory modality because he is almost blind.

15. A 23-year-old male is brought to your office because he was seen busily masturbating in a crowded bus and seemed quite indifferent to people's reactions of shock. You immediately notice facial deformities. You learn that he had sustained a severe craniofacial injury when he was hit by a truck while riding his motorcycle to work some nine months ago. He had been a normal boy before the accident. Mental status examination elicits nothing of significance except some childish features

and inappropriate giggles. Select the best diagnosis and/or treatment from the following.

a. Organic Personality Syndrome, close supervision to minimize the risk of arrest, and jail or custodial care
b. immediate hospitalization, complex differential diagnostic workup
c. Organic Hallucinosis, immediate hospitalization, Valium, and reassurance; no phenothiazines
d. Organic Affective Syndrome requiring custodial care
e. mental retardation requiring special education

16. A 57-year-old man is referred to you by another physician with the following note: Long history of alcohol consumption, insidious onset of memory impairment, confabulations, poor state of nutrition, peripheral neuropathy, and cerebellar ataxia. Not acutely ill and without impairment of attention or consciousness. Your diagnosis is

a. Schizophrenia.
b. diabetic encephalopathy.
c. Korsakoff's Syndrome.
d. Delirium Tremens.
e. Primary Degenerative Dementia.

17. A 19-year-old ingests an unknown but substantial amount of amphetamines. Within a few hours a syndrome characterized by severe inattention, shifting levels of consciousness, disturbances in memory and orientation, insomnia, tactile hallucinations, and increased psychomotor activity emerges. There is also pupillary dilatation and anorexia. According to DSM-III, the diagnosis should be

a. Amphetamine Intoxication.
b. Amphetamine Hallucinosis.
c. Amphetamine Delirium.
d. Amphetamine Dementia.
e. Amphetamine Psychosis.

18. Suppose that the 19-year-old individual in the question above, following the amphetamine ingestion instead had developed the following behaviors: psychomotor excitement, resistance to fatigue, lack of sleepiness that night, exhaustion, and failure to show up for work the following morning. There are tachycardia and chills. No cognitive deficits. The diagnosis then would have been

a. Amphetamine Intoxication.
b. Amphetamine Hallucinosis.
c. Amphetamine Delirium.
d. Amphetamine Dementia.
e. Amphetamine Psychosis.

For the following questions, <u>one</u> or <u>more</u> <u>than</u> <u>one</u> answer may be correct. Circle the correct answer(s).

19. The early phase of Dementia is associated with

    a. loss of memory of recent events.
    b. disorientation as to time, place, and person.
    c. gradually increasing defects of intellectual functioning.
    d. flatness of affect.

20. When given in sufficient dosage, which of the following drugs will cause a condition that <u>most closely</u> mimics Paranoid Schizophrenia?

    a. LSD
    b. mescaline
    c. amobarbital sodium
    d. methamphetamine sulfate

21. In regard to amphetamines, circle true statement(s) (items 21-22).

    a. Isolated amphetamine-induced delusions may persist for a year or more.
    b. Premorbid personalities commonly associated with amphetamine-induced Organic Mental Disorders are the antisocial and the schizoid.
    c. Truck driving and late night studying foster amphetamine abuse.
    d. Visual hallucinations are rare in amphetamine toxicity.

22. a. The amphetamine delusional syndrome is the closest model of Paranoid Schizophrenia.
    b. Amphetamines do not inhibit monoamine oxidase or the reuptake of catecholamines, nor do they release catecholamines from nerve terminals.
    c. A Schizophreniform Paranoid Psychosis is usually seen in chronic amphetamine abusers, but some chronic abusers do not develop this syndrome after 15 years of heavy abuse.
    d. Abrupt withdrawal from cocaine and amphetamines is as lethal as from barbiturates.

23. The differential diagnosis of Delirium most often includes

    a. Schizophrenic Disorders.
    b. Gilles de la Tourette syndrome.
    c. Schizophreniform Disorders.
    d. Panic Disorder.

24. Untreatable Dementia means

    a. palliative or symptomatic treatment is not applicable.
    b. the patient must be cared for in an institution.
    c. further services of a physician are not indicated.
    d. no specific treatment capable of attacking the cause is available.

25. Criteria for diagnosis of Organic Delusional Syndrome include

    a. predominant hallucinations of auditory modality with secondary delusions related to auditory hallucinations.
    b. visual hallucinations and impaired sensorium.
    c. Dementia with demonstrable organic pathology by either history, lab tests, neurodiagnostic procedures, or physical examination.
    d. predominant delusional system associated with organic etiology.

26. The Opioid Abstinence Syndrome and the naloxone-precipitated withdrawal are reminiscent in their clinical manifestations of which of the following?

    a. atropinic toxicity
    b. cholinergic reaction
    c. tricyclic antidepressant toxicity
    d. influenza

27. An infant just born to a methadone-maintained mother

    a. does not develop abstinence reaction because fairly complete emotional and psychological machineries are required for drug-seeking and drug-craving behaviors.
    b. will always develop signs of abstinence because physical dependence has a cellular basis.
    c. should be given naloxone 5 µg/kg daily.
    d. should be observed for signs of withdrawal.

28. A chronic cocaine abuser

    a. should never be withdrawn abruptly.
    b. can be withdrawn immediately without further ado.
    c. develops severe withdrawal 24 hours after cocaine cessation.
    d. will usually have no serious symptoms when the drug is withdrawn.

29. The distinguishing features of glutethimide intoxication include

    a. cholinergic action.
    b. hypoglycemia action.
    c. bone marrow depression.
    d. anticholinergic action.

30. A general rule of narcotic abstinence syndrome includes which of the following?

    a. Agents with shorter duration of action induce withdrawal earlier, but peak and resolution come later.
    b. The shorter the duration of action of the agent, the faster the development of all the stages of withdrawal which means more abrupt transitions and greatest intensity of symptoms.
    c. Agents with longer duration of action cause the briefest withdrawal syndromes.
    d. A naloxone-precipitated withdrawal from methadone is more abrupt and severe than a withdrawal induced by cessation of methadone intake.

31. Substances whose withdrawal syndromes often encompass seizures include

    a. barbiturates.
    b. alcohol.
    c. meperidine.
    d. chlorpromazine.

32. A 23-year-old male is brought to the emergency room in a state of severe agitation, fearfulness, and visually hallucinating combat episodes of his recent Vietnam tour of duty. He is alert and oriented but exhibits the firm delusional conviction that the hallucinated combat flashes are presently real. There are no delusions in any other area. His buddies inform you that recently he has been messing around with LSD and other stuff. Treatment with phenothiazines is not indicated in this case because

    a. LSD panic reactions usually last 12-24 hrs.
    b. Valium and reassurance will probably be sufficient.
    c. phenothiazines may aggravate the hallucinogenic effects of scopalomine and STP.
    d. phenothiazines are ineffective against LSD hallucinosis.

33. The microscopic identification of Alzheimer's disease is based on recognition of

    a. neurofibrillary tangles.
    b. senile plaques.
    c. neuronal loss.
    d. micro-infarcts of mammillary bodies.

34. In regard to Dementia, which of the following statements is/are true?

    a. The cause of Alzheimer's disease is unknown, but the neuropathology is fairly characteristic and identifiable.
    b. The second and third largest groups are due to vascular disease and NPH.
    c. Depression may masquerade as (pseudo-) Dementia in about 4% of those carelessly diagnosed as demented.
    d. Huntington's and Parkinson's diseases, two disorders of the extrapyramidal motor system, have about the same probability of developing Dementia.

35. In regard to Dementias, which of the following statements is/are true?

    a. Progressive Idiopathic Dementia is responsible for cognitive impairment in more than half of all demented patients.
    b. Untreatable Dementias still require services by the physician.
    c. Approximately, a total of 10-15% of demented patients can be helped dramatically by appropriate treatment.
    d. Treatable Dementias refer to Dementias that have specific and effective treatment.

36. Features suggesting Dementia due to multi-infarct etiology include

    a. abrupt onset and step-wise deterioration.
    b. fluctuating course.
    c. history of hypertension and of "strokes."
    d. focal neurological symptoms and signs.

37. Correct phrases pertaining to the course of intoxication with alcohol include which of the following?

    a. average intoxication length: 1-12 hrs
    b. alcohol metabolism rate: 1 oz. of beverage alcohol/hr: 10 oz./10 hrs
    c. signs of intoxication increase as blood alcohol levels increase and vice-versa
    d. short-term tolerance may occur such that less intoxication is possible after many hours of drinking than after a few hours only

38. Correct statements pertaining to the course of intoxication with alcohol include which of the following?

    a. Because of tolerance, intoxication correlates poorly with blood alcohol levels ranging from 30 to 200 mg/100 ml.
    b. Unconsciousness occurs at 400-500 mg/100 ml.
    c. Death occurs at 600-800 mg/100 ml.
    d. Usually unconsciousness supervenes before the individual can drink enough to kill himself.

39. The Alcoholic Withdrawal Syndrome may be mimicked by

    a. familial tremor.
    b. metabolic abnormalities (e.g., hypoglycemia, diabetic acidosis).
    c. withdrawal from sedative-hypnotic drugs.
    d. Barbiturate Withdrawal.

Questions 40-43 pertain to patients with Alcohol Withdrawal Delirium. Select all the correct statements.

40. a. There is always hypoglycemia.
    b. There is always hyperglycemia.
    c. The goal is to suppress all agitation by means of powerfully sedating phenothiazines.
    d. Hospitalize.

41. a. Prophylactic anticonvulsants are a good routine approach.
    b. Antibiotics are always needed.
    c. Dry tongue and mucosae are always clear indication for administration of I.V. fluids.
    d. Thiamine 100-200 mg I.M. or I.V. should always be given immediately and for at least the next few days.

42. a. Paraldehyde is totally innocuous because it is not metabolized by the liver.
    b. Diphenylhydantoin depletes brain stores of folic acid.
    c. Most chronic alcoholics do not have total body potassium depletion.
    d. Potassium chloride plus potassium-retaining diuretics may cause hazardous hyperkalemia.

43. a. Use of aspirin in the alcoholic does not entail any risks.
    b. Most chronic alcoholics are magnesium-deficient regardless of serum concentrations.
    c. Phenothiazines are the best treatment for Delirium Tremens.
    d. I.V. fluids may cause or exacerbate cerebral edema.

44. Concerning hallucinogens, choose the correct statement(s).

    a. None of the hallucinogens are approved drugs; they all fall under the federal narcotic laws; their use or prescription is illicit.
    b. Tolerance to hallucinogens develops rapidly; cross-tolerance from one to another is the rule; tolerance is lost rapidly upon abrupt cessation; and no abstinence syndromes ensue.
    c. Hallucinogens are often euphorohallucinogens, psychotomimetics, psychotogenic agents, illusogens, and psychedelics.
    d. The term psychedelic is usually associated with a "bad trip" and psychotomimetic with "good trip."

Match the following numbered items with the lettered entries. Lettered items may be used once, more than once, or not at all.

_____45. good recall of names of three objects one hour later
_____46. correct six-digit repetition within a few seconds
_____47. good recall of events of 20 years earlier
_____48. failure of digit repetition within a few seconds
_____49. failure to recall the names of three objects at one hour, but correct digit repetition within seconds
_____50. one-hour name recollection intact

a. suggestive of fundamental inattention, immediate memory impairment, and Delirium or Dementia
b. suggests that attention, immediate and short-term memory are all intact, and therefore absence of Amnestic Syndrome
c. Delirium less likely, Amnestic Syndrome still possible
d. tends to rule out Amnestic Syndrome
e. suggests Amnestic Syndrome
f. suggests good remote memory but does not rule out Dementia

Match the following numbered items with the lettered entries below.

_____51. Wernicke's Syndrome
_____52. Korsakoff's Syndrome
_____53. Delirium

a. sudden onset
b. gradual onset usually
c. fundamental inattention

Match the following types of hallucinations with the usually corresponding etiological factors. The lettered items may be used once, more than once, or not at all.

_____54. visual
_____55. auditory
_____56. olfactory
_____57. tactile
_____58. gustatory

a. LSD
b. cocaine
c. uncinate epilepsy
d. Schizophrenia

Match the numbered diagnoses with the lettered descriptions. Lettered items may be used only once.

_____59. secobarbital or pentobarbital poisoning
_____60. phenobarbital intoxication
_____61. severe glutethimide intoxication
_____62. barbiturate intoxication
_____63. alcohol intoxication

a. flaccid coma with reactive pupils, hypothermia, and hypotension
b. flaccid coma with dilated fixed pupils, hypothermia, hypotension, laryngeal spasms, sudden apnea, high mortality
c. blood barbiturate level of 20µg/ml, short coma
d. blood barbiturate level of 115µg/ml, prolonged coma, high mortality
e. flushed face, injected conjuctivae, verbose, cantankerous, aggressive

I.   INTRODUCTION

Dysfunction of the brain is the essential feature of Organic Mental Disorders. This dysfunction can be either transient (reversible) or permanent (irreversible). Evidence for the dysfunction is required from valid information obtained either through history, mental status evaluation, physical examination, or specific laboratory tests, or some combination of these.

The brain is too complex an organ for its dysfunction to be reflected in one single syndrome or for a given syndrome to be pathognomonic of any given etiology or pathogenesis. Etiology means specific causal agent of the condition (the what). Pathogenesis means mechanism by which the disturbance is generated (the how and why). Pathognomonic means that if a given symptom or sign is present, a known disease can be equated with it. There are very few pathognomonic signs or symptoms in medicine in general, and, therefore, no syndrome is itself diagnostic of any single type of etiology, brain pathogenesis, or pathology, particularly in psychiatry.

Mental disorders have traditionally been differentiated into "organic" denoting brain pathology and nonorganic or "functional." This does not mean that functional disorders are independent of brain processes. It only means that, mostly due to deficiencies in our understanding, organic disorders suggest a less ambiguous disturbance in brain processes than do the functional. Also, organic disorders can more often and more readily be demonstrated by classical neuropsychological and neurodiagnostic techniques to be related to some degree and localization of brain pathology, even when the etiology is unknown. Since one cannot adequately account for functional mental disorders on the basis of brain pathology, one tends to see them as a response to psychological, social, or unknown factors-- including nondemonstrable organic factors. Here we have a switch to a different level of understanding. Indeed, most of the intensive research conducted in psychopharmacology, brain neurochemistry, psychiatric genetics, and several other endeavors operates on the general assumption that there are organic (biochemical or molecular) factors involved in the major so-called functional psychoses. This conviction has been pervasively represented throughout most of the history of psychiatry. The best attitude is that for the functional mental disorders, the last word is not yet in and that, from all we know, organic, psychological, and social factors may be etiologically involved.

The first task, therefore, is to present you with the two sections on Organic Mental Disorders in DSM-III. These are provided in Table 5-1 on the following page.

TABLE 5-1

ORGANIC MENTAL DISORDERS
(FROM DSM III)

Section 1

Dementias arising in the senium and
presenium

Primary degenerative dementia,
senile onset,
with delirium
with delusions
with depression
uncomplicated

Primary degenerative dementia,
presenile onset,
Multi-infarct dementia,

Substance-induced

Alcohol
intoxication
idiosyncratic intoxication
withdrawal
withdrawal delirium
hallucinosis
amnestic disorder

Barbiturate or similarly acting
sedative or hypnotic
intoxication
withdrawal
withdrawal delirium
amnestic disorder

Opioid
intoxication
withdrawal

Cocaine
intoxication

Amphetamine or similarly acting
sympathomimetic
intoxication
delirium

delusional disorder
withdrawal

Phencyclidine (PCP) or similarly
acting arylcyclohexylamine
intoxication
delirium
mixed organic mental disorder

Hallucinogen
hallucinosis
delusional disorder
affective disorder

Cannabis
intoxication
delusional disorder

Tobacco
withdrawal

Caffeine
intoxication

Other or unspecified substance
intoxication
withdrawal
delirium
dementia
amnestic disorder
delusional disorder
hallucinosis
affective disorder
personality disorder
atypical or mixed organic
mental disorder

Section 2

Delirium
Dementia
Amnestic syndrome
Organic delusional syndrome
Organic hallucinosis
Organic affective syndrome
Organic personality syndrome
Atypical or mixed organic
brain syndrome

Section One deals with Organic Brain Syndromes whose etiology is related either to aging or the consumption of a drug. Section Two encompasses all other Organic Mental Disorders not listed under Section One. It will be noted that one critical difference between these two sections is that while the pathogenesis or the substance is used as the cornerstone for classification in Section One, the syndrome is used to derive the diagnosis in Section Two, and its etiology or pathogenesis is either unknown or noted as an additional diagnosis. Thus, different criteria are being used.

DSM-III groups Organic Mental Disorders into six categories characterized by:

    a. Relatively global cognitive impairment
        Delirium
        Dementia
    b. Relatively selective areas of cognitive impairment
        Amnestic Syndrome
        Organic Hallucinosis
    c. Resembling the functional disorders, Schizophrenia and Affective Disorders
        Organic Delusional Syndrome
        Organic Affective Syndrome
    d. Features affecting the personality
        Organic Personality Syndrome
    e. Association with administration or cessation of a foreign substance or drug and not meeting the criteria for any of the previous syndromes
        Intoxication
        Withdrawal
    f. A residual category for any other Organic Mental Disorders not classifiable as any of the preceding syndromes

When the syndromes of:

    Organic Hallucinosis
    Organic Delusional Syndrome
    Organic Affective Syndrome, and
    Organic Personality Syndrome

are caused by an ingested substance, they drop the term "organic," the name of the substance is substituted, and the syndromes automatically change from Section Two to Section One, that is substance-induced.

Symptoms and signs are usefully conceived as:

    1) Primary or direct result of the brain disorder itself, or
    2) Secondary or reactive to the brain disorder or associated features

The primary signs are more predictable on the basis of the brain pathology itself, while secondary or reactive manifestations usually depend more heavily on the premorbid personality (before the onset of brain pathology). Primary and secondary manifestations are, however, not always easily distinguished.

QUIZ, Section I.

1. Complete the following definitions.

    a. _____means the specific causal agent of a condition.

    b. _____means mechanisms by which the disturbance is generated.

    c. Mental disorders for which no brain pathology has been demonstrated are called _____.

Circle the letter corresponding to the one correct response.

2. Intoxication and withdrawal are defined

    a. etiologically.
    b. as syndromes.

3. The DSM-III categories of Organic Mental Disorders listed in Section Two are defined

    a. etiologically.
    b. as syndromes.

Upon examining a person who has sustained head trauma you detect the following symptoms. Match these with the lettered categories. The lettered items may be used more than once.

___4. Marked impairment of calculating ability

a. primary or directly due to brain damage

___5. Depression

b. secondary or reactive to the trauma

___6. Memory impairment

___7. Suicidal attempts

II. DSM-III SECTION TWO SYNDROMES

We will now characterize the seven syndromes listed in Table 5-1. Of these, the most frequently observed disorders are Delirium, Dementia, Intoxication, and Withdrawal. But we will follow the order in which they have been listed in Table 5-1, Section Two.

A. DELIRIUM (DSM-III = 293.00)

Common synonyms for acute Delirium are: acute brain syndrome, acute confusional state, toxic psychosis, metabolic encephalopathy.

1. Features.

   The fundamental or most prominent feature of Delirium is a disorder of attention. It is thought that other cognitive disturbances follow the fundamental impairment of attention. These subordinate impairments occur in the following areas:

   a. Memory: short- and long-term, retrograde, and anterograde.
   b. Orientation: time, place, and person.
   c. Thinking: slowing or acceleration, fragmentation, disorganization, loss of train of thought.
   d. Speech: incoherent, difficult to follow.
   e. Wakefulness: reduced (clouded sensorium) or excessive alertness with insomnia, often fluctuates from one extreme to the other or a reversal of the sleep-wake cycle; vivid dreams and nightmares which may merge with visual hallucinations.
   f. Perceptual disturbances: common in the form of misinterpretations, illusions, hallucinations; the latter are typically but not exclusively visual; content of hallucinations may be unformed, or may represent complex scenes of people or animals, as if in motion picture. There is often a delusional conviction of the reality of the hallucinations which, if frightening or threatening, may prompt escape, attack, or exit through the window (accidental suicide).
   g. Psychomotor overactivity or sluggishness, which may range from striking out at nonexistent objects to an attitude reminiscent of catatonic stupor and mutism; often shifts from one extreme to the other, may occur with little warning.
   h. Associated emotional disturbances with stable or rapid and unpredictable changes in:
      Anxiety-fear
      Depression-suicide
      Irritability-attack
      Euphoria-apathy
   i. Associated autonomic arousal: tachycardia, sweating, flushed face, mydriasis, increased systolic blood pressure.
   j. Associated neurological signs are uncommon except for involuntary movements:
      Coarse tremors (common)
      Peculiar flapping tremor of the hyperextended hands ("asterixis")

2. Course.

   Delirium usually has a rapid onset and brief duration (average one week). Wide fluctuations in impairments are typical. The symptoms get worse at night (dark) and improve during the day, particularly in the morning (light). Delirium may be an intermediate stage between coma and full awareness. Thus, patients recovering from coma may pass through a delirious state, in which case Delirium represents a good prognosis. Full recovery from Delirium is the rule, but death or Dementia may rarely result, particularly if the Delirium is allowed to progress untreated. Other complications to guard against are accidents resulting from falling out of bed or

ANSWERS, Section I. _____

1. a. etiology
    b. pathogenesis
    c. functional
2. a
3. b
4. a
5. b
6. a
7. b

---

from attempts to escape, suicidal or homicidal attempts, and agitation which may interfere with medical management.

3. Etiology.
    The causes of Delirium are multiple. The main etiological factors are medical illness such as systemic infection; metabolic imbalance (i.e., hypoxia, hypercarbia, hypoglycemia, electrolyte disturbances); liver or kidney insufficiency; use of drugs or addictive substances and abrupt cessation of their use; brain trauma; seizures; post-operative states; and certain focal lesions of the right hemisphere and of the undersurface of the occipital lobe. Older age, previous brain damage, or history of Delirium are predisposing factors.

4. Differential Diagnosis.
    A differential diagnosis must usually be made with Schizophrenia, Schizophreniform Disorders, and other psychoses.

    Diagnostic criteria for Delirium

    A. Clouding of consciousness (reduced clarity of awareness of environment), with reduced capacity to shift, focus, and sustain attention to environmental stimuli.

    B. At least two of the following:

        (1) perceptual disturbance: misinterpretations, illusions, or hallucinations
        (2) speech that is at times incoherent
        (3) disturbance of sleep-wakefulness cycle with insomnia or daytime drowsiness
        (4) increased or decreased psychomotor activity

    C. Disorientation and memory impairment (if testable).

    D. Clinical features that develop over a short period of time (usually hours to days) and tend to fluctuate over the course of a day.

E.   Evidence, from the history, physical examination, or laboratory tests, of a specific organic factor judged to be etiologically related to the disturbance.

5.   Treatment.

a.   Maintain or restore fluid and electrolyte balance while the etiology is ascertained.   The patient should have an appropriate diet.

b.   Treat all contributing physical abnormalities (i.e., infection, hypoxia, hyperthermia, etc.) promptly and vigorously since the brain cannot wait.

c.   Treat the cause whenever it is known.   This is the primary focus which will vary depending on the cause (i.e., Anticholinergic Delirium is to be treated with physostigmine).

d.   Keep the patient on the medical or surgical ward, and have the psychiatrist act as a consultant.

e.   Provide environmental orientation (i.e., cues as to time, place, and person; radio or television; eyeglasses, hearing-aid, dentures, watch, etc.).   Later, as cognitive function improves, the patient may be offered newspapers, magazines, books, and occupational therapy.

f.   Keep bedrails raised and provide the immediacy of a familiar face by the bedside during the agitated stage; restrict less familiar visitors; keep room with sufficient light to see but windows shut and safe; take advantage of morning lucidity and, if alert, reassure and explain what is happening; the staff should be sympathetic, supportive, and emphatic; leave some light burning at night to help orientation; room should be decorated, pleasant, and comfortable.

g.   Phenothiazines and haloperidol are the drugs of choice to control the agitation, restlessness, delusions, and hallucinations of most deliria except withdrawal syndromes.   Anxiolytics and barbiturates are contraindicated as they may increase the cognitive deficit and confusion.   When sedation is needed, chlorpromazine 25 mg I.M. is very useful unless the patient has cerebrovascular or cardiovascular disease, in which case chlorpromazine may cause hypotension and complicate the above diseases.   Chlorpromazine I.M. may be repeated several times if needed.   The patient can thence be maintained with 50-100 mg of chlorpromazine orally every 4-6 hours.   Haloperidol in doses of 0.5-1 mg can be used instead of thorazine if there is some CNS depression.

B.   DEMENTIA (DSM-III = 294.10)

The term dementia means without a mind (de-mens), or at least without a fully functional mind.

1.   Essential Features.

a.   A deterioration of previously acquired intellectual abilities of sufficient severity to interfere with social or productive functioning. This description excludes mental retardation, in which a mindful stage of cognitive development has never been achieved. Stated differently, one must be normal first to become demented later, while in mental retardation one never reaches the normal stage but is subnormal from childhood or adolescence.

b.   Memory impairment is the most prominent symptom. It is both anterograde (inability to recall information or events following the onset of Dementia) and retrograde (inability to recall events which preceded the onset). The impairment proceeds from the more recent memories (at early stages) to the more remote (at more advanced stages of severeness of the condition). Failure of memory may be responsible for serious accidents (e.g., leaving gas on, engine running, cigarette burning).

c.   Impairment of abstract thinking. The patient cannot generalize from concrete experiences because the capacities for synthesizing, differentiating, logical reasoning, and concept formation are impaired. Novel tasks, complex information, and time pressures are particularly effective stressors in demonstrating this impairment in abstracting capacity.

d.   Impairment in judgement and poor impulse control. The patient's social behavior may be striking because of his coarse language and jokes, sloppiness, and uncleanliness. The "dirty old man" is often a demented patient. A previously cautious and reliable businessman may embark on a reckless business venture which will plunge him and his family into bankruptcy. This type of behavior may present a problem of differential diagnosis with hypomania. The dementia caused by damage of the frontal lobes is particularly prone to exhibit severe impairment in judgement and impulse control.

e.   Personality change. The physician usually learns about this from close relatives who describe him as "not the same." The change may involve accentuation and/or greater rigidity of premorbid personality traits (e.g., "he was always a bit like this, but now he is impossible"). Or his personality may be altered in a way "so unlike himself" (e.g., pious, religious, prudish individual becomes cantankerous, promiscuous, and blasphemous).

2. Associated Emotional Features.

Obviously, the capacity for self-appraisal is one feature of the mind which is also bound to be impaired in Dementia sooner or later. At early stages or in mild Dementia this capacity for self-assessment may often be preserved and allows the patient to realize that his other intellectual abilities are dwindling. This recognition may lead to anxiety, depression, suicide, or social withdrawal. With progression of the dementing process, this capacity for self-evaluation and the resulting awareness of deficiencies may become impaired too, and then the patient will appear less concerned or even blandly self-complacent. In premorbidly compulsive individuals, excessive orderliness and pointless detailed accounts may emerge to compensate for, or mask, the memory defect. In previously suspicious patients, blame may be put on others for his forgetfulness. This may lead to accusations and physical attack. Jealous persons may construe previously insignificant behaviors of the spouse as indicative of marital unfaithfulness.

3. Age at Onset.

The intellectual quotient (IQ) becomes fairly stable by the age of 3-4 years. Therefore, before this age, it would be difficult to rule out mental retardation. Even if apparent mental retardation before age 4 were indeed Dementia, it would usually be advantageous to plan the management as if it were mental retardation. After age 4, it is easier to see an abrupt or slow deterioration of previously acquired intellectual abilities. This, by definition, would be Dementia rather than mental retardation, but the differential diagnosis may still be difficult, and both diagnoses may be appropriate because, although IQ may be stable by age 4, intellectual abilities are not fully developed. Dementia is, however, much more frequent in adulthood or senescence. Indeed, in the elderly the normal process of aging may be associated with some decrement in intellectual functioning. This may pose a problem of differential diagnosis which will be decided on whether or not the deterioration is sufficiently severe to interfere with social or productive functioning. If interference is present, the diagnosis ought to be Dementia rather than normal process of aging.

4. Course.

Dementia may be called progressive if deterioration keeps on increasing, nonprogressive but static if a permanent but fixed degree of impairment sets in, and reversible if the deficits can be cleared away by treatment or natural evolution of the condition. Reversibility is a function of the underlying brain pathology and/or the available and timely application of effective treatment to prevent neuronal death. Deficits ensuing directly from widespread neuronal death will be irreversible; those stemming from temporary blockade of neuronal circuits due to, say, cerebral edema or increased intracranial pressure will be reversed as soon as the causal factors are relieved or eliminated. Most of the direct deficits listed earlier and the associated emotional features are likely to be present from the early stages of Dementia. Other manifestations may emerge as the condition worsens. Some of these are: language disturbance (vague, imprecise, stereotyped, anomic, incomprehensible, or totally absent), difficulty or total impairment in performing complex motor tasks and imitating gestures to the point of inability to dress or shave himself, or manipulate utensils (fork, knife, pen). The course of Dementia, beginning with the onset, largely depends on the underlying etiology.

When impairment becomes very severe, the individual becomes totally oblivious to his surroundings and requires constant custodial and nursing care.

5. Usual Etiologies.
Dementia has the following usual etiologies:

   a. Global neurodegenerative processes: Presenile and Senile Dementias (see p. 187)
   b. Infections: can be bacterial, treponemal, viral, fungal, etc.
   c. Traumatic: head injury, chronic subdural hematoma
   d. Toxic and metabolic: pernicious anemia, folic acid deficiency, pellagra, hypothyroidism
   e. Exogenous intoxication: carbon monoxide, methyl alcohol
   f. Neoplastic lesions: any form of intracranial tumor
   g. Circulatory disorders: multi-infarct
   h. Normal pressure hydrocephalus
   i. Other neurological diseases: Huntington's chorea, multiple sclerosis, etc.

6. Differential diagnosis.
Diagnosis of Dementia should rule out the following disorders:

   a. Normal process of aging: No interference with social or occupational functioning
   b. Delirium: Disturbance in level of awareness
                  Fluctuation in severity of signs
                  Shorter duration
   c. Schizophrenia: Chronic is more of a problem than acute because of its often concomitant intellectual deterioration. Chronic Schizophrenia rather than Dementia will be diagnosed in the absence of identifiable brain pathology.
   d. Depression with cognitive deficits secondary to the affective disturbance (Pseudodementia): If in doubt or at an impasse in diagnostic work-up, resort to a diagnostic-therapeutic trial with tricyclic antidepressant medication, or electroconvulsive therapy may be indicated.

Diagnostic criteria for Dementia

   A. A loss of intellectual abilities of sufficient severity to interfere with social or occupational functioning.

B.　Memory impairment.

C.　At least one of the following:

(1) impairment of abstract thinking, as manifested by concrete interpretation of proverbs, inability to find similarities and differences between related words, difficulty in defining words and concepts, and other similar tasks
(2) impaired judgement
(3) other disturbances of higher cortical function, such as aphasia (disorder of language due to brain dysfunction), apraxia (inability to carry out motor activities despite intact comprehension and motor attention), agnosia (failure to recognize or identify objects despite intact sensory function), "constructional difficulty" (e.g., inability to copy three-dimensional figures, assemble blocks, or arrange sticks in specific designs)
(4) personality change, i.e., alteration or accentuation of premorbid traits

D.　State of consciousness not clouded (i.e., does not meet the criteria for Delirium or Intoxication, although these may be superimposed).

E.　Either (1) or (2):

(1) there is evidence from either physical examination, medical laboratory tests, or the history of a specific organic factor that is judged to be etiologically related to the disturbance
(2) in the absence of such evidence, an organic factor necessary for the development of the syndrome can be presumed if conditions other than Organic Mental Disorders have been reasonably excluded and if the behavioral change represents cognitive impairment in a variety of areas

Once a diagnosis of Dementia has been established, the differential diagnosis must be further refined to arrive at the specific etiology or pathogenesis responsible for the dementia. This is important, because on this basis the clinician can infer whether the dementia is specifically treatable and reversible or untreatable and irreversible. Since Dementia is a syndrome of a number of illnesses, many etiologies or pathogenetic mechanisms have to be considered. The most important consideration is that not all demented patients are "incurables." A second important point is that the term "untreatable," as applied to certain Dementias, does not mean that the physician is free to dismiss the patient, or to ignore or neglect the signs and symptoms presented by the patient or relatives. It only means that no specific or direct treatment capable of attacking the cause is available. But palliative (to mitigate suffering) or symptomatic treatment is usually applicable.

7. Treatment of Dementia.
The treatment of Dementia depends on the diagnosis. Both diagnosis and treatment must be conducted after admission to an inpatient setting. Consultation with specialists (usually neurologist, neurosurgeon, internist, or endocrinologist) is usually needed to arrive at a conclusion of treatable or untreatable Dementia. Table 5-2 below lists the most usual of these two groups of Dementias.

TABLE 5-2

THERAPEUTIC CLASSIFICATION OF DEMENTIAS BASED ON ETIOLOGIES

Treatable	Noncorrectable
Bacterial meningitis	Alcoholic
Benign intracranial masses	Amyotrophic lateral sclerosis
Brain abscess	Brain atrophy, unknown cause
Drug toxicity	Malignant brain tumors
Electrolyte imbalance	Multi-infarct with hypertension
Epilepsy	Neurosyphilis (some cases)
Extracranial vascular disease	Normal pressure hydrocephalus
Hepatic failure	(some)
Neurosyphilis	Parkinson's disease
Normal pressure hydrocephalus	Post-encephalitic Dementia
Pellagra	Post-traumatic Dementia
Pernicious anemia	Slow virus diseases
Post-subarachnoid hemorrhage	
Pseudodementia	
Renal insufficiency	
Thyroid disease	
Wernicke's disease	

While treatable Dementias will often require skills that only other specialists can provide, the primary physician or the psychiatrist should be able to attend to the symptomatic needs of the untreatable Dementias. The outline below provides the basis for helpful measures in the management of demented patients:

a. Psychopharmacotherapy:

   1) For depression: Imipramine, Amitriptyline
   2) For agitation and confusion: Lights on all night, Haloperidol, chlorpromazine, thioridazine, (barbiturates and minor tranquilizers are contraindicated)

3) For insomnia: Barbiturates and benzodiazepines
4) For abulia and apathy: Methylphenidate, dextroamphetamine
5) For extrapyramidal disease: Anti-Parkinsonian Drugs (watch for Atropinic Delirium or psychosis which may be caused by these drugs.)

b. Other measures: Soft diet or tube feeding may be required if there are swallowing difficulties; antispasmodics and anticonvulsants for muscle spasms and seizures respectively; antibiotics for infection; physiotherapy and supportive devices to improve motor capacity; etc.

c. Supportive psychotherapy for patients and relatives:

1) Maximize strengths
2) Encourage to do as much as he can for himself
3) Do not place undue pressures for performance
4) Encourage return to the home after diagnostic work-up has been completed and treatment plan underway if social and family supports are available
5) The physician's primary obligation is to the family after deterioration becomes so severe that the patient requires continued custodial and nursing care in a special facility

****

GO TO VIDEOTAPE

****

C.   AMNESTIC SYNDROME (DSM-III = 294.00)

According to DSM-III the fundamental feature of the Amnestic Syndrome is a short-term memory impairment caused by a specific organic factor in the absence of Delirium or Dementia. This implies that attention must be intact in order to rule out Delirium and that there are no other cognitive or behavioral abnormalities which could be attributed to Dementia. Short-term memory is somewhat arbitrarily but nevertheless empirically defined as the ability to recall events that occurred at least 25 minutes prior to the memory test. The time required to transfer information from immediate memory into memory storage is still uncertain, but most individuals diagnosed as Amnestic Syndrome fail to recall events 25 minutes later while they are quite capable of remembering more immediate events. This description provides a relatively easy way to discriminate immediate from short-term memory.

With the onset of the Amnestic Syndrome the patient cannot retain new information except for very brief intervals (up to 25 minutes). New experiences are retained briefly and then fade away beyond retrieval. This is called anterograde or forward amnesia.

1. Associated Features.
    Anterograde amnesia rarely occurs without some degree of retrograde or backward amnesia; that is, impairment of memory for events prior to the onset of the syndrome. This is probably true because once the pathological factor responsible is at work, it prevents immediately preceding events from consolidating into memory storage for future recall.

    Other associated features may be:

    a. Some disorientation as to time
    b. Confabulation, or covering up the memory defect with pseudo-information
    c. Lack of insight into, or denial of, the memory impairment. Indifference, neglect, and denial of illness are often associated features.

2. Etiological Factors.
    Causes of amnesia can be of any type, but the most common is the thiamine deficiency usually resulting from chronic alcohol abuse. Despite the fact that chronic alcoholism is a widespread problem, it apparently rarely leads to a pure Amnestic Syndrome. Other pathological processes causing bilateral damage of certain limbic structures may also manifest in the form of the Amnestic Syndrome. Components of the so-called Papez Circuit of Emotions in the limbic system such as the hippocampal formation, fornix, mammillary bodies, and nucleus ventralis anterior of the thalamus can be encroached upon by head trauma, surgical intervention, anoxia, posterior cerebral artery infarction, and herpes simplex encephalitis.

3. Differential Diagnosis.
    Before a diagnosis of Amnestic Syndrome can be made, the following processes must be ruled out:

    a. Dementia with other cognitive and behavioral abnormalities.
    b. Delirium with impairment of attention.
    c. Factitious illness with inconsistent findings.
    d. Korsakoff's Syndrome which presents the most difficult differential challenge. In Korsakoff's there is usually a confusional state and confabulation is more frequent, while in the Amnestic Syndrome confabulation may or may not be associated and confusion is lacking. In Korsakoff's there is usually a limited attention span, which is not found in the Amnestic Syndrome. (See more on Korsakoff's in this chapter.)

D.   ORGANIC DELUSIONAL SYNDROME (DSM-III = 293.81)

The presence of delusions or false ideas is the predominant manifestation. Delusions of persecution or of grandeur occur in a normal state of alertness.

1.   Features and Diagnostic Considerations.
     The clinical picture must be clearly attributable to a specific organic
     factor in an individual not suffering from organic hallucinosis (see
     next syndrome), Delirium, or Dementia. The delusions may range
     from simple and poorly organized, such as those occurring in brain
     tumors, to highly structured delusional states such as those seen in
     amphetamine psychoses or in temporal lobe epilepsy. Elaborate
     delusional systems are difficult to distinguish from a Schizophreni-
     form Disorder. The key to the differential diagnosis may be provi-
     ded by other associated features such as hallucinations. In the
     Organic Delusional Syndrome hallucinations are more likely to be
     visual or tactile, while in acute Schizophreniform Disorders they are
     usually found to be auditory. If the predominant manifestations are
     either visual hallucinations or Affective Disorders (depression,
     mania), the syndrome must be diagnosed as Organic Hallucinosis or
     Organic Affective Syndrome, respectively.

     There may be other associated features which do not help, but
     rather confound, the differential diagnosis (d.d.). These are:
     mild cognitive impairment (d.d. with Dementia); communication
     disorder, eccentricity, perplexity, rocking, apathetic immobility
     (d.d. with Schizophreniform); pacing or dysphoric mood (d.d. with
     anxiety or depression).

     The Organic Delusional Syndrome usually leads to severe impairment
     of social and occupational functioning. Persecutory delusions may
     drive the patient to harm himself in attempts to escape or to harm
     others in self-defense. Grandiose delusions may lead to errors of
     judgement usually affecting finances or property.

2.   Etiological Factors and Treatment Considerations.
     There are two main groups of etiologies of organic delusional syn-
     drome. One is exogenous abuse of substances (i.e., amphetamines)
     and the other is represented by a varied assortment of structural
     brain pathologies (i.e., temporal lobe epilepsy, Huntington's chorea,
     general paresis, etc.). The treatment depends on the etiology.
     Sometimes treatment can be fairly specific, but at other times
     neuroleptics may provide the only symptomatic treatment.

E.   ORGANIC HALLUCINOSIS (DSM-III = 293.82)

The predominant feature is persistence or recurrence of hallucinations in
an alert individual in whom organic etiology can be demonstrated, but
criteria for Delirium, Dementia, Organic Delusional or Affective Syndromes
cannot be fulfilled.

1.   Associated features.
     Hallucinogens may produce hallucinations which are experienced
     subjectively as pleasant (psychedelic) or concomitantly with anxiety,
     depression, dysphoria, or fear (psychotogenic or psychotomimetic).
     The patient may have insight into the unreality of the hallucina-
     tions, or he may exhibit a firm delusional conviction that the

hallucinations are real events. As long as this delusion is confined to the existence or content of the hallucinations the syndrome may be diagnosed as Organic Hallucinosis. If the delusions are elaborated beyond this point or if delusions unrelated to the hallucinations emerge, the diagnosis may have to be changed to Organic Delusional Syndrome. The modality of hallucinations usually depends on the etiological agent.

2. Course.
In cases of irreversible pathology of special sense organs the syndrome may be permanent; it may last from weeks to years in Alcoholic Hallucinosis, and is usually very brief when it results from temporary sensory deprivation. Epileptic foci in the temporal or occipital lobes may cause episodic hallucinations throughout life.

F.   ORGANIC AFFECTIVE SYNDROME (DSM-III = 293.83)

Disturbances in mood are the essential and predominant features. These closely resemble the manifestations seen in the nonorganic Affective Disorders (see Bipolar Affective Disorder). But in this syndrome a specific organic factor is presupposed, and physical, historical, or laboratory evidence of this factor must be obtained before the diagnosis can be made. Etiological factors usually include toxic or metabolic insults caused by oral contraceptives, amphetamines, hallucinogens, some antihypertensive agents (clonidine, methyldopa, reserpine, and propranolol), and corticosteroids. Reserpine has been held responsible for causing depression in 5-15% of those taking it and who may have a genetic predisposition to develop depression. Hormonal disturbances causing hyperadrenal corticalism (Cushing's Syndrome) or adrenocortical insufficiency (Addison's Disease) and changes in thyroid or parathyroid function may also be etiological factors. Generalized disease such as systemic lupus erythematosus, uremia, carcinoma of the pancreas or disseminated carcinomatosis, viral infections, and brain trauma or tumor may cause disease-related depression -- or less frequently mania -- as an inherent part of the symptom complex. This Organic Affective Syndrome may range from mild to severe, and is bound to have associated features such as cognitive impairment, excessive somatic concerns, hallucinations, and delusions. Delirium, Dementia, Organic Delusional Syndrome, and Organic Hallucinosis must first be ruled out before this diagnosis can be made. This means that none of the associated features listed above can be seen as the essential and predominant manifestations.

G.   ORGANIC PERSONALITY SYNDROME (DSM-III = 310.10)

A marked change in personality attributable to a clearly identified organic etiology is the essential and predominant feature in this syndrome. Personality is defined by DSM-III as a set of relatively enduring patterns or style of relating to the environment. Personality changes are most often described by relatives and close friends - rather than by the patient - as "not like himself," although sometimes the picture emerges as "he was always a bit like this, but now it is intolerable."

Structural damage to the frontal lobes is the most frequent cause, and a common pattern of personality change involves the following spheres of behavior:

1) Emotional: lability, irritability, temper outbursts, belligerence, sudden bouts of crying, all upon little or no provocation.
2) Impulse control: impaired, sexual indiscretions with little concern for consequences, explosive or dangerous behavior toward self or others.
3) Social judgement: impaired, inappropriate actions (e.g., shoplifting) and interactions often requiring close supervision or even custodial care.

Another pattern of the so-called frontal lobe syndrome is characterized by marked apathy, indifference, and disinterest in usual activities, in events of concern, and in hobbies.

The temporal lobe is the second most important structure whose pathology may cause the syndrome. Temporal lobe (synonym: psychomotor) epilepsy is frequently responsible. The personality change is observable in between ictal episodes. The interictal personality is described as humorless, hyper-emotional, excessively religious, prone to temper outbursts, obsessive, and verbose in speech and writing.

Acute or chronic use of certain drugs (e.g., steroids, amphetamines, LSD, alcohol) or endocrine disorders (e.g., thyroid disease) may also cause temporary or sometimes even permanent personality change.

There may be associated features which in and of themselves will pose problems of differential diagnosis. Obviously, cognitive impairment may be present (differential diagnosis with Dementia). Indeed many types of Dementia begin with mild cognitive impairment and personality change, in which case the diagnosis will have to be changed. The time to change the diagnosis to Dementia is when the cognitive impairment becomes the essential and predominant feature of the clinical manifestations. Temporal lobe epilepsy may closely resemble a Schizophreniform Syndrome.

We have now covered the description of all those syndromes listed in DSM-III Section Two of the Organic Mental Disorders except for the last one called "Other or Mixed Organic Brain Syndrome" (DSM-III = 294.80) which is a residual category reserved for syndromes which do not meet the criteria for any of the Organic Brain Syndromes described above. But the vagaries of the mind encompass more maladaptive changes than we have so far described. This last category is provided to accommodate all these other changes or their mixtures. These other or mixed syndromes will be described after DSM-III Section One has been covered.

You will recall now that we started with Section Two of DSM-III because it provides the main building blocks of the psychopathology of Organic Mental Disorders. We should also remember that the syndromes described in Section Two have general applicability, regardless of the etiology or pathogenesis. Indeed the etiology of the syndromes listed in Section Two may be unknown.

We will now turn to the syndromes of DSM-III Section One. This section is composed of two groups of syndromes. One is made up of the Senile, Presenile and Multi-infarct Dementias of whose pathogenesis we have some understanding, but of the etiology we know very little. The other group is constituted by the substance-induced syndromes whose etiology is completely known but the pathogenesis may not be entirely clear. For purposes of clarity, substance-induced syndromes will be presented under Section IV of this chapter.

QUIZ, Section II.

Complete the following.

1. The fundamental or most prominent feature of Delirium is disorder of _____ .

2. Prominent features of Dementia include: impairment of abstract thinking, impairment in judgement, and in impulse control, personality change and _____ .

3. In early childhood, impairment of intellectual functioning is called _____ .

Circle the letter corresponding to the <u>one</u> correct response.

4. During Delirium the agitation should be managed by using all the following measures <u>except</u>

   a. provide light in the room.
   b. Valium 10 mg qid.
   c. ask family member to remain in room with patient.
   d. Haloperidol 1 mg q 4-6 hours.
   e. provide environmental orientation.

Circle the correct answer(s). <u>One</u> or <u>more</u> <u>than</u> <u>one</u> answer may be correct.

5. The diagnostic criteria for the Amnestic Syndrome are

   a. short-term but not immediate memory impairment.
   b. the amnesia is not part of a Delirium or Dementia Syndrome.
   c. specific organic factor jeopardizing function of some limbic structure.
   d. severe psychic trauma followed by amnesia of the event and a period of time preceding it.

6.   Criteria for diagnosis of Organic Delusional Syndrome are

   a.   predominant delusional system associated with organic etiology.
   b.   predominant hallucinosis of auditory modality with secondary delusions related to auditory hallucinations.
   c.   visual hallucinations and impaired sensorium.
   d.   delusions without demonstrable organic pathology by either history, lab tests, neurodiagnostic procedures, or physical examination.
   e.   no evidence of primary Delirium, Dementia, Schizophreniform, or Affective Disorder.

Case Study.   A 57-year-old male is referred to you by another physician with the following note: Long history of alcohol consumption, insidious onset of memory impairment, confabulations, poor state of nutrition, peripheral neuropathy, and cerebellar ataxia. He is acutely ill and shows no impairment of attention or consciousness.

7.   Your first working diagnosis in the case above should be

   a.   Amnestic Syndrome.
   b.   diabetic encephalopathy.
   c.   Korsakoff's Syndrome.
   d.   Delirium Tremens.

Match the following syndromes with the corresponding descriptions.

___8.   Amnestic Syndrome
___9.   Korsakoff's Syndrome
___10.   Delirium

a.   sudden onset
b.   slow onset usually
c.   fundamental inattention

TRUE or FALSE: Circle the correct answer.

T   F   11. Good short-term memory presupposes good immediate memory.

T   F   12. Good immediate memory warrants good short-term memory.

Consider the concept of stimulus-binding in the following clinical vignettes.

A.   Patient is known to have consumed toxic amounts of LSD. He is hallucinating flashy, exploding, "Star-Wars"-like rockets which pop out of the walls and ceilings of his bare and dimly lit hospital room.

B.   An alcoholic patient complains to you that a male nurse in the next room is calling him homosexual. You were listening and heard the nurse saying to another patient, "turn over so we'll change the sheets now."

T   F   13. Patient A had stimulus-bound hallucinations while patient B betrayed no apparent dependence of his hallucination on external stimuli.

Check your guessing ability to match applicable treatments with etiologies of Organic Delusional Syndromes. Lettered items may be matched once, more than once, or not at all.

___14. Huntington's Chorea
___15. temporal lobe epilepsy
___16. amphetamine delusions
___17. general paresis

a. neuroleptics
b. anticonvulsants or brain surgery
c. penicillin
d. antihypertensives

Match the following hallucinatory modalities on the left with the usually corresponding etiological factors on the right. The numbers may be used once, more than once, or not at all.

___18. visual
___19. auditory
___20. olfactory
___21. tactile
___22. gustatory

a. LSD
b. cocaine
c. uncinate epilepsy
d. Schizophrenia

III. DSM-III SECTION ONE SYNDROMES: PROGRESSIVE IDIOPATHIC AND MULTI-INFARCT DEMENTIAS

A. PRIMARY DEGENERATIVE DEMENTIA; SENILE ONSET, PRESENILE ONSET

These two syndromes constitute a single entity since they cannot be distinguished by clinical or neuropathological analyses. They cannot even be distinguished from brain specimens by the most modern techniques available to the electron microscopist. Yet, because of tradition, DSM-III still lists them as two clinical entities only on the basis of age at onset and gives them different names solely on this basis. Table 5-3 below emphasizes the identity as well as the unremarkable differences.

TABLE 5-3
CHARACTERISTIC FEATURES OF SENILE AND PRE-SENILE DEMENTIAS

	Senile	Pre-senile
Disease Name	Senile Dementia	Alzheimer's Disease
Frequency	Usual	Relative infrequency
	2-4% of population	
Onset	Insidious	Same
Age	65 or over	Before 65
aver. age	74	60
Sex	F = 2:1	Same
Familial prevalence	4X	Same
Course	Progressive	Same
Length	5 years	7 years
Predominant impairments	Memory / Orientation / Intellect	Same
Pathology gross	Cortical atrophy / Wide cortical sulci / Ventricular enlargement	Same
microscopic	Senile plaques / Neurofibrillary tangles / Granular vacuolar degeneration of neurons / Neuronal loss	Same

The diagnosis of Primary Degenerative Dementia is first made on clinical grounds. Table 5-4 below gives the clinical findings in a recent study of 20 patients (Katzman & Karasu, 1975).

TABLE 5-4

CLINICAL FINDINGS IN 20 PATIENTS WITH ALZHEIMER'S DISEASE

Symptoms	%
Memory loss	100
Disorientation	80
Agitation	70
Dysphasia	50
Psychotic factors	40
Incontinence	40
Dyspraxia	35
Hemiparesis or reflex changes	30
Gait disturbances	25
Family history of Dementia	10

The clinical diagnosis is reinforced by special neuroradiological diagnostic procedures such as the pneumoencephalogram, and more recently the CT scan is preferred since it is noninvasive and usually innocuous. These demonstrate generalized cortical atrophy or moderate ventricular dilatation. The electroencephalogram will also suggest the diagnosis if it shows mild to moderate generalized slowing of waveform activity. Definitive identification of Primary Degenerative Dementia can be made only on the basis of histopathological data because this disease has very specific microscopic findings which have been listed in Table 5-3.

There are many other causes of Dementia besides those given for the progressive degenerative type. A rather comprehensive list of Dementias, according to causes, with percentages is provided in Table 5-5 on the following page. This list summarizes the data compiled from a total of over 200 demented patients in a recent review (Wells, 1977).

ANSWERS, Section II.

1.	attention	12.	F
2.	memory impairment	13.	F
3.	mental retardation	14.	a
4.	b	15.	b
5.	a,b,c	16.	a
6.	a,e	17.	c
7.	c	18.	a
8.	a	19.	d
9.	b	20.	c
10.	c	21.	b
11.	T	22.	c

TABLE 5-5

THE RELATIVE INCIDENCE OF DEMENTIAS

Specific Diagnoses	Percent
Atrophy of unknown cause (largely Alzheimer's disease and Senile Dementia)	50.9
Intracranial masses	5.4
Dementia due to vascular disease	7.7
Dementia in alcoholics	5.9
Normal pressure hydrocephalus (NPH)	6.3
Creutzfeldt-Jakob Disease (slow virus infection)	1.4
Huntington's Chorea	4.5
Post-traumatic Dementia	<1
Post-subarachnoid hemorrhage	<1
Post-encephalitic Dementia	<1
Neurosyphilis	<1
Dementia with amytrophic lateral sclerosis	<1
Dementia with Parkinson's disease (Guam's)	<1
Thyroid disease (hypo- or hyper-function)	<1
Pernicious anemia	<1
Hepatic failure	<1
Drug toxicity	3.2
Epilepsy	<1
Depression (Pseudodementia)	4.1
Other psychiatric disease	<1
Not demented - no definite diagnosis	<1
Dementia uncertain	3.2

One might guess that it is this striking combination of hallmarks (overwhelming frequency, unknown etiology, well known neuropathology) which may have led the DSM-III task force to give preferential treatment to Progressive Idiopathic Dementia in a category, actually two categories, all by itself. In a differential diagnosis all the other Dementias listed in Table 5-5 and a few others to be described below and in the last section, must be first ruled out before a diagnosis of progressive Dementia can be made.

You have now seen that the syndrome of Dementia in general (DSM-III = 294.10) afflicts individuals mostly during the senium and less during presenile stages.

Most of the conditions listed in Table 5-5 occur during the presenile years. Yet DSM-III has chosen not to lump them with Alzheimer's disease, a Dementia of presenile onset. DSM-III makes exception of only one Dementia, Pick's disease, which is listed along with Alzheimer's as a progressive idiopathic Dementia of presenile onset.

Pick's disease is exceedingly rare. Many clinicians do not believe that the differential diagnosis with Alzheimer's disease can be made strictly on clinical evidence or even with the aid of neuroradiological studies. Unambiguous differentiation from Alzheimer's disease is only feasible on the basis of characteristic histological findings. Some claims of clinical differences have been made, but, if valid, they still fail to provide a reliable basis for the differential diagnosis. These differences are listed in Table 5-6 on the following page.

TABLE 5-6

CHARACTERISTIC HISTOLOGICAL DIFFERENCES BETWEEN PICK'S AND ALZHEIMER'S DEMENTIAS

	Pick's Dementia	Alzheimer's Dementia
Incidence	Lower	Higher
Personality changes	Tend to precede memory impairment	Follow memory impairment
	More severe than memory impairment	Less severe than memory impairment
Reactive depression	Rare	Often
Insight	Lacking	Often present early
Anxiety	Free	Present early
Speech	Terminal mutism	Disturbed
Extrapyramidal rigidity	Rare	Often
Gait disturbance	Rare	Often
EEG changes	Normal often	↓alpha rhythm, slowing
Pathology		
Gross	More circumscribed	More diffuse
	Fronto-orbito-temporal	Fronto-occipital
Microscopic	No tangles	Neurofibrillary tangles
	Neuronal argyrophilic inclusions	Argyrophilic plaques
	Neuronal loss	Neuronal loss
	Gliosis extensive	

****

GO TO VIDEOTAPE

****

B. MULTI-INFARCT DEMENTIA (DSM-III = 290.4x)

This syndrome is marked by step-wise and patchy deterioration of intellectual functions caused, as the name suggests, by a succession of strokes which leaves patches of ischemic or hemorrhagic infarcts in brain tissue. This affects some cognitive functions and leaves others relatively intact (patchy deterioration). The dementing process becomes more severe and generalized in a step-wise fashion as the number of strokes accumulates. Focal neuro-logical signs and symptoms eventually emerge along with the dementia. This syndrome used to be called Organic Brain Syndrome with Cerebral Arteriosclerosis. It is realized now that there is little correlation between systemic, retinal, and cerebral arteriosclerosis and that the state of the cerebral vessels in and of itself has very little relation to the presence or absence of Dementia. Rather, Dementia depends largely on the severeness, number, and localization of successive strokes. Characteristic clinical differences between Multi-infarct and Alzheimer's Dementia are summarized in Table 5-7.

TABLE 5-7

CHARACTERISTIC CLINICAL DIFFERENCES BETWEEN MULTI-INFARCT AND ALZHEIMER'S DEMENTIAS

	Multi-infarct Dementia	Alzheimer's Dementia
Prevalence	Less common	More common
Onset	Abrupt	Insidious
Course	Step-wise Fluctuating Erratic Rapid changes	Uniformly progressive
Pattern of deficits	Patchy	Diffuse
Focal neurological signs	Frequent	Rare
Vascular disease	Usually present	No association
Hypertension	Usually present	No association
Sex predominance	Male (2:1)	Female (2:1)

QUIZ, Section III.

Circle the letter corresponding to the one correct response.

1.   Of all the differences between Pick's and Alzheimer's listed in Table 5-6, those of most differential-diagnostic value are

    a.   extrapyramidal rigidity and gait disturbance.
    b.   incidence and personality disturbance.
    c.   gross and microscopic pathology.

Circle the correct answer(s). One or more than one answer may be correct.

2.   The microscopic identification of Alzheimer's disease is based on recognition of

    a.   argentophilic neuronal inclusions.
    b.   neurofibrillary tangles.
    c.   senile plaques.
    d.   micro-infarcts of mammillary bodies.
    e.   neuronal loss.

3. Features suggesting Dementia due to cerebral vascular disease include

    a. abrupt onset.
    b. step-wise deterioration.
    c. fluctuating course.
    d. history of presence of hypertension.
    e. history of "strokes."
    f. focal neurological symptoms and signs.

Match the following numbered items with the lettered diseases.

___4. thromboembolic disease of extracranial vessels
___5. neurofibrillary tangles and argyrophilic plaques
___6. circumscribed fronto-temporal atrophy without history of strokes

a. Alzheimer's disease
b. Multi-infarct Dementia
c. Pick's disease

IV. DSM-III SECTION ONE SYNDROMES: SUBSTANCE-INDUCED ORGANIC MENTAL DISORDERS

We are now ready to consider substance-induced Organic Mental Disorders. Again DSM-III has selected nine specific substances or groups of substances on which to base one or various categories of syndromes. A tenth and last group lumps a nameless assortment of substances capable of inducing as many as ten different syndromes. The nine groups of substances are: alcohol, barbiturates and related sedatives, opioids, cocaine, amphetamines and related sympathomimetics, hallucinogens, cannabis, tobacco, and caffeine. All these chemicals have one thing in common - they are substances that individuals tend to use and abuse for psychological or emotional reasons. DSM-III is being responsive to the national concern of the 1960's and the 1970's with abused substances. The syndromes they cause have become the concern of psychiatrists. You will recall that Section Two of Organic Mental Disorders listed seven syndromes. Note that in the last block of substance-induced disorders the number has grown by two additional syndromes. These two new syndromes are intoxication and withdrawal. Not all substances of abuse cause a withdrawal syndrome. Thence, it is missing for those substances. Conceivably every abused substance can cause intoxication, but for some substances intoxication represents an insignificant problem or it takes the form of one of the other syndromes. Thus the syndrome of intoxication may be omitted or is changed depending on the substance. These are the reasons for the variance from one to as many as seven different categories of syndromes ascribed to the nine specific substances. (Study Table 5-1 again.)

We shall now describe the two new syndromes in order to avoid unnecessary repetitiousness later.

A. INTOXICATION

Intoxication has the following essential features:

1) Recent ingestion of the toxicant
2) Presence of toxicant in the body
3) The presence of maladaptive behavior due to effects of the intoxicant on the brain
4) Syndrome does not fit the description of any of the syndromes described in DSM-III, Section Two

Feature 4) above implies that Intoxication as defined by DSM-III is a residual category; that is, it should only be used when the ingestion of an exogenous substance does not cause any of the specific Organic Brain Syndromes described earlier in DSM-III, Section Two. If it does, the syndrome cannot be labeled Intoxication.

Feature 3) of essential features states that maladaptive behavior is required for a diagnosis of Intoxication.

B. WITHDRAWAL

Withdrawal is a syndrome that follows the cessation or intake reduction of a substance that the individual was previously taking regularly. Withdrawal, as Intoxication, is a residual category. This means that if the cessation of substance use causes signs and symptoms that fulfill the criteria for any of the previously described syndromes in DSM-III, Section Two, a diagnosis of Withdrawal cannot be made. Empirically you will find that diagnoses of intoxication by, or withdrawal from, a substance are made when the substance in question induces a milder and less developed syndrome than when the diagnosis would have to be Delirium, Hallucinosis, etc., if it fulfilled the criteria for such syndromes. The most common symptoms of Withdrawal are anxiety, restlessness, irritability, insomnia, and impaired attention. You can see how the last symptom, impaired attention, if it were the essential and predominant manifestation, would force you to consider seriously Delirium rather than Withdrawal as the diagnosis. There are also associated features which may aid in the diagnosis. These partly depend on the nature of the substance. Some examples are:

1) Nausea and vomiting following cessation of alcohol
2) Diffuse malaise following cessation of sedatives
3) Compelling desire to resume use of the substance (for many substances)

The course is usually self-limited and frequently lasts days, rarely weeks. The degree of impairment also varies with the substance. Below are some generalizations:

1) Barbiturate Withdrawal: most severe, can be lethal if untreated
2) Alcohol Withdrawal: very severe
3) Opioid Withdrawal: severe, nonlethal
4) Tobacco Withdrawal: mild

ANSWERS, Section III._____

1.   c
2.   b,c,e
3.   a,b,c,d,e,f
4.   b
5.   a
6.   c

_____

Withdrawal symptoms may drive the victim to get more of the substance by any means at his disposal (e.g., illegal behavior, aggression, murder). These behaviors are considered complications of the withdrawal state. The differential diagnosis also varies with the nature of the substances.

We will now turn to each of the specific substance-induced syndromes which represent different categories in DSM-III. We will follow the same sequence in which they are presented in Table 5-1. It begins with the alcohol-induced Organic Mental Disorders with a total of seven syndromes.

C.   ALCOHOL INTOXICATION (DSM-III = 303.00)

This syndrome is caused by the recent ingestion of a <u>sufficient amount</u> of alcohol which induces essential signs of neurological and psychological impairment and maladaptive behavioral effects, summarized in Table 5-8.

TABLE 5-8

ESSENTIAL FEATURES OF ALCOHOL INTOXICATION

Neurological Signs	Psychological Signs	Maladaptive Behavior
Slurred speech	Mood lability	Fighting
Incoordination	Sexual and aggressive	Impaired judgement
Unsteady gait	disinhibition	Social-job interference
Impaired attention	Irritability	Irresponsibility
and memory	Loquacity	

Associated features often become apparent. These usually involve exaggeration or reversal of personality traits or amnesia for events during the intoxicated state (blackout spells).

The familiarity of most people with alcoholic intoxication should not distract from the fact that other substances, particularly barbiturate and similarly acting sedatives and hypnotics may cause manifestations identical to those of alcohol. Alcoholic breath is no evidence that alcohol is the agent responsible for the behavior. Post-ictal, post-concussional states, and diabetic acidosis may resemble alcohol intoxication. The syndrome to be discussed next (Alcohol Idiosyncratic Intoxication) may not differ behaviorally from Alcoholic Intoxication.

D.   ALCOHOL IDIOSYNCRATIC INTOXICATION (DSM-III = 291.40)

    1.   Essential Features.
        This syndrome does not essentially differ from the preceding one except in one regard: the amount of alcohol ingested is insufficient to induce intoxication in most people. This idiosyncratic pathological reaction to alcohol usually becomes apparent early in life, and the individual ought to be apprised of his proclivity and the dangerous consequences despite the short-lived duration of the episodes. The most striking features are a marked behavioral change usually involving aggressive behavior which is atypical for the individual in the sober state and subsequent amnesia for the intoxicated period. It is not clear why some persons react so dramatically to small amounts of alcohol. In some, it may be a permanent condition possibly correlated with brain damage (e.g., EEG evidence of temporal lobe spiking or epilepsy, trauma, encephalitis). In others, it may be temporary and clearly related to additive or potentiated effects by simultaneous ingestion of tranquilizers or sedatives. Preexisting exhaustion, fasting, or debilitating medical illnesses may also contribute to this pathological Alcohol Intoxication.

E.   ALCOHOL WITHDRAWAL (DSM-III = 291.80)

    1.   Essential features.

        a. coarse tremor of hands, tongue, and eyelids several hours after cessation
        b. nausea and vomiting
        c. malaise, weakness, or dizziness
        d. autonomic hyperactivity:
            1) tachycardia, increased blood pressure, or orthostatic hypotension
            2) sweating, anxiety, irritability, depressed mood
            3) insomnia
        e. grand mal seizures about the third day, earlier or more likely in epileptics
        f. abstinence following heavy drinking for at least several days; it is important to bear in mind, however, that sometimes intercurrent medical problems (e.g., pneumonia, heart failure, malnutrition, subdural hematoma), fatigue, or depression may precipitate the onset of the Withdrawal Syndrome
        g. no delirium
        h. duration: 5-7 days; peak symptom intensity on second or third day

    2.   Associated features.

        a. gastritis, dry mouth
        b. dehydration or
        c. hyperhydration
        d. headache

e. puffy and blotchy complexion
f. mild peripheral edema
g. restless sleep, dreams, nightmares
h. acute anxiety attacks
i. brief unformed visual, auditory, or tactile hallucinations
j. neurological signs
   1) tendon hyperreflexia
   2) myoclonic muscular contractions
   3) spasmodic jerking of extremities
   4) bizarre movement patterns

The Alcoholic Withdrawal Syndrome may be mimicked by:

a. familial tremor
b. metabolic abnormalities (e.g., hypoglycemia, diabetic acidosis)
c. withdrawal from sedative-hypnotic drugs
d. barbiturate withdrawal (almost identical)

3. Treatment.

a. hospitalize
b. thorough physical and neurological examination
c. suspect dehydration only if there are nausea, vomiting, gastritis, and excessive sweating
d. verify and hydrate if necessary
e. avoid routine hydration otherwise, particularly if there are signs of peripheral edema, even if mild
f. take blood tests to determine presence of pancreatitis, infection, and degree of hydration; most alcoholics in withdrawal are overhydrated, even with a dry mouth
g. use diuretics to correct overhydration
h. monitor fluid balance
i. use sedatives (e.g., paraldehyde, chlordiazepoxide) which have cross tolerance with alcohol and cause only mild postural hypotension. Avoid hypotensive neuroleptics such as chlorpromazine and thioridazine. Use these sedatives conservatively to control withdrawal symptoms. Most alcoholics require 200-500 mg/day on the first day. Decrease dose by about 20% per day. Stop by the time the syndrome has cleared away - usually 5-7 days after beginning of treatment.
j. correct hypoglycemia if present, which sometimes may be a complication of Alcoholic Withdrawal and may mask and mimic the Alcohol Withdrawal Syndrome. Hypoglycemia is rare but may occur in individuals who have not eaten in several days.
k. inject thiamine 100 mg I.M. daily for at least one week. Add multiple vitamins in therapeutic, not mega-vitamin or massive doses.

F. ALCOHOL WITHDRAWAL DELIRIUM (DSM-III = 291.00)

1. Essential features.
As implied by the name, the induction of a syndrome of Delirium

within one week after cessation or reduction of heavy alcohol intake is the essential and predominant feature. There is also an autonomic component characterized by hyperactivity in the form of:

1) sweating
2) fever
3) tachycardia
4) elevated blood pressure
5) pupillary dilatation

2. Associated Features.

    a. Tremor is almost consistently present, hence the synonym Delirium Tremens (or DT's).

    b. Rapid fluctuations between the calmness of stupor and the agitation of hyperalertness; these correspond to the characteristic fluctuations in levels of awareness (see Delirium Syndrome).

    c. Hallucinations: typically visual, distressing, and frightening (e.g., rapidly moving small animals), but auditory, olfactory, and tactile modalities may be present.

    d. Stigmata of chronic alcohol abuse such as hepatomegaly, peripheral neuropathy, and cerebellar impairment. The typical case is an individual between 30 and 50 years of age and 5 to 15 years of heavy binge drinking who stopped or reduced drinking three days before he reached the peak of the syndrome and begins to improve by the 5th to 7th day of abstention. But there are many variants including the case of sweet unsuspected little granny who is admitted to the hospital for a routine check-up and develops DT's on the third day post-admission. Concomitant physical disorders predispose to the development of Alcohol Withdrawal with or without delirium. About 5% of patients treated for Alcohol Withdrawal develop the complications of added delirium. If delirium supervenes, the mortality rate due to such complications as hyperthermia or circulatory collapse may range from 4 to 20% depending on the reporting source.

3. Other medical complications.

    a. Respiratory: Pneumonitis, tuberculous infiltrate and cavitation, chronic obstructive pulmonary disease and cor pulmonale, tracheobronchitis, respiratory failure, hyperventilation and respiratory alkalosis.

    b. Gastrointestinal: Gastritis and peptic ulcer with hematemesis; hepatitis and cirrhosis with bleeding from esophageal varices; ascitis and peritonitis; pancreatitis with malabsorption syndrome leading to vitamin D deficiency; hypocalcemia and lowered seizure threshold; vitamin K deficiency and hemorrhage.

c. CNS: Cerebral laceration - epidural and subdural hematoma, cerebral edema, meningitis.

d. Systemic: Severe malnutrition, anemia, vitamin deficiencies (thiamine, D, C, K, folic acid), electrolyte deficiencies, hypoglycemia in the abstinent alcoholic, hyperglycemia in the acute or chronic pancreatitis patient, cardiac arrhythmias with shifts in body potassium, hypomagnasemia leading to weakness, lethargy, or lowered seizure threshold.

e. Iatrogenic: Overhydration and underhydration, oversedation, unnecessary use of diphenylhydantion causing folic acid depletion, unnecessary use of phenothiazines causing postural hypotension or peripheral collapse, overlooked prostatic hypertrophy or neglected Foley catheter causing urinary tract infection, neglect and infection of I.V. catheter.

This list of complications is not exhaustive but points out the major sources of trouble in the treatment of Delirium Tremens. It clearly suggests that generalizations in terms of treatment must be avoided, that each patient requires individualized corrective measures, that Delirium Tremens is a medical emergency, that treatment requires close liaison between internist and psychiatrist, and that certain measures must be taken immediately and consistently because the brain cannot wait.

G.   ALCOHOL HALLUCINOSIS (DSM-III = 291.30)

This is rarely seen in abstaining chronic alcoholics who have recovered from a syndrome of Alcohol Withdrawal with or without delirium. The onset is usually later than that of withdrawal or delirium (1-2 weeks). Duration may encompass weeks, months, or rarely may be longer. If the course is permanent, a differential diagnosis with Schizophrenia, which it resembles most closely, becomes difficult. In the two conditions, auditory hallucinations are the most frequent modality, and delusions may be present. As in Schizophrenia, the sensorium is clear.

H.   ALCOHOL AMNESTIC DISORDER OR KORSAKOFF'S SYNDROME (DSM-III = 291.10)

Short-term memory is impaired following protracted abuse of alcohol. Immediate memory is not impaired. Onset is usually seen after age 35, and it often follows a Withdrawal Syndrome with or without delirium or an acute episode of Wernicke's encephalopathy. Wernicke's is a well-identified neurological syndrome consisting of ataxia of cerebellar and polyneuropathy types, opthalmoplegia involving third and sixth cranial nerves, nystagmus due to damage of the vestibular nuclei, and mental symptoms. The mental symptoms of Wernicke's disease may be mild delirium, but more often take the form of global confusion, dullness, and apathy. Wernicke's disease may clear in a few days or weeks, particularly if it is promptly treated with parenteral thiamine. As Wernicke's disease ameliorates, a Korsakoff's Syndrome emerges usually as permanent sequelae. Usually if the Amnestic Syndrome is not too severe it appears in combination with confabulation or a maneuver to cover up the memory defect by making up stories or inventing pseudoinformation to fill in the memory gaps. When the Amnestic Syndrome is or becomes more severe it does not have the confabulatory component. It looks as if then the patient does not have enough cognitive machinery or resourcefulness to notice the difference or to care to cover up his deficiency. Impairment then is usually so severe that lifelong custodial care is often required. Some patients with Korsakoff's Syndrome do not appear to go through a stage of Wernicke's disease, but the association between the two syndromes is so close as to warrant the joint label Wernicke-Korsakoff Syndrome (W-K). The changing ocular, nystagmic, ataxic, and mental signs appear to be successive stages in the recovery or evaluation from a single disease process.

The responsiveness to thiamine varies for the different signs as follows:

1) Ocular muscle and conjugate gaze palsies - most responsive, within 2 hours to 2 weeks.
2) Horizontal nystagmus and ataxia - intermediate responsiveness, may be permanent even if in milder forms in about 50% of the patients.
3) Initial global confusion and apathy - good to intermediate responsiveness.
4) Memory defect - slow, least, and poorest responsiveness; incomplete recovery in almost 80% of cases.

The major neuropathological damage in the W-K syndrome consists of microscopic vacuolizations, looseness, and destruction primarily of myelinated fibers in the thalamic medial dorsal, anterior medial and pulvinar nuclei; in the mammillary bodies and periaqueductal region; in the floor of the fourth ventricle encompassing the dorsal motor nuclei of the vagus and vestibular nuclei, and the anterior lobe of the cerebellum, particularly the superior cortical vermis. The amnesia appears to be more related to lesions in the thalamic medial dorsal and perhaps pulvinar nuclei than to damage of the mammillary bodies.

The W-K Syndrome is primarily a malabsorptive nutritional disease of the chronic alcoholic patient. Alcohol displaces a variety of foods from the diet which causes deprivation of various vitamins, the most responsible for the syndrome being deficiency of thiamine. Polyneuropathy occurs in over 80% of patients with the W-K Syndrome, but a combination of several deficiencies of the B complex (pyridoxine and/or pantothenic acid or thiamine) is required to cause, in man, manifestations of polyneuropathy.

I.   DEMENTIA ASSOCIATED WITH ALCOHOLISM (DSM-III = 291.2x)

This category is reserved for the rare chronic alcoholics who are not intoxicated or in withdrawal, but exhibit a syndrome of Dementia which persists at least three weeks after cessation of alcohol use. Other manifestations and complications of alcoholism (i.e. cerebellar ataxia, polyneuropathy, cirrhosis) may be present.

****

GO TO VIDEOTAPE

****

J.   BARBITURATE OR SIMILARLY ACTING DRUGS

The next group of substances to be described includes all the barbiturates and similarly acting anxiolytics, sedatives, and hypnotics, even though there are many pharmacological differences between all these substances. They all have, however, one feature in common; that is their capability to cause not only intoxication, but also manifestations of withdrawal which are essentially the same for all the substances in this group. Four syndromes are listed by DSM-III under barbiturate or similarly acting sedatives or hypnotics. These are: Intoxication (305.40), Withdrawal (292.00), Withdrawal Delirium (292.00), and Amnestic Disorder (292.83). The essential and associated features of the four syndromes listed above are almost identical to those described for alcohol. It would, therefore, be unnecessarily repetitious to list them again. Instead, we will emphasize only the differences with alcohol. It should be relatively easy for you now to guess these differences if you remember the organic features associated with alcohol abuse.

The syndromes of intoxication by and withdrawal from barbiturates and related drugs may be serious, even fatal. Aggressive treatment is therefore important and must be conducted in the hospital. A multiple approach and the skills of an intensive care physician are often required. Acute intoxication and withdrawal usually occur independently, but occasionally develop in sequence. A Barbiturate Withdrawal Syndrome is always preceded by decrease or cessation of drug use, whether it is elective or imposed by other circumstances.

1.   Treatment of Acute Barbiturate Intoxication.
Acute Barbiturate Intoxication follows ingestion of an overdose, whether with suicidal intent or accidentally. Severe intoxication in the nonaddicted individual is usually produced by ingestion of 200 to 1000 mg of pentobarbital. A dose slightly higher (1000-1500 mg) is usually fatal. Barbiturates per se do not cause neurological damage if ensuing hypoxia and shock are prevented by adequate supportive measures. In the mildly intoxicated individual who responds to inhalation of 10% CO_2 or to painful pressure to the sternum or supraorbital ridge with an increase in rate and depth of respiration, only symptomatic treatment (i.e., coffee, parenteral caffeine sodium benzoate) and particularly close observation for the possibility of development of signs of deepening coma are indicated. The main complications are: a) respiratory depression leading to cyanosis, shock, and prolonged coma; b) pneumonia; and c) bladder infection. Patients with respiratory insufficiency require immediate endotracheal intubation, suctioning, respiratory assistance, and frequent turning from side to side. Prompt removal of unabsorbed drug from the

gastrointestinal tract is very important in order to prevent deepening coma. Emesis should only be attempted in the fully alert patient and gastric lavage only after insertion of a cuffed endotracheal tube to prevent aspiration of gastric contents. If bowel sounds can be heard after evacuation of the stomach, osmotic cathartics (i.e., sorbital, activated charcoal) can then be administered. If signs of severe respiratory depression (i.e., cyanosis, mydriasis, hypotension, deepening coma) or very high plasma levels of barbiturate are obtained, these are clear features of a serious medical emergency which must be treated vigorously by a skillful intensive care physician. The chief goals then will be correction of hypoxia, hypotension, and removal of already absorbed barbiturate from the body. The hypoxia is usually treated by means of an intermittent positive-pressure respirator in conjunction with judicious use of oxygen and close monitoring of arterial blood gases. The hypotension will usually improve as the state of hypoxia reverses. Additional measures such as elevation of the foot of the bed are helpful. Volume-expanding solutions, whole blood, or plasma may be necessary. But administration of norepinephrine or dopamine is rarely needed. Removal of already absorbed barbiturate may be required if the patient fails to improve in response to all the preceding measures, or if the barbiturate plasma levels remain high. Impaired renal or cardiac function contraindicates forced diuresis to aid in barbiturate removal. Renal or hepatic insufficiency in patients in severe shock or prolonged coma who do not respond to other measures and have ingested lethal amounts or show high plasma levels of barbiturate are requirements for consideration of hemodialysis or peritoneal dialysis. These and forced diuresis are roughly equivalent in effectiveness. Alkalinization of the urine (one standard ampule or 44 mEq of $NaHCO_3$ into each liter of I.V. fluids) combined with 10-20 mEq KCL by the same route has become very popular in recent years in acute phenobarbital intoxication, but is considered to be a poor approach to remove short-acting barbiturates. Hemodialysis is also more effective against the long- and intermediate-acting than the short-acting barbiturates.

A word of caution is appropriate about plasma levels of the offending agent. They are helpful but insufficient in guiding treatment because the drug plasma level may not correlate with the clinical status. Frequent contaminants of this correlation are:

1) Mixed ingestions, particularly alcohol
2) Tolerant, chronically addicted patients
3) Intoxicated patient who is given parenteral caffeine sodium benzoate

Therefore, use Table 5-9, which follows, with caution as a general guide.

TABLE 5-9

POTENTIALLY FATAL SERUM LEVEL OF BARBITURATES AND RELATED DRUGS

Drug	$(\mu g/ml)$
Barbiturates	
Short-acting	≥ 35
Pentobarbital	
Secobarbital	
Long-acting	100-120
Barbital	
Phenobarbital	
Methaqualone	8
Glutethimide	20
Methyprylon	40
Meprobamate	100
Ethchlorvynol	100

The similarities of therapeutic and toxic action between the drugs in Table 5-9 are more impressive than the differences. Some of the distinguishing features may be clinically useful, however, in case of intoxication:

1) Alcohol: Flushed face
   Suffused conjunctivae
2) Glutethimide: Fluctuating course
   Paralytic ileus
   Dilated pupils
   Tachycardia
   Laryngeal spasms
   Sudden apnea
3) Chloral hydrate: May produce constricted pupils
4) Ethchlorvynol: Characteristic odor of body fluids

2. Treatment of Chronic Barbiturate Intoxication (Barbiturate Addiction) and of Barbiturate Withdrawal.

The treatment of barbiturate addiction consists of a systematic step-wise withdrawal of the barbiturate without causing the signs and symptoms of abrupt barbiturate cessation which may be fatal. The first step, therefore, is the determination of the daily dose of barbiturate to which the patient is addicted. This information can be obtained from the history (if reliable) or estimated from the effects of the so-called "test dose" of 200 mg of pentobarbital. The test dose procedure is based on the generally verifiable assumption that in a normal, nonaddicted person it usually induces sleep from which he can be aroused. On the contrary, a person who, through chronic abuse, has developed tolerance to, and dependence on, the barbiturate may experience nothing, or mild, or moderate intoxication following the test dose. It is generally agreed that:

1) No effect means addiction of about 5-6 times the test dose (= 1000-2000 mg daily).

2) Mild effect such as fine lateral nystagmus means addiction of about four times the test dose (=800 mg daily).

3) Moderate effect such as drowsiness, ataxia, slurred speech, and coarse lateral nystagmus means that the individual is addicted to about 2-3 times the test dose (=400-600 mg daily).

This test is crude and should not be rigidly adhered to the disregard of all else. For example, if the patient under test is already intoxicated or suffering from the Withdrawal Syndrome, the test results obviously may be disastrous or cannot be valid. These possibilities alone drastically reduce the usefulness of the test.

Once the addicting dose has been determined, it is given in equally divided doses every 4-6 hours for 24 hours. The step-wise, systematic but flexible withdrawal begins by decreasing the total daily dose by 10% each successive day. As stated above, flexibility will require a decrease of 5% instead of 10% should increasing signs of abstinence emerge. There are many variants of this procedure, but they are all based on the same general assumption. For example, withdrawal may be conducted with phenobarbital instead of pentobarbital if one uses a substitution ratio of 30 mg of phenobarbital for each 100 mg of pentobarbital. Other useful equivalences of 200 mg pentobarbital are: 3-4 ounces of whiskey, 400 mg of meprobamate, 500 mg of glutethimide.

QUIZ, Section IV, A-J.

Circle the letter corresponding to the <u>one</u> correct response.

A 19-year-old ingests an unknown but substantial amount of amphetamine. Within a few hours a syndrome emerges which is characterized by severe inattention, shifting levels of consciousness, disturbances in memory and orientation, insomnia, tactile hallucinations, and increased psychomotor activity. There is also pupillary dilatation and anorexia.

1. According to DSM-III, the diagnosis should be

    a. Amphetamine Intoxication.
    b. Amphetamine Hallucinosis.
    c. Amphetamine Delirium.
    d. Amphetamine Dementia.

2. If the 19-year-old individual in the question above exhibits the following behaviors: psychomotor excitement, resistance to fatigue, lack of sleepiness that night, exhaustion, and failure to show up for work the following morning; there is tachycardia and chills; no cognitive deficits. The diagnosis then would have been

    a. Amphetamine Intoxication.
    b. Amphetamine Hallucinosis.
    c. Amphetamine Delirium.
    d. Amphetamine Dementia.

3. The distinguishing features of glutethimide intoxication suggest

    a. cholinergic action.
    b. hypoglycemia action.
    c. anticholinergic action.
    d. bone marrow depression.

4. Any patient sufficiently recovered from an intentionally suicidal overdose of barbiturates or related drugs

    a. should be left alone unless he tries again.
    b. can be discharged since most overdose patients are hysterical and inconsequential.
    c. should have a thorough psychiatric evaluation since many are depressed, very angry, or frustrated.
    d. should receive pharmacological education because most overdose patients are only confused and can be conceptualized as involuntary suicides.

Circle the correct answer(s). One or more than one answer may be correct.

5. The treatment outlined for alcohol withdrawal maximizes your chances of guarding against

    a. withdrawal grand mal seizures.
    b. full blown Delirium Tremens.
    c. high mortality rate.
    d. chronic alcohol dependence.

6. Select two correct answers.

    a. Korsakoff's is a chronic disease.
    b. Korsakoff's is an acute disease.
    c. Wernicke's is more treatable than Korsakoff's.
    d. Wernicke's is less treatable than Korsakoff's.

Match the following syndromes with the corresponding levels of severity.

___7.	Alcohol Idiosyncratic Intoxication	a. least severe, nonlethal
___8.	Alcohol Withdrawal	b. moderately severe
___9.	Alcohol Withdrawal Delirium (Delirium Tremens)	c. most severe, potentially lethal

Match the sites of lesions with their deficits.

___10. vestibular nuclei
___11. third and sixth cranial nerve nuclei
___12. superior cortical vermis

a. horizontal nystagmus
b. ataxia
c. ocular palsies and disconjugate gaze

Match the descriptions below with the most appropriate lettered diagnosis.

___13. flaccid coma with reactive pupils, hypothermia, and hypotension
___14. flaccid coma with dilated fixed pupils, hypothermia, hypotension, laryngeal spasms, sudden apnea, high mortality
___15. blood barbiturate level of 20μg/ml, short coma
___16. blood barbiturate level of 115 μg/ml, prolonged coma, high mortality
___17. flushed face, injected conjunctivae, verbose, cantankerous, aggressive

a. secobarbital or pentobarbital poisoning
b. phenobarbital intoxication
c. severe glutethimide intoxication
d. Barbiturate Intoxication
e. Alcohol Intoxication

K.   OPIOID INTOXICATION (DSM-III = 305.50)

The Opioid Organic Mental Disorders are caused by a group of naturally occurring and synthetic narcotic analgesics with morphine-like action. The pain relief induced by narcotics may be partly due to blunting of the affective component usually concomitant with pain. Morphine is the prototype of these agents, although not the most frequently abused or responsible for Intoxication and Withdrawal Syndromes. Agents in this group are shown in Table 5-10 below:

TABLE 5-10

RELATIVE ADDICTIVE ABILITIES OF NARCOTICS

Narcotic Agent	Addictiveness
Pentazocine (Talwin)	Low
Propoxyphene (Darvon)	Low
Codeine (Methylmorphine)	Medium
Meperidine (Demerol)	High
Morphine	High
Heroin	High
Methadone (Dolophine)	High
Hydromorphine (Dilaudid)	High
Oxycodone (Percodan)	High
Levorphanol (Levo-Dromoran)	High

The two most frequently abused narcotics are heroin and methadone. The high incidence of addiction to these agents is also responsible for their deliberate (suicidal) or accidental induction of acute poisoning. Accidental intoxication may be due to errors in calculation of dose, naivete about narcotics, ignorance about the potency of the sample supplied, murderous intent on the part of drug pushers, unusual sensitivity to the drug, or loss of tolerance to previously acquired tolerance levels following a period of withdrawal. The mildest manifestations of acute intoxication include sedation, relief of anxiety, analgesia, euphoria, or dysphoria. With dysphoria there may be nausea, vomiting, and anorexia. An inhibitory effect of the drug on gastrointestinal motility may cause constipation. Apathy, psychomotor retardation, and loss of sexual interest are frequent. The mental status examination at this stage will reveal drowsiness, slurred speech, and impaired attention and memory. Maladaptive behavioral manifestations often appear in the form of impaired judgement, interference with social or occupational functioning, and failure to meet responsibilities. Moderate severeness of intoxication is manifested by varying degrees of unresponsiveness, depressed consciousness, depressed respiration (i.e., slow rate, periodic pattern), bradycardia, hypotension, pulmonary congestion, hypothermia, and miosis. Pinpoint pupils may cause reduced visual acuity. In the most severe cases pulmonary edema, cyanosis of the skin and mucosae, circulatory failure, and pupillary dilatation due to anoxia will supervene. Complications at this stage are shock, coma, cardiorespiratory arrest, or even death. Survival in these cases may be accompanied by anoxic encephalopathy or hemiplegia.

1. Associated Features.
    A characteristic "rush" sensation localized in the abdominal region which addicts compare to a sexual orgasm is often experienced concomitantly with the bolus injection of the "fix." This may be followed later by itching sensation and flushing of the skin. Old and fresh needle marks are often apparent all along the veins among "mainliners." The injection of crude adulterants (quinine, sugar, flour, powdered milk, etc.) and contaminants in unsterile needles are often responsible for infectious complications (i.e., abscess, cellulitis, septic thrombophlebitis, hepatitis, periarteritis). Quinine adulteration of heroin has been thought to be responsible for amblyopia. Other neurological complications include: a) transverse myelopathy causing paraplegia with a sensory level of deficit in the trunk whose pathogenesis is obscure; b) peripheral neuropathies usually due to damage at injection sites, compression during coma, or prolonged sitting while "stoned" in the lotus position; and c) acute generalized myopathy and myoglobinuria with renal failure may follow intravenous injection of adulterated heroin, or circumscribed myopathy with brawny edema (Volkmann's contracture) may follow subcutaneous and intramuscular injections.

2. Differential Diagnosis.
    The differential diagnosis of Opioid Intoxication includes:
    a. Other causes of coma in severe overdose
    b. Barbiturates and alcohol (no miosis)
    c. Cocaine, amphetamines, hallucinogens (pupillary dilatation without cyanosis)

3. Treatment.
   Treatment of acute Opioid Intoxication includes:
   a. Hospitalize and support or restore circulation and respiration.
   b. Prevent aspiration of vomitus.
   c. Insert cuffed endotracheal tube if necessary, always if the patient is comatose or gastric lavage is contemplated.
   d. Start an intravenous route and proceed with blood determinations; then inject a 50% glucose solution which will rule out hypoglycemic coma and will not hurt.
   e. Gastric lavage if the drug was ingested; opiates cause severe pylorospasm and lavage, therefore, may be effective many hours after ingestion.
   f. If no response is obtained to lavage or if route of overdose was parenteral, use an opioid antagonist. Naloxone hydrochloride (Narcan®) is the antagonist of choice to induce reversal of respiratory depression. The usual dose ranges from 0.4 to 1.2 mg I.V., but higher doses may be required, or the usual dose may have to be repeated several times during the first day to antagonize long-acting narcotics such as methadone. A therapeutic response to naloxone is manifested by prompt reversal of respiratory depression, improvement of the level of consciousness, and decreased miosis or normalization of pupillary size. If the chosen dose is ineffective, it should be repeated at five minute intervals. If still no improvement is observed, assume that other causes of respiratory depression are at work (i.e., drugs other than narcotics, trauma, etc.). Thus, this very rewarding response within minutes is also of tremendous diagnostic value since it is specific for intoxication by opioid and synthetic analgesics only. Following an adequate respiratory response to naloxone, observation for 24 hours or over is still necessary because the offending narcotic may be long-acting (e.g., methadone: 24-28 hours) and the action of naloxone lasts only from 30 minutes to two hours. Relapse into respiratory depression and coma can be prevented by further doses of naloxone given intramuscularly at regular intervals and at doses 50% higher than those found effective earlier by the intravenous route. There is no risk of aggravating respiratory depression by excessive use of naloxone because this drug is a pure opioid antagonist without agonistic action. There is the risk, however, that excessive naloxone administration may induce a severe withdrawal syndrome in a chronically addicted individual who has overdosed. Since this is most often the case, such possibility must always be kept in mind. Therefore, naloxone therapy must always be individualized.

L. OPIOID WITHDRAWAL (DSM-III = 292.00)

This is a characteristic syndrome of drug-seeking behavior, lacrimation, rhinorrhea, pupillary dilatation, piloerection (cold turkey skin), sweating, nausea, vomiting, diarrhea, yawning, increased blood pressure, tachycardia, tachypnea, fever, tremor, anorexia, irritability, weakness, abdominal cramps, involuntary muscle spasms, weight loss, orgasms, and insomnia, following recent cessation or reduction of opioid administration in a chronically addicted individual. The duration of addiction varies with the narcotic. It may be 7-10 days for morphine. The time of onset after cessation and course also depends on the agent. The onset of morphine or heroin withdrawal occurs within 6-8 hours from the previous dose, reaches a peak on the second or third day, and disappears in 7-10 days. The withdrawal syndrome from meperidine begins more quickly, reaches a peak 24 hours earlier than for morphine, and is over within 4-5 days. Methadone withdrawal may not begin for 1-3 days, and the course may be mild. Although methadone withdrawal typically ends by the 10-14th day, it may last up to three weeks or even more. Table 5-11 below summarizes these features of typical withdrawal syndromes.

TABLE 5-11

A SUMMARY OF FEATURES OF TYPICAL WITHDRAWAL SYNDROMES

Narcotic Agent	Duration of Action	Onset (hours)	Peak (hours)	Resolution (days)
Meperidine	Short	3-4	8-12	4-5
Morphine and heroin	Medium	6-16	48-72	7-10
Methadone	Long	24-72	72 or >	10-21 or >

1. Differential Diagnosis.
   The diagnosis of Opioid Withdrawal is based on the history, drug-seeking and craving behaviors, blood and urine tests (heroin is excreted in the urine as morphine), needle tracks, and the clinical manifestations listed earlier. But none of these inquiries provides incontrovertible evidence of addiction or withdrawal with the very resourceful and unreliable narcotic user who may not be suffering from withdrawal and is just seeking a "fix" from the physician. Third party confirmation may be valuable but not necessarily always reliable. A positive urine test only means that the drug has been consumed within the last 24 hours but not necessarily that the individual is physiologically dependent on the drug. If there is no

physical dependence, there can be no withdrawal syndrome. It is very important to arrive at a certain diagnosis of physical addiction because institution of treatment in a nondependent individual would be unfortunate. Although the narcotic withdrawal syndrome is very unpleasant, contrary to that from barbiturates, it is not fatal. The most reliable way to ascertain signs of abstinence is by precipitating or exacerbating them by means of naloxone. This antagonist should be injected only with the permission of the patient in the presence of another professional. A slow intravenous injection of 0.4 mg is started and stopped when a cholinergic response is obtained (pupillary dilatation, tachypnea, lacrimation, rhinorrhea, sweating, yawning). A second injection may be given 5-10 minutes later if no response to the first was obtained. Failure of the second injection to obtain the suspected response or to obtain signs of abstinence rules out physical dependence upon opiates and therefore also withdrawal. The naloxone precipitated withdrawal will evolve very rapidly (onset at 5, peak at 20, decline at 60, and resolution at 180 minutes or 3 hours). Naloxone does not precipitate abstinence symptoms in individuals physically dependent upon meperidine unless the daily dose exceeds 1600 mg. Addiction to and withdrawal from meperidine are frequent among physicians and nurses. Another unique feature of meperidine withdrawal is its propensity to course with seizures. These are unusual in abstinence from other narcotics.

2. Management of Opioid Dependence and Withdrawal.
    The ideal approach to the problem of opioid dependence is avoidance or prevention. This entails the application of complex measures geared toward influencing the psychological, emotional, and socio-economic orientation of prone individuals. They are discussed in detail in the following section entitled Substance Use Disorders. The emphasis here will be on the medical and pharmacological management of the Organic Mental Disorders caused by the dependence and withdrawal syndromes. The general view is that individuals who are physically dependent on opioids are in a state of chronic intoxication which they have reached through the development of tolerance and gradually increasing requirements of the opioid to experience euphoria, relief from pain, or blunting of the discomforts of mild or more severe withdrawal manifestations. Another general, if not unanimous, view is that such individuals should be encouraged or sometimes coerced to wean themselves from the dependence. The most popular approach is to substitute one opioid, methadone, for the abused drug. This procedure has been carefully controlled by federal regulations since 1972. Physicians are not free to prescribe methadone or any other opioid for an addict merely in order to prevent withdrawal manifestations. On an outpatient basis, this can only be done legally with a special license and within the setting of a federally authorized methadone program. The method used now almost exclusively consists of substituting methadone according to the following ratio:

    1 mg methadone for 1 mg heroin
                        3 mg morphine
                       20 mg meperidine
                       30 mg codeine

Usually, however, 40 mg of methadone daily in two equal oral doses is sufficient as a starting dose to prevent violent withdrawal. The patient is stabilized at this dose for 3-5 days and then rapidly reduced and withdrawn over the next 3-5 days. The most uncomfortable and painful effects of "cold turkey" withdrawal are those of cholinergic nature.

Propoxyphene napsylate (Darvon N®) may be used to prevent distressing or painful withdrawal reaction instead of methadone. There are no federal restrictions or penalties against the use of propoxyphene for this purpose. Propoxyphene has considerable cross-tolerance with the opiates. Indeed, its chemical configuration remarkably resembles that of methadone. Some well-motivated addicts may prefer propoxyphene to methadone because it is easier to "kick" this habit. However, a recently released FDA Drug Bulletin draws attention to the growing incidence of fatalities due to propoxyphene. This product has become a widely used prescription analgesic. It is estimated that it is the most frequently prescribed, with over 30 million prescriptions written in 1978. A major hazard associated with propoxyphene use is death. Propoxyphene alone or in combination with other substances has been associated with an estimated one to two thousand deaths per year. The majority of these appear to be suicides; these estimates make propoxyphene rank second only to the barbiturates as the leading prescription drug associated with drug fatalities. Some of these deaths occur among drug abusers who try to get a "high" with propoxyphene in high doses. Others are not habitual drug abusers but use propoxyphene in conjunction with other CNS depressants without an understanding of the dangers of drug interactions.

Propoxyphene, if taken for a protracted period of time in daily doses of 500-800 mg (hydrochloride) or 800-1200 mg (napsylate salt), produces morphine-type physical dependence. The usual cause of death due to propoxyphene overdose is respiratory depression, although cardiac toxicity due to nor-propoxyphene, the major metabolite, may be a contributing factor. The FDA's current claim is that propoxyphene in the usual dose of 32-65 mg is approximately two-thirds as potent as codeine and no more effective analgesically than the usual doses of aspirin or acetaminophen. In view of all these considerations, the FDA is currently reevaluating propoxyphene and the determination may well be withdrawal of the drug from the market.

The short-term prognosis for remaining abstinent from heroin after methadone has been completely discontinued is very poor because most patients in their younger years revert to opioids within weeks. The long-term prognosis, however, may not be as discouraging because this opioid proclivity seems to "burn out" with age in some individuals.

During the last two decades heroin addiction and methadone substitution have become widespread. Thus many individuals may require surgery while they are on methadone maintenance. In such cases the methadone schedule ought to be continued, with the last dose administered shortly before the anesthetic is given. Surgical problems, medical illness, or acute infection may increase opiate tolerance and the severity of withdrawal symptoms, in which case higher initial doses of methadone and a longer period of withdrawal may be necessary. If vomiting, which is a sign of the withdrawal syndrome, becomes distressing or debilitating, trimethobenzamide (Tigan®) or hydroxyzine (Vistaril®) may be given to correct it if increasing the dose of methadone to prevent withdrawal symptoms is contraindicated. If there is concurrent depression, doxepin administration may be indicated.

M.   COCAINE INTOXICATION (DSM-III = 305.60)

This is the only syndrome of importance caused by cocaine because cocaine produces little, if any, physical dependence; therefore, cocaine withdrawal symptomatology is not seen. Thus, it is usually safe to withdraw the patient immediately from cocaine. Cocaine is usually taken subcutaneously or by sniffing the crystalline flakes or powder. Chronic sniffing may cause perforation of the nasal septum, a sign to look for in an individual suspected of cocainism. Intravenous administration is often preferred by heroin mainliners. This mixture of cocaine and heroin is called "speedball." By this route, the effects are most intense (characteristic "rush"), but brief (minutes). The user experiences well-being and a sense of confidence.

1.   Features.
     The features of cocaine intoxication vary with the premorbid personality, state of physical health, environment, number and amount of other drugs mixed with cocaine, route of administration, and dose. The essential features can be classified into physical, psychological, and maladaptive behaviors. Physical signs are: tachycardia, increased blood pressure, pupillary dilatation, perspiration or chills, hyperthermia, nausea, vomiting, decreased appetite or anorexia, decreased sleep or insomnia, tremulousness, convulsive fits, itching, picking. Excoriation and pallor of the skin may occur as well as pallor of the nasal mucosa (nasal septum perforation). The patient may present a haggard look and veins show needle marks.

     Psychological manifestations are: first psychomotor excitement, elation, euphoria, grandiosity, loquacity, sense of well-being and confidence, feelings of immunity to fatigue and great muscle power, heightened awareness of sensory input; these are followed by loose associations, paranoid ideation, restlessness, pacing about, vivid auditory and visual hallucinations often frightening, haptic or tactile hallucinations of small animals crawling on or under the skin (formication, from formica = ant), illusions, dream-like twilight states, broodiness, irritability, and apprehension.

Maladaptive behaviors are often forced by paranoid ideation, or by frightening hallucinations, or a strong desire to take more cocaine one hour or longer after the euphoria has passed and the individual feels the "crashing" aftermath of anxiety, tremulousness, irritability, fatigue, lethargy and depression. Under such pressures, violent or assaultive behavior may emerge and impaired judgement and failure to meet responsibilities may be exhibited.

Other associated features may include confusion, rambling or incoherent speech, and even convulsions, respiratory failure and coma if the intoxication is sufficiently severe. Characteristically, however, the sensorium remains clear.

The course of the kaleidoscopic manifestations listed above is self-limited and brief because the stimulating effects may wear off within one hour. Cocaine has a very short half-life due to its rapid metabolism by the liver. Full recovery usually takes place within 24 hours.

Complications may occur in cases of poor physical health or massive intravenous doses. Chest pain, cardiac arrhythmia, syncope, convulsion of a temporal lobe seizure pattern, delirium, respiratory paralysis, coma, and death have been reported.

2. Differential Diagnosis.
The diagnosis of Cocaine Intoxication must be made on the basis of the history and the clinical manifestations listed above. Attempts to determine cocaine or its metabolites in urine are often of little consequence six hours or more after usage, due to its rapid metabolism. This syndrome must be differentiated from other drug intoxications, particularly those caused by amphetamines and related sympathomimetics which mimic cocaine action, but are of longer duration than cocaine. The onset of manifestations is also earlier with cocaine than with amphetamines. Many other disorders (anxiety, affective, Schizophrenia, epilepsy, and Alcohol Delirium Tremens) pose questions of differential diagnosis.

The student should note that although cocaine can induce hallucinations, delusions, depression, and delirium along with other manifestations (see above), DSM-III provides a single category of intoxication under this substance and makes no provisions for syndromes of hallucinosis, delusional, affective, or delirious disturbances. The reason for this is that these specific manifestations in Cocaine Intoxication are always transient and do not extend beyond the time of direct substance effect.

Appreciation of the immediate onset and short duration of manifestations in Cocaine Intoxication is the best way to distinguish it clinically from acute Amphetamine Intoxication which is otherwise identical in terms of signs and symptoms. The persistence of disturbances beyond the time of direct amphetamine action furthermore explains in part why in DSM-III there are four different syndromes under amphetamines and similarly acting sympathomimetics. There are many names to become acquainted with that "speed freaks" use to refer to some of these amphetamine-like substances (e.g., bennies, bombitas, crank, crystal, dexies, splash, speed, uppers).

Rather than repeating most of the clinical manifestations listed under Cocaine Intoxication, which also apply to the four amphetamine syndromes, only the defining features of each one of these syndromes will be emphasized.

N.   AMPHETAMINE INTOXICATION (DSM-III = 305.70)

The manifestations of this syndrome are identical to those caused by cocaine. Corroboration of this diagnosis may be provided by urine tests for amphetamines. Delusions and hallucinations may persist beyond the time of direct substance effect. In that case, the diagnosis is changed to Amphetamine Delusional Syndrome.

O.   AMPHETAMINE DELIRIUM (DSM-III = 292.81)

This is a delirious syndrome occurring within 24 hours of intake of an amphetamine. The onset is usually seen within one hour, and the episode is usually over in about six hours, but it may last up to 24 hours. Intravenously, it may be induced almost immediately. In any case, the delirium disappears when other pharmacological effects wear off. Delirium is not as common as intoxication. Obviously delirium implies a greater impairment than intoxication. There is no cognitive impairment in intoxication. Indeed clouding of consciousness, disorientation, and attention and memory impairment are typical in any delirium and, therefore, should be present in Amphetamine Delirium but are typically absent in Amphetamine Intoxication. Rarely the delirium follows a period of intoxication.

P.   AMPHETAMINE DELUSIONAL DISORDER (DSM-III = 292.11)

This is more common than delirium. The essential feature is development of an Organic Delusional Syndrome triggered by a recent dose of amphetamine in a long-term abuser. It is felt that this syndrome does not follow a single, even if large, dose unless preceded by chronic abuse. Although the syndrome develops rapidly, the paranoid delusions, which are the characteristic ingredient, may persist and linger for a week or longer after cessation of amphetamine intake and therefore beyond the time of direct substance effect. Thus, although the serum half-life is several days, these toxic symptoms may persist sometimes for over a year. There may be tactile or visual hallucination of bugs or vermin crawling on or under the skin similar to those of Cocaine Intoxication. These are often accompanied by itching, scratching, and skin excoriations. No syndrome of amphetamine hallucinosis is available in DSM-III. The paranoid ideation with delusions of persecution and auditory hallucinations often overshadow and outlast the other types of hallucinations. When voices convey derogatory comments, criticisms, threats, and accusations or command the patient to commit violent acts, hospitalization is often required. Assaultive behavior may be precipitated by such experiences.

Q. AMPHETAMINE WITHDRAWAL (DSM-III = 292.00)

This is clearly an unfortunate choice of terms by the DSM-III Task Force because true physical dependence in the sense of barbiturates, opioids, or alcohol ("BOA") does not follow chronic abuse of amphetamines. The term withdrawal should have been reserved for the "BOA" group. Some kind of loosely defined withdrawal syndrome does follow cessation or reduction of amphetamine abuse, but it would have been less confusing to call it an after-effect of amphetamine abuse. These physical sequelae are presumably due to the extrusion and depletion of brain catecholamines. Characteristically, this syndrome always involves a depressed mood, pronounced fatigue, apathy, and flattening of affect, which are often more severe than in the depressions of Affective Disorders and capable of leading to suicide. This depression is grossly equivalent to the "crashing" following Cocaine Intoxication. Another characteristic of this syndrome is hypersomnia. The patient spends increasing amounts of time in sleep, sometimes 18 to 20 hours daily for up to three days. The sleep is mostly of rapid eye movement or REM stage. This increase in percentage of REM or dream sleep represents a rebound phenomenon following the REM suppression caused by the amphetamine. The hypersomnia begins within a day of cessation or reduction of substance abuse and may last for weeks. The depression sets in somewhat later, reaches a peak at 2-4 days after cessation of amphetamines, or may increase over the next two weeks. The depression may often persist for months if it is not treated. Depressive features for more than several weeks call for differential diagnostic work-up.

These patients should be hospitalized because they often develop bizarre delusions, suspiciousness, overwhelming fear of threats or of being watched and followed. Their hallucinations are integrated into their delusions of persecution, and they often arm themselves in response and defense against imagined persecutors. Rapid improvement usually follows hospitalization. Acute toxic syndromes clear between 12 and 36 hours later. But agitation, acute psychosis, and violence may require protection, restraint, and sedation. This is best accomplished with reassurance in a quiet room. Diazepam 10-20 mg orally or intramuscularly may be helpful. If antipsychotics are required for acute psychosis or severe agitation, chlorpromazine 50-100 mg orally or intramuscularly may be given initially and every 30 minutes if needed, and later every 4-6 hours prn. Chlorpromazine should not be given in smaller doses because it may paradoxically potentiate the effects of the amphetamine. Chlorpromazine is contraindicated if anticholinergic agents are partly responsible for the syndrome. Haloperidol 2.5-5 mg orally or intramuscularly tid may be given instead of chlorpromazine. Antipsychotics are specific antidotes of amphetamines, presumably due to their central antiadrenergic and antidopaminergic properties. Antipsychotics are usually not required beyond the first few days.

There is no need to taper the amphetamines. Indeed, they should be discontinued immediately, and the patient should be watched closely for the possibility of surreptitious consumption of the drug while in the hospital. Unabsorbed drug should be removed by means of emesis, lavage, and catharsis. These measures should be beneficial even several hours after ingestion. Absorbed drug in cases of severe intoxication can be eliminated more rapidly by acidifying the urine with NH_4Cl orally or intravenously. The dose may range from 4 to 16 gm daily. Urine pH must be monitored and kept at 4-5. NH_4Cl is contraindicated if there is shock, systemic acidosis, hepatic failure, or portosystemic shunting.

Hyperpyrexia is best treated by physical manipulation (i.e., cooling blanket, tepid water-wet towels vigorously applied to the skin), rather than by antipyretics.

Moderate hypertension will respond favorably to chlorpromazine, whereas severe hypertension requires use of alpha-adrenergic blocking agents such as phentolamine (Regitine®). Nitrites may also be effective.

Hypersomnia should be allowed to run its course with close observation and maintenance of hydration and nutrition. The degree of malnutrition and sleeplessness that preceded the acute episode contributes significantly to the severity of the syndrome.

The depression and delusions may exhibit the longest endurance and may require tricyclic antidepressants or antipsychotics for 1-2 months or longer. Exploratory psychotherapy or group therapy with other "speed freaks" should be considered once the acute episode is under control.

R.   HALLUCINOGEN MENTAL DISORDERS

The Hallucinogen Organic Mental Disorders are caused by two types of substances with primary hallucinogenic properties. These agents are related to either 5-hydroxy-tryptamine (i.e., lysergic acid diethylamine or LSD, dimethyltryptamine or DMT, diethyl-tryptamine or DET, psilocybin) or to phenyl-ethylamine (i.e., mescaline or peyote). Note that many other substances capable of causing hallucinations (i.e., phencyclidine, marijuana, Jimson seed, etc.) are not included in this group of hallucinogens. Marijuana is the subject of the next section (see p. 218), and its identity as a hallucinogen is unsettled. Indeed, its adverse reactions are less frequent and less dramatic. Phencyclidine (PCP, Sernyl or angel's dust) causes pure hallucinosis very rarely. Jimson seed is a new hallucinogen on the horizon which pertains to the belladonna alkaloids and as such, has powerful anticholinergic properties which lead to delirium. Both phencyclidine and Jimson seed, as well as many other new euphorohallucinogens and psychotogens, will have to be categorized under the last heading of substance-induced Organic Mental Disorders called "Other or Unspecified Substance."

1.   Essential Features.
     Those hallucinogens that we are considering here are usually taken orally. Their effects are comparable and difficult to distinguish. The essential features are characteristic perceptual changes, often involving subjective intensification of percepts, depersonalization, derealization, illusions, hallucinations, or synesthesias (i.e., smells have color, fingertips can hear). The illusions often involve

distortions of the patient's body image. The hallucinations, sometimes called pseudohallucinations, are usually visual and of geometric patterns which the user knows are unreal. Auditory hallucinations are rare, despite the presence of hyperattention and hyperacusis. Consciousness remains clear, despite the presence of confusion, difficulty in expressing thoughts, and distortions of the sense of time (events happen more slowly).

Physical concomitants include pupillary dilation, tachycardia, palpitations, sweating, blurred vision, tremors or incoordination. There is a slight rise in body temperature and blood pressure, but in contrast to cocaine and amphetamines, severe hyperthermia and hypertension are usually not observed.

Frequently, with low doses of the offending agent, the perceptual changes do not include hallucinations. But DSM-III chooses to call the syndrome described above, with or without hallucinations, Hallucinogen Hallucinosis (305.30) if the syndrome follows recent ingestion of the hallucinogen, if the patient realizes that all the perceptual changes are due to the effects of the hallucinogen, even if, more rarely, the patient is convinced that he has irretrievably lost his sanity, and even though the patient may exhibit ideas of reference and paranoid ideation.

The Hallucinogen Delusional Disorder (292.11) and the Affective Disorder (292.84) are viewed by DSM-III as more rare and emerging sometimes as complications of hallucinosis and other times as syndromes that persist beyond the period of direct effect of the hallucinogen. If the patient reaches the delusional conviction that the perceptual and thought disturbances, described above, correspond to reality, it is called Delusional Syndrome. If depression, elation, or anxiety dominate the clinical picture, it is called Affective Syndrome for as long as preoccupation with thoughts and fears of irreparable brain destruction, going crazy, etc., do not have the conviction that would make them delusional. Thus, a prerequisite for this diagnosis, Affective Syndrome, is absence of delusions. Note: If you, the student, feel that we are splitting hairs too thinly, you are not alone.

2. Treatment of Hallucinogen Organic Mental Disorders.
The most important measures are the provisions of a quiet room, the company of a trusted and dependable friend or relative, and appropriate reassurance. The patient must be sheltered from intrusive, inquisitive, and aggressive people, from noises or too much sensory stimulation, and from panic by reassurance that he is not insane, that there is no evidence of irreparable brain or chromosomal damage, and that he is experiencing the effects of the substance ingested. Do not carry your reassurance to the point of promise of well-being in a day or two because, although the panic reactions most likely last only up to 12-24 hours, psychotic symptoms may last for months to years, particularly in individuals with pre-existing schizophrenic illness or severe borderline personality characteristics.

Provide frequent contact and orienting cues as needed (i.e., where he is, the time, what is happening to him, etc.) and instruct his companion to reinforce and repeat the cues.

There are no specific antidotes against these hallucinogens and indeed drugs are best avoided if the above measures suffice. If the panic reaction requires medication, the benzodiazepines are the best choice (diazepam 15-30 mg or chlordiazepoxide 25-50 mg orally or intramuscularly). If there is no response in one hour, repeat the dose. If the patient is not already hospitalized and panic attacks have not abated with the benzodiazepine in six hours, hospitalization then becomes mandatory. Phenothiazines or other antipsychotics can be used initially if benzodiazepines have failed to control panic and agitation and if there is certainty that no other unknown hallucinogens or drugs have been mixed with the presumed offending agent. The phenothiazines are remarkably effective in counteracting the central effects of LSD, for example, but this degree of certainty that LSD is the sole offending agent is not always possible because toxicological screening is not reliable and "drug heads" will often take anything that they can lay their hands on. Thus, STP - which is another amphetamine-derived hallucinogen not included in this section - scopolamine, phenothiazines of potent anticholinergic action, and various other drugs may have been mixed and may react adversely with, or complicate the clinical picture caused by, the hallucinogen in question. Barbiturates should not be used because they may cause respiratory depression and obtundation of the sensorium. Should a protracted Delusional or Affective Syndrome persist, a regime of neuroleptics or tricyclic antidepressants must be entertained.

Flashbacks are spontaneous recurrences of the original LSD experience or bits of it which are triggered by unknown factors long after cessation of use of the agent. They may be precipitated by smoking marijuana, by dietary irregularities and malnutrition, by weight loss, or by trauma. They are usually brief (minutes) and attenuated in intensity, but they may last for hours and be quite severe and frightening. The patient may believe that now he is really going crazy since he has been "clean" for months or years. He may become depressed and conclude that suicide is the only alternative to madness. The treatment for flashbacks does not differ from that outlined above for the more acute episodes.

S.   CANNABIS MENTAL DISORDERS

The Cannabis Organic Mental Disorders include the intoxication and the delusional syndromes induced by substances derived from the cannabis plant. Marijuana, hashish, and the powerful purified product - tetrahydrocannabinol - are the usual substances smoked or ingested in the United States. Folklore terms are bhang, grass, MJ, Mary Jane, and pot. Hashish is often quite potent but some "grass" -- as one writer has put it -- is just that with no tetrahydrocannabinol (or THC), the active substance.

1. Cannabis Intoxication (DSM-III = 305.20).

   It is very difficult to distinguish this syndrome, on the basis of signs and symptoms, from hallucinosis induced by a low dose of a hallucinogen which, as stated in the preceding section, may not include hallucinations. On the other hand, although very high blood levels of cannabis may cause hallucinations, such experiences are rare in Cannabis Intoxication and for this reason cannabis hallucinosis is not a diagnosis in DSM-III. It will therefore be more profitable to point out the salient features of Cannabis Intoxication. Tachycardia, reddened eyes due to conjunctival injection often concealed with dark glasses, increased appetite often for "junk food," and the characteristic sweet smell of burned cannabis on clothing fit the stereotype of the marijuana "tripper." In low doses Cannabis Intoxication resembles mild ethanol intoxication. The distinction can be made on the basis of the differences summarized in Table 5-12 below:

TABLE 5-12

FEATURES OF CANNABIS AND ALCOHOL INTOXICATION

Psychophysiological Response	Cannabis	Alcohol
Appetite	Increased	Decreased
Aggressiveness	Not usually	Increased
Smell	Burned cannabis	Ethanolic breath
Neurological signs	Not usually	Nystagmus, ataxia

2. Cannabis Delusional Disorder (DSM-III = 292.11).

   It is very doubtful that the creation of this diagnostic category is justified, and DSM-III recognizes this with unambiguous half-heartedness. This is because the presence of delusions is required for this diagnosis, but they may have been already apparent in intoxication (!). Furthermore, this syndrome supposedly develops during the course of intoxication or immediately following cannabis use; it does not persist beyond a few hours (up to six following cessation of use), which is no more than the usual duration of intoxication. Obviously there is no need to multiply syndromes in this manner, but there it is! The treatment of cannabis-induced disturbances does not essentially differ from that outlined for hallucinogens.

QUIZ, Section IV, K-S.

Circle the letter corresponding to the one correct response.

1. Appropriate coadjuvant treatment of concomitant or lingering opioid abstinence symptoms (depression) may include

    a. phenobarbital.
    b. haloperidol.
    c. amphetamine.
    d. doxepin.
    e. physostigmine.
    f. none of the above.

2. Propoxyphene-induced death in combination with other CNS depressants may occur at doses

    a. only slightly higher than the upper limit of the recommended dose.
    b. twice as high as the usual therapeutic dose because the drug metabolizing liver enzyme systems are induced by the other concomitantly administered drugs.

Circle the correct answer(s). One or more than one answer may be correct.

3. The Opioid Abstinence Syndrome and the naloxone-precipitated withdrawal are reminiscent in their clinical manifestations of which of the following?

    a. atropinic toxicity
    b. cholinergic reaction
    c. tricyclic antidepressant toxicity
    d. influenza

4. Cocaine Intoxication resembles amphetamine toxicity in the following:

    a. The substance should never be withdrawn abruptly.
    b. It can be withdrawn immediately without further ado.
    c. Severe withdrawal occurs 24 hours after cessation of substance.
    d. No serious symptoms develop when the drug is withdrawn.
    e. Convulsions following an overdose usually respond to anticonvulsants.
    f. Overdose can effectively be treated by forced diuresis or acidification of the urine.

5. Table 5-11 illustrates a general rule of narcotic abstinence syndromes; based on it select all the correct statements among those offered below.

    a. Agents with shorter duration of action induce withdrawal earlier, but peak and resolution come later.
    b. Agents with longer duration of action cause the briefest withdrawal syndromes.

c. The shorter the duration of action of the agent, the faster the development of all the stages of withdrawal which means more abrupt transitions and greatest intensity of symptoms.

d. A naloxone-precipitated withdrawal from methadone is more abrupt and severe than a withdrawal induced by cessation of methadone intake.

Match the following lettered items with the numbered entries.

___6. 5-hydroxytryptamine   a. tricyclic antidepressant
___7. phenylethylamine   b. serotonin
___8. amitriptyline   c. catecholamine

TRUE or FALSE: Circle the correct letter.

T   F   9. Isolated amphetamine-induced delusions may persist for a year or more.

T   F   10. Premorbid personalities commonly associated with amphetamine-induced Organic Mental Disorders are the antisocial and the schizoid.

T   F   11. Visual hallucinations are rare in amphetamine toxicity.

T   F   12. Truck driving and late night studying (medical students) may foster amphetamine abuse.

T   F   13. The Amphetamine Delusional Syndrome is the closest model of paranoid Schizophrenia.

T   F   14. Amphetamines do not inhibit monoamine oxidase or the reuptake of catecholamines, nor do they release catecholamines from nerve terminals.

T   F   15. A Schizophreniform Paranoid Psychosis is usually seen in chronic amphetamine abusers, but some chronic abusers do not develop this syndrome after 15 years of heavy abuse.

T   F   16. Acute Cocaine Intoxication is more persistent than Acute Amphetamine Intoxication.

T   F   17. Abrupt withdrawal from cocaine and amphetamine is as lethal as from barbiturates.

T   F   18. Marijuana's effects are normally short-lived (up to 5-8 hours).

T   F   19. Most marijuana smokers do not seek medical assistance.

T   F   20. Marijuana causes physiological dependence, addiction, and withdrawal manifestations as strong and severe as opioids.

21. Name three types of substances whose withdrawal syndromes often encompass seizures.

_____

_____

_____

_____

T. TOBACCO WITHDRAWAL (DSM-III = 292.00)

Psychological and physiological disturbances are observed in some smokers, but not in all, when tobacco smoking is abruptly interrupted. Even among those who react there is great individual variability which is not well-understood. This reaction is called Tobacco Withdrawal. It is assumed, but not completely proven, that the withdrawal reaction is caused by nicotine abstinence because this is the most important, but not the sole, pharmacologically active alkaloid in tobacco. The diagnosis of withdrawal rarely becomes a problem; your clients will come to you with a diagnosis already made. Following cessation of smoking they may complain of any of the following symptoms: a need or craving for tobacco, irritability, restlessness, anxiety, dullness, drowsiness, sleep and gastrointestinal disturbances, headache, amnesia, various impairments (concentration, judgement, performance), increased appetite, weight gain. Concomitant signs are: decrease in heart rate and blood pressure, the EEG alpha rhythm decreases and slower and sleep-like patterns increase, increase in REM sleep and dreaming, and increase in jaw clenching due to increased frequency of masseter muscle contraction. The onset of some of the withdrawal phenomena can be detected within two hours after the last cigarette, a peak of craving occurs up to about 24 hours, and it gradually declines over the next few days or several weeks. The amount of nicotine intake or the duration of the habit required to produce physical dependence is not known, but DSM-III has chosen these criteria: use of tobacco for at least several weeks at a level equivalent to more than 10 cigarettes per day of at least 0.5 mg of nicotine each. Your patient may ask you for help or advice to quit smoking with the most tolerable degree of withdrawal phenomenology. Various measures have been advocated and none is very successful in preventing relapse, but it behooves you to provide help or guidance if asked. Over 30 million Americans have stopped smoking during the past 15 years without any formal help. This should be the preferred approach in strong and seriously motivated individuals, but those do not usually ask for help. Use of benzodiazepines may be helpful during the peak intensity of withdrawal symptoms. Lobeline up to 55 mg/day by injection has been used in many pharmacological therapies. Lobeline is the chief alkaloid of Indian tobacco and has a pharmacological action similar to, but weaker than, that of nicotine. Psychotherapy and behavior modification may also be effective. The mean initial success rates for populations with no formal treatment, medication, psychotherapy, and behavior modification have been reported to be 7, 37, 45, and 45 respectively.

U. CAFFEINE INTOXICATION OR CAFFEINISM (DSM-III = 305.90)

The primary sources of ingested caffeine are coffee, tea, cola, chocolate, cocoa, and prescription and over-the-counter medications. A cup of coffee contains 100-150 mg of caffeine. Tea is 1/2, and cola about 1/3 as strong. Most caffeine-containing prescription doses are 1/2-1/3 the strength of a cup of coffee, but some prescriptions and over-the-counter medications may contain as much caffeine per tablet as a cup of coffee. Excessive ingestion of caffeine-containing substances or drugs may lead to overdosage symptomatology which is rarely fatal but nonetheless important to recognize.

Caffeinism is characterized by a subjective feeling of nervousness, restlessness, excitement, insomnia, flushing, gastrointestinal complaints, diuresis, and fine tremor of fingers. In some individuals, the above manifestations may be seen with as little as 250 mg of caffeine per day (2-3 cups). More than 1 gm/day may cause tachypnea, palpitations, tachycardia, extrasystoles, cardiac arrhythmia, muscle twitches, hyperesthesias, hyperreflexia, exuberance, inexhaustibility, increased psychomotor activity, rambling flow of thought and incoherent speech (d. diagnosis with mania). Greater daily ingestions may additionally cause special sense disturbances (i.e., tinnitus, light flashes) and delirium. Doses in excess of 10 gm/day will cause grand mal seizures, respiratory failure, and death. Patients with cardiovascular and gastrointestinal incompetence may have serious complications (i.e., circulatory failure, hematemesis) with excessive caffeine ingestion. The excitatory action of caffeine can be controlled with barbiturates. But reduction or withdrawal of caffeine intake and supportive encouragement should suffice in the management of caffeinism, and for the control of the Caffeine Withdrawal Syndrome. Withdrawal includes: irritability, restlessness, nervousness, lethargy, decreased performance, and headache.

V.   OTHER OR UNSPECIFIED SUBSTANCE

We are near the end of the section entitled Substance-Induced Organic Mental Disorders. Nine different substances or groups of substances encompassing 25 different syndromes have been described and their treatments outlined in the preceding pages. Any other substances not specifically mentioned earlier may induce one or various of the general syndromes described in Section One. For these substances the last group of categories of Section One will be used. It is entitled "Other or Unspecified Substance-Induced Mental Disorders." It would be nearly impossible and of dubious usefulness to describe here the innumerable varieties of compounds capable of inducing a kaleidoscope of Organic Mental Disorders. DSM-III tabulates in this section a list of 66 other commonly used substances in medical practice and their frequently associated Organic Mental Disorders. A simplified version of this list is given in Table 5-13.

ANSWERS, Section IV, K-S.

1. d	13. T
2. a	14. F
3. b,d	15. T
4. b,d	16. F
5. c,d	17. F
6. b	18. T
7. c	19. T
8. a	20. F
9. T	21. barbiturates, alcohol, meperidine
10. T	
11. F	
12. T	

TABLE 5-13

COMMONLY USED SUBSTANCES IN MEDICAL PRACTICE and ASSOCIATED ORGANIC MENTAL DISORDERS

Chemical or Generic Name	INTOXICATION	DELIRIUM	DEMENTIA	O. DELUSIONAL	O. HALLUCINOSIS	O. AFFECTIVE	WITHDRAWAL	PERSONALITY
Acetophenazine	X					X		
Amantadine	X					X		
Anticholinesterases	X							
Antihistamines	X	X						
Antimalarials		X				X		X
Antineoplastics		X	X			X		X
Atropine	X	X						
Bromides	X		X	X				
Butaperazine	X					X		
Carbamazepine	X	X						
Cardiac Glycosides	X	X						
Chlorpromazine	X					X		
Chlorprothixene	X					X		
Cholinesterase Blockers	X							
Corticosteroids		X				X	X	X
Corticotropin					X	X	X	X
Dehydrobenzperidol	X					X		
Desmethylimipramine	X	X						
Disulfiram	X							
Doxepin	X	X						
Estrogens						X		
Ethosuximide	X							
Fluphenazine	X					X		
Haloperidol	X					X		
Imipramine	X	X						
Indomethacin		X				X		
Isocarboxazid	X	X						
Isoniazid	X	X						
L-Dopa	X	X			X	X		
Lithium Carbonate	X	X						
Loxapine	X					X		
Mercurial Diuretics		X			X	X		X
Mesoridazine	X					X		

Chemical or Generic Name	INTOXICATION	DELIRIUM	DEMENTIA	O. DELUSIONAL	O. HALLUCINOSIS	O. AFFECTIVE	WITHDRAWAL	PERSONALITY
Methotrimeprazine	X					X		
Methyldopa	X					X		
Methysergide	X					X		
Molindone	X					X		
Nialamide	X	X						
Nortriptyline	X	X						
Pargyline	X	X						
Perphenazine	X					X		
Phenelzine	X	X						
Phencyclidine	X	X		X		X		
Phenylbutazone						X		
Phenytoin	X	X			X			
Piperacetazine	X					X		
Primidone	X							
Prochlorperazine	X					X		
Procyclidine	X	X						
Progestins						X		
Promazine	X					X		
Promethazine	X					X		
Propranolol	X					X		
Protriptyline	X	X						
Quinidine		X						
Reserpine	X					X		
Salicylates	X	X						
Scopolamine	X	X						
Thiocyanates	X	X						
Thiopropazate	X					X		
Thioridazine	X					X		
Thiothixene	X					X		
Tranylcypromine	X	X						
Triflupromazine	X					X		
Trihexyphenidyl	X	X						
Trimethadione	X							

QUIZ, Section IV, T-V.

TRUE or FALSE: Circle the correct letter.

T   F   1. Judging from the available statistics, there appears to exist a paradox about the habit of heavy smoking: great interindividual variability of withdrawal phenomenology, yet great relapse rate.

T   F   2. In terms of rationale, lobeline is to nicotine what methadone substitution is to heroin addiction.

T   F   3. Social acceptance for the abused substances below is, from most to least, as follows: heroin > caffeine = nicotine > alcohol.

T   F   4. Mild versions of the "coffee drinker's" syndrome are probably very pervasive.

T   F   5. Every psychiatric patient nonrespondent to usual anxiolytics, hypnotics, or other psychotherapeutic agents ought to be suspected, not diagnosed, of caffeinism.

T   F   6. The differential diagnosis of caffeinism need not include anxiety neurosis, mania, or epilepsy.

It is apparent from Table 5-13 and the preceding material on Organic Mental Disorders tabulated in Table 5-1 that:

T   F   7. By far the most frequent substance-induced syndrome is that of Intoxication; this is followed by Delirium, Organic Affective Disorder, and Withdrawal in that order.

T   F   8. Alcohol can induce the largest number of syndromes available (6/9).

T   F   9. Comparatively very few substances produce Dementia, Organic Hallucinosis, and Personality Disorders.

T   F   10. Listed as dementing agents are alcohol, antineoplastics, and bromides.

T   F   11. Listed as capable of inducing Organic Hallucinosis are alcohol, mercurial diuretics, phenytoin, and L-Dopa.

T   F   12. Listed with potential for causing a Personality Disorder are mercurial diuretics, corticosteroids, ACTH, antimalarials, and antineoplastics.

T   F   13. Dementia and Organic Personality Disorders should be suspected secondarily to the use of antineoplastics.

T   F   14. One distinguishing feature between Substance-Induced Organic Mental Disorders and the next chapter entitled Substance Use Disorders is the presence of an Organic Brain Syndrome in the former and its absence in the latter.

ANSWERS, Section IV, T-V.

1. T	8. T
2. T	9. T
3. F	10. T
4. T	11. T
5. T	12. T
6. F	13. T
7. T	14. T

POST-TEST

For the following questions, circle the letter corresponding to the <u>one</u> correct response.

1. Dementia characteristically includes all the following features <u>except</u>

    a. memory impairment.
    b. impairment of abstract thinking.
    c. impairment in judgement.
    d. personality change.
    e. autonomic arousal.

2. Differential diagnosis of Dementia includes all the following <u>except</u>

    a. Schizophrenia.
    b. depression with cognitive deficit.
    c. normal process of aging.
    d. Somatization Disorder.
    e. Delirium.

3. Usual features of the Alcohol Amnestic Syndrome include all of the following <u>except</u>

    a. attention is intact.
    b. short-term memory is intact.
    c. confabulation.
    d. apathy and emotional blandness.
    e. some disorientation as to time.

4. A 24-year-old man comes to the emergency room in a state of agitation and restlessness. He complains of loss of appetite and insomnia. Examination shows an elevated blood pressure, tachycardia, a clear sensorium, and paranoid delusions. Of the following the most likely cause is

    a. Anxiety Disorder.
    b. cocaine withdrawal.
    c. Barbiturate Intoxication.
    d. Delirium Tremens.
    e. Amphetamine Intoxication.

5. Among the following, visual hallucinations are most common in

    a. Schizophreniform Disorder.
    b. Bipolar Affective Disorder.
    c. Delirium.
    d. Catatonic Schizophrenia.
    e. Amnestic Syndrome.

6. The most fundamental feature of Delirium is

   a. disorder of attention.
   b. anxiety.
   c. fine tremor of hands.
   d. auditory hallucinations.
   e. pressure of speech.

7. The usual course of Delirium may best be described as

   a. slow onset with rapid recovery.
   b. rapid onset and progressively deteriorating.
   c. chronic and unremitting.
   d. rapid onset and brief duration.
   e. gradual onset with periodic recurrence at biweekly intervals.

8. The management of Delirium includes all the following except

   a. provide light in the room.
   b. Valium, 10 mg qid.
   c. haloperidol, 1 mg q 4-6 hrs.
   d. provide environmental orientation.
   e. ask family members to remain in room with patient.

9. A 28-year-old man is hospitalized for pneumonia. He states that he is addicted to heroin and is going into withdrawal. This can be verified by

   a. presence of needle tracks.
   b. detection of hepatitis.
   c. detection of opiates in urine during the first hospital day.
   d. presence of rhinorrhea, restlessness, and muscle twitches.
   e. intravenous injection of naloxone.

10. Which of the following is not characteristic of a patient with Dementia?

    a. neologisms
    b. emotional lability
    c. impairment of social judgement
    d. neglect of personal appearance
    e. disorientation to time

11. Delirium is characterized by all the following except

    a. memory impairment.
    b. emotional lability.
    c. normal sleep patterns.
    d. perceptual disturbances.
    e. autonomic arousal.

12. Any patient sufficiently recovered from an intentionally suicidal overdose of barbiturates or related drugs

    a. should be left alone unless he tries again.
    b. can be discharged since most overdose patients are hysterical and inconsequential.
    c. should have a thorough psychiatric evaluation since many are depressed, very angry, or frustrated.
    d. should receive pharmacological education because most overdose patients are only confused and can be conceptualized as involuntary suicides.
    e. should be discouraged from discussing the idea of suicide.

13. A known male heroin addict has just been admitted to your licensed inpatient facility, and he begins to develop signs of abstinence (i.e., tachypnea, sweating, lacrimation, rhinorrhea, yawning, piloerection). You know for a fact that his last IV "fix" of heroin was about 16 hours earlier, but you do not know the amount he injected. You choose to give him 20 mg of methadone orally. Following that, he becomes somnolent. The next dose that evening should be

    a. less than 20 mg.
    b. 20 mg again.
    c. more than 20 mg.
    d. withheld indefinitely; allow patient to go "cold turkey."
    e. based on the amount the patient usually takes.

14. You examine a 23-year-old male college graduate with skull depression on left frontal region, enophthalmos and total blindness of the eye on the same side, poor vision in the right eye, great difficulty reading optotype paragraphs of large size. History reveals severe craniofacial injury two years earlier resulting from a fight with an individual who was trying to rape the patient's fiancee. He has been unable to return to school to get his Master's Degree, to find a job, or to retain his fiancee's interest in him. He appears severely depressed and seriously considering suicide. There are no major cognitive deficits, delusions, or hallucinations. The most likely diagnosis in this case is

    a. Traumatic Dementia.
    b. Affective Syndrome.
    c. Delirium.
    d. Organic Personality Syndrome.
    e. Organic Hallucinosis of auditory modality because he is almost blind.

15. A 23-year-old male is brought to your office because he was busily masturbating in a crowded bus and quite indifferent to people's reactions of shock. You immediately notice facial deformities. You learn that he had sustained a severe craniofacial injury when he was hit by a truck while riding his motorcycle to work some nine months ago. He had been a normal boy before the accident. Mental status examination elicits nothing of significance except some childish features and inappropriate giggles. Select the best diagnosis and/or treatment from the following.

    a. Organic Personality Syndrome, close supervision to minimize the risk of arrest, and jail or custodial care
    b. immediate hospitalization, complex differential diagnostic workup
    c. Organic Hallucinosis, immediate hospitalization, Valium, and reassurance; no phenothiazines
    d. Organic Affective Syndrome requiring custodial care
    e. mental retardation requiring special education

16. A 57-year-old man is referred to you by another physician with the following note: Long history of alcohol consumption, insidious onset of memory impairment, confabulations, poor state of nutrition, peripheral neuropathy, and cerebellar ataxia. Not acutely ill and without impairment of attention or consciousness. Your diagnosis is

    a. Schizophrenia.
    b. diabetic encephalopathy.
    c. Korsakoff's Syndrome.
    d. Delirium Tremens.
    e. Primary Degenerative Dementia.

17. A 19-year-old ingests an unknown but substantial amount of amphetamines. Within a few hours a syndrome characterized by severe inattention, shifting levels of consciousness, disturbances in memory and orientation, insomnia, tactile hallucinations, and increased psychomotor activity emerges. There is also pupillary dilatation and anorexia. According to DSM-III, the diagnosis should be

    a. Amphetamine Intoxication.
    b. Amphetamine Hallucinosis.
    c. Amphetamine Delirium.
    d. Amphetamine Dementia.
    e. Amphetamine Psychosis.

18. Suppose that the 19-year-old individual in the preceding question, following the amphetamine ingestion instead had developed the following behaviors: psychomotor excitement, resistance to fatigue, lack of sleepiness that night, exhaustion, and failure to show up for work the following morning. There are tachycardia and chills. No cognitive deficits. The diagnosis then would have been

    a. Amphetamine Intoxication.
    b. Amphetamine Hallucinosis.
    c. Amphetamine Delirium.
    d. Amphetamine Dementia.
    e. Amphetamine Psychosis.

For the following questions, one or more than one answer may be correct. Circle the correct answer(s).

19. The early phase of Dementia is associated with

    a. loss of memory of recent events.
    b. disorientation as to time, place, and person.
    c. gradually increasing defects of intellectual functioning.
    d. flatness of affect.

20. When given in sufficient dosage, which of the following drugs will cause a condition that most closely mimics Paranoid Schizophrenia?

    a. LSD
    b. mescaline
    c. amobarbital sodium
    d. methamphetamine sulfate

21. In regard to amphetamines, circle true statement(s) (items 21-22).

    a. Isolated amphetamine-induced delusions may persist for a year or more.
    b. Premorbid personalities commonly associated with amphetamine-induced Organic Mental Disorders are the antisocial and the schizoid.
    c. Truck driving and late night studying may foster amphetamine abuse.
    d. Visual hallucinations are rare in amphetamine toxicity.

22. a. The amphetamine delusional syndrome is the closest model of Paranoid Schizophrenia.
    b. Amphetamines do not inhibit monoamine oxidase or the reuptake of catecholamines, nor do they release catecholamines from nerve terminals.
    c. A Schizophreniform Paranoid Psychosis is usually seen in chronic amphetamine abusers, but some chronic abusers do not develop this syndrome after 15 years of heavy abuse.
    d. Abrupt withdrawal from cocaine and amphetamines is as lethal as from barbiturates.

23. The differential diagnosis of Delirium most often includes

    a. Schizophrenic Disorders.
    b. Gilles de la Tourette Syndrome.
    c. Schizophreniform Disorders.
    d. Panic Disorder.

24. Untreatable Dementia means

    a. palliative or symptomatic treatment is not applicable.
    b. the patient must be cared for in an institution.
    c. further services of a physician are not indicated.
    d. no specific treatment capable of attacking the cause is available.

25. Criteria for diagnosis of Organic Delusional Syndrome include

    a. predominant hallucinations of auditory modality with secondary delusions related to auditory hallucinations.
    b. visual hallucinations and impaired sensorium.
    c. Dementia with demonstrable organic pathology by either history, lab tests, neurodiagnostic procedures, or physical examination.
    d. predominant delusional system associated with organic etiology.

26. The Opioid Abstinence Syndrome and the naloxone-precipitated withdrawal are reminiscent in their clinical manifestations of which of the following?

    a. atropinic toxicity
    b. cholinergic reaction
    c. tricyclic antidepressant toxicity
    d. influenza

27. An infant just born to a methadone-maintained mother

    a. does not develop abstinence reaction because fairly complete emotional and psychological machineries are required for drug-seeking and drug-craving behaviors.
    b. will always develop signs of abstinence because physical dependence has a cellular basis.
    c. should be given naloxone 5 μg/kg daily.
    d. should be observed for signs of withdrawal.

28. A chronic cocaine abuser

    a. should never be withdrawn abruptly.
    b. can be withdrawn immediately without further ado.
    c. develops severe withdrawal 24 hours after cocaine cessation.
    d. will have no serious symptoms when the drug is withdrawn.

29. The distinguishing features of glutethimide intoxication include

    a. cholinergic action.
    b. hypoglycemia action.
    c. bone marrow depression.
    d. anticholinergic action.

30. A general rule of narcotic abstinence syndrome includes which of the following?

    a. Agents with shorter duration of action induce withdrawal earlier, but peak and resolution come later.
    b. The shorter the duration of action of the agent, the faster the development of all the stages of withdrawal which means more abrupt transitions and greatest intensity of symptoms.
    c. Agents with longer duration of action cause the briefest withdrawal syndromes.
    d. A naloxone-precipitated withdrawal from methadone is more abrupt and severe than a withdrawal induced by cessation of methadone intake.

31. Substances whose withdrawal syndromes often encompass seizures include

    a. barbiturates.
    b. alcohol.
    c. meperidine.
    d. chlorpromazine.

32. A 23-year-old male is brought to the emergency room in a state of severe agitation, fearfulness, and visually hallucinating combat episodes of his recent Vietnam tour of duty. He is alert and oriented but exhibits the firm delusional conviction that the hallucinated combat flashes are presently real. There are no delusions in any other area. His buddies inform you that recently he has been messing around with LSD and other stuff. Treatment with phenothiazines is not indicated in this case because

    a. LSD panic reactions usually last 12-24 hrs.
    b. Valium and reassurance will probably be sufficient.
    c. phenothiazines may aggravate the hallucinogenic effects of scopalomine and STP.
    d. phenothiazines are ineffective against LSD hallucinosis.

33. The microscopic identification of Alzheimer's disease is based on recognition of

    a. neurofibrillary tangles.
    b. senile plaques.
    c. neuronal loss.
    d. micro-infarcts of mammillary bodies.

34.   In regard to Dementia, which of the following statements is/are true?

    a.   The cause of Alzheimer's disease is unknown, but the neuropathology is fairly characteristic and identifiable.

    b.   The second and third largest groups are due to vascular disease and NPH.

    c.   Depression may masquerade as (pseudo-) Dementia in about 4% of those carelessly diagnosed as demented.

    d.   Huntington's and Parkinson's diseases, two disorders of the extra-pyramidal motor system, have about the same probability of developing Dementia.

35.   In regard to Dementias, circle true statement(s).

    a.   Progressive Idiopathic Dementia is responsible for cognitive impairment in more than half of all demented patients.

    b.   Untreatable Dementias still require services by the physician.

    c.   Approximately, a total of 10-15% of demented patients can be helped dramatically by appropriate treatment.

    d.   Treatable Dementias refer to Dementias that have specific and effective treatment.

36.   Features suggesting Dementia due to multi-infarct etiology include

    a.   abrupt onset and step-wise deterioration.

    b.   fluctuating course.

    c.   history of hypertension and of "strokes."

    d.   focal neurological symptoms and signs.

37.   Correct phrases pertaining to the course of intoxication with alcohol include which of the following?

    a.   average intoxication length: 1-12 hrs

    b.   alcohol metabolism rate: 1 oz. of beverage alcohol/hr: 10 oz./10 hrs

    c.   signs of intoxication increase as blood alcohol levels increase and vice-versa

    d.   short-term tolerance may occur such that less intoxication is possible after many hours of drinking than after a few hours only

38.   Correct statements pertaining to the course of intoxication with alcohol include which of the following?

    a.   Because of tolerance, intoxication correlates poorly with blood alcohol levels ranging from 30 to 200 mg/100 ml.

    b.   Unconsciousness occurs at 400-500 mg/100 ml.

    c.   Death occurs at 600-800 mg/100 ml.

    d.   Usually unconsciousness supervenes before the individual can drink enough to kill himself.

39. The Alcoholic Withdrawal Syndrome may be mimicked by

   a. familial tremor.
   b. metabolic abnormalities (e.g., hypoglycemia, diabetic acidosis).
   c. withdrawal from sedative-hypnotic drugs.
   d. barbiturate withdrawal.

Questions 40-43 pertain to patients with Alcohol Withdrawal Delirium.

40. a. There is always hypoglycemia.
    b. There is always hyperglycemia.
    c. The goal is to suppress all agitation by means of powerfully sedating phenothiazines.
    d. Hospitalize.

41. a. Prophylactic anticonvulsants are a good routine approach.
    b. Antibiotics are always needed.
    c. Dry tongue and mucosae are always clear indication for administration of I.V. fluids.
    d. Thiamine 100-200 mg I.M. or I.V. should always be given immediately and for at least the next few days.

42. a. Paraldehyde is totally innocuous because it is not metabolized by the liver.
    b. Diphenylhydantoin depletes brain stores of folic acid.
    c. Most chronic alcoholics do not have total body potassium depletion.
    d. Potassium chloride plus potassium-retaining diuretics may cause hazardous hyperkalemia.

43. a. Use of aspirin in the alcoholic does not entail any risks.
    b. Most chronic alcoholics are magnesium-deficient regardless of serum concentrations.
    c. Phenothiazines are the best treatment for Delirium Tremens.
    d. I.V. fluids may cause or exacerbate cerebral edema.

44. Concerning hallucinogens, choose the correct statement(s).

   a. None of the hallucinogens are approved drugs; they all fall under the federal narcotics laws; their use or prescription is illicit.
   b. Tolerance to hallucinogens develops rapidly; cross-tolerance from one to another is the rule; tolerance is lost rapidly upon abrupt cessation; and no abstinence syndromes ensue.
   c. Hallucinogens are often euphorohallucinogens, psychotomimetics, psychotogenic agents, illusogens, and psychedelics.
   d. The term psychedelic is usually associated with a "bad trip" and psychotomimetic with "good trip."

Match the following numbered items with the lettered entries. Lettered items may be used once, more than once, or not at all.

_____ 45. good recall of names of three objects one hour later
_____ 46. correct six-digit repetition within a few seconds
_____ 47. good recall of events of 20 years earlier
_____ 48. failure of digit repetition within a few seconds
_____ 49. failure to recall the names of three objects at one hour, but correct digit repetition within seconds
_____ 50. one-hour name recollection intact

a. suggestive of fundamental inattention, immediate memory impairment, and Delirium or Dementia
b. suggests that attention, immediate and short memory are all intact, and therefore absence of Amnestic Syndrome
c. Delirium less likely, Amnestic Syndrome still possible
d. tends to rule out Amnestic Syndrome
e. suggests Amnestic Syndrome
f. suggests good remote memory but does not rule out Dementia

Match the following numbered items with the lettered entries below.

_____ 51. Wernicke's Syndrome
_____ 52. Korsakoff's Syndrome
_____ 53. Delirium

a. sudden onset
b. gradual onset
c. fundamental inattention

Match the following types of hallucinations with the usually corresponding etiological factors. The lettered items may be used once, more than once, or not at all.

_____ 54. visual
_____ 55. auditory
_____ 56. olfactory
_____ 57. tactile
_____ 58. gustatory

a. LSD
b. cocaine
c. uncinate epilepsy
d. Schizophrenia

Match the numbered diagnoses with the lettered descriptions. Lettered items may be used only once.

_____ 59. secobarbital or pentobarbital poisoning
_____ 60. phenobarbital intoxication
_____ 61. severe glutethimide intoxication
_____ 62. barbiturate intoxication
_____ 63. alcohol intoxication

a. flaccid coma with reactive pupils, hypothermia, and hypotension
b. flaccid coma with dilated fixed pupils, hypothermia, hypotension, laryngeal spasms, sudden apnea, high mortality
c. blood barbiturate level of 20µg/ml, short coma
d. blood barbiturate level of 115µg/ml, prolonged coma, high mortality
e. flushed face, injected conjuctivae, verbose, cantankerous, aggressive

PRE-TEST ANSWERS

1.	e	22.	a,c	43.	b,d
2.	d	23.	a,c	44.	a,b,c
3.	b	24.	d	45.	b,d
4.	e	25.	d	46.	c
5.	c	26.	b,d	47.	f
6.	a	27.	d	48.	a
7.	d	28.	b,d	49.	e
8.	b	29.	d	50.	b,d
9.	e	30.	b,d	51.	a
10.	a	31.	a,b,c	52.	b
11.	c	32.	a,b,c	53.	c
12.	c	33.	a,b,c	54.	a
13.	a	34.	a,b,c	55.	d
14.	b	35.	a,b,c,d	56.	c
15.	a	36.	a,b,c,d	57.	b
16.	c	37.	a,b,c,d	58.	c
17.	c	38.	a,b,c,d	59.	c
18.	a	39.	a,b,c,d	60.	d
19.	a,c	40.	d	61.	b
20.	d	41.	d	62.	a
21.	a,b,c	42.	b,d	63.	e

POST-TEST ANSWERS

1.	e	22.	a,c	43.	b,d
2.	d	23.	a,c	44.	a,b,c
3.	b	24.	d	45.	b,d
4.	e	25.	d	46.	c
5.	c	26.	b,d	47.	f
6.	a	27.	d	48.	a
7.	d	28.	b,d	49.	e
8.	b	29.	d	50.	b,d
9.	e	30.	b,d	51.	a
10.	a	31.	a,b,c	52.	b
11.	c	32.	a,b,c	53.	c
12.	c	33.	a,b,c	54.	a
13.	a	34.	a,b,c	55.	d
14.	b	35.	a,b,c,d	56.	c
15.	a	36.	a,b,c,d	57.	b
16.	c	37.	a,b,c,d	58.	c
17.	c	38.	a,b,c,d	59.	c
18.	a	39.	a,b,c,d	60.	d
19.	a,c	40.	d	61.	b
20.	d	41.	d	62.	a
21.	a,b,c	42.	b,d	63.	e

REFERENCES

Adams, R. D., & Victor, M. Principles of neurology. New York: McGraw-Hill, 1977.

Arieti, S., et al. American handbook of psychiatry (Vol. 4). In M. F. Resier (Ed.), Organic disorders and psychosomatic medicine. New York: Basic Books, Inc., 1975.

Benson, D. F., & Blumer, D. (Eds.) Psychiatric aspects of neurologic disease. New York: Grune & Stratton, 1975.

Dale, A. J., et al. Organic brain syndrome. In A. M. Freedman, H. I. Kaplan, & B. Sadock (Eds.), Comprehensive textbook of Psychiatry III (Vol. I). Baltimore: The Williams & Wilkins Co., 1975.

Greenblatt, D. J., & Shader, R. I. Treatment of the Alcohol Withdrawal Syndrome. In R. I. Shader (Ed.), Manual of psychiatric therapeutics. Boston: Little, Brown, & Co., 1975.

Katzman, R., & Karasu, T. B. Differential diagnosis of Dementia. In W. S. Fields (Ed.), Neurological & sensory disorders in the elderly. Chicago: Year Book Publishers, Inc., 1975.

Quinker, R. B., & Sahs, A. L. Neurology. Springfield, Ill.: Charles C. Thomas, 1966.

Sagar, S. M. Toxic and metabolic disorders. In M. A. Samuels (Ed.), Manual of neurologic therapeutics. Boston: Little, Brown, & Co., 1978.

Torack, R. M. The pathologic physiology of dementia. New York: Springer-Verlag, 1978.

Vaillant, G. F. Alcoholism and drug dependence. In A. M. Nicholi (Ed.), The Harvard guide to modern psychiatry. Cambridge, Mass.: The Belknap Press of Harvard University Press, 1978.

Victor, M., Adams, R. D., & Cellins, G. H. The Wernicke-Korsakoff Syndrome. Philadelphia: F.A. Davis Company, 1971.

Wells, C. E. Diagnostic evaluation and treatment in dementia. In C. E. Wells (Ed.), Dementia. Philadelphia: F.A. Davis Company, 1977.

CHAPTER 6

Substance Use Disorders

Douglas F. Crane, M.D.
Patricia B. Sutker, Ph.D.
Carol M. Randall, Ph.D.
Jay W. Birnbaum, M.D.

Chapter Outline

Learning Objectives

Pre-Test

Post-Test

Pre-Test/Post-Test Answers

References

Learning Objectives

Upon completion of this chapter the student will be able to:

1. Identify the diagnostic criteria for Substance Use Disorders.

2. Distinguish between the substance use disorders and substance-induced organic mental disorders.

3. Recognize the nine categories of substances of abuse; the clinical picture produced by intoxication by these substances and withdrawal syndromes associated with them and their pharmacologic properties.

4. Describe the treatment approaches and management of both intoxication and withdrawal syndromes.

5. Develop indices of suspicion and casefinding strategies.

6. Name the treatment options for the substance use disorders.

7. Recognize the importance of a multidisciplinary approach to the management of addicted patients.

8. Recognize the common patterns of drug use and the variations in patterns depending on the drug used.

9. Recognize the prevalence and the pervasiveness of the effects of substance use disorders.

PRE-TEST

For the following questions, <u>one</u> or <u>more</u> <u>than</u> <u>one</u> answer may be correct. Circle the correct answer(s).

1. Which of the following conditions is/are among the criteria for the diagnosis of Substance Dependence?

    a. tolerance
    b. medical complications of use
    c. withdrawal
    d. daily use for three weeks

2. Catabolism of alcohol occurs mainly in the

    a. lungs.
    b. intestines.
    c. brain.
    d. liver.

3. Which of the following treatment strategies is/are reasonable approaches for a newly diagnosed alcoholic?

    a. referral to a subacute detoxification unit for supervised detoxification
    b. immediate hospitalization
    c. referral to AA
    d. outpatient detoxification

4. Which of the following statements is/are true of treatment outcome of alcohol dependence ?

    a. Total abstinence is the only legitimate goal.
    b. Abstinence almost always leads to improved social functioning.
    c. If the patient drinks, even a little, treatment has failed.
    d. The spontaneous remission rate of alcoholics is about 20%.

5. Major classes of sedative-hypnotic drugs include

    a. barbiturates.
    b. benzodiazepines.
    c. carbamate derivatives.
    d. phenothiazines.

6. Which of the following statements is/are true about barbiturates ?

    a. Development of functional tolerance involves noradrenergic neurons.
    b. Some are clinically useful in the treatment of epilepsy.
    c. The use of barbiturates in suicide attempts has declined.
    d. They are useful as adjuncts in the management of pain.

7. Risk factors for drug automatism include

    a. minor head injury in the past.
    b. increased age.
    c. various Organic Mental Disorders.
    d. substance abuse.

8. From the following, select true statements in reference to tolerance to sedative-hypnotic drugs.

    a. Both pharmacodynamic and metabolic tolerance develop with use of sedative-hypnotic drugs.
    b. Tolerance develops more rapidly to short-acting barbiturates than to the more long-acting compounds.
    c. There is cross-tolerance among compounds of this class of drugs.
    d. Tolerance not only develops to the hypnotic effects of these drugs, but also increases the limits of a lethal dose.

9. True statements about opiate abuse in the U.S. include which of the following?

    a. It has always been limited in occurrence to minority and low socioeconomic groups.
    b. Because of high availability and easy access to opiates, the groups at highest risk for opiate abuse are medical personnel, including physicians, nurses, and their spouses.
    c. The epidemic of heroin addiction continues to accelerate.
    d. The addiction rate for the general population is approximately 0.3%.

10. Opiate-induced pupillary miosis

    a. is blocked by atropine.
    b. results from stimulation of the Edinger-Westphal nucleus of cranial nerve III.
    c. is not induced by meperidine.
    d. diminishes as tolerance develops.

11. Factors predisposing a person to Opiate Abuse or Dependence Disorders include(s)

    a. a Conduct or Antisocial Personality Disorder.
    b. a period of intensive polydrug experimentation and use.
    c. an inability to handle strong negative affects in an interpersonal setting.
    d. lower socioeconomic origins, unemployment, minority group membership.

12. Which of the following criteria is/are diagnostic for Opiate Dependence ?

    a. social complications of use
    b. daily use for two months
    c. tolerance to opiates
    d. the presence of a deviant lifestyle

13. Complication(s) of narcotic dependence include

    a. osteomyelitis.
    b. hepatitis.
    c. endocarditis.
    d. death by homicide.

14. Which of the following is(are) acute effect(s) of low to medium doses of cocaine taken intranasally?

    a. local anesthesia at the site of application
    b. increased muscle tone and metabolic rate
    c. mydriasis
    d. production of a subjective euphoric feeling

15. Chronic use of cocaine can result in

    a. cachexia.
    b. a paranoid psychosis.
    c. Magnan's sign.
    d. tolerance.

16. Neurochemical effect(s) of amphetamine include(s)

    a. release of acetylcholine.
    b. release and depletion of norepinephrine.
    c. MAO substrate.
    d. release and depletion of dopamine.

17. Legitimate medical use(s) of amphetamines is/are limited to the

    a. treatment of narcolepsy.
    b. treatment of depression.
    c. enhancement of Attention Deficit Disorders.
    d. treatment of obesity.

18. Although setting and expectation strongly influence the experience when hallucinogenic substances are ingested, certain phenomena are consistently reported. These phenomena, in the presence of a clear sensorium, include

    a. synesthesia.
    b. depersonalization.
    c. heightened sensory perception.
    d. pseudohallucinations.

19. Pharmacologic effect(s) of nicotine result from an initial, transient stimulation and subsequent, more persistent, depression of all autonomic ganglia and would include

    a. increased heart rate, vasoconstriction and elevated blood pressure.
    b. discharge of epinephrine from the adrenal medulla.
    c. increased tone and motor activity of bowel.
    d. inhibition of salivary and bronchial secretions.

Circle the letter corresponding to the <u>one</u> correct response.

20. The U.S. <u>per capita</u> consumption of beverage alcohol has

    a. increased over the past 200 years.
    b. decreased over the past 200 years.

21. Concomitant administration of disulfiram and phenytoin in an epileptic alcoholic is

    a. indicated.
    b. contraindicated.

I. INTRODUCTION TO SUBSTANCE USE DISORDERS

The DSM-III specifies 14 Substance Abuse or Dependence Disorders involving the use of nine categories of substances (Table 6-1). Five residual categories may be used for specified, unspecified, or combined substance abuse or dependence. The substances included in this group of psychiatric disorders are CNS active and produce mood and/or behavioral changes. Some drugs such as cocaine, opioids, sedative-hypnotics, amphetamines (and other sympathomimetics), and inhalants (nitrous oxide and halothane), are used medically. Alcohol and tobacco are accepted as substances of recreational use. At this time neither the hallucinogens nor cannabis has accepted medical or recreational uses in our society. This section of the classification, then, "deals with behavioral changes resulting from taking substances that affect the central nervous system and that in almost all subcultures would be viewed as undesirable" (DSM-III, 1980).

TABLE 6-1

DSM-III SUBSTANCE USE DISORDERS

305.0X	Alcohol Abuse
303.9X	Alcohol Dependence (Alcoholism)
305.4X	Barbiturate or Similarly Acting Sedative or Hypnotic Abuse
304.1X	Barbiturate or Similarly Acting Sedative or Hypnotic Dependence
305.5X	Opioid Abuse
304.0X	Opioid Dependence
305.6X	Cocaine Abuse
305.7X	Amphetamine or Similarly Acting Sympathomimetic Abuse
304.4X	Amphetamine or Similarly Acting Sympathomimetic Dependence
305.9X	Phyncyclidine (PCP) or Similarly Acting Arylcyclohexylamine Abuse
305.3X	Hallucinogen Abuse
305.2X	Cannabis Abuse
304.3X	Cannabis Dependence
305.1X	Tabacco Dependence
305.9X	Other, mixed, or Unspecified Substance Abuse
304.6X	Other Specified Substance Dependence
304.9X	Unspecified Substance Dependence
304.7X	Dependence on Combination of Opioid and Other Nonalcoholic Substance
304.8X	Dependence on a Combination of Substances, Excluding Opioids and Alcohol

To consider the diagnosis of a Substance Use Disorder, some distinctions must be kept in mind. The Substance Use Disorders refer to the maladaptive behaviors consequent to the use of a substance, whereas the substance-induced Organic Mental Disorders described in Chapter 4 refer to the direct effects of substance use or sequelae on the CNS. The distinction to be made, then, is between the behavioral and pharmacologic toxicity of the substance in question. The former is required for a diagnosis of a Substance

Use Disorder, the latter may well be a concomitant of a Substance Abuse Disorder. The phenomenon of pharmacologic tolerance and/or withdrawal is required to diagnose a Substance Dependence Disorder. The issue of the behavioral toxicity of a substance serves also to help make the distinction between unwanted sequelae of the recreational or legitimate medical use of a substance and the presence of a Substance Use Disorder.

A brief review of pharmacologic phenomena and concepts will be useful for understanding the diagnostic concepts of substance abuse and dependence . Tolerance to a given drug is defined as reduced response to a given dose, usually, but not always, following chronic administration of that given dose. Thus, increased doses will be required to effect a given response. Metabolic tolerance is a result of decreased availability of the drug to receptor sites because of an increase in the rate of drug metabolism, thus leading to a more rapid inactivation of the drug. The underlying mechanisms here are induction of enzyme synthesis and more efficient operation of alternate metabolic pathways. Cellular or pharmacodynamic tolerance, on the other hand, is the result of diminished response to the drug at a cellular level. The mechanisms are not known. However, it is speculated that alterations in number, response, configuration or availability of receptor sites, or alterations in neurotransmitter systems and cell membranes may underlie this form of tolerance. Pharmacodynamic tolerance must be present for cessation of drug intake to result in an abstinence syndrome. Although tolerance is usually associated with <u>chronic</u> administration of a given dose, implying that duration of exposure is needed, acute CNS tolerance to alcohol and barbiturates has been demonstrated in humans.

Cross-tolerance can occur when drugs share common mechanisms of action and/or metabolic pathways. It results in a markedly less than expected effect of a given dose of a drug that has not been taken regularly. Cellular and metabolic cross-tolerance exist among alcohol, barbiturates, and nonbarbi- turate sedative-hypnotic drugs including the minor tranquilizers, the pro- panediols (meprobamate, tybamate) and the benzodiazepines (diazepam, chlordiazepoxide, lorazepam). Cellular, if not metabolic, cross-tolerance exists between all of the naturally occurring semisynthetic and synthetic opioids. They are, therefore, opiate receptor site agonists. Two synthetic opioids, pentazocine (Talwin) and butorphanol (Stadol), are agonist/antago- nists. Administration of either to a person with opioid tolerance will result in the onset of the Opioid Withdrawal Syndrome, in addition to the agonist effects of analgesia, respiratory depression, etc.

General criteria for Substance Use Disorders as conceptualized in DSM-III are outlined in Table 6-2 on the following page.

TABLE 6 - 2

DIAGNOSTIC CRITERIA FOR SUBSTANCE USE DISORDERS*

Substance Abuse	Dependence
Pattern of pathological use	Tolerance or withdrawal
Impairment in social or occupational functioning due to substance use	(For Alcohol Dependence and Cannabis Dependence a pattern of pathological use or impairment in social or occupational functioning is also required. Tobacco depenis an exception).
Minimal duration of disturbance of at least one month	

*From DSM III, 1980, p. 163.

Social complications of use as described in the DSM-III manual include: failing to meet important obligations, inappropriate expression of aggressive feelings, erratic and impulsive behavior, and disruption of interpersonal relationships in any or all of several areas (social, familial, marital). Deterioration in occupational functioning (including excessive absences, decreased efficiency and/or productivity) and job termination for behaviors related to substance use are diagnostic considerations. Legal difficulties associated with substance use, except for possession or sale, may also be used in the diagnosis. Thus, arrests for driving under the influence, disorderly conduct, public intoxication, and criminal activity aimed at obtaining drugs either directly or indirectly may be considered.

Finally, signs of the disturbance as described above must last at least one month. Such need not be present continuously throughout the month, but should be sufficiently frequent for a pattern of pathological use to be apparent.

To review, Substance Use Disorder criteria focus primarily on the behavioral and social toxicity of substance use over a specified period of time. The medical complications or sequelae of prolonged, compulsive use of a substance are not discussed or considered necessary to diagnose Substance Abuse or Dependence. This omission may well be a serious shortcoming of DSM-III substance use concepts.

Inspection of Table 6-1 reveals that there are five classes of substance associated with both abuse and dependence: alcohol, barbiturates or similarly acting sedatives or hypnotics, opioids, amphetamines or similarly acting sympathomimetics, and cannabis. Cocaine, phencyclidine, and hallucinogens are associated with abuse only because no clear-cut tolerance or withdrawal states have been documented. The final, specific Substance Use Disorder, Tobacco Dependence, is a new category with its own separate criteria.

QUIZ, Section I.

1. Which of the following conditions are among the criteria for the diagnosis of a substance dependence disorder?

   a. tolerance
   b. medical complications of use
   c. withdrawal
   d. daily use for three weeks

2. Which of the following are included in the criteria for substance abuse?

   a. daily use for one month
   b. medical complications of use
   c. pathological pattern of use
   d. impairment in social or occupational functioning

II.   ALCOHOL

Alcohol is a source of fuel for the body that provides calories, as well as a drug with distinct pharmacologic properties. In the context of this chapter, the focus is on beverage alcohol formed through fermentation of sugar from a number of products, including fruit and grain.

Although per capita consumption of alcohol has decreased over the past 200 years, current levels of per capita alcohol consumption in the United States are estimated by Grossman (1977) to be 0.7 oz/day spirits, 0.5 oz/day wine, and 7 oz/day beer. Noble (1978) calculated the national average for alcohol consumption per day to be .94 ounces. Alcoholic beverages are commonplace in the home and readily available at social gatherings. Alcohol is legally and socially sanctioned. Although it is an accepted fact that alcohol has addicting properties and is associated with adverse physiological and psychosocial complications, alcohol use continues to represent an important facet of American life. The only qualification which societal pressure may exert is that continual drunkenness is frowned upon and alcoholism scorned. Certainly, the misuse of alcohol is no small problem. The number of alcoholics in the United States is conservatively estimated to be 11 million people, and alcoholism is listed as the third most important national health problem. Of the approximately 100 million people who use beverage alcohol, 5-10% do so irresponsibly and with negative consequences for themselves and others. It is no exaggeration to cite figures attributing 20-30% of medical-surgical admissions to complications of excessive alcohol use and 50% of violent crimes (e.g., murder, rape) and highway fatalities to alcohol intoxication.

The most common route of administration for alcohol is oral ingestion. Alcohol passes from the stomach into the small intestine where it is readily absorbed into the blood stream and freely distributed in body water. Since alcohol is a simple nonpolar compound, it readily enters all body tissues.

Distribution throughout the body is proportional to the water content of the tissues. Most organs contain 70-80% of the plasma concentration at equilibrium. Adipose tissue will contain only 10-20% of plasma concentrations because of its low water content and poor blood supply. It is important to note that food in the stomach delays absorption and that not all alcoholic beverages are absorbed at the same rate. Sugar slows absorption, while carbon dioxide and bicarbonate (characteristic of sparkling wines) accelerate the process. Alcohol is rapidly absorbed through the lungs but not significantly through the skin. The duration of effect from alcohol depends upon its elimination from the body. The rate of elimination, in turn, depends upon individual variability.

Alcohol is usually considered to have negligible nutritional value. However, when 1 gm of ethanol is metabolized in the body, 7.1 calories are released, and a significant portion of this chemical energy can be utilized to maintain cellular metabolism. Unfortunately, even though ethanol can be considered an excellent source of calories, and certain alcohol beverages contain other nutrients, the intake of ethanol interferes with normal metabolism of the nutrients contained in alcoholic beverages or other foods. Ethanol interferes with nutrient absorption by inhibiting gastric emptying, increasing acid secretion in the stomach, and producing changes in the motility of the jejunum and ileum. In addition, ethanol directly inhibits the energy-coupled processes involved in the transport of amino acids, vitamins, and minerals across the intestinal mucosa and thus, the transport of these compounds.

The major catabolic pathway of ethanol is via the zinc-containing liver enzyme alcohol dehydrogenase, which in the presence of nicotinamide-adenine dinucleotide (NAD^+), dehydrogenates ethanol to acetaldehyde. It is the rate-limiting step and follows zero-order kinetics. It causes the blood alcohol concentration to fall at the uniform, predictable rate of approximately 100-200 mg/kg per hour, irrespective of plasma concentrations and gives rise to the common estimate that humans can metabolize about 1 oz whisky/hr (Westerfeld & Schulman, 1959). The acetaldehyde is converted to acetate by mitochondrial acetaldehyde dehydrogenase and to acetyl coenzyme A which enters the citric acid cycle. There are two other enzyme systems, the microsomal ethanol oxidizing system and catalase, which comprise lesser pathways of ethanol metabolism in the liver (Isselbacker, 1977).

Disulfiram (Antabuse) competes with NAD^+ for sites on the aldehyde dehydrogenase, interfering with the metabolism of acetaldehyde. This results in accumulation of acetaldehyde and produces an unpleasant syndrome of flushing, diaphoresis, dyspnea, hyperventilation, tachycardia, nausea, and vomiting in individuals not innately sensitive to alcohol. There is initially an increase in blood pressure in response to the accumulated acetaldehyde followed by hypotension, which can be severe enough to result in a potentially lethal state of shock. Inhibition of alcohol metabolism, causing minor disulfiram-like, acetaldehyde reactions, has been reported for several drugs including tolbutamide (Orinase) and other antidiabetic drugs, phentolamine (Regitine), chloramphenicol, furazolidone (Tricofuron vaginal suppositories), griseofulvin, quinicrine (Atabrine), and metronidazole (Flagyl). Disulfiram also interferes with the metabolism of phenytoin (Dilantin), leading to accumulation and the risk of phenytoin toxicity.

The pharmacologic and metabolic effects of alcohol are exerted on almost every organ system, although the most marked impact is on the CNS, where alcohol acts as a sedative-hypnotic depressant. The extent of the effect parallels the rise in blood levels. As with other anesthetics, low blood alcohol levels result in an initial stimulation secondary to the cortical release produced by the depression of lower, inhibitory pathways in the reticular activating system. Moderate levels of alcohol (50-100 mg/dl) often result in slurred speech, euphoria or emotional lability, loss of inhibition, increased sexual desire, and impaired coordination and memory. More severe intoxication (100-200 mg/dl) may be associated with ataxic gait, nystagmus, garrulousness, emotional lability, decreased judgment, and poor impulse control. The effect of alcohol on mood states is a complex function of pre-consumption emotional states and predispositions, dose level and rate of consumption, expectancy set, and other person and context factors. Ingestion raising blood alcohol levels above 200 mg/dl may result in the emergence of anesthetic states, including delirium, stupor, and coma. At levels above 500 mg/dl, respiration becomes depressed and death ensues. Finally, it must be noted that alcoholics develop tolerance to the behavioral effects of alcohol such that overt signs of intoxication are minimized. Large amounts of alcohol may be tolerated, and alcoholics with blood alcohol levels near 300 mg/dl may seem only slightly impaired.

Highly intoxicated patients may represent a source of danger to themselves and others, and their management may be difficult, as illustrated in the case study presented below.

Case Study: Mr. D., a 40-year-old longshoreman, is brought to the emergency room (E.R.) by his friends following a fall which occurred when he attempted to negotiate a narrow flight of stairs and sustained a laceration of the forehead. Although hemostasis was accomplished with pressure applied to the wound with a hand towel, the patient's shirt was covered with blood. In the E.R., he is belligerent and frightened and refuses to allow the Triage Nurse to obtain vital signs. She manages to cajole him into an examining room and calls for a house officer. You respond to the call. After explaining the immediate situation, she provides you with the reassuring history that on the occasion of Mr. D.'s last E.R. visit, six city policemen were required to subdue him after he had assaulted the physician and partially wrecked the examining room.

At this juncture, you might consider:

a. Calling the police and having Mr. D. removed from the premises immediately.
b. Getting together the hospital guards and some orderlies to form a six-man team to be immediately available, but out of sight, should you need assistance.
c. Going into the examining room and demanding that Mr. D. comply with E.R. routine and "cut out the nonsense."
d. Approaching Mr. D. in a nonthreatening, friendly fashion, avoiding prolonged eye contact with him and sitting in a slightly slumped posture, hands open and unclenched.

ANSWERS, Section I._____

1.   a,c
2.   a,c,d
_____

e.   Inquiring about his injury in a sympathetic, nonurgent fashion.
f.   Offering to get him coffee or a soft drink.
g.   Attempting to sedate him with chlorpromazine or thioridazine oral con-
     centrate or administer it IM.
h.   Inquiring if he is feeling anxious and offering a benzodiazepine tran-
     qulizer administered orally in low dose.

Case Study continued: Ejecting Mr. D. from the premises and avoiding
further disruption of the ER does not address the patient's needs. The
extent of his injury has not been assessed and, while it may be minor, you
have no basis for that assumption. If later complications arise, you are
probably legally at risk. Option A is viable only if other measures have
failed. Aggressive or even assertive confrontation, as in option c, may well
escalate his belligerence into an attack on your person. The strategy
outlined in options b, d-f will assure your protection by having a
team close by if needed and will, by your nonthreatening behavior,
de-escalate the situation to the point that a proper assessment can be
carried out. Never attempt to subdue a patient alone; this can lead to
injury to yourself and the patient. If physical restraint is necessary,
at least five people are needed. Medicating Mr. D. with a phenothiazine
tranquilizer could result in a potentially lethal hypotensive episode. If
sedation is needed, a low dose of a benzodiazepine is more appropriate.
One must remember, however, that the sedative effects of minor tranquilizers
and alcohol are synergistic, and alcohol speeds the absorption of diazepam.
Once his condition has been assessed and his lesion attended to, Mr. D.
could be discharged from the ER. Hospitalization is not indicated. Retaining
him in an observation area or sending him to a subacute detoxification unit
(if he is willing) to sleep it off under supervision would be preferable.

Chronic ingestion of alcohol is often associated with serious medical sequelae
as well as deteriorating personal and social behaviors. Probably one of the
earlier long-term effects is suppression of REM sleep with increased Stage 4
sleep. Depression of the supraoptico-hypophyseal system results in
suppression of ADH secretion. In addition, depression of hippocampal and
thalamic areas involved in short-term memory produces an acute anterograde
amnesia with no formation of long-term memory. This is experienced by the
drinker as a "blackout spell."

A common nervous system abnormality seen frequently among alcoholics is
peripheral neuropathy manifested by painful paresthesia and diminished deep
tendon reflexes, particularly of the lower extremities. The earliest sign is
loss of the Achilles reflex which is generally attributed to a direct toxic
effect. Recovery is slow and sometimes incomplete. Wernicke's encephalopathy and the Alcohol Amnestic Disorder (Korsakoff's psychosis),
described in Chapter 5, are thiamine deficiency disorders and, thus, secondarily related to alcohol abuse. Among Korsakoff's index cases were nonalcoholic, pregnant women whose nutritional deficiencies resulted from intractable hyperemesis gravidarum. It is important to remember that thiamine

reserves can be depleted by excessive glycolysis. Infusion of glucose into a malnourished, debilitated patient prior to administration of thiamine can precipitate Wernicke's encephalopathy (Vogel, 1977). Thiamine HCl, 100-200 mg IV or IM should suffice as a prophylactic dose, as well as in the acute management of the disorder; the dose should be continued, either PO or IM, for approximately one week. Victor, Adams, and Collins (1971) reported that of patients with Korsakoff's syndrome in their series, 21% recovered, 53% recovered to some extent, and 26% showed no recovery.

The hypermetabolic state produced by chronic alcohol consumption has a role in the development of alcoholic hepatitis (Isselbacker, 1977). Its clinical findings include fever, hepatomegaly often associated with right upper quadrant tenderness, leukocytosis, elevated bilirubin, and jaundice. There are moderate elevations in serum SGOT and SGPT levels. Alcoholic hepatitis may be the precursor state of alcoholic cirrhosis. It has been shown that the latter will develop in primates despite adequate nutrition (Rubin & Lieber, 1974). Cirrhosis of the liver is the ninth-ranked cause of death in the U.S. and the fourth leading cause among men over 40 years old. Alcohol and/or its metabolite acetaldehyde have direct toxic effects on both skeletal and cardiac muscles. Alcoholic myopathy results in weakness and frequently myoglobinuria. The latter can, when severe, result in acute renal failure. Finally, alcoholic overindulgence may be the leading cause of pancreatitis in the United States among men and is associated with cancer of the head and neck (Williams & Horm, 1977), as well as obstetrical and gynecological problems among women (Sokol, Miller, & Reed, 1980).

Alcoholics of both sexes appear to have higher death rates than the general population. There is also a well-established association between alcoholism and suicide, with rates between 6 and 20 times those for the general population (Goodwin, 1973). Several studies report a greater-than-expected rate of excessive drinking among patients with diagnosed Affective Disorder (Reich, Davies, & Himmelhoch, 1974). In American society, the use of alcohol is significantly related to accidental physical injury and the expression of violence. For example, alcohol is related to half of all traffic fatalities, 40% of fatal industrial accidents, 69% of drownings, 83% of fire fatalities, and 70% of deaths resulting from falls (Noble, 1978). Studies also show high involvement of alcohol in crimes of robbery, rape, assault, and homicide.

The following case illustrates how the various direct and indirect effects of heavy alcohol consumption can combine with catastrophic results.

Case Study: Ms. R. is a single, unemployed, 29-year-old female who was brought by ambulance to the E.R. after her cousin discovered her bed-ridden and "out of her head" in her apartment. The cousin's visit was serendipitous, and he could supply little history beyond stating that, as far as he knew, she had been in good health. He thought she was em-ployed, or had been until recently, and the only untoward thing he could remember was that on a visit a year and a half ago he felt that she was drinking too much beer, "at least a 6-pack a day." The patient's vital signs were T 97, P 85, R 18, BP 120/70 supine and 100/55, in the sitting position. Physical exam revealed her to be a greatly dishevelled, thin, white woman who appeared malnourished. Significant findings were tangled, unwashed, brittle, dry hair; a coarse horizontal nystagmus; moderate decrease in skin turgor; a flaccid paralysis of the distal portions of all extremities with profound weakness, allowing some voluntary movement of the proximal extremities. Her truncal musculature was similarly involved, and she could not sit up without support. Deep tendon reflexes were 1-2+ and symmetric. There was no Babinski sign. Her mental state was such that she could not cooperate with the eye exam. Initially apathetic, Ms. R. became agitated during the exam. She insisted that she was at the Veterans Hospital and had no idea of the time or date. She complained of abdominal pain and insisted that she was in labor. She became frightened at one point and insisted that "the Indian over there wants to kill me." After this, she relapsed into an alert, but apathetic state. Laboratory studies were unremarkable except for hypomagnesemia, elevated CPK, a moderate hypochromic, macrocytic anemia, and a slightly elevated sedimentation rate.

She was hospitalized for both psychiatric and neurologic evaluation. The differential diagnostic list included porphyria, Guillain-Barre syndrome, Wernicke's encephalopathy, conversation paralysis, and hysterical psychosis.

Further tests required to make the diagnosis would include electromyography (EMG), EEG, urine urobilinogen, CSF studies, serum folate levels, and serum B^{12} levels. Further history and nerve conduction studies should also be obtained.

EMG and nerve conduction studies revealed slow conduction and abnormal action potentials indicative of peripheral nerve and skeletal muscle damage. EEG showed diffuse slowing consistent with global delirium. Urinary uro-bilinogen, serum folate and B_{12} levels were within normal limits. History revealed that Ms. R. had been drinking up to a case of beer a day for the past 18 months. The global confusion took two weeks to clear. She retained a profound Alcohol Amnestic Disorder with an anterograde amnesia that left her unable to remember events or information for more than five minutes. There was a patchy retrograde amnesia for events of the previous six months. The anterograde amnesia diminished over the ensuing five-month hospitalization. By the end of the first month, muscle strength and movement had improved such that she was transferred from the neurology service to physical medicine. At the time of discharge, she was ambulatory with the aid of a walker, and her memory deficits could only be elicited by formal testing. Still lacking fine motor control of her hands, she went to live with relatives.

Within the past decade, a pattern of birth defects has been observed in children of alcoholic women that has been named the Fetal Alcohol Syndrome (FAS). The primary features of the FAS are prenatal and postnatal growth disturbances, mental retardation, craniofacial peculiarities, CNS deficits, and major organic anomalies. More specifically, offspring of alcoholic women are small and short for gestational age and do not exhibit postnatal catch-up growth; they have a unique cluster of facial peculiarities such as short palpebral fissures, elongated philtrum, narrow vermilion border, and epicanthal folds; mental retardation and impaired fine motor coordination have been observed in over 80% of the cases, and cardiac and urogenital defects have been recorded to a somewhat lesser degree. The estimate of the FAS is 1-2/1000 live births (Clarren & Smith, 1978). Milder forms of the FAS that exhibit only partial expression of the syndrome have been documented in children of nonalcoholic mothers and are reported to occur at the rate of 3-5/1000 live births. A safe limit of alcohol consumption during pregnancy has not been established. The contribution to FAS of confounding variables frequently associated with maternal alcohol abuse is not known, but it is clear that alcohol per se is sufficient to produce the FAS.

There have been documented cases of neonatal alcohol withdrawal at birth. For the most part, the withdrawal syndrome is less severe than that occurring from opiates. It includes hyperexcitability, tremors, crying, and hyperactivity. Although the syndrome does not appear to be life-threatening, it is important that it be recognized. It should be emphasized that the neonate has only about one fourth the capacity to metabolize alcohol as the adult. For this reason, blood alcohol levels will fall slowly. Additional sedative drugs are, therefore, contraindicated.

So-called "behavioral tolerance" to the effects of alcohol seen in heavy alcohol users results from development of both cellular and metabolic tolerance. However, with continued alcohol abuse and as pathology of the liver develops, metabolic tolerance diminishes. Then, even small amounts of alcohol can produce intoxication. It should be noted that even though alcoholics can tolerate a great deal of alcohol without the appearance of intoxication, the lethal dose remains similar to that in nonalcoholics. This appears to be the case with most CNS depressants. With the development of tolerance, the heavy user of alcohol becomes at risk for experiencing a mild to potentially lethal withdrawal syndrome when intake is suddenly stopped or decreased for more than 12-24 hr. This Organic Mental Disorder is described in Chapter 5.

Withdrawal seizures are self-limited, and in patients who report a negative history for seizures other than those associated with withdrawal, placement on long-term seizure prophylactic medication is not indicated. By the same token, the pharmacokinetics of phenytoin are such that administration in usual doses (e.g., 100 mg tid) to prevent withdrawal seizures is futile because effective steady-state blood levels take 5-7 days to be reached. If a seizure occurs, the usual first-aid measures to protect the patient during the seizure -- protecting the head from trauma and turning the head to avoid aspiration of vomitus -- should suffice. Phenobarbital 60-120 mg IM acutely and then 2-3 mg/kg PO over the next 3-4 days will offer protection in the withdrawal-seizure prone patient. If phenytoin is to be used, then a loading dose of 1000 mg PO or 11-17 mg/kg IV slowly, while monitoring for arrhythmias with the EKG, will result in adequate blood levels (Penry & Newmark, 1979). Oral phenytoin 3-5 mg/kg should be continued for the next 3-4 days. Rarely, a patient will develop status epilepticus for which the treatment is IV diazepam and immediate hospitalization.

There are two main approaches to the treatment of alcohol withdrawal: nonmedical "drug-free" milieu treatment and medical treatment. Nonmedical approaches emphasize a therapeutic regimen of one-on-one support, fluids, and nutrients, but no medications are administered during the withdrawal. Patients are generally accepted only after careful screening for concurrent medical problems. Program proponents believe that sharing in the suffering of the patient establishes a bond which is critical in helping the patient maintain sobriety. It must be emphasized, however, that careful screening is critical because untreated Alcohol Withdrawal Delirium is associated with a mortality rate of 10-25%, depending upon the age and physical status of the person. A second and more common approach to treatment of alcohol withdrawal is medical, that is carried out in hospitals or in subacute detoxification units. Again, certain patients are not appropriate for such units; those with fully developed Alcohol Withdrawal Delirium should be hospitalized as should those with GI bleeding or severe heart, pulmonary, or renal disease. The principle of treatment is based on the phenomenon of cross-tolerance. A wide spectrum of agents have been used: chloral hydrate, paraldehyde, and phenobarbital are old standbys. More recently, the benzodiazepines, chlordiazepoxide (Librium), and diazepam (Valium) have become the drugs of choice because of their low toxicity, wide therapeutic index, and favorable pharmacokinetics. Typical protocols for these drugs are given below.

	Diazepam	Chlordiazepoxide	Oxazepam
Day 1	10 mg PO tid	50 mg PO qid	30 mg PO q 6 hrs
Day 2	10 mg-5 mg-10 mg PO	50 mg PO tid	30 mg PO q 6 hrs
Day 3	5 mg PO bid	50 mg PO bid	30 mg PO q 6 hrs
Day 4	--------------	50 mg PO hs	-----------------

These protocols are merely guidelines. Dose, frequency of administration, and rapidity of tapering the dose-frequency schedule should be tailored to the individual response of the patient. Serax, (Oxazepam) with a single metabolite and a half-life of 8-10 hours, is preferred by many clinicians since it is glucuronidated by tissue, excreted by the kidney, and is therefore not particularly hepatotoxic. The main disadvantage of these medications is that they are very poorly and erratically absorbed by IM route; thus if a patient is nauseated and vomiting, titration of doses given IM will be difficult. If parenteral medication is needed, Lorazepam (Ativan), with a single metabolite and a half-life of 6-8 hrs, may be given since it has the advantage of reliable, complete IM and sublingual absorption.

Alcohol abuse and dependence are hidden disorders; only about 5% of alcoholics fit the stereotype of the street bum or "revolving door alcoholic." Hence, casefinding is made difficult by denial attendant upon the disorder and by family cover-up motivated by shame and disgust. Unless the family physician's index of suspicion is high, the problem often goes undetected. Therefore, the physician must be sensitive to early or frank signs of medical sequelae of heavy alcohol use, including moderate nontender hepatomegaly; frequent bruising or easy bruisability in the nonelderly; ulcer disease apparently refractory to usual treatment; elevation in serum uric acid and triglycerides; and persistent unexplained elevations in liver function tests. Such problems may provide important cues for the physician to uncover, diagnose, and coordinate treatment of alcohol use disorders. In addition, social or personal complications such as DUI arrests, work absenteeism, and weight loss may suggest need for concern and carefully planned interviewing.

Knowledge of possible predisposing factors to Alcohol Abuse adds to the casefinding armamentarium. For example, alcoholism is more common among Scandinavians, Irish, American Indians, and Eskimos than among Italians, Jews, Greeks, or Orientals. Biologic, rather than cultural factors, may predominate in the latter groups. Last-borns are over-represented among alcoholics, as are children of total abstainers or alcoholics. Certain occupations and social settings such as bartending, the armed services, other mobile work situations, and college seem to be associated with heavy drinking. The rate of alcohol-associated problems among physicians is somewhat higher than that for the general population, or 15-18%, as opposed to roughly 10%.

Although it is certainly difficult to tease apart the contributions of genetics or biology, learning and environment, and the combined effects of these factors in influencing the development of alcoholism, evidence exists to suggest that heritability is an important factor in determining drinking behavior, innate tolerance or sensitivity, ethanol metabolic rate, acquired tolerance (metabolic and/or CNS), physical dependence, and susceptibility to medical complications (Li, 1977). In a series of studies of Danish adoption and intemperance registers, Goodwin and colleagues have found that adopted-away sons of alcoholics, separated from their parents early in life, are four times more likely to become alcoholic than adoptees whose biologic parents were not alcoholic (Goodwin, Schulsinger, Hermansen, Guze, & Winokur, 1973). These workers could not demonstrate a similar effect for the daughters of alcoholics (Goodwin, Schulsinger, Knop, Mednick, & Guze, 1977).

Factors which might alert the clinician to alcohol use problems include attention to crises associated with developmental stages and life changes, e.g., adolescence, menopause, retirement, etc. Special concerns are centered around the alcohol problems of adolescents, women, and the elderly. The trend is for adolescents to begin drinking at earlier ages and in greater quantities. Most studies show that adolescent girls no longer drink less often than boys; however, boys still drink more alcohol. There is also rising concern over alcohol problems among women and their special biological vulnerabilities, e.g., changes related to the sexual cycle, menopause, pregnancy (Hill, in press), as well as for the elderly who, forming an ever-enlarging proportion of population, have shown increased alcohol and drug consumption. Still, the highest rates of alcoholism, according to a 1973 HEW report, were found among urban single and divorced men under age 25.

The medical practitioner is faced with detecting a disorder that the patient would rather keep hidden. Although not diagnostic, a screening device such as the Michigan Alcoholism Screening Test or MAST (Moore, 1972; Selzer, 1971) provides a useful casefinding tool. The MAST is presented in Table 6-3. An aggregate score greater than 5 is considered highly indicative of alcoholism. As a screening test, the MAST tends to be over-inclusive;

however, it is adequate for screening. The actual diagnosis must rest on the clinical judgment of the medical professional in applying the DSM-III criteria:

Diagnostic Criteria for Alcohol Abuse (DSM-III 305.0x)

A. Pattern of pathological alcohol use: need for daily use of alcohol for adequate functioning; inability to cut down or stop drinking; repeated efforts to control or reduce excess drinking by "going on the wagon" (periods of temporary abstinence) or restricting drinking to certain times of the day; binges (remaining intoxicated throughout the day for at least two days); occasional consumption of a fifth of spirits (or its equivalent in wine or beer); amnesic periods for events occurring while intoxicated (blackouts); continuation of drinking despite a serious physical disorder that the individual knows is exacerbated by alcohol use; drinking of nonbeverage alcohol.

B. Impairment in social or occupational functioning due to alcohol use: e.g., violence while intoxicated, absence from work, loss of job, legal difficulties (e.g., arrest for intoxicated behavior, traffic accidents while intoxicated), arguments or difficulties with family or friends because of excessive alcohol use.

C. Duration of disturbance of at least one month.

Diagnostic Criteria for Alcohol Dependence (DSM-III 303.9x)

A. Either a pattern of pathological use or impairment in social or occupational functioning due to alcohol use.

Pattern of pathological alcohol use: daily use of alcohol is a prerequisite for adequate functioning; inability to cut down or stop drinking; repeated efforts to control or reduce excess drinking by "going on the wagon" (periods of temporary abstinence) or restriction of drinking to certain times of the day; drinks non-beverage alcohol; goes on binges (remains intoxicated throughout the day for at least two days); occasionally drinks a fifth of spirits (or its equivalent in wine or beer); has had two or more "blackouts" (amnesic period for events occurring while intoxicated); continues to drink despite a serious physical disorder that the individual knows is exacerbated by alcohol use.

Impairment in social or occupational functioning due to alcohol use: e.g., violence while intoxicated, absence from work, loss of job, legal difficulties (e.g., arrest for intoxicated behavior, traffic accidents while intoxicated), arguments or difficulties with family or friends because of excessive alcohol use.

B.　Either tolerance or withdrawal:

　　(1) Tolerance:　need for markedly increased amounts of alcohol to achieve the desired effect, or markedly diminished effect with regular use of the same amount.

　　(2) Withdrawal:　development of Alcohol Withdrawal (e.g., morning "shakes" and malaise relieved by drinking) after cessation of or reduction in drinking.

TABLE 6-3

MICHIGAN ALCOHOLISM SCREENING TEST

Questions	Answers with Weighted Scoring	
1. Do you feel you are a normal drinker? (If patient denies any use of alcohol, check here _____.)	Yes __	No _2_
2. Have you ever awakened the morning after some drinking the night before and found that you could not remember a part of the evening before?	Yes _2_	No __
3. Does your spouse (or parents) ever worry or complain about your drinking?	Yes _1_	No __
4. Can you stop drinking without a struggle after one or two drinks?	Yes __	No _2_
5. Do you ever feel bad about your drinking?	Yes _1_	No __
6. Do friends or relatives think you are a normal drinker?	Yes __	No _2_
7. Do you ever try to limit your dinking to certain times of the day or to certain places?	Yes _0_	No __
8. Are you always able to stop drinking when you want to?	Yes __	No _2_
9. Have you ever attended a meeting of Alcoholics Anonymous (AA)?	Yes _5_	No __
10. Have you gotten into fights when drinking?	Yes _1_	No __
11. Has drinking ever created problems with you and your spouse?	Yes _2_	No __
12. Has your spouse (or other family member) ever gone to anyone for help about your drinking?	Yes _2_	No __
13. Have you ever lost friends or girlfriends/boyfriends because of drinking?	Yes _2_	No __
14. Have you ever gotten into trouble at work because of drinking?	Yes _2_	No __
15. Have you ever lost a job because of drinking?	Yes _2_	No __
16. Have you ever neglected your obligations, your family, or your work for two or more days in a row because you were drinking?	Yes _2_	No __
17. Do you ever drink before noon?	Yes _1_	No __
18. Have you ever been told you have liver trouble? Cirrhosis?	Yes _2_	No __
19. Have you ever had delirium tremens (DT's), severe shaking, heard voices, or seen things that weren't there after heavy drinking?	Yes _2_	No __
*20. Have you ever gone to anyone for help about your drinking?	Yes _5_	No __
*21. Have you ever been in a hospital because of drinking?	Yes _5_	No __
*22. Have you ever been a patient in a psychiatric hospital or on a psychiatric ward in a general hospital where drinking was part of the problem?	Yes _2_	No __
*23. Have you ever been seen at a psychiatric or mental health clinic, or gone to a doctor, social worker, or clergyman for help with an emotional problem in which drinking had played a part?	Yes _2_	No __
24. Have you ever been arrested, even for a few hours, because of drunk behavior?	Yes _2_	No __
25. Have you ever been arrested for drunk driving or driving after drinking?	Yes _2_	No __

*Do not include this hospital episode or any outpatient consultation that led to this hospital episode.

In addition to the diagnosis of the Alcohol or other Substance Use Disorders, the course may be subtyped using the following definitions in Table 6-4. They would be coded as a fifth digit.

TABLE 6-4

SUBTYPES OF ALCOHOL OR OTHER SUBSTANCE USE DISORDERS

Code	Course	Definition
1	Continuous	More or less regular maladaptive use for over six months
2	Episodic	A fairly circumscribed period of maladaptive use, with one or more similar periods in the past
3	In remission	Previously exhibited maladaptive use, but not using substance at present
0	Unspecified	Course unknown or first signs of illness with course uncertain

What do you do when you have decided upon a diagnosis of alcoholism? The first order of business is to share the diagnosis with the patient in a non-judgmental fashion. To judge may serve to alienate the individual. Attempting to engender fear by describing all the terrible sequelae could back-fire. That is, if you scare the patient, anxiety levels will increase, contributing to further drinking "to calm down." In the office setting outpatient detoxification would most likely be fruitless and possibly dangerous. The patient would be at risk for combining a benzodiazepine with drinking, a potentially lethal combination. Outpatient detoxification should only be attempted when the patient has a strong supportive family system, e.g., a spouse or other relative will dispense the medication only as directed. For the most part, your role is to attend to the medical needs of the patient while at the same time allying yourself with the person so that he will allow you to coordinate a broad-based treatment plan that will, in most cases, involve referral to specialized treatment modalities. Treatment approaches for Alcohol Dependence cover a broad spectrum of modalities including self-help groups; residential treatment such as therapeutic communities; psychotherapy including individual, group, and family approaches; behavioral therapies, and combined approaches. Any of these may be supplemented by pharmacologic, ancillary approaches using disulfiram, minor or major tranquilizers, or antidepressant medications depending upon medical indications and the philosophic stance of the modality. Not every approach is appropriate for every patient.

The oldest and best known of the self-help groups is Alcoholics Anonymous (AA), founded in 1935 by an alcoholic physician and an alcoholic stockbroker. Chafetz, Hertzman, and Berenson (1974) estimated there are 450,000-500,000 alcoholic participants in AA worldwide. The goal of the AA program is sobriety through mutual help, support, and submission to a higher power. Members are urged to attend weekly meetings, to read the book Alcoholics Anonymous, and to participate in a network of self-help activities. Sponsors (old timers) are virtually always available to the beginner. AA collects little outcome data, but its effectiveness is thought to be well above the spontaneous remission rate (20%) for alcoholics. Direct outgrowths in approach and philosophy are Al-Anon and Al-Ateen, independent organizations aimed at the relatives, spouses, and teenage children of alcoholics.

Residential treatment for alcoholics is provided by a broad spectrum of programs and facilities in both the public and private sectors. The Veterans Administration Medical Center system offers over 20 specialized alcohol treatment units. Some states provide specialized alcohol and drug addiction treatment facilties. There are also privately funded facilities such as Fenwick Hall in Charleston, S.C. and Willingway in Statesboro, Georgia. On a local level, there are increasing numbers of subacute detoxification facilities which offer a diversity of outpatient services including group and individual counseling, as well as halfway house facilities for recently detoxified alcoholics.

Traditional individual psychotherapy has a poor track record in the treatment of alcoholism. This approach is predicated on the hypothesis that substance abuse is symptomatic of underlying psychopathology: if the patient achieves insight, the conflict will be manifest on a conscious level and amenable to logical problem-solving techniques. This system works well for a host of problems. That it may not be effective for alcoholics as a group is likely related to several factors: (1) Persons diagnosed Alcohol Dependent constitute a very heterogeneous group; (2) A multiplicity of learning factors reinforce and perpetuate abuse in a given case irrespective of the intrapsychic conflicts; and, (3) The historical focus of traditional psychotherapy frequently diverts attention away from the behavior itself and at times even provides further rationalizations for continued abuse. For that group of alcoholics whose dependence arises from their attempts to alleviate the symptoms of a major psychiatric disorder, a psychopharmacologic approach in combination with a therapeutic alliance, has much to offer. There has been a fairly recent shift in focus from the individual alcoholic as if in vacuo to the individual's context, the family. Helping the identified patient and the family understand the communications, strategies, and behaviors which reinforce the maladaptation has potential not only for altering the substance abuse but for strengthening the family system in a healthier direction.

Behavioral approaches to treatment of alcoholism also cover a broad spectrum. Proponents of behavioral strategies conceptualize alcohol or other substance abuse as learned behavior patterns determined by reinforcing consequences. Those conditions associated with a high probability that the behaviors will occur are considered antecedents of the behaviors. The various strategies attempt to identify the antecedents and reinforcers and then help the patient to learn new responses to antecedents and/or new ways of obtaining reinforcement, to reduce the number of antecedents, and to alter consequences of substance abuse. A variety of techniques are used alone or in combination: relaxation training, assertiveness training, and instruction in controlled use. This latter, controversial idea raises the question of treatment outcome. The traditional goal has been abstinence in and of itself, at times without regard to overall social functioning. Just as alcohol use occurs in a continuum, so too should treatment outcome be considered as subtending a broad spectrum of intervention consequences.

QUIZ, Section II.

Circle the letter corresponding to the one correct answer.

1. The U.S. per capita consumption of beverage alcohol has

    a. increased over the past 200 years.
    b. decreased over the past 200 years.

2. Catabolism of alcohol occurs mainly in the

    a. lungs.
    b. intestines.
    c. brain.
    d. liver.

Circle the correct answer(s). One or more than one answer may be correct.

3. Absorption of alcohol occurs through the

    a. intestines.
    b. hair.
    c. lungs.
    d. stomach.

4. The rate-limiting step in alcohol catabolism is mediated by and requires

    a. catalase.
    b. NAD^+.
    c. acetaldehyde dehydrogenase.
    d. alcohol dehydrogenase.

5. Antabuse is used as an adjunctive measure in the treatment of alcoholism by making the individual intolerant to alcohol. This intolerance is the result of the accumulation of _____ by disulfiram interfering with the function of _____.

6. Concomitant administration of disulfiram and phenytoin in an epileptic alcoholic is

    a. indicated.
    b. contraindicated.

7. A 24-year-old married woman comes to your Family Practice office for her prenatal care. She inquires about the use of alcohol during pregnancy. You inform and advise her that

    a. alcohol does cross the placenta.
    b. given our limits of knowledge, it would be best to forego alcohol while pregnant.
    c. alcohol withdrawal has been reported in neonates.
    d. three cocktails a night would probably not be deleterious to the fetus.

8. As a pediatric consultant to the local school district, you are asked to evaluate a six-year-old boy whose lack of growth and poor scholastic progress are of concern. After obtaining a thorough developmental history, performing a physical exam including neurologic testing, and obtaining psychometric testing, you entertain the diagnosis of Fetal Alcohol Syndrome. Which of the following support(s) your diagnosis?

    a. low birth weight and length for gestational age with continued small stature for his age, in a thin child with parents of average build
    b. his face has short palpebral fissures, hypoplastic philtrum and maxilla, thinned upper vermilion and micrognathia
    c. testing reveals moderate mental retardation
    d. his mother is a heavy drinker with a history of multiple hospitalizations for detoxification over the past eight years

9. Mr. P., a 50-year-old alcoholic, is admitted to your ward from jail after 12 hours of incarceration for drunken and disorderly conduct when it was ascertained by the jail physician that he has pneumonia. A call to the local detoxification center, with his permission, reveals that he regularly has seizures when withdrawing and that he has had two documented episodes of Alcohol Withdrawal Delirium in the past three years. Appropriate medications for this man, besides his antibiotics would include

    a. 500 mg phenytoin po.
    b. 1 gm phenytoin po.
    c. chlorpromazine.
    d. thiamine 100 mg tid.

10. Match the diagnosis in the left hand column with the postulated effect of alcohol on the right.

    1. Amnestic (Korsakoff's) Disorder   a. direct toxic effect
    2. alcoholic polyneuropathy   b. indirect toxic effect
    3. alcoholic myopathy

III. BARBITURATE OR SIMILARLY ACTING SEDATIVE OR HYPNOTIC ABUSE AND DEPENDENCE

Use of sedative-hypnotic medications in the United States equals, if not exceeds, that of antibiotics. Major classifications of sedative-hypnotic drugs include the benzodiazepines, barbiturates, and carbamate derivatives. Recent testimony before a congressional committee indicated that 44 million prescriptions for Valium (diazepam) were filled in 1978. However, a recent Institute of Medicine study revealed a 39% decrease in prescriptions of sedative-hypnotics for insomnia. Barbiturates, which accounted for 47% of these prescriptions in 1971, only accounted for 7% in 1977. The extent of sedative-hypnotic misuse is not easily represented by available statistics, because a sizable segment of individuals using and dependent upon these drugs is covert and solitary in their drug taking. Certainly, misuse of these compounds is more widespread than that of the opiates and cocaine and may compare with stimulant abuse.

Sampling a cross-section of over 2,500 household adults, Parry, Balter, Mellinger, Cisin, and Manheimer (1973) found widespread medical and nonmedical use of prescription and over-the-counter (OTC) agents among women and men. Use of sedative-hypnotics among women is strongly associated with high rates of ER and medical examiner contacts as compared to those recorded for men. Figures reflect an association between life-threatening complications and nonmedical use of tranquilizers, non-narcotic analgesics, barbiturate and nonbarbiturate sedative, alcohol, and drugs in combination. Adolescents constitute a high risk group for barbiturate use, and a recent National Youth Polydrug Study report (Friedman, Farley, Santo, & Speck, 1978) revealed that of 2,750 youths, 12-18 years old and in treatment for drug abuse, approximately 40% reported current or past use of barbiturates.

Administered in low doses, the drugs in this category exert sedating effects and induce a calm or tranquil state. The barbiturates are prototypic of drugs which produce progressive depression of function in the CNS and other organs. Distributed to all tissues and fluids, if present in plasma sufficiently long, barbiturates readily cross the placental barrier. Although the effects of barbiturates on CNS function are of primary importance for their abuse, drugs in this class also have a depressant effect on skeletal, smooth, and cardiac muscles as well as on the activity of nerves and respiration. Drug distribution is varied, but heavy concentrations are found in the liver and kidney.

Consideration of the half-life of these compounds is important from two aspects. First, steady-state levels of a drug, regularly administered at a particular dose, are attained over a period of time, five to seven times the duration of the half-life. Adequate steady-state levels of phenobarbital for seizure control may take 11 to 30 days to achieve -- a disadvantage if rapid stabilization is needed. By the same token, tolerance develops slowly. In contrast, regular administration of suggested doses of meprobamate will achieve steady-state levels in 2½ days. With escalation of dose, tolerance occurs, concomitant with the risk of withdrawal reactions. For purposes of detoxification, the prolonged half-life of phenobarbital becomes an advantage; the extended excretion time makes it less likely that withdrawal reactions will occur. The second consideration involves using drugs in this class with long half-lives for their hypnotic effects. Although steady-state levels take longer to achieve, accumulation of the drug is more rapid--a disadvantage in the treatment of sleep disorder. Thus, less than half of a recommended hypnotic dose of flurazepam taken at bedtime will have been eliminated by the following morning. More drug is, therefore, available to interfere with mental functioning and to interact with other sedatives, such as alcohol, during the next day. Gradual oversedation with the development of delirium has been reported in geriatric patients administered sedative-hypnotics with prolonged half-lives.

CNS regions depressed by sedative-hypnotics include the cerebral cortex limbic system, hypothalamus, and ascending reticular formation. Effects are thought to be mediated by release of neurotransmitters as well as by interference with neurotransmitter effects at the post-synaptic membrane. The most commonly reported reactions to sedative doses of barbiturates include slowness, drowsiness, mild euphoria, and weakness. As doses increase, speech is impaired, coordination and visual acuity are affected,

ANSWERS, Section II. _____

  1. b
  2. d
  3. a,c,d
  4. b,d
  5. acetaldehyde, aldehyde dehydrogenase
  6. b
  7. a,b,c
  8. a,b,c,d
  9. b,d
 10. 1. b
      2. a
      3. a

_____

and reaction time is slowed. Sedative doses may also potentiate the mood-elevating and euphoric effects of d-amphetamine and diminish the excitement produced by that drug. Hypnotic doses of short-acting barbiturates may be used to induce sleep; however, barbiturate-induced sleep is characterized by reduction of REM activity. After regular use for a period of time, discontinuation of the barbiturate will result in REM-rebound. Barbiturate-induced drowsiness may last only a few hours, but the residual effects on mood and judgment and the impairment of fine motor skills may be observed several hours later.

Basically, the acute and chronic effects of mild sedative-hypnotic intoxication resemble alcohol inebriation. There is evidence of cognitive confusion, general sluggishness, impaired speech and comprehension, memory impairment, faulty judgment, narrowed range of attention, emotional lability, and exaggeration of personality characteristics. Neurological effects include thick, slurred speech; strabismus; diplopia; nystagmus; vertigo; ataxia; hypotonia; and decreased superficial reflexes. Unlike narcotic analgesics, barbiturates do not seem to alleviate the experience of pain and may produce hypalgesia. However, they are effective in inhibiting convulsions, and phenobarbital exerts a selective anticonvulsant effect useful in the symptomatic therapy of major motor epilepsy. Even in nonsedative doses, phenobarbital may be useful in eliminating major motor seizure activity without producing drowsiness.

As noted above, larger doses of barbiturates produce a picture of intoxication. In severe cases, the patient may become comatose -- a not uncommon major therapeutic problem in large urban medical centers. Although barbiturates may be used deliberately to commit suicide, drug overdose is often accidental. Self-administered overdose resulting from "drug automatism" occurs when a patient forgets how many tablets have been consumed to fall asleep and repeats drug ingestion. Increased age; barbiturate, alcohol, or other drug abuse and withdrawal; epilepsy; dementia; and even minor head injury predispose one to drug automatism which may be preceded by sleep or altered wakefulness (Good, 1976). Respiratory and cardiovascular complications are usually the cause of death. Death is most often attributed to direct drug toxicity, and rarely is one drug present in isolation. Finkle, McCloskey, and Goodman (1979) found that of 1,239 cases of drug-related deaths involving diazepam, only two cases used diazepam alone.

Chronic use of sedative-hypnotics results in tolerance to the effects of the drug, physical and psychological dependence. That the body compensates for the presence of these drugs is well established, and there is evidence of activation of drug-metabolizing enzyme systems manifested by more rapid detoxification, decrease in sleeping time, and increase in average dose required to maintain a given concentration in tissue. Sedative-hypnotic users are often tolerant to the hypnotic effects of the drugs, although as with alcohol their tolerance may not extend to increase the limit of a lethal dose. Attempts to discover the neurochemical bases of tolerance to sedative-hypnotics are as yet inconclusive.

Withdrawal from sedative-hypnotics is similar to that from alcohol, with a range of symptoms including tremor, anxiety, weakness, insomnia, abdominal discomfort, grand mal seizures, and delirium. With short-acting barbiturates, withdrawal symptoms reach their peak during the second and third days of abstinence. However, for the longer-acting drugs the peak of symptoms may not be reached for up to seven or eight days. Those patients who experience seizures may well progress to exhibit delirium, frightening dreams, visual hallucinations, and disorientation. During the period of delirium, agitation and hyperthermia may lead to exhaustion and cardiovascular collapse. Treated or untreated, a full-blown sedative-hypnotic withdrawal syndrome carries a mortality rate of roughly 10%. See Chapter 5 for further information regarding sedative-hypnotic withdrawal.

Development of sedative-hypnotic abuse or dependence may be generally classified in terms of two different patterns described. Since sedative-hypnotics are prescription drugs, much abuse and dependence are iatrogenic. Drugs are secured initially from physicians for therapeutic purposes, such as sleep induction, and the user may become psychologically dependent on them for daily relief of insomnia and anxiety. The pattern of use is continuous with gradual dose escalation, sometimes to high levels. Members of this group of users tend to be older (30-60 years), middle-income individuals not associated with the "drug culture" who obtain their drugs through licit channels. Women may predominate. Longer-acting sedatives such as phenobarbital and butabarbital, as well as shorter-acting hypnotics, are used. The route of administration is almost always limited to oral ingestion. Sedative-hypnotic abuse in this group is covert and is subject to high levels of denial. Persons in this group are under-represented in drug treatment programs and are therefore not counted in CODAP* compilations.

---

*Client Oriented Data Acquisition Process, operated by NIDA, collects data from drug treatment programs.

A second pattern of developing drug abuse occurs in persons of young age (teens-20's) who are looking for a "high." The drugs are purchased "on the street" through illicit channels. Short-acting sedative-hypnotics are preferred. Generically referred to as "Downers," drugs such as methaqualone ("'Ludes", "Sopers", "714's"), secobarbital ("Reds," "Red devils"), pentobarbital ("Yellow jackets," "Nembies"), and a proprietary combination of amobarbital and secobarbital, trade name Tuinal ("Tooies"), are current favorites. At this time methaqualone is the drug of choice. A pattern of intense binge use over several days, interspersed with periods of abstinence or use of other substances, usually cannabis and/or alcohol, is most common. Some barbiturate users may prefer to combine their use with such stimulants as amphetamines or the hallucinogens, whereas others ingest barbiturates exclusively. Administration of these drugs IV is not uncommon. A significant proportion of these individuals combine the use of alcohol and sedative-hypnotic drugs. Drug overdose can occur when alcohol is taken concurrently with barbiturates, even though the dose of each individual drug is sublethal. The combination of the two drugs results in synergistic effect that can be lethal. In such instances, drug ingestion may result in intoxication, anesthesia, coma, and death.

The DSM-III lists two disorders involving the use of these compounds: Barbiturate or Similarly Acting Sedative or Hypnotic Abuse and Dependence, and the criteria are as follows:

Barbiturate or Similarly Acting Sedative or Hypnotic Abuse (DSM-III 305.4x)

A. Pattern of pathological use: inability to cut down or stop use; intoxication throughout the day; frequent use of the equivalent of 600 mg or more of secobarbital or 60 mg or more of diazepam; amnesic periods for events that occurred while intoxicated.

B. Impairment in social or occupational functioning due to substance use: e.g., fights, loss of friends, absence from work, loss of job, or legal difficulties (other than a single arrest due to possession, purchase or sale of the substance).

C. Duration of disturbance of at least one month.

Barbiturate or Similarly Acting Sedative or Hypnotic Dependence (DSM-III 304.1x)

Either tolerance or withdrawal:

Tolerance: need for markedly increased amounts of the substance to achieve the desired effect, or markedly diminished effect with regular use of the same amount.

Withdrawal: development of Barbiturate or Similarly Acting Sedative or Hypnotic Withdrawal after cessation of or reduction in substance use.

QUIZ, Section III.

Circle the correct answer(s). <u>One</u> or <u>more</u> <u>than</u> <u>one</u> answer may be correct.

1. Major classes of sedative-hypnotic drugs include

    a. barbiturates.
    b. benzodiazepines.
    c. carbamate derivatives.
    d. phenothiazines.

2. If treatment is initiated at standardized doses of a **sedative-hypnotic** drug, _____ half-lives are required for the **drug concentration to** nearly reach steady state (select one).

    a. 2-3
    b. 5-7
    c. 8-10
    d. 12-15

3. Which of the following are acute and residual **effects of sedating doses** of barbiturates?

    a. drowsiness from effects on the ascending reticular formation
    b. wild euphoria from effects on the limbic system **and the cerebral** cortex
    c. incoordination from effects on the cerebellum
    d. irritability from limbic system and cerebral **cortical effects**
    e. impaired judgments from effects on the cerebral cortex
    f. excitement from effects on the limbic system **and cerebral cortex**
    g. hypothermia from effects on the hypothalamus

4. True statement(s) about barbiturates include(s) **which of the following?**

    a. Some are clinically useful in the treatment of **epilepsy.**
    b. The use of barbiturates in suicide attempts has **declined.**
    c. They are useful as adjuncts in the management **of pain.**

5. Risk factor(s) for drug automatism include(s) **which of the following?**

    a. minor head injury in the past
    b. increased age
    c. various Organic Mental Disorders
    d. substance abuse

6. Which of the following statements are true in reference to tolerance to sedative-hypnotic drugs?

 a. Both pharmacodynamic and metabolic tolerance develop.
 b. Tolerance develops more rapidly to short-acting barbiturates than to the more long-acting compounds.
 c. There is cross-tolerance among compounds of this class of drugs.
 d. Tolerance does not only develop to the hypnotic effects of these drugs, but also increases the limits of lethal dose.

7. The withdrawal syndrome associated with barbiturate or other sedative-hypnotic dependence

 a. resembles alcohol withdrawal.
 b. is more benign than alcohol withdrawal.
 c. is managed principally by preventing development of the syndrome by establishing the degree of tolerance before withdrawal is attempted.
 d. can easily be managed on an outpatient basis.

8. A dose of 1800 mg/24 hr of pentobarbital is equivalent to a stabilization dose requirement of _____ mg phenobarbital/24 hr.

 a. 1800 mg
 b. 900 mg
 c. 540 mg
 d. 135 mg

IV. OPIATES

Prior to passage of the Harrison Narcotics Act in 1914, the population of opiate using and dependent individuals was predominantly composed of women and the "sickly" who required the drug for pain or psychological malady. Opiates could be easily obtained by prescription or, in some cases, over the counter. Hence, systems of law enforcement, treatment, and criminal justice personnel were not required to function in relation to the use of opiates and other drugs defined as illicit. Once possession and/or sales of opiate drugs became nonsanctioned and defined as criminal, except as prescribed by physicians for specific purposes, different groups of individuals experimented with these drugs and/or became opiate dependent. After passage of the act, heroin use went underground. Heroin dependence was found in urban dwelling minority groups, often those with "bohemian" lifestyles in their late 20's and 30's. In the mid-1960's a dramatic shift in the pattern of heroin addiction occurred. The mid- to late-teenage years became the highest risk period for those who were primarily minority-group, inner city dwellers, unemployed, single, male, high school drop-outs who frequently had a criminal history that antedated their involvement with heroin.

As drug use of all types became practically epidemic from 1965 to 1975, opiate use infiltrated all social groups across boundaries of age, gender, and race (Domestic Council Drug Abuse Task Force, 1975). It was reported, for instance, that up to 20% of U.S. servicemen stationed in Viet Nam used opiate derivatives on a regular basis (Robins, Helzer, & Davis, 1975). The figure 0.3% is accepted as the risk for the population at large. This is small in comparison to the 1-2% for the highest risk population -- the medical profession. The rate among returning Viet Nam veterans proved to be 1%. Persons with psychological profiles which meet DSM-III criteria for Conduct Disorders and/or Antisocial Personality Disorder are also at higher risk.

The opioids include narcotic analgesics produced naturally by the opium poppy, semisynthetics derived from the natural alkaloids, and synthetics derived from coal tar and petroleum products. Stimulated by awareness of the epidemic proportions of opiate use during the 1960's, pharmacologic research on opiates and their actions has blossomed. Among the more important investigatory trends are those which have (1) attempted to specify the effect of opiates on CNS functioning, (2) promoted discovery and actions of endogenous morphine-like peptides and pentapeptides (endorphins and enkephalins), and (3) developed narcotic agonists and antagonists (see Goldstein, 1978). Aspects of opiate action suggest that effects are exerted on highly specific opiate receptor sites neuronal membranes in the brain and spinal cord. Although there is marked variation in opiate receptor density throughout the CNS, opiate receptors have been found to be highly concentrated in such brain structures as the amygdala, hypothalamus, thalamus, and striatum -- that is, in areas involved in pain transmission, respiration, motor activity, endocrine control, and mood.

The sedative effect of opiates results from depression of the sensory area of the cerebral cortex. Low or initial doses of narcotics in naive subjects stimulate the medullary chemoreceptive trigger zone (CTZ), resulting in emesis. Higher doses or repeated use results in depression of the vomiting center. The analgesia produced by narcotics results from effects on many areas of the neuraxis. Nociceptive reflexes are depressed at the spinal cord level. The mid-brain tegmentum is involved, and the activity or responsiveness of such limbic system structures as the amygdala and hippocampus is depressed. The affective response to opiates is also mediated by effects on limbic structures. Pupillary constriction or, more accurately, over-reacting to light, is thought to be the result of stimulation of the Edinger-Westphal nucleus. The miotic effect is not seen with meperidine and is blocked by atropine and other anticholinergic agents. Opiates increase the resting tone of gastrointestinal smooth muscle, thereby slowing peristalsis, increasing the tone of the ileocecal valve and anal sphincter, and resulting in constipation. Atropine partially blocks this effect. Use of opiates in high doses may result in extreme sedation. Toxic doses (200 mg of morphine in naive subjects) may elicit coma, shock, pinpoint pupils, depressed respiration, and death by respiratory arrest. Rapid reversal of overdose can, however, be accomplished by administration of a narcotic antagonist such as naloxone, if no other drugs have been ingested.

Development of tolerance to the effects of opiates is closely associated with development of physical dependence. Nevertheless, there are acute effects of opiates such as pupillary constriction and constipation to which the body does not become tolerant. Takemori (1975) indicated that a change in the opiate receptor occurs after exposure to morphine and continues to change as long as narcotics are available. Thus, he attributed tolerance to a change in quality of the receptors rather than quantity. It is well documented that, with repeated administration of opiates, both tolerance and physical dependence are established. Certainly, the organism compensates for the presence of the drug and for many of its effects, and withdrawal is a rebound phenomenon. In this context, the demonstration by Gold, Redmond, and Kleber (1978) that clonidine, a centrally acting, sympatholytic antihypertensive agent, blocks opiate withdrawal symptoms is interesting. In addition to tolerance and/or dependence, chronic use of opiates is associated with legal, social, and medical complications, as well as increased dysphoria and negative mood states. Chronic users of opiates are seen as deviant and marginal in a society which tolerates neither opiate use nor dependence. Individuals with a history of opiate addiction often constitute sizable percentages of inmate populations throughout the country. Criminal behavior, difficulties in interpersonal adjustment, and occupational problems are common among addicts in prison or treatment. Of course, one of the more perplexing questions is whether deviant behavior is antecedent to or a consequent of drug-taking patterns. Although criminal behavior may increase as pressures to support drug use become greater, studies indicate that more often than not delinquency predated drug use and that criminality and drug dependence appeared as expressions of general deviance or social nonconformity.

Although tolerance and physical dependence cannot be discounted as important factors maintaining drug use, psychological and social factors may be far more powerful determinants in compulsive opiate use. Preble and Casey (1969) concluded that more than the temporary euphoric and analgesic effects of intermittent doses of heroin, addicts were desirous of and dependent upon the active, challenging, and career-oriented lifestyle necessitated by its illicit use. However, not all opiate addicts exhibit behavior patterns characteristic of the addict street lifestyle, and studies of users who do not become physically dependent provide interesting information about those factors which control or mitigate against physical or psychological dependence.

In humans, narcotic self-administration can be seen to serve adaptive functions by augmenting ego defenses by direct pharmacological efficacy or psychological expectancy effects. For many individuals, self-medication motives for opiate use can be differentiated from use prompted by sensation or pleasure seeking. Opiate use may also alleviate anxiety in interpersonal relationships, and the comfortable detachment of a heroin high could prove especially appealing to those who are fearful of interpersonal involvement. It has been suggested that opiate dependence, by reducing libidinal urges, is an effective defense against expression of adult sexuality. Wurmser (1978) described the compulsive use of narcotics as a defense compromise-formation in managing overwhelming feelings of disappointment, rage, shame, hurt, and terror as grandiose illusions of nurturance collapse in individuals whose narcissistic defects are such that no one "significant other" could ever care or nurture enough.

To diagnose Opiate Abuse or Dependence, the patterns and sequelae of drug use must be assessed. According to DSM-III, opioid abuse or dependence follows a period of polydrug use which may involve cigarettes, alcohol, marijuana, and other drugs and comes to dominate an individual's lifestyle. It is estimated that approximately one-half of those who abuse opiates go on to become opioid dependent and that situational variables are highly important in influencing this outcome. Indeed, drug use patterns seem to be complexly related to situational factors, general environmental variables, physiological and genetic dimensions, personality traits, and emotional states (see Sutker & Archer, 1982). The following DSM-III criteria were established to arrive at a diagnosis of Opioid Abuse and Dependence.

Opioid Abuse (DSM-III 305.5x)

A. Pattern of pathological use: inability to reduce or stop use; intoxication throughout the day; use of opioids nearly every day for at least a month; episodes of opioid overdose (intoxication so severe that respiration and consciousness are impaired).

B. Impairment in social or occupational functioning due to opioid use: e.g., fights, loss of friends, absence from work, loss of job, or legal difficulties (other than due to a single arrest for possession, purchase, or sale of the substance).

C. Duration of disturbance of at least one month.

Opioid Dependence (DSM-III 304.0x)

Either tolerance or withdrawal:

Tolerance: need for markedly increased amounts of opioid to achieve the desired effect, or markedly diminished effect with regular use of the same amount.

Withdrawal: development of Opioid Withdrawal after cessation of or reduction in substance use.

Generally speaking, four patterns of nonmedical opiate use can be described. First, one or two-time experimental use is reported frequently by polydrug abusers and individuals in treatment for other Substance Use Disorders. Recreational opiate use, known as "chipping" in the addict subculture, is a second pattern. The number of chippers is unknown in that their drug of choice forces them to be clandestine, and they rarely require treatment or incarceration. Zinberg and Jacobson (1976) described chipping as a relatively stable use pattern and discussed the rituals and rules by which opiate use is controlled among such individuals. This overt structure is analogous to and serves the same function as the unconsciously internalized alcohol use education to which members of our society are exposed as a matter of course. Chipping is usually not associated with physiological or psychological dependence.

A third pattern of narcotic use is intensified use with significant potential for abuse and dependence. Intensive users have more in common with those who abuse barbiturates than individuals who occupy an entire lifesyle with opiates. Indeed, the beginnings of narcotic use are sometimes iatrogenic in both opiate and barbiturate users with drugs obtained through licit channels and oral intake patterns. Narcotic use by physicians and other medical personnel often falls into this category as well as drug use incidental to accident or injury. Brotman, Myer, and Freedman (1965) found that 23% of addicts in treatment at the East Harlem Municipal Hospital were "conform-ists," e.g., married, regularly employed, and uninvolved with criminal ac-tivities. Hence, intensive use patterns often describe socially conforming individuals who resort to "drugstore dope" to manage life crises or physical illness and become addicted to the drug. The following case studies il-lustrate this pattern.

Case Study 1: Mrs. S. is a 26-year-old LPN, referred for evaluation and treatment by her nursing supervisor who had caught Mrs. S. administering meperidine (Demerol) to herself IV. Mrs. S. states that she first used oral meperidine (Mepergan fortis) nine months ago following extraction of impacted and abscessed wisdom teeth. She found that the Mepergan capsules not only relieved her pain, but made it easier to tolerate the stresses associated with her deteriorating marriage and her new job. Her use gradually intensified, and four months ago she found that when she went more than 12 hr. without it she became increasingly "nervous" and uncomfortable with muscular twitching and moderate muscular and abdominal cramping. She escalated use to two to three times daily; to do this, she intensified her pilfering of hospital supplies of Demerol.

Case Study 2: Mr. M. is a 40-year-old social worker who has been ingesting 5-8 Percodan tablets a day (oxycodone, aspirin, phenacetin, and caffeine) for the past 20 yr. He states that he initially started using them to relieve the severe, daily headaches which he has had since early adolescence. "Percodan has been my 'friend' all these years, relieving my headaches and making the daily grind more bearable." His family physician initially prescribed them. When his physician died, Mr. M. attempted to get along without the drug. "After two days I was desperately ill; my headaches returned. I went to a privately run sanitorium for help. I stayed off the pills for four months, but my headaches made life hell, I couldn't do my job...I found myself hating my clients, their problems unbearable. I finally found Dr. E. who wrote prescriptions for me for years."

A fourth pattern of opiate use is that typical of the "lifestyle" user who is occupied on the streets with "taking care of business." Basically, "taking care of business" is a phrase which encompasses all the daily activities related to drug use, e.g., obtaining the money required to purchase narcotics, finding a connection or someone from whom to make the purchase, locating a safe place to ingest the drugs or "get off," and repeating the sequence. Quite obviously, if one considers the price of opiate drugs and the pressures of continual illegal activity, this process becomes a full-time obsession and occupation. "Hustling" is the rubric used to describe the activities necessary to raise the capital for the drug, and the range of possiblities include: pilfering, shoplifting, running con games, breaking and entering, burglary, and other felony crimes. Prostitution is frequent among female users and may predate opiate use.

Many addicts "work doctors" for prescriptions, and an eroded tooth with accompanying peridontal disease could provide narcotics for weeks. Some addicts have learned to fake a variety of disorders; a favorite is renal colic. Feigning the appropriate symptoms and pricking a finger to produce a microscopic hematuria will often earn an enterprising user a shot of Demerol. Forging prescriptions is also common. Many physicians and dentists err in ordering prescription blanks printed with their DEA license number, making forgery of prescriptions for legend substances easy. A few, highly self-inimical, opiate-dependent individuals will go so far as to inflict injury upon themselves to get drugs.

Drug use is not limited to heroin sold on the street. Legal narcotics are frequently available either through diversion of drugs or by robbery of physicians' offices or drug-stores. Hydromorphone (Dilaudid), meperidine (Demerol), oxycodone (Percodan), morphine, and methadone (Dolophine) are frequently used. Licit opiates are also fraudulently obtained from legitimate channels.

Case Study 3: Mr. L. is a 30-yr-old multiple drug abuser who prefers "downers" and narcotics. During a "dry spell" in narcotic availability on the streets, he felt that he was not obtaining sufficient relief from his "Jonesing" (withdrawal) using a variety of minor and major tranquilizers (Valium, Mellaril and Elavil). He tried cooked-down paregoric (camphorated tincture of opium) with only moderate relief. He then resorted to burning his left arm over a kitchen range, producing a large 2° burn which sufficed to get IM Demerol in the emergency room.

Complications of Opiate Abuse and Dependence fall into two broad categories: medical and social. Death by homicide, suicide, and injuries resulting from drug-related activities, in addition to the various medical complications, are associated with shortened life expectancy and an annual death rate estimated to be about 2% each year (Vaillant, 1970). The majority of medical complications are, however, related to the route of drug administration and adulterants contained in street heroin rather than use of the narcotics per se.

Medical complications related to unsterile conditions and to microbial and non-narcotic substance contamination can involve any major organ system; most are infections. Viral hepatitis, usually Hepatitis B, is common. Evidence is beginning to accumulate that non-Group A - non-Group B is also a problem in addict populations. In any event, the usual course is fairly benign. Louria, Hensle, & Rose (1967) reviewed some 40 cases of bacterial endocarditis: 42% were due to coagulase-positive Staphylococcus aureus; 19% were due to enterococci; 17.5% were due to species of Candida;

and 17.5% were due to coagulase-negative Staph. aureus or gram-negative species, E. coli, Klebsiella-Nerobacter and Pseudomonas aeruginosa. The aortic and tricuspid valves were most often infected. The source of such infections is often subcutaneous abscesses or purulent thrombophlebitis. Tuberculosis is all too common in addicts. Treatment of tuberculosis can be complicated in methadone-maintained addicts by the induction of a withdrawal syndrome by rifampin (Kreek, Garfield, Gutjahr, & Giusti, 1976). Cutaneous problems are those predictable from unsterile technique: cellulitis, subcutaneous abscess, vasculitis with sclerosing of the veins. Deeper infections also occur with pyomyositis and fascitis. Osteomyelitis also occurs. The most commonly involved bones are those of the lumbar and sacral spine. Pseudomonas aeruginosa is the most common organism. Tetanus has been reported fairly frequently in addict populations. The disease in this group is fulminant and usually fatal in spite of careful medical management.

Noninfectious complications related to adulterants or the narcotic itself include a variety of syndromes. Quinine amblyopia has been reported. There are reports of rhabdomyolysis with myoglobinuria and acute renal failure associated with IV heroin use (Koffler, Friedler, & Massry, 1976). Pastan, Silverman, and Goldenberg (1977) reported a syndrome of fever, paraspinal myalgia, and periarthritis with no evidence of infection. The syndrome was self-limited and associated with the IV use of Mexican brown heroin. Several syndromes are more directly related to heroin or other opiates. The nephrotic syndrome, sometimes associated with renal amyloidosis, is thought to be an immunologically mediated phenomenon with the narcotic perhaps acting as a hapten (Scholes, Derosena, Appel, Jao, Boyd, & Pirani, 1979). The term heroin or narcotic overdose is used so loosely when death associated with narcotic use cannot be explained that it is almost meaningless. True overdose deaths do occur. The context is usually a naive, nontolerant experimenter who uses too much of the drug or an addict who has lost tolerance. Death ensues, after a period of coma, from respiratory depression and failure. The mechanism of the rapid, highly fatal "heroin overdose" is obscure. At autopsy, the most striking finding is marked pulmonary edema. It has been hypothesized that this may represent an anaphylactic-type reaction to the heroin or adulterants. Often, it is not an overdose in the pharmacologic sense.

The role of the physician in managing of the opiate dependent patients can be difficult. Attempting to meet the legitimate medical needs whether related to complications of narcotic use or not, is complicated by patients' hidden agendas, as well as by federal and state regulations strictly limiting the role of the physician in managing addiction problems. For example, an addict hospitalized for treatment of a medical or surgical problem may legitimately be maintained on a narcotic, preferably methadone, for the duration of the illness. He or she must then be either detoxified in less than 21 days or referred to a federally licensed program. To maintain an addict on an outpatient basis by prescribing opiates for nonexistent medical conditions is forbidden by law.

There are three main approaches to the long-term treatment of Opiate Dependence: drug-free residential milieu or therapeutic community programs, methadone maintenance detoxification and outpatient programs, and multimodality programs including drug-free outpatient options. Proponents of the therapeutic community approach hold to the assumption that the irresponsible and deviant behavior of addicts is probably more binding than dependence on the drug itself. Hence, clients accepted into such programs face a prolonged therapeutic plan which mandates personal responsibility and behavioral control. Close supervision, careful structuring of activities, peer pressure, group therapy and confrontation, reward for accomplishments, and a stratified system of levels of progress constitute essentials of most residential programs.

The rationale for methadone maintenance treatment of Opiate Dependence, originally proposed by Dole and Nyswander (1965), is that Opiate Dependence represents an altered biochemical state of the CNS, perhaps permanent. They postulated that the social rehabilitation of addicts could be accomplished if they were maintained on a narcotic which could be ingested orally, lacks the euphoriant effects of heroin, and lasts long enough so that the daily threat of withdrawal would not be a problem. Extinction of drug-seeking and drug-taking for the euphoriant effects would be accomplished by administering "blocking doses" of methadone. "Shooting up" then to exper- ience the drug would represent a futile exercise and therefore diminish or extinguish. After a period of stability and concomitant changes in lifestyle, addicts might then be slowly weaned from methadone to lead a narcotic-free existence. It is important to note, that for such programs to be successful, they must offer more than cheap, legal "dope." Individual and/or group counseling and active referral and collaboration with other social agencies such as vocational rehabilitation, mental health clinics, family planning clinics, health service delivery systems, and educational institutions are also essential. To be placed on methadone maintenance, an individual must have a documented two-year history of nearly daily use of an opiate and be physically and psychologically dependent upon the drug. Persons not meeting these basic criteria may be placed on methadone for detoxification for a maximum of 21 days.

Over the past decade, active research has been undertaken to develop a long-acting opiate antagonist which could be used more effectively in drug abuse treatment. One example is the antagonist/agonist cyclazocine which was administered frequently in the early 1970's as a substitute for methadone. The drug was poorly accepted by clients who complained of its unpleasant side effects. More recently, pilot programs have tested the long-lasting narcotic antagonist naltrexone. The strategy has been to offer naltrexone to detoxified methadone maintenance clients as a form of "insurance" against narcotics should they impulsively "slip up" and self-administer drugs. Naltrexone is not as yet FDA-approved for general use and is undergoing phase-three studies.

QUIZ, Section IV.

Circle the correct answer(s). One or more than one answer may be correct.

1. True statement(s) about opiate abuse in the U.S. include(s) which of the following?

    a. It has always been limited in occurrence to minority group and low socioeconomic groups.
    b. Because of high availability and easy access to opiates, the groups at highest risk for opiate abuse are medical personnel, including physicians, nurses, and their spouses.
    c. The epidemic of heroin addiction continues to accelerate.
    d. The addiction rate for the general population is 0.3%.

2. Opiate-induced pupillary miosis

    a. is blocked by Atropine.
    b. results from stimulation of the Edinger-Westphal nucleus of cranial nerve III.
    c. is not induced by meperidine.
    d. diminishes as tolerance develops.

3. Acute effect(s) of narcotic agonists include(s)

    a. stimulation of the CTZ.
    b. decrease in gastrointestinal smooth muscle tone with concomitant slowing of peristalsis.
    c. depression of nociceptive reflexes and certain limbic structures.
    d. a state of sympathetic dominance.

4. Which of the following factors increase the risk that a person will develop Opiate Abuse or Dependence Disorders?

    a. Conduct or Antisocial Personality Disorder
    b. period of intensive polydrug experimentation and use
    c. inability to handle strong negative affects in an interpersonal setting
    d. lower socioeconomic origins, unemployment, minority group membership

5. Which of the following is/are diagnostic criterion(a) for Opiate Abuse and/or Dependence?

    a. social complications of use
    b. daily use for two months
    c. tolerance to opiates
    d. the presence of a deviant lifestyle

6. Which of the following patterns of nonmedical opiate use is consistent with a diagnosis of Opiate Abuse?

   a. experimental use
   b. recreational use
   c. lifestyle use
   d. polydrug use

7. Which of the following is/are true about nonmedical opiate use?

   a. Recreational use, or chipping, is usually a stable pattern.
   b. For the lifestyle user, the excitement and challenge of life on the streets are often as reinforcing, if not more so, than the actual drug use.
   c. Opiate users are always dysfunctional.
   d. Opiate dependent persons are over-represented in prison populations.

8. Complications of narcotic dependence include(s)

   a. osteomyelitis.
   b. hepatitis.
   c. endocarditis.
   d. death by homicide.

9. Which of the following factors result(s) in complications of narcotic dependence?

   a. adulterated black market drugs
   b. high risk lifestyle
   c. unsterile conditions of use
   d. the legal status of this disorder

10. Which of the following statements about the complications of narcotic abuse or dependence is/are true?

   a. Lower back pain or localized bone pain in an opiate addict should be considered osteomyelitis until proven otherwise.
   b. The majority of direct street heroin related deaths are due to pharmacologic overdose.
   c. Seemingly minor cellulitis at an injection site bears close observation because fascitis and pyomyositis with rhabdomyolisis and myoglobinemia leading to acute renal failure can develop rapidly.
   d. Nephrotic syndrome in addicts may be related to the hyperimmune state produced by the constant immunologic challenge of IV drug use with the opiates acting as haptens.

V. COCAINE

The coca plant, <u>Erythroxylon</u> <u>coca</u>, is a shrub grown in the Andes Mountains, 1,500 to 6,000 feet above sea level, and cultivated in Bolivia, Peru, and Columbia. Origins of its use are lost in preliterate history, but for 2,000 years Indians in this region have chewed the leaves of coca for their euphoric-, strength-, and endurance-increasing properties. The active alkaloid was isolated by Albert Niemann in 1860 and named cocaine. Both Schroff, in 1862, and Anrep, in 1880 observed its local numbing properties.

Much in the same manner as heroin, cocaine became a commonly used drug in the United States during the early 1900's. Many forms of cocaine were available including vin Mariani, a wine with cocaine, and Coca-Cola, which contained the drug until 1903. By 1914 the majority of states passed laws to control the sale and use of cocaine. So in the same year as passage of the Harrison Narcotics Act, the public was warned that use of cocaine, heroin, and other illicit substances could be extremely dangerous and, in fact, criminal. It was not surprising then that the recreational use of cocaine fell out of vogue between the 1930's and the late 1960's. Cocaine is yet listed on Schedule II of controlled substances. It continues to have limited application as a topical anesthetic and vasoconstrictor in ENT and ophthalmologic surgery.

In 1979, the editor of the Medical Letter estimated that as many as two million Americans have experimented with cocaine. Abelson and Fishburne's (1976) nationwide survey of reported use (within the month prior to questioning) showed affirmative answers for cocaine from 0.7% of adults age 18 and over, 2.0% of young adults 18-25 yrs., and 1.0% of youth 12-17 years. Friedman, Farley, Santo, and Speck (1978) also reported that 25.8% of 2,750 youths in treatment for drug abuse admitted use of cocaine. Street prices in 1980 ranged from $100 to $150 a gram for a sample containing, in addition to cocaine, such substances as lactose, other local anesthetics (such as lidocaine, procaine, and tetracaine), or amphetamine.

The acute effects of cocaine are anesthesia at the site of application, sympathetic excitement, vasoconstriction, and feelings of mild euphoria and well-being. Cocaine, a catecholamine-facilitating agent, is one substance which can, under certain conditions, provide potent reinforcement for self-administration behavior in animals. The acute effects of cocaine resemble those of amphetamine euphoria with accompanying physiological changes such as increased metabolic rate, increased muscle tone, mydriasis, constriction of peripheral blood vessels, hyperthermia, and hyperglycemia. Cocaine exerts a sympathomimetic, principally catecholaminergic action. It potentiates the effects of norepinephrine, dopamine, and serotonin by blocking re-uptake into the presynaptic ending. Other direct effects have also been described.

In low doses, cocaine seems to reduce hunger, thirst, and fatigue, and to promote feelings of improved cognitive and physical prowess and a sense of heightened sexual interest. In moderate doses, these effects become more exaggerated and may be accompanied by dysphoria, marked irritability, and appetite reduction. Van Dyke, Jatlow, Ungerer, Barash and Byck (1978) determined plasma levels of cocaine after applying 1.5 mg/kg topically to nasal mucosa. Blood levels were measurable within 3 min., increased over the next 15-20 min., and peaked in 15-60 min. Levels decreased gradually over the next 3-5 hr. They found evidence from in vitro studies suggesting that cocaine is hydrolysed by plasma cholinesterase in humans. In high doses, cocaine may be associated with restlessness, racing thoughts, paranoia, aggression, and stereotypic behavior such as chewing or bruxism. At higher doses, cocaine can also produce pallor, tremors, cold sweat, headache, weak pulse, Cheyne-Stokes respiration, nausea, vertigo, convulsions, unconsciousness, and ultimately death. Toxic doses may cause cardiac standstill or ventricular fibrillation. Convulsions and then paralysis of the medullary brain center controlling respiration most frequently cause death from overdose.

If cocaine is administered chronically, frequently, and at high doses in humans, cocaine psychosis may develop, particularly among individuals who are marginally adjusted psychologically. In such cases, feelings of anxiety, paranoia, and extreme excitement obliterate whatever positive effects may have been associated with the drug, and aggression or violence may occur. Post (1975) described an orderly progression of clinical syndromes -- euphoria, dysphoria, paranoid psychosis -- related to dose and chronicity of use.

The phenomenon of tolerance has not been demonstrated with continued use of cocaine. Abrupt cessation of cocaine use after continued exposure produces mild physical discomfort but not necessarily a predictable physiological withdrawal syndrome. Negative psychological states are often sequelae of drug use cessation and include lethargy, irritability, and depression.

According to DSM-III, the criteria for Cocaine Abuse include:

Cocaine Abuse (DSM-III 305.6x)

A. Pattern of pathological use: inability to reduce or stop use; intoxication throughout the day; episodes of cocaine overdose (intoxication so severe that hallucinations and delusions occur in a clear sensorium).

B. Impairment in social or occupational functioning due to cocaine use: e.g., fights, loss of friends, absence from work, loss of job, or legal difficulties (other than due to a single arrest for possession, purchase, or sale of the substance).

C. Duration of disturbance of at least one month.

Because neither tolerance nor a predictable withdrawal syndrome has been clearly delineated for cocaine, no diagnosis of cocaine dependence is possible using DSM-III criteria. This poses a diagnostic problem for classifying an individual with a chronically relapsing pattern of heavy, compulsive use. The most frequent pattern of cocaine use today is recreational, usually in some specific social setting. Use of the drug cuts across socioeconomic lines and is not confined to the "jet set" and drug culture stereotype users. Since black market cocaine is highly expensive, cost is a frequently

1. b,d	6. c
2. a,b,c	7. a,b,d
3. a,c	8. a,b,c,d
4. a,b,c,d	9. a,b,c,d
5. a,c	10. a,c,d

cited determinant for the common binge pattern of cocaine use. The following case studies and vignettes are provided to illustrate the range of problems seen with cocaine use and abuse.

Case Study 1: Mr. K. is a 28-year-old single architect whose business is moderately successful. He presents requesting help "for my addiction to cocaine." He is a well-developed thin man who appears to have lost weight recently. He is moderately agitated and tearful and sits slumped in his chair, wringing his hands. He avoids eye contact and speaks haltingly, although spontaneously, with adequate elaboration. "I tried cocaine at a party about eight months ago. I liked the way it made me feel." Up until three months ago his use was confined to weekends. "For some reason I just wanted to do more and more, and I began doing it during the week -- often every night after work. Three weeks ago I did four ounces by myself over a period of three days. The only reason I stopped was because I got scared. I started seeing lights and patterns, and I began to think that my neighbors were somehow after me. Since then I've tried to cut down and stop using coke. That last binge nearly wiped out my savings. I'm scared that I won't be able to stop."

Case Study 2: Ms. W. is a 22-year-old, single, intermittent college student, referred for treatment by her parents. She is under threat of civil commitment by them if she does not stop her use of cocaine. Her father describes her recent behavior: "Over the past seven months I have had to make good close to $18,000 in overdrawn and forged checks. She has continually overdrawn her account and when I closed it out, she stole checks from me and my wife. She has borrowed money all over town and even sold some of her jewelry."

Ms. W. is a thin, intense, well-dressed and groomed young woman who sits nervously on her chair. Her speech is rapid, almost pressured, as she describes her use of cocaine for the past 10 months. "I really don't like what cocaine has done to me...I mean I feel just rotten about the stealing and lying I've done...I try to keep it in mind...but somehow it doesn't matter when I get going on it. I keep going usually three to four days at a time. Usually, I finally burn out. Lately I've tried to stop. But the longest I've gone without is 10 days." She agrees to enter a residential treatment program.

Although the diagnosis of cocaine abuse is appropriate for the cases of Mr. K. and Ms. W., the seriousness of the compulsion to use, particularly in Ms. W.'s case, is probably not adequately described by the term "abuse."

As no formal programs exist for cocaine users _per se_, therapeutic approaches must be tailored to individual patient needs and implemented within available therapeutic resources.

QUIZ, Section V.

Circle the correct answer. One or more than one answer may be correct.

1. True statement(s) about cocaine include(s) which of the following?

    a. It is legally classified as a Schedule II narcotic.
    b. Illicit use in the U.S. seems to be increasing.
    c. Cocaine preparations were available over-the-counter at one time.
    d. Cocaine has been used to treat people with alcohol dependence.

2. Acute effect(s) of low to medium doses of cocaine taken intranasally include(s)

    a. local anesthesia at the site of application.
    b. increased muscle tone and metabolic rate.
    c. mydriasis.
    d. production of a subjective euphoric feeling.

3. Pharmacologically, cocaine

    a. is a sympathomimetic stimulant.
    b. is inactivated by gastric secretions.
    c. acts by blocking re-uptake of catecholamine neurotransmitter.
    d. is effective when given orally.

4. Chronic use of cocaine can result in

    a. cachexia.
    b. a paranoid psychosis.
    c. Magnan's sign.
    d. tolerance.

VI.   AMPHETAMINES

Ephedrine was first isolated and synthesized in 1887 by the Japanese scientist Yamanishi. Rediscovering his work, Chen and Schmidt isolated this compound from a plant and noted that it relieved symptoms of asthma, prompting exploration for more effective congeners (Kelleher, 1977). Amphetamine was among the sympathomimetic amines synthesized, and in addition to its sympathomimetic effects, amphetamine was found to be a psychomotor stimulant and appetite suppressant. The first clinical use of amphetamine for its central stimulatory effects was that of Prinzmetal and Bloomberg (1935) who used a racemic mixture of the d and l forms of amphetamine to treat narcolepsy. The main impetus to widespread use of amphetamine and other congeners, such as methamphetamine, was World War II. As a matter of policy, amphetamine and later methamphetamine were dispensed to German troops. The Japanese dispensed amphetamine to both troops and factory workers, and the British army used amphetamines as well. Some 80 million tablets were supplied to U.S. servicemen by the British. Intravenous use of the drug probably first occurred among U.S. troops stationed in Korea during the early 1950's (Smith, 1969).

Amphetamine was advocated as useful in the treatment of morphine and codeine addictions in addition to the treatment of nicotinism (tobacco smoking) and caffeinism. Benzedrine was also touted for the treatment of head injuries, heart block, irradiation sickness, hypotension, infantile cerebral palsy, sea sickness, persistent hiccup, as well as a host of other ailments. Oral ingestion of amphetamines became a pattern of drug abuse for college students, long distance truckers, and others. Widespread intravenous use of methamphetamine began to appear among heroin users on the West Coast in the early 1960's and rapidly spread to other groups.

Structurally, the sympathomimetic amines are derivatives of β-phenethylamine. Substitutions on the ring and side-chain alter activity. Amphetamine itself is an MAO inhibitor and catecholamine neurotransmitter releaser. The sensitivity of these amines to amphetamine is: norepinephrine > dopamine > serotonin. In addition to being catecholamine releasers and depleters, amphetamine and some of its congeners may exert direct effects on post-synaptic neurons, through metabolites acting as "false" neurotransmitters.

Because of their mood-, mind-, and energy-altering effects and their status as legally prescribed agents, sympathomimetic drugs such as amphetamine and methamphetamine have been subject to abuse among heterogeneous population subgroups. Stimulant drugs have been prescribed for appetite reduction and weight loss and for treatment of depression and fatigue. Such use is no longer acceptable medical practice and prescription of amphetamines and cogeners is now limited to treatment of narcolepsy and attentional disorders. Although not by prescription, many college students are introduced to amphetamines to counteract fatigue, increase alertness, and enhance concentration when studying for examinations. Athletes may also be exposed to stimulant drugs to improve their physical performance and increase endurance. Thus, therapeutic or self-imposed purposive uses of these licitly prescribed drugs may be extended to misuse or abuse for their physical and psychic effects. CNS stimulants are also favorites among street addicts who use them exclusively to enjoy the high or combine them with "downers" for contrast effects. Because stimulant drugs, with the exception of cocaine, may be obtained legally, detection of hidden abusers such as housewives or teenagers is difficult and may be delayed until serious medical attention is required.

Generally, the effects of sympathomimetic drugs resemble responses to stimulation of adrenergic nerves, and drugs in this class may exert peripheral excitatory and inhibitory effects, specific effects on heart and metabolism, and/or CNS excitatory action. Effects of amphetamines include increased systolic and diastolic blood pressures, stimulation of the medullary respiratory center, facilitation of monosynaptic and polysynaptic transmission in the spinal cord, and behavioral activation. Psychic effects observed are increased wakefulness and alertness, decreased fatigue, feelings of initiative and confidence, seeming enhanced ability to concentrate, euphoria and elation, and increased motor activity and speech. Even in low to moderate doses, however, amphetamines may result in report of headache, dizziness, flight of ideas, expansiveness, heart palpitation, emotional apprehension, feelings of dysphoria, agitation, and/or confusion. Amphetamines also interfere with the normal cycles of sleep by reducing REM sleep to almost half its normal occurrence.

Prolonged use or large doses of amphetamines may result in psychological and physical complications. Acute Amphetamine Intoxication or toxic Delirium may be signaled by such signs as restlessness, dizziness, tremor, hyperactive reflexes, talkativeness, irritability, weakness, insomnia, fever, and mood changes. In patients who have a history of mental illness, the probability of more severe psychiatric signs is increased and would include confusion, combativeness, panic, hallucinations, increased libido, and delirium. In acute intoxication, cardiac symptoms of palpitation, arrhythmias, anginal pain, and pallor or flushing may be observed. There will also be hyperactivity, tremulousness, loquacity, diaphoresis, mydriasis, tachycardia, hypertension, and confused thinking. The lethal dose for a nontolerant adult is 20-25 mg/kg, and life-threatening symptoms include delirium, cardiac arrhythmias, hyperpyrexia, convulsions, disseminated intravascular coagulation, circulatory collapse, and coma. Acute cardiovascular complications of high dose IV amphetamine administration are the stroke syndromes of either occlusive vascular disease with gradual onset of focal neurological deficits or intracerebral hemorrhage with rapid onset of stupor and coma. Death or permanent neurologic deficits are frequent outcomes of these complications. Intravenous methamphetamine has been shown to cause necrotizing angiitis.

Tolerance to amphetamines and other sympathomimetic drugs may be greatly pronounced, although a predictable constellation of physiological withdrawal signs suggestive of physical dependence may not be easily observed in all cases. Tolerance develops to many of the physiologic and behavioral effects of amphetamines and other stimulant drugs. Most certainly, tolerance to the anorectic effects of amphetamines as well as behavioral activation and euphoria develops within a few weeks. Individuals will express a psychological craving for stimulants. Upon sudden cessation of amphetamine use, there is a fairly predictable withdrawal state consisting of lassitude, lethargy, sleep disturbance, and an associated disturbance of REM sleep. In addition, there develops a depressive state, frequently profound. Suicidal behavior may occur.

Diagnosis of Amphetamine or Similarly Acting Sympathomimetic Abuse/Dependence requires consideration of drug use patterns and their consequences.

ANSWERS, Section V. _____

1.   a,b,c
2.   a,b,c,d
3.   a,c,d
4.   a,b,c

Amphetamine or Similarly Acting
Sympathomimetic Dependence (DSM-III 304.4x)

Either tolerance or withdrawal:

Tolerance: need for markedly increased amounts of the substance
to achieve the desired effect or markedly diminished effect with
regular use of the same amount.

Withdrawal: development of Amphetamine or Similarly Acting
Sympathomimetic Withdrawal after cessation of or reduction in
substance use.

QUIZ, SECTION VI.

Circle the correct answer(s). One or more than one answer may be correct.

1.   Sympathomimetic compound(s) sharing the basic phenethylamine struc-
     ture include(s)

     a.   norepinephrine.
     b.   amphetamine.
     c.   dopamine.
     d.   serotonin.

2.   Neurochemical effect(s) of amphetamine include(s)

     a.   release of acetylcholine.
     b.   release and depletion of norepinephrine.
     c.   MAO substrate.
     d.   release and depletion of dopamine.

3.   Stimulant drugs may be used nonmedically to

     a.   combat fatigue and improve alertness.
     b.   improve physical performance.
     c.   enjoy the high.
     d.   increase appetite.

4. Legitimate medical use of amphetamines is limited to the

   a. treatment of narcolepsy.
   b. treatment of depression.
   c. treatment of Attention Deficit Disorders.
   d. treatment of obesity.

5. Which of the following is/are signs of acute Amphetamine Intoxication?

   a. hyperactivity and excitement
   b. cardiac arrhythmias and anginal pain
   c. mydriasis and diaphoresis
   d. mood changes and disorientation

6. The IV administration of 25 mg/kg of methamphetamine to a nontolerant adult could produce

   a. cerebrovascular accident.
   b. hyperpyrexia.
   c. disseminated intravascular coagulation
   d. necrotizing angiitis.

Use the following case study to answer question 7.

As the physician for a small college you receive a call one evening from a dormitory counselor requesting your help with a student who is suicidal. You have him brought to the infirmary. T. is a 20-year-old sophomore. His facies reflect fatigue and sadness. He is mildly agitated, intermittently tearful. He is thin and appears to have lost weight recently. Physical exam and vital signs are unremarkable except for fresh and resolving needle marks in the right antecubital fossa. T.'s roommate W. reports that up until two days ago, T. had been "full of energy, on the go all the time, going two or three days at a time without sleep." This had been occurring quite regularly over the past two months. T. himself complains of fatigue; hyper-somnolence; intense, unpleasant dreams; sadness; and helplessness that puzzle and frighten him. He admits to suicidal thoughts. His sensorium is clear.

7. The differential diagnosis in this young man's case includes which of the following?

   a. depresson.
   b. Sedative or Hypnotic Intoxication.
   c. Amphetamine Withdrawal.
   d. opiate abstinence syndrome.

Use the following case study to answer question 8.

Further history elicited both from the patient and his roommate reveals that although T. had been "riding high," he had virtually stopped attending classes, had attempted to study for exams by "pulling all-nighters." For the week prior to admission to the infirmary, T. had kept himself locked in his room. His roommate, the only one he allowed in the room, describes T.

as "really paranoid at times. He finally got so scared that he wouldn't go out even to get more speed. He ran out two days ago and really crashed hard."

8.   With this data you can now make the diagnosis of

   a. Amphetamine Dependence.
   b. Amphetamine Abuse.
   c. Amphetamine Withdrawal.
   d. Amphetamine Delirium.

VII. PHENCYCLIDINE

A substance encountered in ER situations and substance abuse programs all too frequently is phencyclidine [1-(1-phenylcyclohexyl) piperidine], also known as PCP, angel dust, hog, "the peace pill," and "T." This compound was marketed in 1963 as an intravenous anesthetic. Although effective, the incidence of untoward side effects in humans was such that in 1965 the product was withdrawn by the company. Street use of the drug was noted in San Francisco in 1967; however, the high incidence of untoward reactions was such that its popularity was shortlived. In 1967 it was marketed again, under the name Sernylan, for veterinary use only. As of April 1, 1979, all legal manufacture of PCP in the USA ceased (Garey, 1979). PCP began to appear on the streets in the 1970's, and use has climbed fairly steadily. Friedman, Farley, Santo, & Speck (1978) report PCP to be the 7th most popular drug among youths in their study with 31.8% reporting use. Continued use was reported by 67% of those who ever used it. These are knowing users of PCP. PCP frequently is mixed with other drugs, particularly marijuana, LSD, cocaine, and heroin. PCP is also often misrepresented as "pure THC," the active substance in marijuana, mescaline, or other hard-to-get exotic drugs (Garey, 1979; Schuckit, 1979; Sioris & Krenzelok, 1978). There are, therefore, many unknowing PCP users whose numbers may be reflected in the increasing number of PCP intoxication reports appearing in the medical literature. The frequency of such events led Tong, Benowitz, Becker, Forni, & Boerner (1975) to comment that "PCP abuse has become so increasingly common that PCP toxicity should be considered in patients with unexplained acute psychosis, dystonic reaction, status epilepticus, or coma."

The pharmacology of phencyclidine is complex. PCP is a competitive inhibitor of acetylcholinesterase (Maayani, Weinstein, Cohen, & Sokolovsky, 1973). In the peripheral nervous system it has been shown to block re-uptake of norepinephrine and to have anticholinergic properties at muscarinic receptors (Nedergaard, 1973; Weinstein, Maayani, Srebrenik, Cohen, & Sokolousky, 1973). Centrally, it has been shown to affect the metabolism of serotonin, norepinephrine, and dopamine. PCP competitively inhibits uptake of dopamine into presynaptic terminals and causes release of dopamine (Garey & Heath, 1976; Smith, Meltzer, Arora, & Davis, 1977). These findings are intriguing in light of the dopamine hypothesis of Schizophrenia (Snyder, Unger, Blatchley, & Barfknecht, 1974; Tamminga, Schaffer, Smith, & Davis, 1978) as well as suggestive of a mechanism for the drug-induced psychosis.

The clinical effects of PCP are dose-dependent and range from mild euphoric or dysphoric states, distortions of body image, and catatonia to prolonged coma. Mild symptoms result from low dose exposure (5-10 mg), with progressively more severe symptoms as the dose is increased through moderate (10-20 mg) to high dose (> 20 mg) (Sioris & Krenzelok, 1978). However, PCP in even low doses can induce a toxic psychosis which may be maintained as long as two-three weeks past the period of acute intoxication.

TABLE 6 - 5

SYMPTOMS OF PCP INTOXICATION
(Showalter and Thornton, 1977; Sioris and Krenzelok, 1978; Garey, 1979)

Symptom	Comment
Psychological Changes	
Euphoria	Low dose or early effect
Giddiness	Low dose or early effect
Changes in body image, distortion	Low to medium dose
Anxiety	Low to medium dose
Depersonalization	Medium dose
Depression	Medium dose
Negativism	Medium dose
Disorganization of thought;	
Concrete thinking with diminished symbolic thinking	
Impairment of sequential thinking	
Blocking	
Neologisms	
Cataleptic state - a state of dissociative anesthesia	Obtained with a dosage of 0.25 mg. kg
Anterograde amnesia	Frequently appears as a post-intoxication finding
Neurological Changes	
Hyperactive deep tendon reflexes	Low to anesthetic doses
Sensory impairments;	Early to low dose
Diminished two point discrimination, Restricted visual fields, Diminished auditory acuity	
Loss of position sense, taste, and visual acuity	Later, medium to high dose
Eye findings: Mydriasis	Early, transient
Nystagmus, Horizontal and vertical	Persistent 3-4 days
Diploplia	Low to high doses
Diminished light reflex	
Absent corneal reflex	
Bilateral ptosis	
Pharyngeal and laryngeal hypertoxicity	Medium to high doses
Clonic movements, opisthotonos, acute dystonia	Medium to high dose
Ataxia	Medium to high dose
Dysarthria	Medium to high dose
Depressed reflexes	High doses, polysynaptic affected more than monosynaptic
Convulsions	High dose
Coma	High dose, may be quite prolonged at doses >100 mg
Status epilepticus	Doses >100 mg
Physiological Changes	
Systolic and diastolic hypertension	Seen with low doses, increases with increasing dose and may persist for a time (2 - 3 days) post-intoxication
	Not blocked by ganglionic blockers but is by α-blockers such as phentolamine
Potentiation of pressor responses to epinephrine, norepinephrine and serotonin	
Increased bronchial and salivary secretions	
Lacrimation	
Diaphoresis	
Tachycardia	
Cardiac arrhythmias	
EEG abnormalities; rhythmic theta activity, interrupted by periodic slow or sharp wave complexes	
Beta activity is suppressed	
Cardiovascular collapse	High dose
Acute renal failure	Associated with high dose

PCP psychosis occurs with low to medium doses in about 15 to 20% of users. As would be predicted on the basis of the pharmacologic actions, the manifestations of PCP-induced psychosis are like the primary symptoms of Schizophrenia. Disordered thinking and affect are usually evident. Garey (1979) described the course of a PCP psychosis as a tri-phasic phenomenon: "1) initial violent, aggressive and/or disorganized behavior with or without paranoid ideation lasting from less than 4 hr to as long as several days; 2) restless and combative behavior for 24 to 48 hr but in some cases up to 7 days; and 3) personality reintegration and restoration of normal behavioral and thought patterns usually complete in one week but requiring 12 to 18 mo to return to predrug status." Allen and Young (1978) described a time course of 6 to 90 days in their subjects. Fauman and Fauman (1979) found that chronic PCP use was associated with violent behavior; those who became violent with chronic use did not necessarily have a history of violence during drug-free periods. Marked depression, often resulting in suicidal ideation and behavior, is also associated with chronic PCP use.

Management of the PCP-toxic individual, particularly when psychosis is a part of the picture, can be difficult. Because exteroceptive input appears to play a role in the psychotomimetic effects of PCP, attempts to "talk the patient down," as with an LSD reaction, frequently serve only to agitate the patient further. A supportive, quiet atmosphere is therefore important. Agitation and apprehension may be calmed by judicious use of diazepam and psychotic symptoms by haloperidol. Diazepam will also help reduce increased muscle tone. Diphenhydramine would serve to treat the PCP-induced dystonia, if present. Reactions manifested by increasing dominance of neurologic and physiological effects, ingestion of > 20 mg of PCP, and psychotic manifestations lasting over four hours would indicate a need for hospitalization. In addition to the acute episode resulting from either a single or chronic ingestion, Garey (1979) reported an approximate 20% occurrence rate for flashbacks which appear after a single dose for as long as 30 days. These flashbacks are associated with measurable PCP in the urine and have been found to appear in the absence of repeated ingestion. Recycling of PCP, a function of its physical-chemical properties may explain the phenomenon.

The DSM-III criteria for Phencyclidine (PCP) or Similarly Acting Arylcyclohexylamine Abuse follow.

Phencyclidine (PCP) or Similarly Acting
Arylcyclohexylamine Abuse (DSM-III 305.9x)

A. Pattern of pathological use: intoxication throughout the day; episodes of Phencyclidine or Similarly Acting Arylcyclohexylamine Delirium or Mixed Organic Mental Disorder.

B. Impairment in social or occupational functioning due to substance use: e.g., fights, loss of friends, absence from work, loss of job, or legal difficulties (other than due to a single arrest for possession, purchase, or sale of the substance).

C. Duration of disturbance of at least one month.

ANSWERS, Section VI.

1. a,b,c,d
2. b,d
3. a,b,c
4. a,c
5. a,b,c,d
6. a,b,c,d
7. a,c
8. a,c

QUIZ, Section VII.

Circle the correct answer(s). One or more than one answer may be correct.

1. Symptoms and signs of PCP Intoxication include

    a. depersonalization.
    b. concrete thinking with diminished symbolic thinking.
    c. loss of position sense.
    d. acute dystonia.

2. Management of acute PCP Intoxication would include

    a. talking the patient down.
    b. use of Diphenhydramine for dystonia.
    c. administration of Chlorpormazine for PCP induced psychosis.
    d. administration of diazepam, and if necessary, haloperidol to help ease agitation and psychotic symptoms.

VIII. HALLUCINOGENS

The use of hallucinogenic compounds of plant origin is ancient and world-wide. Best known of the plants is the cactus Lophophora williamsii Lemaire also known as Anhalonium lewinii of northern Mexico which was familiar to the Aztecs as peyotl. This plant, containing mescaline, was, and continues to represent, an integral part of religious ceremonies to the natives of the region where it grows. There are several classes of drugs which by altering CNS function can induce hallucinations, delusions, paranoia, and ideas of reference: they include bromides, cocaine, corticosteroids, and amphetamines. However, the unique characteristic of hallucinogens is their capacity to induce or compel states of altered perception, thought, and feeling that are not (or cannot be) experienced otherwise except in dreams, or at times, during religious exaltation.

The first European to describe experiences associated with an hallucinogen was the German toxicologist and pharmacologist Louis Lewin. He described the effects of peyote (mescaline) in 1888. Albert Hoffman, a Swiss scientist, also provided an unbiased account of drug-related sequelae. On April 16, 1943, while working with the compound lysergic acid diethylamide (LSD) at the Sandoz laboratories in Basel, Switzerland, Hoffman accidentally consumed a small quantity of LSD. His resulting experience was so peculiar that three days later he ingested 0.25 mg of LSD with the intent of studying its effects. He wrote about the process as follows (Hoffman, 1970, pp. 93-94):

I decided to conduct some experiments on myself with the substance in question. I started with the lowest dose that might be expected to have any effect, i.e., 0.25 mg LSD. The notes in my laboratory journal read as follows:

4:20 P.M.: 0.5 cc (0.25 mg LSD) ingested orally. The solution is tasteless.

4:50 P.M.: No trace of any effect.

5:00 P.M.: Slight dizziness, unrest, difficulty in concentration, visual disturbances, marked desire to laugh . . .

At this point the laboratory notes are discontinued: The last words were written only with great difficulty. I had great difficulty in speaking coherently, my field of vision swayed before me, and objects appeared distorted like images in curved mirrors. I had the impression of being unable to move from the spot. . .

As far as I remember, the following were the most outstanding symptoms: vertigo; visual disturbances; the faces of those around me appeared as grotesque, colored masks; marked motoric unrest, alternating with paralysis; an intermittent heavy feeling in the head, limbs, and the entire body, as if they were filled with lead; dry, constricted sensation in the throat; feeling of choking; clear recognition of my condition, in which state I sometimes observed, in the manner of an independent, neutral observer, that I shouted half insanely or babbled incoherent words. Occasionally I felt as if I were out of my body.

. . . . Six hours after ingestion of the LSD my condition had already improved considerably. Only the visual disturbances were still pronounced. Everything seemed to sway and the proportions were distorted like the reflections in the surface of moving water. Moreover, all objects appeared in unpleasant, constantly changing colors, the predominant shades being sickly green and blue. When I closed my eyes, an unending series of colorful, very realistic, and fantastic images surged in upon me. A remarkable feature was the manner in which all acoustic perceptions (e.g., the noise of a passing car) were transformed into optical effects, every sound evoking a corresponding colored hallucination constantly changing in shape and color like pictures in a kaleidoscope. At about one o'clock I fell asleep and awoke next morning feeling perfectly well.

_____

The range of compounds capable of producing alterations in perceptual and cognitive functioning is extensive. Most common are the indole alkylamines. All compounds in this group are characterized by an indole nucleus structure similar to serotonin. The indole alkylamines include: the semisynthetic ergot derivative d-lysergic acid diethylamide (LSD); N, N-dimethyltryptamine (DMT, contained in Cohoba snuff); 5-hydroxy-N, N-dimethyltryptamine (Bufotenine, from the skin and parotid glands of the marine toad, Bufo marinus); and O-phosphoryl-4- hydroxy-N, N-dimethyltryptamine (Psilocybin, from the mushroom Psilocybe mexicana). The next group is the phenylalkylamines containing mescaline and several synthetic amphetamine derivates such as DOM (STP) and MDA.

LSD produces CNS alterations at dose levels beginning at .20-.25 mg. Most somatic effects are related to the sympathomimetic characteristics of the drug: pupillary dilation, increased blood pressure, tachycardia, hyper-reflexia, tremor, nausea, piloerection, and muscular weakness. Within minutes of ingestion the LSD user may experience dizziness, weakness, drowsiness, nausea, paresthesias, and periods of laughing or crying which seem to be a response to inner tension. Two to four hours following ingestion, visual illusions may appear as well as other perceptual changes, fear of self-disintegration and synesthesia. Time is seen to pass slowly, and extreme mood swings are common. The entire experience, including CNS and somatic effects, begins to abate at about 12 hours, though the half-life of the drug is about 3 hours.

Sequelae of repeated hallucinogen use include development of tolerance to the drug and possible psychological and physical complications. That rapid development of tolerance to the effects of LSD occurs in humans when an effective dose, 1 mg/kg, is given on a daily basis has been known for over 20 years (Isbell, Belleville, Fraser, Wikler, & Logan, 1956). Sensitivity to LSD in humans returns after a short drug-free period, however. Cross-tolerance has been demonstrated between LSD, mescaline, and psilocybin, but not between LSD and amphetamine derivatives.

Among the biomedical complications associated with long-term psychedelic use is necrotizing angiitis (Citron, Halpern, McCarron, Lundberg, McCormick, Pincus, Tatter, & Haverback, 1970) subsequent to IV injections, resulting in severe renal, gastrointestinal, cardiac, and neurologic involvement. Possible chromosomal damage has been claimed, as well as pancreatitis, renal failure, hypertension, pulmonary edema, and neuropathy. No withdrawal syndrome has been described for any of the psychedelic substances, and death as a result of the direct pharmacologic effect of an hallucinogen has not been reported.

Patterns of hallucinogen use tend to be defined by the classes of individuals who incorporate these drugs into their lifestyle. Hallucinogens are favored among college students, the affluent, and the artistic rather than by those in the lower socioeconomic classes. The one- to two-time experimental use pattern is probably most common. Even among more intensive hallucinogen users, the pattern is more often episodic than that seen with marijuana or other drugs of abuse. Generally, weeks or months separate "trips." Although the overall use of these agents appears to have declined markedly since the late 1960's, Friedman, et al. (1978) in their survey of drug-abusing adolescents in treatment found that 40% reported having used hallucinogens, and of this group 58% admitted continued use. Finally, there are small numbers of chronic users of psychedelics, but even among these, two to three trips a week appear to be maximal.

The DSM-III diagnostic criteria for Hallucinogen Abuse are:

Hallucinogen Abuse (DSM-III 305.3x)

A.   Pattern of pathological use: inability to reduce or stop use; intoxication throughout the day (possible only with some hallucinogens); episodes of Hallucinogen Delusional Disorder.

B.   Impairment in social or occupational functioning due to hallucinogen use: e.g., fights, loss of friends, absence from work, loss of job, or legal difficulties (other than due to a single arrest for possession, purchase, or sale of the substance).

C.   Duration of disturbance of at least one month.

QUIZ, SECTION VIII.

Circle the correct answer(s). One or more than one answer may be correct.

1.   Although setting and expectation strongly influence the experience when hallucinogenic substances are ingested, certain phenomena are consistently reported. These phenomena, in the presence of a clear sensorium, include

     a. synesthesia.
     b. depersonalization.
     c. heightened sensory perception.
     d. pseudohallucinations.

Use the following case study to answer question 2.

A disheveled young man in his early 20's is brought to the ER by two police officers. Although quite agitated and frightened, he offers no resistance to them. He had approached them requesting help, stating that he felt he was going crazy because "I can't get separate from the moonlight music" and then burst into tears. The officers have brought him in because they believe "he's high on something and shouldn't be wandering around like that." Vital signs upon admission to the triage area are T 99.8, P 104, BP

110/70, R 15-18. Physical exam is unremarkable except for mydriasis, excessive salivation, and episodic piloerection. He is oriented in all spheres. He states that about four hours prior to admission he ingested some "purple microdot." He states that while the increased perception of light and sound is "O.K.," he is frightened by the "split off" feeling. "I keep feeling like there's two of me and I hate it. It feels like this has been going on forever. I'm afraid I'll never get back together."

2. At this point, you should

    a. diagnose probable LSD Delusional Disorder
    b. diagnose LSD abuse.
    c. obtain a urine for drug screen.
    d. hospitalize for observation.
    e. have him call a close friend to be with him.
    f. place him in a small counseling room just off of the main E.R. with an experienced mental health counselor.
    g. give 50 mg chlorpromazine IM.
    h. assure him that his perceptions are being distorted as the result of the drug and that the effect is temporary.
    i. give diazepam 10 mg P.O.

Complete the following.

3. Because no withdrawal syndrome has been documented for hallucinogens in this section on Substance Abuse Disorders, DSM-III allows only the diagnosis of Hallucinogen Abuse for which the criteria are

    a. continuous or episodic use for at least _____ .
    b. impairment in _____ or _____ functioning, and
    c. pattern of _____ use.

IX. CANNABIS

Cannabis sativa is the sole species of the herbaceous annual hemp plant (Linnaeus, 1753). Distribution is worldwide in the tropical and temperate zones. Cultivation is extensive in Jamaica, Columbia, Mexico, Africa, and the Middle East. As its name implies, the plant has been cultivated for the fibers of its stem (hemp) and the uses of its seeds for feed and paint. All parts of the plant contain psychoactive compounds, but the highest concentration of cannabinoids is in the flower clusters and leaves. Hashish is prepared from the sticky yellow resin secreted by the flowering tops of the female plant.

In the 1930's the United States Congress enacted the Marijuana Tax Act which declared illegal all use of marijuana, medicinal or otherwise. Nevertheless, marijuana use remains worldwide in prevalence, particularly in Asia and the Near East. In 1956, the U.N. Commission on Narcotic Drugs estimated that regular users of marijuana numbered in excess of 200 million persons worldwide (Tashkin, Soares, Hepler, Shapiro, & Rachelefsky, 1978).

With the trend toward increasing drug use in the 1960's, however, marijuana smoking spread from inner city ghettos to suburbia and college campuses.

Current marijuana use in the United States is widespread. A survey of some 60,000 people between the ages of 18 and 25 years (Abelson & Fishburne, 1976) revealed that 53% of the total had used marijuana and 25% were current users. Numerous recent surveys have shown a general trend toward greater use among older adults across all socioeconomic classes. Consistent findings from studies include: urban residents use at a higher rate than those in rural areas; rates of use increase with higher levels of education and income, and use is more frequent in the Northeast and Western regions of the United States where smoking tends to be less censured from a legal standpoint (Greene, Nightingale, & DuPont, 1975). Friedman and his colleagues (1978) surveyed adolescent drug treatment clients and showed that 90.4% admitted current or past use of marijuana. Of those reporting use, 96% revealed continued smoking. The mean age of first use of marijuana was 12.9 years for boys and 13.1 years for girls.

Cannabis has many cannabinoid derivatives and metabolites, but the most psychoactively potent for humans is the delta-9-Tetrahydrocannabinol, or THC. The pharmacokinetics of THC and its metabolites described by Garrett (1979) differ whether intake is oral or by smoking. Smoking results in a biovailability 5 to 10 times greater than ingestion. The pharmacokinetics of fat-soluble THC are not dose-dependent but are characterized by rapid disappearance from plasma followed by a lingering for days, indicating varying rates of penetration into and return from numerous body compartments. It is known now that daily or frequent smoking of marijuana results in a high body accumulation and that 30 days are required for a single THC dose to be eliminated. Its half-life in tissues is seven days, and approximately 20% of THC is eliminated by kidneys with the rest excreted in the feces.

An average marijuana cigarette delivers 5 to 10 mg THC. Among the acute effects of smoking are stimulation of cardiovascular, ocular, and CNS structures, and mood-altering changes. Immediate effects of THC -- tachycardia and dilation of scleral capillaries -- are well known. Ocular effects of the THC in normal humans include: slight pupillary constriction with no effect on responses to light or accomodation, reduced lacrimal secretion, conjunctival hyperemia, and dramatic decrease in intraocular pressure (Tashkin et al., 1978). Marijuana has also been documented to decrease intraocular pressure in patients with glaucoma with no alteration in visual function, cumulative effects, or tolerance (Taskin et al., 1978).

Moderate doses of THC also produce notable effects on mood, memory, motor coordination, cognitive ability, sensorium, time sense, and self-perception. Users have reported euphoria, relaxation, sleepiness, and spontaneous laughter. As the dose increases to a level equivalent to several cigarettes, short-term memory may be impaired, and performance on tasks of increasing complexity and number of steps may show signs of deterioration. Temporal disintegration, e.g., confusion of past, present, and future also begins to be in evidence. Decreased muscle strength and hand unsteadiness may be demonstrated, although performance on simple motor tasks and simple

ANSWERS, Section VIII. _____

1.   a,b,c,d
2.   a,c,e,f,h,i
3.   a.   one month
     b.   social, occupational
     c.   pathological

_____

reaction times remains relatively unimpaired.   Marijuana smokers report increased hunger and dry mouth and throat. Visual and auditory stimuli, previously ignored, become vivid, may take on a novel quality.   The nondominant senses of touch, smell, and taste seem to be enhanced. Additionally, time is said to pass more slowly, such that minutes may seem like hours.   Further increases in dose can induce hallucinations and paranoid delusions with disorganized thinking, depersonalization, and accentuated altered sense of time. When high enough doses are reached, the clinical picture of toxic psychosis may occur. However, psychiatric emergencies related to marijuana use are relatively uncommon (Drug Abuse Warning Network, 1978).

Many investigators have attempted to identify possible long-term effects of chronic marijuana use. As noted in a review by Nahas (1979), studies have focused on cellular metabolism, lung function, the reproductive system, the developing embryo and fetus, and brain behavior relationships.

Looking at lung function, studies by Tashkin, Shapiro, Lee, and Harper (1976) focused on potential long-term effects of marijuana in 23 subjects who smoked a mean of 5 marijuana cigarettes a day for 47-59 days as compared to controls.   These investigators found that lung volumes, Forced Expiratory Volume 1 sec maximum mid expiratory flow rate, and closing volumes were similar.   However, an index of central airway obstruction, specific airway conductance, was lower in the marijuana using group, suggesting functional impairment.   Further, studies by Huber, Pochay, Shea, Hinds, Weker, First, and Sornberger (1979) at Harvard Medical School indicate that marijuana smoke is more destructive to the defense system of the lung protecting against bacteria than is tobacco smoke.

Among the brain/behavior relationship which may be disrupted as a consequence of long-term marijuana smoking are those related to the experience and expression of emotions, general psychological functioning, and cognitive efficiency. Impairments in memory functioning, including acquisition, storage, and retrieval components, have been discussed by Clark, Goetz, McCarthy, Bemporad, and Zeidenberg (1979) who found organizational process impairment, storage deficits, acquisition loss, and retrieval deficiency in humans, the range depends upon the extent and duration of THC use.

DSM-III criteria for Cannabis Abuse are similar to those for other Substance Use Disorders.

Cannabis Abuse (DSM-III 305.2x)

    A.   Pattern of pathological use: intoxication throughout the day; use of cannabis nearly every day for at least one month; episodes of Cannabis Delusional Disorder.

    B.   Impairment in social or occupational functioning due to cannabis use: e.g., marked loss of interest in activities previously engaged in, loss of friends, absence from work, loss of job, or legal difficulties (other than a single arrest due to posession, purchase, or sale of the substance).

Demonstration of tolerance to cannabis is necessary for diagnosis of dependence. In test animals, tolerance develops to the lethal, hypothermic, and some of the behavioral effects of THC. Both in animals and in humans, large doses of the THC are required over long periods of time for tolerance to develop. Nevertheless, narrative accounts indicate that chronic marijuana users may show little effect from moderate doses and tend to increase consumption to achieve similar levels of intoxication. Evidence is not as clear-cut as it could be, albeit the preponderance of findings support the notion that marijuana tolerance develops in man.

Cannabis Dependence (DSM-III 304.3x)

    A.   Either a pattern of pathological use or impairment in social or occupational functioning due to cannabis use.

        Pattern of pathological use: inability to reduce or stop use; repeated efforts to control use with periods of temporary abstinence or restriction of use to certain times of the day; is intoxicated throughout the day; uses cannabis nearly every day for at least one month; has had two or more episodes of Cannabis Delusional Disorder.

        Impairment in social or occupational functioning due to cannabis use: e.g., marked loss of interest in activities previously engaged in, loss of friends, absence from work, loss of job, or legal difficulties (other than due to a single arrest for possession, purchase, or sale of an illegal substance).

    B.   Tolerance: need for markedly increased amounts of cannabis to achieve the desired effect or markedly diminished effect with regular use of the same amount.

Although there is no generally recognized or well-defined cannabinoid withdrawal syndrome, a constellation of features including irritability, discomfort, hyperkinesis, and nausea may characterize individuals suddenly removed from marijuana use. Certainly, in this case there is a subtle blurring of physiological and psychological sequelae, but for the individual in discomfort they may be both stressing and unanticipated.

Patterns of cannabis use are not well specified. Surveys provide information on the users, quantities, and frequency of use, but little data exist regarding the patterning of use among various population subgroups. The overall impression is that by far the most common pattern of use in the United States after occasional, sporadic, or experimental uses, is regular, recreational use of the drug in social settings. Obviously, any use is illegal, putting all users at risk for societal censure. Finally, it might be noted that there are certain subgroups of individuals for whom marijuana use is both unwise and hazardous. Nahas (1979) summarized the findings by pointing to the following five vulnerable types of persons: 1) patients with lung disease or heart disorder; 2) adolescents whose neurohormonal regulatory systems are developing and integrating; 3) epileptics for whom the CNS stimulating effects may induce seizure; 4) persons with tendencies toward Schizophrenia and mental illness; and 5) women of childbearing age.

Individuals whose patterns of cannabis use meet DSM-III criteria for abuse or dependence are often quite conflicted and/or character disorders. Often, the cannabis use pattern is that of self-medication. Frequently the dysfunctional use of cannabis is in the setting of multiple substance use and abuse.

QUIZ, Section IX.

Circle the correct answer(s). One or more than one answer may be correct.

1.   Which of the following are true statements about cannabis ?

   a.   Cannabis is used to make rope.
   b.   Cannabis use has been strictly limited to recreational use because of its psychoactive properties.
   c.   Cannabis is the most prevalent illicit drug in use today.
   d.   Cannabis use was banned in the U.S.A. in 1937.
   e.   Cannabis use is more frequent in individuals from higher educational and socioeconomic groups.

2.   You are asked by the PTA to answer questions by concerned parents about substance abuse. One parent asks for some signs she can use to tell if her child has been smoking marijuana. Which of the following clues would you consider accurate and reliable?

   a.   tachycardia with rates up to 140/min
   b.   euphoria, intoxicated behavior
   c.   odor of marijuana smoke on breath or in clothing
   d.   hyperemia of sclerae and conjunctiva

3.   Another parent of the audience challenges your last statement, saying that he knows he's caught his son high on pot but he did not see the "red eyes." You explain this by stating

   a.   conjunctival hyperemia isn't all that common.
   b.   that this effect is common knowledge and that common over-the-counter eyedrops will eliminate this sign.

Use the following case studies to answer questions 4-5.

Case Study 1: Anne F. is a 16-year-old high school student referred for treatment by her school adviser, at Anne's request. She has been doing fairly well in school, although over the past four months she has dropped from all A's to C's. Anne reports that she began using marijuana at age 13. Her pattern of use up until 6 months ago was to smoke "a few joints with my friends at parties on weekends." She is concerned because now, "I'm smoking five or six joints a night...staying high is the only way I can stand being at home, the hassle I get from my Mom and Dad doesn't matter so much." She describes herself as anxious and tense most of the time; "The pot does help me relax." She complains that at times her parents are over-controlling and at others distant, uninvolved and uncaring. She is particularly upset by the change in her relationship with her father. "We used to be so close, now he acts like he's angry with me most of the time." Added now to her worries over her family problems is her concern that her use of marijuana has gotten out of hand. "I can't seem to leave it alone and I know that if I keep it up, not only will I get caught but my school work will be hurt more. As it is now I get behind 'cause I just don't study as well when I'm high. At first I thought I did, but I don't really." Anne denies use of alcohol beyond "a beer once in a while at a party" and denies use of any other drug or substance. She does not smoke tobacco.

Case Study 2: Joe M. is a 20-year-old, intermittently employed carpenter's helper, referred for treatment by his lawyer following his third arrest for driving under the influence (DUI) and driving without a valid driver's license. He states that he has been "smoking reefer since I was 12 years old." He describes daily use by age 13, stating that by then he and his friends would skip out of school after homeroom and "get stoned." The excessive truancy resulted in failure of the school year so that by the time he was 16 years old and could legally drop out he was still in the ninth grade.

After losing a job for being "stoned" at work, he curtailed his cannabis use, restricting it to the evening. His pattern of substance use expanded to include beer and wine on a regular basis along with the marijuana. He reports, in retrospect, that "by the time I was 17, even 6 or 7 joints didn't do much for me and I began using 'ludes (methaqualone), usually one or two Roerig 714's to really mellow out."

He experimented with a variety of "chemicals"; but decided that both "tripping" and "speeding" were unpleasant for him. "I prefer the downers; the high is better; and I feel calmer." His most recent DUI, as with the other two, followed an evening with his friends during which he had smoked 6 joints, had 4 beers, and 2 tablets of methaqualone.

4.   Which of the following statements is/are true about Anne F.?

    a.   A diagnosis of Cannabis Abuse is warranted.
    b.   A diagnosis of Cannabis Dependence is warranted.
    c.   Family Therapy would be an appropriate part of her treatment plan.
    d.   Because she realizes that cannabis is a problem for her, a psychiatric diagnosis is not indicated.
    e.   From a developmental perspective, her conflicts with her parents are atypical.

5.   Which of the following statements is/are true with regard to Joe M.?

    a.   He seems to meet the criteria for a diagnosis of Cannabis Dependence.
    b.   Barbiturate or Similar Acting Sedative Hypnotic Abuse would be a second Axis I diagnosis.
    c.   Joe will need detoxification from cannabis.
    d.   He will need careful evaluation of his degree of tolerance to both alcohol and methaqualone to find out if a supervised detoxification is warranted.

X. TOBACCO

The practice of inhaling smoke produced by burning dried leaves of the plant Nicotiana tabacum and its cultivation date to the early years of the Age of Exploration. At the close of the 15th century, Portuguese, Spanish, and English mariners carried tobacco on their voyages and taught those they came in contact with its use and cultivation. By 1542, tobacco had been introduced to lands as distant from Europe as Japan; on the continent, use had spread through central Europe by mid-17th century.

By the 18th century, tobacco use was almost universally accepted if not officially sanctioned, whether smoked, inhaled as snuff, or chewed. Cigars and pipes were the sole sources of tobacco smoke until the mid-1880's when advances in paper technology and automatic manufacturing machinery resulted in development and marketing of cigarettes. The first decade of the 20th century, 4.2 billion cigarettes were produced a year, and by 1970 the figure was 583 billion (Brecher, 1972).

Although hundreds of tobacco smoke constituents have been described, the major pharmacologic effects of tobacco use are produced by the potent cholinomimetic alkaloid nicotine. The pharmacology of this compound is complex and beyond the scope of this chapter. Nicotine has both stimulant and depressant phases of action, so that the ultimate response of a structure or system will represent the algebraic summation of the various and opposing effects of nicotine. Nicotine is a CNS stimulant, and with high doses the stimulant effects are followed by depression. Death will result from both central paralysis and peripheral blockade of the respiratory musculature.

With continued use, tolerance develops to the effects of nicotine as do physical and psychological dependence. The withdrawal syndrome associated with reduction or cessation of nicotine intake is described in Chapter 5. A number of psychological symptoms may also be evidenced during withdrawal, many of which are likely exaggerated responses to stress unique to the individual. Continued tobacco use, primarily cigarette smoking, has been implicated as a significant risk factor or etiologic contributor to many diseases. Many of these complications were described in 1964 by the Surgeon General's Advisory Committee on Smoking and Health. The information disseminated and the public debate engendered by this and other reports have, after 15 years, resulted in shifts in public attitudes toward and acceptance of tobacco use. Statutes restricting public smoking are abundant, and an ever-increasing array of private and governmental bodies are engaged in activities designed to diminish or eliminate tobacco use. The public and most smokers included seem to have accepted that cigarette smoking is hazardous to overall health.

Cognizance of growing public concern about the effects of smoking is reflected by inclusion of the category, Tobacco Dependence, in DSM-III. Criteria for determining this disorder are different from those of the other Substance Use Disorders. Tobacco use is so common in our culture that it is considered normative. The withdrawal reaction is not considered "illness." Tobacco use per se rarely produces a definable state of intoxication as does alcohol. For these reasons, tobacco use would be difficult to define as a disorder if the usual criteria applied to other Substance Use Disorders in DSM-III were used. Hence, the criteria specify:

Tobacco Dependence (DSM-III 305.1x)

A. Continuous use of tobacco for at least one month.

B. At least one of the following:

   (1) serious attempts to stop or significantly reduce the amount of tobacco use on a permanent basis have been unsuccessful
   (2) attempts to stop smoking have led to the development of Tobacco Withdrawal
   (3) the individual continues to use tobacco despite a serious physical disorder (e.g., respiratory or cardiovascular disease) that he or she knows is exacerbated by tobacco use

In American society, patterns of tobacco use usually begin in adolescence. Equal numbers of girls and boys seem to experiment with the drug, but among older smokers, use is somewhat more prevalent among men (Abelson, Fishburn & Cisin, 1977). Tobacco smoking occurs more frequently in individuals with other substance abuse problems, often involving alcohol or the opioids. Some smokers extend the habit over a brief course and report relatively little discomfort upon quitting. More commonly, others find it exceedingly difficult to quit. Because of the extent of the problem and its seeming resistance to change, a wide range of treatment approaches have

ANSWERS, Section IX. _____

1. a,c,d,e
2. a,c,d
3. b
4. a,c
5. a,b,d

_____

been developed for application to individual needs. These include behavior modification strategies, psychotherapy, group therapy, hypnotism, and meditation techniques. There have also been attempts to use lobeline to wean people from nicotine. Regardless of the approach, treatment results have been discouraging, and recidivism rates may be as a great as 50% at six months and 70% or higher at one year. The high incidence of failure is related to a secondary use pattern of smoking among individuals who have tried to stop smoking and failed. Often such persons become secretive smokers and hide their behavior from family and colleagues. In addition, a loss in self-esteem, guilt, and depression may be experienced.

_____

QUIZ, Section X.

Circle the correct answer. One or more than one answer may be correct.

1. Pharmacologic effect(s) of nicotine result from an initial, transient stimulation and subsequent, more persistent, depression of all autonomic ganglia and would include

    a. increased heart rate, vasoconstriction, and elevated blood pressure.
    b. discharge of epinephrine from the adrenal medulla.
    c. increased tone and motor activity of bowel.
    d. inhibition of salivary and bronchial secretions.

Use the following case study to answer questions 2-3.

During his years in medical school and as a house officer, Dr. F. had developed the habit of smoking up to 20 cigars daily. At the age of 38, he noted onset of severe chest pain associated with smoking cigars. The angina persisted. He consulted a colleague who ascertained that Dr. F. developed a transient arrhythmia on some occasions when he smoked a cigar. He was advised to stop smoking. Dr. F. attempted to do so. He reported that, "soon after giving up smoking there were tolerable days...Then there came suddenly a severe affliction of the heart, worse than I ever had when smoking...And with it an oppression of mood in which images of dying and farewell scenes replaced the more usual fantasies." After 7 weeks he resumed smoking. Later he was able to maintain abstinence for 14 months, but at such an emotional cost to him, he capitulated and began smoking again. When he was 67 years old, he noted sores on his right palate and jaw that failed to heal. Over the next 16 years he underwent 33 operations for cancer of the jaw and oral cavity. He continued to use cigars. At age 73 he again attempted to stop; this lasted 23 days. At 81, he was still smoking 20 cigars a day. He died at age 83 in 1939. The physician's name was Sigmund Freud.

2. Which of the following criteria for a diagnosis of Tobacco Dependence is/ are met?

    a. continuous use of tobacco for at least one month
    b. serious attempts to stop or reduce tobacco use on a permanent basis were unsuccessful
    c. social complications of use
    d. the presence of a serious physical disorder in which tobacco smoking is a significant etiological or exacerbating factor

3. In this case a diagnosis of Tobacco Use Dependence _____ warranted.

    a. is
    b. is not

XI. RESIDUAL CATEGORIES

The DSM-III provides for five residual diagnostic categories of Substance Use Disorders. Other, Mixed, or Unspecified Substance Abuse, (305.9x) categories would be used if the substance of abuse or dependence cannot be classified in any other category or is as yet unknown. Mixed Substance Abuse involves abuse of substances from more than one nonalcoholic substance category and should be used only when the specific substance cannot be identified or when so many substances are abused that it would be preferrable to indicate a combination of substances rather than list each separately. A second residual category, Other Specified Substance Dependence, 304.6x, should be used when the person is dependent on a substance such as Toluene which is not classified in any other category. Another diagnostic category, 304.9X, Unspecified Substance Dependence, would be used as an initial diagnosis when the specific substance is not yet known. The last two categories, 304.7x, Dependence on a Combination of Opioid and Other Nonalcoholic Substances, and 304.8x, Dependence on a Combination of Substances, Excluding Opioids and Alcohol, would be used when several substances are being abused at the same time. These categories should be used only when the specific substances cannot be identified or when the dependence involves so many substances that it would be preferable to indicate a combination of substances rather than list each specific substance.

There are several substances or groups of substances, not classified elsewhere, that are used with enough frequency to merit brief discussion here. The first is the inhalants, divided into two subgroups: 1) the industrial volatiles or organic solvents and 2) gaseous anesthetics.

The volatile anesthetic agents include ether, chloroform, nitrous oxide and, more recently, halothane. Historically, recreational use predated medicinal use of the first three agents. Ether and chloroform are seldom used for recreational purposes today, but nitrous oxide and halothane continue to be used nonmedically. Acute effects resulting from the use of these substances include irritation of the eyes, sensitivity to light, double vision, ringing in the ears, irritation of the lining or mucous membrane of the nose and mouth, and a cough. An abuser may also complain of nausea, vomiting, and diarrhea, and become faint or demonstrate arrhythmias (Schuckit, 1979). In spite of the fact that these agents are safe anesthetics, their abuse frequently leads to toxicity. Recently, Kaplan, Bakken, Quadracci, and Schubach (1979) reported three cases of halothane abuse in ancillary operating room personnel. All three demonstrated clinical signs of hepatotoxicity; one person developed fulminant centrolobular hepatitis with acute yellow atrophy, and one person died.

In addition to inhalation of anesthetic agents, "huffing" organic solvents such as toluene, paint, or airplane glue for the purpose of intoxication is a phenomenon of the 1960's. As with the volatile anesthetics, a solvent high may occur unintentionally in the course of employment. Toxic effects have been reported in chronic recreational users (Taher, Anderson, & McCartney, 1974). It is of interest to note that recreational users of organic solvents are primarily adolescents. Cohen (1977) reported that about five times as many adolescents experiment with solvents as those who become regular users. Concurrent experimentation with other substances, particularly cannabis and alcohol, usually results in a switch from inhalants to other drugs. Huffing becomes viewed as childish, and the uncontrolled, transient high derived from inhalants is considered inferior to the more sustained effects of the new drug of choice.

The following case vignettes illustrate the range often seen in exclusive solvent use.

Case Study 1: Robert S. is a 13-year-old, eighth grade student, in good standing, brought in for treatment by his mother. Mrs. S. explains that the previous Saturday afternoon she had noted her son acting strangely. "He was giddy and couldn't seem to walk right. He didn't seem to notice me watching him. I ran inside to call my husband. By the time he got home 15 minutes later Robbie seemed O.K. When we asked him what was wrong he looked a little puzzled but said he was all right and finished mowing the lawn. Then yesterday, we caught him out in the shed sniffing a gasoline-soaked rag. He got sick to his stomach and threw up. We took him to the emergency room. The doctors there said he was all right and recommended that we bring him here. Robbie claims he only remembers going to the shed." Robbie is a slender, neatly groomed, bespectacled adolescent who appears younger than his stated age. Physical and mental status exams are entirely within normal limits except for a lacunar, retrograde amnesia for the events described by his mother. He describes feeling "funny" that Saturday; "I was putting gas in the lawn mower out in the shed and spilled some. I started feeling strange as I was cleaning it up. I got O.K. pretty quick. I thought it might have been the gasoline, so I tried it out Sunday.   I feel kinda bad that I got my folks so upset; I don't think I'll do this again.   I know now that it was the gasoline."   Follow-up at 6 months reveals that Robert is doing well.   There have been no further incidents of "huffing."

Case Study 2:   Michael Q. is a 15-year-old resident of a runaway shelter, admitted to the brief-stay, intensive care, psychiatric unit following a suicide attempt while in a severe confusional state.   He had been found by the shelter manager in a basement storage closet, crying, delirious, and bleeding from both wrists.   There were two cans of spray paint and a plastic bag in the room with him.   The delirium cleared in a few hours.   Michael states that he began "huffing" paint 3 yr ago.   He and two friends would cut school and get high.   "Getting high is better than being in school. At least I can feel good when I'm high.   All my troubles just aren't there." Psychological evaluation reveals Michael to be operating in the dull-normal range of intelligence.   There is evidence of difficulty with verbal processing. Although Michael is homesick he agrees to enter a residential treatment unit for adolescents with drug use problems.

The final group of substances to be considered here is the deliriants. Members of this group often are lumped with the hallucinogens, although hallucinations occur as a part of the intoxication, most often in the absence of a clear sensorium.   The intoxicating properties of nutmeg, the seed of an aromatic evergreen tree, Myristica fragrans, have been recognized since the 16th century.   Abuse of this spice is usually on an experimental basis, and going on "nutmeg jags" is a fairly common practice in prisons when other drugs are unavailable.   Even in moderate amounts, the taste of nutmeg is unpalatable.   Its effects are most often unpleasant and similar in manifestation to atropine poisoning (Faquet & Rowland, 1978).   Fatal fatty degeneration of the liver has been reported from extended use.

Similar in symptomatology, and more common than nutmeg abuse, are the effects of a variety of anticholinergic compounds and mixtures of compounds; the latter usually of plant origin.   Abuse of anticholinergic medications, used to treat the extrapyramidal side effects of neuroleptic drugs, has been reported by MacVicar (1977) and Goggin and Solomon, (1979).   These authors report use of trihexy-phenidyl (Artane) for its euphoriant effect; high doses (24-50mg) produce a toxic psychosis which may be misinterpreted as an exacerbation of a preexisting schizophrenic process. Goggin and Solomon (1979) also provided anecdotal reports of misuse of benztropine (Congentin) and biperiden (Akineton) for euphorogenic effects.

The flowers, leaves, and seeds of the hardy, annual, solanaceous herbs of the genus Datura contain a potent mixture of alkaloids including: atropine, hyoscyamine, and scopolamine.   The deliriant effects of Datura stramonium L., also called Jimson weed, Thornapple, devil's apple, and locoweed, have been known since the late 1600's.   Intoxication produced by ingestion of tea made from flowers and leaves of the ornamental plant Angel's trumpet (Datura sauveolens) has also recently been reported (Hall, Popkin, & McHenry, 1977).   Symptoms of Datura intoxication, are reviewed in Table 6 on the following page (also seen in tricyclic antidepressant overdose.)

ANSWERS, Section X. _____

1.   a,b,c,d
2.   a,b,d
3.   a

_____

TABLE 6 - 6

SIGNS OF DATURA INTOXICATION: THE ANTICHOLINERGIC SYNDROME
(Modified from: Hall, Popkin and McHenry, 1977; Baldessarini, 1977; Mikolich, Paulson
and Cross, 1975)

_____

Neuropsychiatric Signs:
    Mydriatic pupils with reduced or absent response to light
    Restlessness
    Anxiety
    Agitation/combativeness
    Purposeless overactivity
    Impairment of immediate recall and recent memory
    Predominantly visual hallucinations
    Dysarthria
    Ataxia
    Myoclonus
    Hyperactive deep tendon reflexes
    Marked muscular weakness
    Major motor seizures
    Delirium
    Coma
    Babinski's sign present
    Decerebrate posturing
Systemic Signs
    Hyperpyrexia
    Flushed, warm, dry skin
    Decreased mucosal secretions
    Scleral injection
    Tachycardia
    Tachypnea
    Hypertension with wide pulse pressure
    Reduced bowel motility
    Urinary retention

_____

Mikolich, Paulson, and Cross (1975) cited elevations in serum SGOT and
LDH, prolongation of the prothrombin time, and EEG abnormalities in their
cases of Jimson weed poisoning. This syndrome can be treated effectively by
intravenous administration of 1-2 mg physostigmine salicylate and supportive

measures. Repeated doses may be required at 1-2 hr intervals because of the rapidity with which physostigmine is metabolized. For all the severity of the symptoms, the course of Datura intoxication is remarkably benign with most of the neuropsychiatric and systemic signs clearing over a 24-hr period. Mydriasis and transient episodes of hallucinosis may persist for a few days. Short-term memory deficits and processing difficulties may persist for a week or so.

QUIZ, Section XI.

Indicate which symptoms most closely fit with PCP intoxication or Datura intoxication, both or neither, for questions 1-11.

  a. PCP intoxication
  b. Datura intoxication
  c. Both
  d. Neither

_____ 1. decreased mucosal secretions
_____ 2. increased mucosal secretions
_____ 3. hyperactive deep tendon reflexes
_____ 4. hypertension
_____ 5. reduced bowel activity
_____ 6. absent corneal reflex
_____ 7. restlessness, anxiety
_____ 8. cataleptic state
_____ 9. hyperpyrexia
_____ 10. symptoms clear when physostigmine is given
_____ 11. atropine clears symptoms

Use the following case study to answer question #12.

A young adolescent male is brought to the emergency room by the police. His agitation is such that he is placed in a Posey belt and four point restraints. He is grossly hallucinating and incoherent for the most part. Vital signs are T 42°C, P 128, BP 170/110. His skin is flushed, dry, and hot. Oral secretions are greatly diminished and he complains of thirst. Bowel sounds are absent. His pupils are mydriatic and unresponsive to light. The only history obtained by the police is that the patient ingested an unknown quantity of an unknown substance 2 hr ago. An IV line is put in place. A nasogastric tube is passed and the stomach contents aspirated. The decision to administer physostigmine is made on the basis of

  a. the symptom complex of "mad as a hatter, red as a beet and dry as a bone."
  b. hyperpyrexia.
  c. some small, black, pock-marked seeds are obtained in an otherwise unremarkable gastric aspirate.
  d. absent bowel sounds.

ANSWERS, Section XI. _____

1. b	7. c
2. a	8. a
3. c	9. b
4. c	10. b
5. b	11. d
6. a	12. a,b,c,d

POST-TEST

For the following questions, <u>one</u> or <u>more</u> <u>than</u> <u>one</u> answer may be correct. Circle the correct answer(s).

1. Which of the following treatment strategies is/are reasonable approaches for a newly diagnosed alcoholic?

    a. referral to a subacute detoxificaton unit for supervised detoxification
    b. immediate hospitalization
    c. referral to A.A.
    d. outpatient detoxification

2. Which of the following statements is/are true about barbiturates?

    a. Development of functional tolerance involves noradrenergic neurons.
    b. Some are clinically useful in the treatment of epilepsy.
    c. The use of barbiturates in suicide attempts has declined.
    d. They are useful as adjuncts in the management of pain.

3. Which of the following conditions is/are among the criteria for the diagnosis of Substance Dependence?

    a. tolerance
    b. medical complications of use
    c. withdrawal
    d. daily use for three weeks

4. Major classes of sedative-hypnotic drugs include

    a. barbiturates.
    b. benzodiazepines.
    c. carbamate derivates.
    d. phenothiazines.

5. Catabolism of alcohol occurs mainly in the

    a. lungs.
    b. intestines.
    c. brain.
    d. liver.

6. Which of the following statements is/are true of treatment outcome of alcohol dependence?

    a. Total abstinence is the only legitimate goal.
    b. Abstinence almost always leads to improved social functioning.
    c. If the patient drinks, even a little, treatment has failed.
    d. The spontaneous remission rate of alcoholics is about 20%.

7. True statements about opiate abuse in the U.S. include which of the following?

   a. It has always been limited in occurrence to minority and low socioeconomic groups.
   b. Because of high availability and easy access to opiates, the groups at highest risk for opiate abuse are medical personnel, including physicians, nurses, and their spouses.
   c. The epidemic of heroin addiction continues to accelerate.
   d. The addiction rate for the general population is approximately 0.3%.

8. Which of the following criteria is/are diagnostic for Opiate Dependence?

   a. social complications of use
   b. daily use for two months
   c. tolerance to opiates
   d. the presence of a deviant lifestyle

9. Factors predisposing a person to Opiate Abuse or Dependence Disorders include(s)

   a. a Conduct or Antisocial Personality Disorder.
   b. a period of intensive polydrug experimentation and use.
   c. an inability to handle strong negative affects in an interpersonal setting.
   d. lower socioeconomic origins, unemployment, minority group member-ship.

10. Risk factors for drug automatism include

   a. minor head injury in the past.
   b. increased age.
   c. various Organic Mental Disorders.
   d. substance abuse.

11. From the following, select true statements in reference to tolerance to sedative-hypnotic drugs.

   a. Both pharmacodynamic and metabolic tolerance develop with use of sedative-hypnotic drugs.
   b. Tolerance develops more rapidly to short-acting barbiturates than to the more long-acting compounds.
   c. There is cross-tolerance among compounds of this class of drugs.
   d. Tolerance not only develops to the hypnotic effects of these drugs, but also increases the limits of a lethal dose.

12. Opiate-induced pupillary miosis

   a. is blocked by atropine.
   b. results from stimulation of the Edinger-Westphal nucleus of cranial nerve III.
   c. is not induced by meperidine.
   d. diminishes as tolerance develops.

13. Although setting and expectation strongly influence the experience when hallucinogenic substances are ingested, certain phenomena are consistently reported. These phenomena, in the presence of a clear sensorium, include

    a. synesthesia.
    b. depersonalization.
    c. heightened sensory perception.
    d. pseudohallucinations.

14. Chronic use of cocaine can result in

    a. cachexia.
    b. a paranoid psychosis.
    c. Magnan's sign.
    d. tolerance.

15. Complication(s) of narcotic dependence include

    a. osteomyelitis.
    b. hepatitis.
    c. endocarditis.
    d. death by homicide.

16. Which of the following is/are acute effect(s) of low to medium doses of cocaine taken intranasally?

    a. local anesthesia at the site of application
    b. increased muscle tone and metabolic rate
    c. mydriasis
    d. production of a subjective euphoric feeling

17. Neurochemical effect(s) of amphetamine include(s)

    a. release of acetylcholine.
    b. release and depletion of norepinephrine.
    c. MAO substrate.
    d. release and depletion of dopamine.

18. Legitimate medical use(s) of amphetamines is/are limited to the

    a. treatment of narcolepsy.
    b. treatment of depression.
    c. treatment of Attention Deficit Disorders.
    d. treatment of obesity.

19. Pharmacologic effect(s) of nicotine result from an initial, transient stimulation and subsequent, more persistent, depression of all autonomic ganglia and would include

   a. increased heart rate, vasoconstriction and elevated blood pressure.
   b. discharge of epinephrine from the adrenal medulla.
   c. increased tone and motor activity of bowel.
   d. inhibition of salivary and bronchial secretions.

Circle the letter corresponding to the one correct response.

20. Concomitant administration of disulfiram and phenytoin in an epileptic alcoholic is

   a. indicated.
   b. contraindicated.

21. The U.S. per capita consumption of beverage alcohol has

   a. increased over the past 200 years.
   b. decreased over the past 200 years.

PRE-TEST ANSWERS

1.	a,c	12.	a,b,c
2.	d	13.	a,b,c,d
3.	a,b,c	14.	a,b,c,d
4.	d	15.	a,b,c
5.	a,b,c	16.	b,d
6.	a,b	17.	a,c
7.	a,b,c,d	18.	a,b,c,d
8.	a,b,c	19.	a,b,c,d
9.	b,d	20.	b
10.	a,b,c	21.	b
11.	a,b,c,d		

POST-TEST ANSWERS

1.	a,b,c	12.	a,b,c
2.	a,b	13.	a,b,c,d
3.	a,c	14.	a,b,c,
4.	a,b,c	15.	a,b,c,d
5.	d	16.	a,b,c,d
6.	d	17.	b,d
7.	b,d	18.	a,c
8.	a,b,c	19.	a,b,c,d
9.	a,b,c,d	20.	b
10.	a,b,c,d	21.	b
11.	a,b,c		

REFERENCES

Abelson, H. I., & Fishburne, P. Non-medical use of psychoactive substances. Princeton, N.J.: Response Analysis Corporation, 1976.

Abelson, H. I., Fishburne, P., & Cisin, I. National survey on drug abuse: 1977. Princeton, N.J.: Response Analysis Corporation and the Social Research Group of the George Washington University, 1977.

Baldessarini, R. J. Chemotherapy in psychiatry. Harvard University Press: Cambridge, Mass., 1977.

Brecher, E. M. Licit and illicit drugs. Boston: Little, Brown, and Company, 1972.

Brotman, R. E., Myer, A. S., & Freedman, A. M. An approach to treating narcotic addicts based on a community mental health diagnosis. Comprehensive Psychiatry, 1965, 61, 104.

Chafetz, M. E., Hertzman, M., & Berenson, D. Alcoholism: A positive view. In S. Arieti & E. B. Brody (Eds.), American handbook of psychiatry, Vol. III. New York: Basic Books, Inc., 1974.

Citron, B. P., Halpern, M., McCarron, M., Lundberg, G. G., McCormick, R., Pincus, I. J., Tatter, D., & Haverback, B. J. Necrotizing angiitis associated with drug abuse. New England Journal of Medicine, 1970, 283, 1003-1011.

Clark, W. C., Goetz, R. R., McCarthy, R. H., Bemporad, B., & Zeidenberg, P. Effects of marijuana on pain and verbal memory: A sensory decision theory analysis. In G. G. Nahas & W. D. M. Paton (Eds.), Marihuana: Biological effects. New York: Pergamon Press, 1979.

Clarren, S. K., & Smith, D. W. The fetal alcohol syndrome. New England Journal of Medicine, 1978, 298, 1063-1067.

Cohen, S. Abuse of inhalants. In S. N. Pradham & S. N. Dutta (Eds.), Drug abuse clinical and basic aspects. St. Louis: C. V. Mosby Co., 1977.

Dole, V. P., & Nyswander, M. A medical treatment for diacetylmorphine (heroin) addiction: A clinical trial with methadone hydrochloride. Journal of the American Medical Assocation, 1965, 193, 646-650.

Domestic Council Drug Abuse Task Force. White paper on drug abuse: A report to the President from the Domestic Council Drug Abuse Task Force. Washington, D.C.: U.S. Government Printing Office, 1975.

Drug Abuse Warning Network: Phase V report. Ambler, Pa.: I.M.S. America, 1978.

Faquet, R. A., & Rowland, K. R. "Spice cabinet" intoxication. American Journal of Psychiatry, 1978, 135, 860-861.

Fauman, M. A., & Fauman, B. J. Violence associated with phencyclidine abuse. American Journal of Psychiatry, 1979, 136, 1584-1586.

Finkle, B. S., McCloskey, K. L., & Goodman, L. S. Diazepam and drug-associated deaths. Journal of the American Medical Association, 1979, 242, 429-434.

Friedman, A. S., Farley, E., Santo, Y., & Speck, D. Phencyclidine use among youths in drug abuse treatment. N.I.D.A. Services Research Report. DHEW Publication No. (HDM) 78-635, 1978.

Garey, R. E. PCP: An update. Journal of Psychedelic Drugs, 1979, 11, 265-275.

Garey, R. E., & Heath, R. G. The effects of phencyclidine on the uptake of 3H-catecholamines by rat striatal and hypothalamic synaptosomes. Life Sciences, 1976, 18, 1105-1110.

Garrett, E. R. Pharmacokinetics and disposition of 9-tetrahydrocannabinol and its metabolites. In G. G. Nahas & W. D. M. Paton (Eds.), Marihuana: Biological effects. New York: Pergamon Press, 1979.

Goggin, D.A., & Solomon, G.F. Trihexyphenidyl abuse for euphorigenic effect. American Journal of Psychiatry, 1979, 136, 459-460.

Gold, M. S., Redmond, D. E., Jr., & Kleber, H. D. Clonidine in opiate withdrawal. Lancet, 1978, 1, 929-930.

Goldstein, A. Opiate receptors and opioid peptides: A ten-year overview. In M. A. Lipton, A. DiMascio, & K. F. Killam (Eds.), Pharmacology: A generation of progress. New York: Raven Press, 1978.

Good, M. I. The concept of drug automatism. American Journal of Psychiatry, 1976, 133, 948-952.

Goodwin, D. W., Schulsinger, F., Hermansen, L., Guze, S.B., & Winokur, G. Alcohol problems in adoptees raised apart from alcoholic biologic parents. Archives of General Psychiatry, 1973, 28, 238-243.

Goodwin, D. W., Schulsinger, F., Knop, J., Mednick, S., & Guze, S.B. Alcoholism and depression in adopted-out daughters of alcoholics. Archives of General Psychiatry, 1977, 34, 751-755.

Greene, M. H., Nightingale, S. L., & DuPont, R. L. Evolving patterns of drug use. Annals of Internal Medicine, 1975, 83, 402-411.

Grossman, H. J. Grossman's guide to wines, beers and spirits. Revised by Harriet Lambeck. New York: Scribner, 1977.

Hall, R. C. W., Popkin, M. K., & McHenry, L. E. Angel's trumpet psychosis: A central nervous system anticholinergic syndrome. American Journal of Psychiatry, 1977, 134, 312-314.

Hoffman, A. The discovery of LSD and subsequent investigations on naturally occurring hallucinogens. In T. J. Ayd & B. Blackwell (Eds.), Discoveries in biological psychiatry. Philadelphia: Lippincott, 1970.

Huber, G. L., Pochay, V. E., Shea, J. W., Hinds, W. C., Weker, R. R., First, M. W., & Sornberger, G. C. An experimental animal model for quantifying the biologic effects of marijuana on the defense system of the lung. In G. G. Nahas & W. D. M. Paton (Eds.), Marihuana: Biological effects. New York: Pergamon Press, 1979.

Isbell, M., Belleville, R.E., Fraser, H.F., Wikler, A., & Logan, C.R. Studies on lysergic acid diethylamide (LSD-25) I. Archives of Neurology and Psychiatry, 1956, 76, 468-478.

Isselbacker, K. J. Metabolic and hepatic effects of alcohol. New England Journal of Medicine, 1977, 296, 612-616.

Kaplan, H. G., Bakken, J., Quadracci, L., & Schuback, W. Hepatitis caused by halothane sniffing. Annals of Internal Medicine, 1979, 90, 797-798.

Kelleher, R.T. Psychomotor stimulants. In S.N. Pradham & S.N. Dutta (Eds.), Drug abuse: Clinical and basic aspects. St. Louis: Mosby, 1977.

Koffler, A., Friedler, R. M., & Massry, S. G. Acute renal failure due to nontraumatic rhabdomyolysis. Annals of Internal Medicine, 1976, 85, 23-28.

Kreek, M. J., Garfield, J.W., Gutjahr, C.L., & Giusti, L.M. Rifampin-induced methadone withdrawal. New England Journal of Medicine, 1976, 294, 1104-1106.

Li, T-K. Enzymology of human alcohol metabolism. In A. Meister (Ed.), Advances in enzymology and related areas of molecular biology. New York: John Wiley & Sons, 1977.

Linnaeus, C. L. Species plantarum. Stockholm, Sweden, 1753.

Louria, D. B., Hensle, T., & Rose, J. The major medical complications of heroin addiction. Annals of Internal Medicine, 1967, 67, 1-22.

Maayani, S., Weinstein, H., Cohen, S., & Sokolovsky, M. Acetylcholine-like molecular arrangement of psychotomimetic anticholinergic drugs. Proceedings of the National Academy of Sciences of the U.S., 1973, 70, 3103-3107.

MacVicar, K. Abuse of antiparkinsonian drugs by psychiatric patients. _American Journal of Psychiatry_, 1977, 134, 809-811.

Mikolich, J. R., Paulson, G. W., & Cross, C. J. Acute anticholinergic syndrome due to Jimson seed ingestion. _Annals of Internal Medicine_, 1975, 83, 321-325.

Moore, R. A. The diagnosis of alcoholism in a psychiatric hospital: A trial of the Michigan Alcoholism Screening Test (MAST). _American Journal of Psychiatry_, 1972, 128, 1565-1569.

Nahas, G. G. A biological indictment of marijuana. _The U.S. Journal of Drug and Alcohol Dependence_, March 1979, p.7.

National Commission on Marijuana and Drug Abuse. _Drug use in America: Problems in perspective._ Washington, D.C.: U.S. Government Printing Office, 1973.

Nedergaard, O. A. Cocaine-like effect of ketamine on vascular adrenergic neurones. _European Journal of Pharmacology_, 1973, 23, 153-161.

Noble, E. P. (Ed.). _Third special report to the U.S. Congress on alcohol and health._ Rockville, Md.: National Institute on Alcohol Abuse and Alcoholism, 1978.

Parry, H. L., Balter, M., Mellinger, G., Cisin, I. H., & Manheimer, D. I. National patterns of psychotherapeutic drug use. _Archives of General Psychiatry_, 1973, 28, 769-783.

Pastan, R. S., Silverman, S. L., & Goldenberg, D. L. A musculoskeletal syndrome in intravenous heroin users: Association with brown heroin. _Annals of Internal Medicine_, 1977, 87, 22-29.

Penry, J. K., & Newmark, M. E. The use of antiepileptic drugs. _Annals of Internal Medicine_, 1979, 90, 207-218.

Post, R. M. Cocaine psychosis: A continuum model. _American Journal of Psychiatry_, 1975, 132, 225-231.

Preble, E., & Casey, J. J., Jr. Taking care of business: The heroin user's life in the street. _International Journal of the Addictions_, 1969, 4, 124.

Prinzmetal, M., & Bloomberg, W. The use of benzedrine for the treatment of narcolepsy. _Journal of the American Medical Association_, 1935, 105, 2051-2054.

Reich, L. H., Davies, R. K., & Himmelhoch, J. M. Excessive alcohol use in manic-depressive illness. _American Journal of Psychiatry_, 1974, 131, 83-86.

Robins, L. N., Helzer, J. E., & Davis, D. H. Narcotic use in Southeast Asia and afterward: An interview study of 898 Vietnam returnees. Archives of General Psychiatry, 1975, 32, 955-961.

Rubin, E., & Lieber, C. S. Fatty liver, alcoholic hepatitis and cirrhosis produced by alcohol in primates. New England Journal of Medicine, 1974, 290, 128-135.

Scholes, J., Derosena, R., Appel, G. B., Jao, W., Boyd, M. T., & Pirani, L. L. Amyloidosis in chronic heroin addicts with the nephrotic syndrome. Annals of Internal Medicine, 1979, 91, 26-29.

Schuckit, M. A. Drug and alcohol abuse: A clinical guide to diagnosis and treatment. New York: Plenum Publishing Co., 1979.

Selzer, M. L. The Michigan Alcohol Screening Test: The quest for a new diagnostic instrument. American Journal of Psychiatry, 1971, 127, 1653-1658.

Showalter, C. V., & Thornton, W. E. Clinical pharmacology of phencyclidine toxicity. American Journal of Psychiatry, 1977, 134, 1234-1238.

Sioris, L. J., & Krenzelok, E. P. Phencyclidine intoxication: A literature review. American Journal of Hospital Pharmacy, 1978, 35, 1362-1367.

Smith, R. C. The marketplace of speed: Violence and compulsive methamphetamine abuse. In E.M. Brecher, Licit and illicit drugs. Boston, Mass.: Little, Brown and Company, 1972.

Smith, R. C., Meltzer, H. Y., Arora, R. C., & Davis, J. M. Effects of phencyclidine on [3H] catecholamine and [3H] serotonin uptake in synaptosomal preparations from rat brain. Biochemical Pharmacology, 1977, 26, 1435-1439.

Snyder, S. H., Unger, S., Blatchley, R., & Barfknecht, C. F. Stereospecific actions of DOET (2, 5-dimethoxy-4-ethylamphetamine) in man. Archives of General Psychiatry, 1974, 31, 103-106.

Sokol, R. J., Miller, S. I., & Reed, G. Alcohol abuse during pregnancy: An epidemiologic study. Alcoholism: Clinical and Experimental Research, 1980, 4, 134-145.

Sutker, P.B., & Archer, R.P. Drug abuse and dependence disorders: Psychopathology and deviance. In H.E. Adams & P.B. Sutker (Eds.), Comprehensive handbook of psychopathology. New York: Plenum, 1982.

Taher, S. M., Anderson, R.J., & McCartney, R. Renal tubular acidosis associated with toluene "sniffing." New England Journal of Medicine, 1974, 290, 765-768.

Takemori, A. E. Commentary: Neurochemical bases for narcotic tolerance and dependence. Biochemical Pharmacology, 1975, 24, 2121-2126.

Tamminga, C. A., Schaffer, M.H., Smith, R.C., & Davis, J.M. Schizophrenic symptoms improve with apomorphine. Science, 1978, 200, 567-568.

Tashkin, D. P., Shapiro, B.J., Lee, Y.E., & Harper, C.E. Subacute effects of heavy marijuana smoking on pulmonary function in healthy men. New England Journal of Medicine, 1976, 294, 125-129.

Tashkin, D.P., Soares, J.R., Hepler, R.S., Shapiro, B.J., & Rachelefsky, G.S. Cannabis, 1977. Annals of Internal Medicine, 1978, 89, 539-549.

Tong, T. G., Benowitz, N. L., Becker, C. E., Forni, P. J., & Boerner, U. Phencyclidine poisoning. Journal of the American Medical Association, 1975, 234, 512-513.

Vaillant, G.E. The natural history of narcotic drug addiction. Seminars in Psychiatry, 1970, 2, 486-498.

Van Dyke, C., Jatlow, F., Ungerer, J., Barash, P.G., & Byck, R. Oral cocaine: Plasma concentrations and central effects. Science, 1978, 200, 211-213.

Victor, M., Adams, R. D., & Collins, G. H. The Wernicke-Korsakoff Syndrome. Philadelphia: F. A. Davis Co., 1971.

Vogel, F. S. Concerning the pathogenesis of central pontine myelinolysis and Wernicke's encephalopathy: Associates of chronic alcoholism. Alcoholism: Clinical and Experimental Research, 1977, 2, 67-72.

Weinstein, H., Maayani, S., Srebrenik, S., Cohen, S., & Sokolovsky, M. Psychotomimetic drugs as anticholinergic agents. Part II. Journal of Molecular Pharmacology, 1973, 9, 820.

Westerfeld, W. W., & Schulman, M. P. Metabolism and caloric value of alcohol. Journal of the American Medical Association, 1959, 170, 197-203.

Williams, R. R., & Horm, J. W. Association of cancer sites with tobacco and alcohol consumption and socioeconomic status of patients: Interview study from the Third National Cancer Study. Journal of the National Cancer Institute, 1977, 58, 525-547.

Wurmser, L. The hidden dimension: Psychodynamics in compulsive drug use. New York: Jason Aronson, 1978.

Zinberg, N. E., & Jacobson, R. C. The natural history of "chipping." American Journal of Psychiatry, 1976, 133, 37-40.

CHAPTER 7

Schizophrenic Disorders, Psychoses Not Elsewhere Classified and Paranoid Disorders

Patricia M. Randels, M.D.
Luis A. Marco, M.D.
Darlene L. Shaw, Ph.D.

CHAPTER OUTLINE

Learning Objectives

Pre-Test

LEARNING OBJECTIVES

After completing this chapter, you will be able to:

1. List the important contributions to our current concept of Schizophrenia of E. Bleuler, Kraepelin, and Schneider.

2. Define and recognize characteristic symptoms occurring in Schizophrenia including: looseness of associations, neologisms, poverty of content of speech, blocking, delusions, hallucinations, flatness of affect, inappropriate affect, ambivalence, and abnormal motor behavior.

3. Define: Schizophrenia, psychosis, autism, vagueness, tangentiality, catatonia, prodromal, residual.

4. Differentiate Schizophrenia from Schizophreniform Disorders, Schizoaffective Disorders, and Brief Reactive Psychosis.

5. Diagnose Schizophrenia including the subtypes, paranoid, catatonic and undifferentiated.

6. Recognize Schizophreniform Disorder and Brief Reactive Psychosis.

7. Recognize genetic risks for Schizophrenia.

8. List two current biochemical theories for the cause of Schizophrenia and cite evidence to support these theories.

9. Recognize the clinical features commonly seen in the Paranoid Disorders.

10. Identify the DSM-III diagnostic criteria for Paranoia, Acute Paranoid Disorder, and Shared Paranoid Disorder.

11. Recognize facts regarding the course and etiology of the Paranoid Disorders.

PRE-TEST

For the following questions, <u>one</u> or <u>more</u> <u>than</u> <u>one</u> answer may be correct. Circle the correct answer(s).

1. Argument(s) in support of the serotonin or methylation theory of Schizophrenia include which of the following?

    a. LSD and other hallucinogens include EEG patterns typical of arousal.
    b. Serotonin content of platelets in chronic schizophrenics is high.
    c. MAO activity of platelets in chronic schizophrenics is low.
    d. Good therapeutic results with nicotinic acid (a methyl receptor) are seen in treatment of Schizophrenia.

2. If an endogenous hallucinogen were to be found to be the cause of Schizophrenia, it would have to meet which of the following criteria?

    a. Tolerance to the compound does not develop.
    b. It would have to be a compound that could be synthesized by the body.
    c. It should be possible to discover the compound in body fluids.
    d. The compound should chemically resemble amphetamines.

3. Drug(s) that support(s) the dopamine theory of Schizophrenia because they indirectly increase dopamine and can be associated with Schizophreniform Psychoses, is/are

    a. nicotinic acid.
    b. levodopa.
    c. lysergic acid diethylamide.
    d. amphetamines.

4. Factor(s) that suggest the involvement of dopamine in Schizophrenia are related to which of the following antipsychotic drug effects?

    a. dopamine receptor blockade
    b. extrapyramidal side effects
    c. increased dopamine turnover
    d. a sedative effect

5. Which of the following criteria is/are essential for a diagnosis of Schizophrenia?

    a. characteristic symptoms
    b. disorganization of a previous level of functioning
    c. duration of at least six months
    d. early age of onset

6. Which of the following statements is/are true?

   a. Schizophrenia can be reliably diagnosed if catatonic symptoms are present.
   b. Schizophrenia can be reliably diagnosed if looseness of associations is present.
   c. Schizophrenia can be reliably diagnosed if autism is present.
   d. A diagnosis of Schizophrenia based on signs and symptoms is unreliable.

7. Which of the following disorders commonly occur(s) in Schizophrenia?

   a. impaired intelligence
   b. impaired orientation
   c. impaired memory
   d. autism

8. Which of the following clinical features is/are consistent with a diagnosis of Paranoid Disorder?

   a. Persecutory delusions or delusional jealousy is present.
   b. The daily functioning of the individual is severely disrupted.
   c. The delusions are not due to another psychiatric or organic syndrome.
   d. The emotional response to the delusions is inappropriate.

9. In Acute Paranoid Disorder

   a. the onset is usually gradual.
   b. the duration of the illness is less than six months.
   c. there are prominent hallucinations.
   d. changes in the person's environment such as immigration or prison are often precipitating factors.

10. The DSM-III diagnostic criteria for Paranoid Disorders include

   a. persistent persecutory delusions or delusional jealousy.
   b. not due to Organic Mental Disorder.
   c. duration at least one week.
   d. prominent hallucinations.

11. The Paranoid Disorders are divided into

   a. Paranoia.
   b. Shared Paranoid Disorder.
   c. Acute Paranoid Disorder.
   d. Conjugal Paranoid Disorder.

12. With regard to Paranoia,

    a. the onset is usually gradual.
    b. it is a rare disorder.
    c. the course is usually chronic with few cures.
    d. few patients with this disorder seek treatment on their initiative.

For the following questions, circle the letter corresponding to the one correct response.

13. Prognostic factors in Schizophrenia include all except

    a. type of clinical symptom.
    b. age at onset.
    c. mode of onset.
    d. premorbid adjustment.
    e. cultural background.

Use the following case study to answer questions 14 and 15.

A 28-year-old man states that he has invented a device that could be used to monitor the thoughts of world leaders. Because of the sensitive nature of this invention, the Patent Office has tried to steal it and the FBI has scrutinized his activities, including wire tapping his telephone. The FBI has also developed subtle ways of brain washing which it has employed on the patient for the past two years.

14. Here we have an example of

    a. thought insertion.
    b. grandiose and persecutory delusions.
    c. thought withdrawal.
    d. superstitiousness.
    e. religiosity.

15. According to DSM-III, symptoms of this nature are highly suggestive of

    a. manic depressive illness.
    b. Paranoid Schizophrenia.
    c. Schizoid Personality.
    d. amphetamine psychosis.
    e. none of the above.

16. All the following are among Bleuler's 4 A's except

    a. anhedonia.
    b. ambivalence.
    c. looseness of associations.
    d. affect.
    e. autism.

Use the following case study to answer questions 17 and 18.

A 27-year-old single, white female who had been employed as a clerk-typist until 10 days ago was brought to the hospital by her parents who reported progressive withdrawal until she became mute, negativistic, and refused to eat. There was no history of previous mental illness.

The patient appeared as a withdrawn, immobile person who did not gesture or move her body and who was difficult to understand because she would only whisper a few words. She did state that she felt thoughts were being put into her mind which she could not decode, and as a result she could not talk. She laughed after she said this.

17. The most likely diagnosis would be

    a. Briquet's syndrome.
    b. Catatonic Schizophrenia.
    c. Paranoid Schizophrenia.
    d. Schizophreniform Disorder.
    e. amphetamine psychosis.

18. The patient exhibited all of the following symptoms <u>except</u>

    a. hallucinations.
    b. delusions.
    c. autism.
    d. motor disturbance.
    e. inappropriate affect.

19. All of the following are useful in the treatment of Schizophrenic Disorders <u>except</u>

    a. psychoanalysis.
    b. antipsychotic drugs.
    c. milieu therapy.
    d. behavioral modification.
    e. supportive psychotherapy.

Matching: Lettered items may be used once, more than once, or not at all.

Match the following risks for Schizophrenia with the corresponding percentages.

___20.	risk for monozygotic twin	a.	1%
___21.	risk in general population	b.	3%
___22.	risk for fraternal twin	c.	10%
___23.	risk for other siblings	d.	25%
___24.	risk if both parents schizophrenic	e.	40%
		f.	50%
		g.	90%

Match the following terms with the corresponding examples.

___25. delusion of influence
___26. neologism
___27. superstition
___28. delusion of grandeur
___29. somatic delusion

a. a woman believes that her every move is controlled by unseen agents
b. the brakish-brack waters scalidify the snails
c. "My horoscope says I am under the influence of Mars and Pluto today."
d. a postmenopausal woman believes she is pregnant
e. "I am the Virgin Mary."

Match the following terms and definitions.

___30. vagueness
___31. concreteness
___32. poverty of content of speech
___33. derailment
___34. hallucination
___35. autism
___36. neologism

a. responses that are literal rather than abstract
b. obscure or unclear responses
c. ideas do not proceed logically
d. an undefined, made-up word
e. failure to convey much information, although there is an adequate amount of speech
f. perceptual experience without a stimulus
g. preference for fantasy over reality

I. DEFINITIONS AND HISTORY

Schizophrenia is not a single syndrome, but a group of disorders. These disorders are classified as being psychotic. They are chronic and are characterized by deterioration of a previous level of functioning and by distinctive symptoms involving multiple psychological processes.

The term "psychotic" has been defined variously in the past so that the meaning has become diffuse and imprecise. In DSM-III psychotic is redefined to denote impaired reality testing and is manifested by any of the following psychotic symptoms: delusions, hallucinations, incoherence, looseness of associations, marked poverty of content of thought, marked illogicality, and behavior that is grossly disorganized or catatonic. As we shall see, psychotic symptoms do occur in Schizophrenia, and they also occur in other psychotic disorders such as Affective Disorders, Organic Brain Syndromes, and drug abuse disorders. Therefore, in diagnosing Schizophrenia, it is important to exclude other disorders which manifest psychotic symptoms.

Until the late nineteenth century, psychoses were described in terms of many separate syndromes. Kraepelin observed common denominators among diverse conditions and categorized functional psychoses into two groups, mania and Dementia Praecox. Dementia Praecox corresponds to what we now call Schizophrenia. Kraepelin was emphasizing the tendency toward a deteriorating course (Dementia) and the usual onset in early adult life (praecox). Today the concept of Schizophrenia is not limited to illnesses with a progressively deteriorating course, but does imply chronicity (a minimum of six months existence of symptoms and a tendency toward recurrence) and a deterioration of a previous level of functioning when symptoms are present. The concept of onset in early adult life has also withstood the test of time.

Eugen Bleuler studied patients with Dementia Praecox and renamed the condition Schizophrenia. "Schizo" means split, and "phrenia" refers to the mind. Thus, the term implies a splitting of the functions of the mind; i.e., an idea and the mood that corresponds do not occur at the same time. This split contrasts with the lay term "split personality" (DSM-III - "multiple personality"), a dissociative disorder, in which separate but intact personalities may occur at different times, with amnesia in one state for the other.

Bleuler observed that in Schizophrenia several mental functions such as orientation, memory, and consciousness were not disturbed, and thus found the term, Dementia, inappropriate.

Bleuler thought that certain mental functions were impaired in all patients with Schizophrenia at some time in the course of the illness. These manifestations of impairment included disordered associations, a loss of contact with reality, disordered affect, and ambivalence. These symptoms are sometimes called Bleuler's "four A's." Bleuler called his first basic symptom of Schizophrenia, looseness of associations, which denotes that associations are not connected in a logical sequence. The second fundamental symptom described by Bleuler referred to patients' disordered relationship to reality. For this symptom he coined a term, autism, which denotes the schizophrenic's withdrawal from reality and preference for fantasy. The third basic symptom described by Bleuler was an abnormal emotional or feeling tone or a disorder of affect. The fourth symptom of Schizophrenia which Bleuler deemed fundamentally important was ambivalence. Everyone has ambivalences, and pathological ambivalence exists in other psychiatric disorders, but Bleuler thought the schizophrenic felt two ways about almost everything. In other conditions one attitude is often conscious and the opposing attitude unconscious but indirectly expressed. In Schizophrenia both attitudes, though contradictory, may be conscious at the same time.

Bleuler thought that hallucinations and delusions were derived from the four fundamental symptoms, and he designated hallucinations and delusions as secondary or accessory symptoms. DSM-III nosology tends to take a reverse position from Bleuler's by terming certain delusions and hallucinations as being characteristic features of Schizophrenia with the "four A's" being considered more or less accessory symptoms. The current approach is strongly influenced by Schneider who has designated certain types of delusions and hallucinations as being characteristically found in Schizophrenia. He called these "First Rank Symptoms." Some of the Schneiderian First Rank Symptoms will be described below under Characteristic Psychological Symptoms.

QUIZ, Section I.

Circle the letter corresponding to the one correct response.

1.   All of the following are true about Schizophrenia except:

    a.   It is a chronic disease.
    b.   It is a psychotic disorder.
    c.   It may be acute or chronic.
    d.   It is manifested by distinctive symptoms.
    e.   It is manifested by a deterioration in a previous level of functioning.

2.   Psychotic means

    a.   the patient has a Schizophrenic Disorder.
    b.   impaired reality testing.
    c.   the patient is unable to function.
    d.   an irreversible mental impairment.
    e.   the individual should be committed.

3.   The schizophrenic is frequently preoccupied with his idiosyncratic world view rather than with dealing with the real world. This symptom is called

    a.   ambivalence.
    b.   autism.
    c.   looseness of associations.
    d.   disorder of affect.

Circle the correct answer(s).   One or more than one answer may be correct.

4.   Which of the following concepts derived from Kraepelin does modern psychiatry retain about Schizophrenia?

   a.   chronicity and deterioration of functioning
   b.   onset in early adult life
   c.   Dementia (Organic Mental Disorder)

5.   A symptom necessary for the diagnosis of Schizophrenia is

   a.   impaired reality testing.
   b.   splitting of thought content and mood.
   c.   impaired orientation.
   d.   impaired memory.
   e.   deterioration of a previous level of functioning.

Complete the following.

6.   The four symptoms of Schizophrenia which Bleuler observed are referred to in a shorthand fashion as "Bleuler's four A's."   They are

   a.   looseness of _____.
   b.   a preference for fantasy over reality which is called _____.
   c.   mixed feelings or _____.
   d.   a disorder of emotional tone or _____.

Match the following names with the concepts they espouse.

7. chronicity and deterioration	a. Schneider
8. disturbances in psychological processes	b. Bleuler
9. first rank symptoms	c. Kraepelin

II.   CHARACTERISTIC PSYCHOLOGICAL SYMPTOMS

There are a number of psychological features that are characteristic of Schizophrenia, some of which can be objectively demonstrated and can provide direct evidence of Schizophrenia.   Others might be considered "soft" signs; these may be somewhat obscure, and examiners may have difficulty in agreeing on the presence of these features.   In order to try to categorize a group of disorders that can be identified worldwide as Schizophrenia, current nosology insists on the existence of the more objective signs at some time during the course of the illness.   It is thought that this group of disorders is relatively homogeneous in regard to response to treatment, presence of a familial pattern, onset in early adult life, tendency toward recurrence, and impairment of the level of functioning.

A. THOUGHT DISORDERS

Disturbances of thinking are one of the objective signs. Disorders of thinking include disorders of language and communication (disorders of form or formal thought disorder) and disorders of content of thought. DSM-III recommends avoidance of these general terms, and rather, usage of the term for the specific disorder which the patient exhibits.

Language and communication disorders result from failure to follow grammatical rules or from deviations in rate or from an illogical association of ideas. Although very characteristic of Schizophrenia, language and communication disorders occurring alone are not sufficient to make the diagnosis of Schizophrenia, but rather must be accompanied by certain other signs such as disturbances in affect.

1. Looseness of Associations.
   One of the interesting and common disorders seen in Schizophrenia is looseness of associations, also called derailment. As described by Bleuler:

   > "In this malady the associations lose their continuity
   > . . . thinking operates with ideas and concepts
   > which have no, or a completely insufficient, connec-
   > tion with the main idea and should therefore be ex-
   > cluded from the thought-process. The result is that
   > thinking becomes confused, bizarre, incorrect, ab-
   > rupt." (Bleuler, 1950)

   Looseness of associations means that associations do not proceed in a logical sequence.

2. Neologisms.
   A neologism is an invented word with autistic meaning.

3. Poverty of Content of Speech.
   Poverty of content of speech commonly occurs in Schizophrenia but is not limited to this condition. Although adequate in amount, little information is conveyed. The lack of information may be related to other characteristics of schizophrenic speech such as vagueness, tangentiality, concreteness, or stereotypy (perseveration of ideas). Vagueness means obscure or unclear responses. Tangentiality means that responses veer off to a subject that appears unrelated to the topic of discussion. Concreteness means responses that are literal rather than abstract. Stereotypy - Bleuler (1950): "The tendency to stereotype produces the inclination to cling to one idea to which the patient then returns again and again. Generally, there is a marked dearth of ideas to the point of mono-ideaism."

4. Blocking.
   Sometimes the chain of thought is totally interrupted; after such "blocking," ideas may emerge which have no recognizable connection with preceding ones.

ANSWERS, Section I.

1.	d	6.	a. associations
2.	b		b. autism
3.	b		c. ambivalence
4.	a,b		d. affect
5.	e	7.	c
		8.	b
		9.	a

---

5. Delusions.
   Delusions are a type of thought disorder. They are false beliefs which are not culturally determined and which are not subject to alteration by logical proof.

   Superstitiousness, belief in clairvoyance, telepathy, or other peculiar ideas are borderline examples that could represent prodromal or residual symptoms of Schizophrenia. Belief in astrology is currently widespread and therefore should probably be considered culturally determined. Over-valued ideas such as preoccupation with the special significance of particular dietary habits, prejudices, or extreme political beliefs may also be prodromal or residual symptoms but are not generally considered to be delusions.

6. Delusions of Being Controlled (or Influenced).
   The individual believes that his feelings, impulses, or actions are not his own, and are imposed on him from some external force. The delusion of being controlled is one of Schneider's First Rank Symptoms. Delusion of passivity is a synonym.

7. Thought Withdrawal and Insertion.
   Thought withdrawal is the belief that thoughts have been removed from one's head. Thought insertion is the belief that thoughts, which are not one's own, have been inserted into the mind. These are two additional First Rank Symptoms of Schneider.

8. Thought Broadcasting.
   This is the belief that an individual's thoughts are broadcast as they occur, from his mind into the external world so that others can hear them. It is another of Schneider's First Rank Symptoms.

9. Somatic and Nihilistic Delusions.
   Somatic delusions occur in Schizophrenia and other psychotic disorders, principally depression. Somatic delusions pertain to the body of the individual. He usually believes that some part is abnormal or decaying; there is a growth in the stomach; the bones have turned to liquid or the heart to stone. Bizarreness distinguishes these delusions from mere hypochondriasis.

Nihilistic delusions are beliefs that the individual is doomed or that the world is coming to an end. Nihilistic delusions occur in psychotic depression as well as in Schizophrenia. Somatic delusions may also be nihilistic delusions if belief concerns the nonexistence of the body or a body part.

10. Grandiose, Persecutory and Religious Delusions.
Grandiose delusions are seen often in Schizophrenia and in mania. Individuals with this type of delusion exhibit an exalted self-opinion, feeling they are the wealthiest, the most famous individuals, the most accomplished musicians or artists, the best fighters, etc. Rarely seen any longer is a delusion in which the patient believes that he is some important individual such as Napoleon. Grandiose delusions occur in the paranoid subtype of Schizophrenia and are often combined with delusions of persecution. A persecutory delusion is one in which the individual believes that he is being persecuted, harassed, or conspired against. Dynamically the persecution is thought to be because of the individual's (exaggerated) importance.

Religious delusions also occur in the paranoid subtype of Schizophrenia and occasionally in mania. Religious delusions may be closely akin to grandiose delusions; for example, the belief that one is Jesus or the Virgin Mary. It is sometimes necessary to be familiar with the patient's cultural background in order to differentiate religious beliefs from delusions. Delusions are beliefs that are not accepted by other members of the patient's culture.

B. PERCEPTION

The first type of psychological symptom occurring in Schizophrenia was disorders of thinking; the second type is disorders of perception, of which hallucinations are the only important example. Hallucinations are perceptions without an external stimulus. Hallucinations are usually described in terms of the sensory modality affected. Hallucinations occurring in Schizophrenia are usually auditory. Other kinds of hallucinations should make you first think of an organic disorder rather than Schizophrenia, although all types of hallucinations can occur in Schizophrenia. A voice which keeps up a running commentary about the patient's actions or two voices conversing with each other are said by some to occur only in Schizophrenia. These two types of hallucinations are among Schneider's First Rank Symptoms.

C. AFFECT

Affective disturbance is a third type of psychological symptom found in Schizophrenia. The term "affect" is generally equivalent to "emotions," although in psychiatry, affect is usually restricted to the subjective aspects and emotion to the objectively determinable components (biochemical, physiological or behavioral). In Schizophrenia a disturbance in affective expression may be noted in that there is a deficiency in the capacity to modulate or adapt affect to changing thought content. There appears to be inadequate depth of affect. These abnormalities are referred to as blunted, flattened, or inappropriate affect. The patient with blunted affect may appear to be indifferent to all situations; the intensity of affective expression is severely limited. Flatness of affect is more extreme, there being virtually no evidence of affective expression. Inappropriate affect means that the feeling tone is not congruent with what the patient is talking about; for example, the patient may laugh when describing something sad or painful. Lability of affect also sometimes occurs; this implies sudden changes in affect for which no environmental provocation is apparent.

D.   SENSE OF SELF

Another psychological symptom occurring in Schizophrenia is a disturbance in the sense of self. Patients with Schizophrenia sometimes describe the experience of being unable to determine where they leave off and the world begins. This experience is also termed "loss of ego boundaries" or "oceanic feelings," and commonly leads to problems of identity. The development of the sense of self begins in early childhood. In Schizophrenia there is said to be a dissolution of the ego boundaries with a return to an infantile-like ego state. Regression is the defense mechanism involved.

E.   VOLITION

A disturbance in volition means a disturbance in motivation or will. Schizophrenia is described as a disorder in which there is a deterioration of a previous level of functioning. There is impairment in ability to work or to care for oneself. The disturbance in ability to function may in part be related to a disturbance in self-initiated goal directed activity, lack of interest or motivation; that is, a disturbance in volition. In part, this may be due to ambivalence, and in part to anhedonia. Anhedonia means the inability to experience pleasure from activities that ordinarily produce pleasure. Anhedonia is thought by some to be a central problem in Schizophrenia. The deterioration in level of functioning may also be attributable to autism. Ambivalence, anhedonia, and autism are symptoms that may contribute to the disturbance in ability to function. Disturbance in ability to function is an objective finding required for the diagnosis of Schizophrenia.

F.   DIMINISHED RELATIONSHIP TO EXTERNAL WORLD (AUTISM)

In Schizophrenia there is a tendency to withdraw from the external world and to become preoccupied with fantasies. Reality may be ignored or distorted. This is called autism. Autism means an inward preoccupation with one's own idiosyncratic world view, rather than dealing with the real external world.

G.   MOTOR BEHAVIOR

Disorders of motor behavior are prominent in catatonic syndromes.

1) Catatonic stupor - There is a marked decrease in reactivity to the environment, with a reduction in spontaneous movements and activity, and the individual may appear unaware of his surroundings.

2) Catatonic rigidity - The individual may maintain a rigid posture.

3) Catatonic excitement - The individual may exhibit apparently purposeless, stereotyped and excited motor activity.

4) Catatonic posturing - The individual may assume inappropriate or bizarre postures.

5) Flexibilitas cerea (waxy flexibility) - The individual maintains postures in which he is placed by others. Not seen much nowadays.

Mannerisms and grimacing are also disturbances of motor behavior, not confined to catatonic syndromes. Other less extreme forms of motor behavior are also seen in other types of Schizophrenia, pacing and rocking, for example. Apathy may lead to decreased movement. Tardive dyskinesia is a movement disorder linked to chronic antipsychotic medication. It is further described in Chapter 16, Psychopharmacology.

****

GO TO VIDEOTAPE

****

QUIZ, Section II.

Circle the correct answer(s). <u>One</u> or <u>more</u> <u>than</u> <u>one</u> answer may be correct.

1. DSM-III attempts to bring together, under the heading of Schizophrenia, a group of disorders that have in common

   a. acute onset.
   b. family pattern.
   c. onset in early adult life.
   d. tendency toward recurrence.
   e. impairment of level of functioning.

2. Looseness of associations is (all of the following are correct <u>except</u>)

   a. one of Bleuler's "four A's."
   b. diagnostic of Schizophrenia.
   c. a condition in which ideas do not follow a logical sequence.
   d. a type of thought disorder.

3. An undefined, made-up word is called

   a. clang association.
   b. neologism.
   c. a word salad.
   d. looseness of associations.

4. Symptoms of Schizophrenia include all of the following <u>except</u>

    a. blocking.
    b. neologisms.
    c. vagueness.
    d. loquaciousness.
    e. looseness of associations.

5. A veteran is suing the VA because he believes that while in the VA hospital the dentist replaced a molar with a powerful radio transmitter so that now at unexpected times his innermost thoughts can suddenly be heard by everyone around him. This is an example of

    a. persecutory delusion.
    b. thought broadcasting.
    c. somatic delusion.
    d. tactile hallucination.

6. A 28-year-old man states that he has invented a device that could be used to monitor the thoughts of world leaders. Because of the sensitive nature of this invention the Patent Office has tried to steal it and the FBI has scrutinized his activities, including wire tapping his telephone. The FBI has developed subtle ways of brain washing which it has employed on the patient for the past two years. Here we have an example of

    a. thought insertion.
    b. grandiose and persecutory delusions.
    c. thought withdrawal.
    d. superstitiousness.
    e. religiosity.

7. Schneiderian First Rank Symptoms include all <u>except</u>

    a. flatness of affect.
    b. delusions of influence.
    c. voices commenting on the patient's behavior.
    d. thought broadcasting.
    e. thought insertion.

8. The defense mechanism involved in returning to an earlier developmental stage is called

    a. reaction formation.
    b. regression.
    c. projection.
    d. introjection.
    e. displacement.

9. Psychological symptoms occurring in Schizophrenia include all the following except

   a. looseness of associations.
   b. disturbance in volition.
   c. hallucinations.
   d. loss of ego boundaries.
   e. disorientation.

10. All of the following are true about autism except:

    a. implies a withdrawal from reality
    b. is one of Bleuler's "four A's"
    c. according to DSM-III is found only in Schizophrenia
    d. means a preference for the fantasy world over the real world

11. From the following list of examples, identify the delusion(s).

    a. A four-year-old girl expects Santa Claus to bring her a bike.
    b. A 35-year-old Christian Scientist refuses an appendectomy.
    c. A 25-year-old black male refuses to be inducted into the military service because he doesn't believe in killing.
    d. A 30-year-old white woman with a sixth grade education believes that thoughts that are not her own are being put into her mind.
    e. A 42-year-old man with rheumatoid arthritis says he hears the voice of God telling him he will be healed.

12. Delusions are

    a. disorders of perception.
    b. false beliefs not culturally determined.
    c. exclusively found in Schizophrenia.
    d. due to memory impairment.
    e. necessary to make a diagnosis of Schizophrenia.

13. From the following list, identify the somatic delusion(s).

    a. the persistent fear that one has cancer
    b. a postmenopausal woman believes that she is pregnant
    c. the conviction that the brain is rotting
    d. the persistent belief that one has no intestines

Match the following terms with the correct definitions.

____14. impairment of abstraction   a. neologism
____15. obscure responses   b. concreteness
____16. an invented word with autistic   c. vagueness
         meaning

Match the following terms with the corresponding descriptions.

____17. a woman believed that sexual feelings were being put into her body by unknown forces

____18. "My horoscope says I am under the influence of Mars and Pluto today."

____19. "They always infortiate the spirits at night."

a. delusion of influence
b. neologism
c. superstition

Match the following terms with the appropriate descriptions:

____20. delusions of persecution
____21. somatic delusion
____22. delusions of influence
____23. delusions of grandeur

a. A 30-year-old woman believes that sexual feelings are being put into her body.
b. "My brain is on fire."
c. "I am the Virgin Mary."
d. "The CIA has my house wired."

Match the following types of hallucinations with the appropriate diagnosis.

____24. Organic Disorder more likely
____25. Schizophrenia more likely

a. visual hallucinations
b. auditory hallucinations

III.   COURSE OF ILLNESS

A particularly confusing terminology in relationship to Schizophrenia is the use of "acute" which has sometimes been used to refer to types of symptoms, and at other times to a renewed exacerbation of severe symptoms, and at still other times the term has been reserved for a single episode of symptoms. "Acute" has also often been used to refer to those syndromes thought to have a good prognosis. The DSM-III terminology deletes the term "acute." Brief nonrecurring episodes of schizophrenia-like symptoms are classified as "schizophreniform".

One purpose of the DSM-III classification is to attempt to differentiate "true," "process," or "chronic" Schizophrenia which is thought to have a poor prognosis from "reactive" (acute) Schizophrenia which is thought to have a better prognosis. Evidence suggesting hereditability of Schizophrenia applies to the true or chronic forms of Schizophrenia and not to schizophreniform (acute) types. So there are good empirical reasons for not linking these two disorders.

The diagnosis of Schizophrenia has long been associated with an expectation of poor outcome. You will recall that Kraepelin used a deteriorating course as a part of his definition of Dementia Praecox. More recently the belief that a deteriorating course is an essential pattern has been challenged. However, this challenge has often been countered by the view that a properly made diagnosis of Schizophrenia based on characteristic or nuclear symptoms would identify a group of patients with poor outcome (truly schizophrenic). Some investigators have suggested that particular symptoms, either alone or in combination, are of major importance in diagnosing "true" Schizophrenia and therefore give strong implication of poor outcome. Langfeldt (1971) has been particularly influential in stressing prognostic implication of certain symptom clusters combined with other patient characteristics. Studies of outcome have been reported that support Langfeldt's distinction between true and Schizophreniform Psychoses. Other reports offer conflicting evidence. The International Pilot Study of Schizophrenia (IPSS) is a transcultural psychiatric investigation involving countries from four continents (Sartorius et al., 1978). The United States group has issued several reports that address the question of whether or not outcome is predicted by various sign and symptom criteria. Using two-year and five-year followup evaluations in U.S. diagnosed Schizophrenia patients, they determined that patients with Schneider's First Rank symptoms had the same outcome as the less stringently diagnosed patients with no first rank symptoms. When the same schizophrenic patients were assigned to two groups according to Langfeldt's criteria, no difference in outcome was found between the true schizophrenic and schizophreniform patients. Thus, symptomatology does not appear to predict chronicity or recovery.

There has long been general agreement that diagnosed schizophrenic patients who manifest symptoms of depression, anxiety, mania, or confusion tend to have good prognoses, while similarly diagnosed patients with flatness of affect have poor prognosis. The IPSS has recently reported finding only one sign that predicted poor outcome: flatness of affect. Thus the only sign that discriminates between good prognosis and bad prognosis Schizophrenia appears to be flatness of affect. Unfortunately, unless this feature is severe, it is not reliably assessed by psychiatrists or other trained observers.

DSM-III resolves the problem of Schizophrenia vs. Schizophreniform by length of time that symptoms last. If schizophrenic symptoms last less than six months then the illness is called Schizophreniform.

Studies that have tried to divide Schizophrenia into chronic and schizophreniform types have done so on the basis of pathognomonic symptoms, as well as the presence or absence of affectivity. In addition, features in the clinical history, such as premorbid adjustment and mode of onset have been examined. Bleuler (1950) stated: "The onset of schizophrenia is usually an insidious one, though the relatives of the patients generally insist that it first started acutely ... However, whenever we have a thorough case history, it is an exception if we are unable to detect the previous earlier signs of disease whether it be nervous symptoms, character changes, or even direct overt schizophrenic manifestations. It is certainly difficult to evaluate personality changes when they do not point directly to the disease, or when the later manifest illness did not evolve from this character. Yet, it is impossible to say whether the personality changes had already belonged to the disease picture itself or not ... Thus, when we speak of the initial symptoms of schizophrenia, we must limit ourselves to the first symptoms which come to notice. All too often we do not know the first real manifestations."

The onset is most often during adolescence or early adulthood. The later the onset the better the prognosis is thought to be. The patient's

ANSWERS, Section II. _____

1.	b,c,d,e	10.	c	18.	c
2.	b	11.	d	19.	b
3.	b	12.	b	20.	d
4.	d	13.	b,c,d	21.	b
5.	b	14.	b	22.	a
6.	b	15.	c	23.	c
7.	a	16.	a	24.	a
8.	b	17.	a	25.	b
9.	e				

prepsychotic personality and adjustment also affect the prognosis. For example, being married or employed are adjustments that improve the outlook for recovery.

Recent evidence suggests that cultural background also may affect the outcome of Schizophrenia. For example, the risk of chronicity is greatest in those cultures where insanity is viewed as a permanent disability. Recovery appears as a more likely outcome when the society views insanity as curable, or alternatively, as caused by some external agent. These outcomes are independent of the views of the staff treating the patient; rather they are expectations internalized by the patient. The behavior of the public toward the patient appears to be of key importance.

There are few long-term follow-up studies of Schizophrenia to determine what is the natural course of the disease. Most observations have concerned only those patients who remain chronically ill; the recovered are lost sight of because they are not treated again. However, Manfred Bleuler, the son of Eugene Bleuler, has kept records on 2,000 patients for 30 years. His review of the life histories of these patients reveals that about 25% achieve full remission, 50% make at least a partial social remission, and 25% remain social invalids or hospitalized.

In summary, no individual clinical symptom, including any particular category of delusion or hallucination is pathognomonic for Schizophrenia. Such symptoms may be seen in Schizophreniform illness, Schizoaffective Disorders, Primary Affective Disorders, as well as a variety of drug intoxications.

The diagnosis of Schizophrenia by DSM-III standards requires that continuous symptoms of Schizophrenia have lasted for six months at some time during the person's life. An active phase with psychotic symptoms must be a part of this six-month period. Part of the six-month period may be prodromal or residual symptoms. Active psychotic symptoms could be present for the entire six months.

Prodromal and residual symptoms are similar and include social isolation or withdrawal, marked impairment in role functioning or self-care, markedly eccentric or peculiar behavior, blunted, flat or inappropriate affect, speech that is tangential, vague, circumstantial, over-elaborate or metaphorical, odd or bizarre ideas, and perceptual experiences. At least two of these symptoms must be present for a chronic or subchronic phase of Schizophrenia to be diagnosed.

The course is coded in the fifth digit and is divided into:

1) Subchronic - Duration is less than two years but at least six months.
2) Chronic - Duration is more than two years.
3) Subchronic with acute exacerbation - Re-emergence of prominent psychotic symptoms in an individual with a subchronic course (duration less than two years) who has been in the residual phase of the disorder.
4) Chronic with acute exacerbation - Re-emergence of prominent psychotic symptoms in an individual with a chronic course (duration more than two years) who has been in the residual phase of the illness.
5) In remission - This should be used when the individual met full criteria for Schizophrenia in the past and is now free of all clinical signs of the illness (whether or not on medication).

Remember there is no "acute Schizophrenia." A first episode of a schizophrenia-like illness is classified as Schizophreniform Disorder. If an episode of Schizophreniform Disorder lasts for six months or more, the diagnosis is changed to Schizophrenia. Based on a cross-sectional evaluation of a patient, Schizophreniform Disorder and Schizophrenia are indistinguishable.

It is important that the student be aware of another point of view besides that represented by DSM-III. DSM-III has adopted primarily the Schneiderian symptoms as criteria for diagnosis of Schizophrenia, and it is this type of symptom that is a weak prognostic indicator. Wing (1978) identified positive symptoms (delusions, hallucinations, looseness of associations) and negative symptoms (flatness of affect, poverty of speech and loss of volition) as occurring in Schizophrenia. Crow (1980) has proposed that the positive and negative symptoms reflect two different underlying processes. He has labelled the positive symptoms the Type I syndrome and the negative symptoms the Type II syndrome, also called the defect state. The importance of this distinction is that the two syndromes predict different things. The Type I syndrome predicts potential response to antipsychotic drugs, while the presence of the Type II syndrome predicts poor outcome regardless of drug treatment. Recall that the IPSS reported finding only one sign that discriminated between good prognosis and bad prognosis Schizophrenia: flatness of affect (a negative symptom), but for the most part the IPSS was based on positive symptoms. Recent reports (Johnstone et al., 1978) indicate that in some chronic schizophrenic patients there is CT scan evidence of increased ventricular size, and in these patients increased ventricular size is correlated with intellectual impairment and the presence of negative symptoms. If Type I and Type II syndromes represent different dimensions of psychopathology, they nevertheless do not constitute separate diseases, because they are often associated together. Episodes of Type I syndrome not uncommonly progress into the Type II syndrome, with or without the persistence of positive symptoms. Or either syndrome may occur alone. A Type I syndrome corresponds with a schizophreniform psychosis. The pure Type II syndrome would have been called simple Schizophrenia, a diagnosis that has been dropped by DSM-III. Although DSM-III represents advances in the reliability of psychiatric diagnoses, in this instance it may have ignored a real and very frequent outcome of the disease. Morel's coinage of the label "Dementia Praecox" for Schizophrenia was probably not adopted fortuitously by such an astute observer as Kraepelin, and it may be premature to discard the entity described as Type II syndrome, "chronic," process, defect or simple Schizophrenia. Table 7-1 summarizes growing evidence for retention of the distinction of Type I (acute) and Type II (chronic) forms of Schizophrenia.

TABLE 7-1

*COMPARISON OF CLASSICAL AND SCHNEIDERIAN SCHIZOPHRENIA

	Classical Schizophrenia (Kraepelin/Bleuler)	Schneiderian Psychosis
Crow classification	Type II	Type I
Clinical phenomena	Negative symptoms the defect state, Simple schizophrenia (flatness of affect, poverty of speech, loss of volition)	First-rank, Florid symptomatology (delusions, hallucinations, thought disorder)
Type of illness in which most frequently seen	Chronic schizophrenia	Acute schizophrenia
Potential for response to anti-psychotic drugs	Poor	Good
Presence if intellectual impairment	Sometimes	Absent
Outcome	? Irreversible	Reversible
Pathological process	Cell loss and structural changes in the brain Dilated cerebral ventricles (CT scan)	Increased dopamine receptors
Time-course and pattern	Chronic (by definition)	Acute breakdown, sometimes in the setting of the defect state

*adapted from Crow (1980) and Mackay (1980)

This growing evidence indicates that "chronic Schizophrenia" is sometimes an Organic Mental Disorder - Dementia, but that the many patients suffering from the disorder are difficult to diagnose by DSM-III criteria because of the requirement of the presence of active psychotic symptoms.

QUIZ, Section III.

Circle the letter corresponding to the one correct response.

1. A diagnosis of Schizophrenia based on signs and symptoms

    a. is reliable.
    b. is not reliable.

2. When an individual gives a long history of personal and social maladjustment, especially if schizoid features have been prominent and it is difficult to tell when the psychotic phase of the illness began because no obvious precipitating factors are evident, the prognosis tends to be poor, or in other words, the ultimate diagnosis is more likely

    a. Schizophrenia.
    b. Schizophreniform Disorder.

3. Prognostic factors in Schizophrenia include all the following except

    a. type of clinical symptom.
    b. age at onset.
    c. mode of onset.
    d. premorbid adjustment.
    e. flatness of affect.

4. By deleting acute (and certain other types of disorders) formerly classified as Schizophrenia, DSM-III identifies as Schizophrenia a group of disorders that have in common which of the following?

    a. response to treatment
    b. onset in early adult life
    c. tendency toward recurrence
    d. impairment of level of functioning
    e. all of the above

Complete the following.

5. If the symptoms last longer than six months, the diagnosis is changed from Schizophreniform to _____.

6. In order to make a diagnosis of Schizophrenia, signs of the illness must have persisted continuously for at least _____ months at some time during the individual's life and there are currently some signs of the illness.

Matching: Lettered items may be used once or more than once.

Match the following numbered items with the corresponding disorders.

___7.	hereditable	a.	Schizophreniform
___8.	good prognosis	b.	chronic Schizophrenia
___9.	poor prognosis		

Match the following diagnoses and case histories.

a.   Schizophreniform Disorder
b.   Chronic Schizophrenia, acute exacerbation
c.   Schizoid Personality
d.   none of the above

___10.   M.L., a 33-year-old mother of twins, was first hospitalized at age 25 with florid psychotic symptoms including the belief that her feelings were not her own and that she was being forced to think obscene thoughts. She was hospitalized for a period of 3 months and attended a day care treatment program for an additional 6 months. She was maintained on Stelazine for approximately 18 months and appeared somewhat improved. However, she remained socially isolated, her speech was vague and confused, and her affect was blunted. Six months ago her husband filed for divorce and one month ago he obtained custody of the children. Two weeks later M.L. was again hospitalized, at which time she appeared unkempt, was mute, and exhibited bizarre posturing.

___11.   S.D. is an 18-year-old white male, high school drop-out who was apparently well according to family informants until two weeks ago, at which time he was fired from his job as a carpenter's helper and began staying up all night. One week ago he began reading the Bible aloud and preaching to his family until 2 or 3 a.m. The parents stated that his girlfriend had broken off with him about a month ago and from that time he had appeared preoccupied and withdrawn. The patient stated that two individuals from work were continually following him around, talking about him constantly, and describing his thoughts even before he thought them. He was described as previously disinterested in religion and as always having "plenty of friends."

IV.   DIAGNOSTIC CRITERIA FOR A SCHIZOPHRENIC DISORDER

Schizophrenia is a chronic, disabling, psychotic disorder. A + B + C (below) must be present and D and E must be absent to make a diagnosis of Schizophrenia.

Criterion A.   Characteristic psychotic symptoms. One or more of the following symptoms has been present during an active phase of the illness:

(1) Bizarre delusions, such as delusions of being controlled, thought broadcasting, insertion, or withdrawal.

(2) Somatic, grandiose, religious, nihilistic, or other delusions without persecutory or jealous content.

(3) Delusions with persecutory or jealous content if accompanied by hallucinations of any type.

(4) Auditory hallucinations in which either a voice keeps up a running commentary on the individual's behavior or thoughts as they occur or two or more voices converse with each other.

(5) Auditory hallucinations on several occasions without affective content and not limited to one or two words.

(6) Looseness of associations, marked illogicality or marked poverty of content of speech if accompanied by flat or inappropriate affect, delusions or hallucinations or behavior that is grossly disorganized or catatonic.

Criterion B. Deterioration of a previous level of functioning. During the active phase of the illness the characteristic symptoms have been associated with significant impairment in two or more areas of daily functioning such as work, social relations and self-care.

Criterion C. Chronicity. The diagnosis of Schizophrenia cannot be made on the basis of a cross-sectional evaluation of a patient; rather, symptoms must have persisted for at least six months at some time during that person's life. Thus, a longitudinal assessment is required.

Criterion D. Manic or depressive symptoms not present or developed after the schizophrenic symptoms.

Criterion E. Not due to any Organic Mental Disorder.

The diagnosis of Schizophrenia requires that continuous signs of the illness have existed for at least six months during the person's life, and this time period must include an active period of psychotic symptoms from those listed in Criterion A. The psychotic symptoms associated with the active phase are those listed in Criterion A. The six-months requirement may be met by the persistence of the active phase for six months or by any combination of active and prodromal and/or residual symptoms so long as the total duration of symptoms was for at least six months.

ANSWERS,   Section   III._____

1.	b	7.	b
2.	a	8.	a
3.	a	9.	b
4.	e	10.	b
5.	Schizophrenia	11.	a
6.	six		

_____

_____

QUIZ, Section IV.

Complete the following.

1. The diagnosis of Schizophrenia requires that continuous signs of the illness have existed for at least _____months during the person's life, and this time period must include an active period of psychotic symptoms from those listed in Criterion A.

2. At least _____of the Criterion A symptoms must have occurred at some time during the individual's life, and in addition the individual now has some sign of Schizophrenia in order to make a diagnosis of Schizophrenia.

3. A schizophrenia-like illness that lasts for less than six months is called _____.

4. The essential positive features in diagnosing Schizophrenia are:

    A =
    +
    B =
    +
    C =

_____

V.   PHENOMENOLOGICAL SUBTYPES

A.   DISORGANIZED (HEBEPHRENIC) 295.1X

This subtype is characterized by disorganized thinking, shallow and inappropriate affect, silly, unpredictable and regressive behavior and mannerisms, and frequent hypochondriacal complaints. The onset is usually early and insidious. The prognosis is poor, the course usually being chronic, unremitting and deteriorating. This type of Schizophrenia is rarely seen today.

The diagnostic criteria for the disorganized type of Schizophrenia include:

    A. Frequent incoherence
    B. Absence of systematized delusions
    C. Affect is silly, incongruous or flat

****

GO TO VIDEOTAPE: Disorganized Type

****

B.   CATATONIC 295.2X.

The word "catatonia" means a lowering of tension and refers to the muscular flexibility that is sometimes seen in the catatonic schizophrenic patient. Catatonia is perhaps a misnomer because the patient often exhibits muscular rigidity. Four types of catatonia are distinguished: the withdrawn, excited, rigid and posturing types. A patient generally manifests only one type, but sometimes patients pass rapidly from the withdrawn to the excited phases. Both of these phases require careful monitoring. In the excited phase, the patient may be dangerous to himself or others, perhaps being driven to obey hallucinatory commands. In the severely withdrawn phase, the nutritional status requires careful attention because the patient might starve.

Catatonic Schizophrenia was once reported to be common; it is now relatively rare. The prognosis of Schizophrenia, Catatonic Type is fair.

The diagnostic criterion for the catatonic type of Schizophrenia is:

> During the active phase of the illness one or more of the following symptoms dominate the clinical picture: catatonic stupor or mutism, catatonic negativism, catatonic rigidity, catatonic excitement or catatonic posturing.

C.   PARANOID SCHIZOPHRENIA

This subtype of Schizophrenia is characterized by the presence of persecutory or grandiose delusions often associated with hallucinations. Sometimes delusions of jealousy occur. Excessive religiosity is sometimes seen. Paranoid schizophrenic behavior is frequently hostile and aggressive but this behavior tends to be consistent with the delusions. Although the prognosis is poor for recovery, most patients with Paranoid Schizophrenia when medicated are able to function outside the hospital.

The diagnostic criteria for Paranoid Schizophrenia are:

    A.   Meets the criteria for Schizophrenia.
    B.   During the active period of the current episode the clinical picture is dominated by one or more of the following: delusions of persecution, grandiosity or

ANSWERS, Section IV.

1. six
2. one
3. Schizophreniform
4. A = characteristic symptoms
   B = deterioration of a previous level of functioning
   C = chronicity (at least six months)

---

jealousy or hallucinations with persecutory or grandiose content.

****

GO TO VIDEOTAPE

****

D. UNDIFFERENTIATED SCHIZOPHRENIA

This diagnosis is made when the episode of illness is manifested by psychotic symptoms that do not fit categories previously listed or when the symptoms are mixed and the patient could be classified in more than one category.

E. RESIDUAL

Patients who at some previous time had an episode involving psychotic symptoms from Criterion A and who now have signs of Schizophrenia such as blunted affect, eccentric behavior, or communication disorder are classified here. Perhaps Type II Syndrome of Crow best fits here.

VI. GENETICS AND BIOCHEMISTRY OF SCHIZOPHRENIA

People have always been looking for the cause of Schizophrenia and have at various times ascribed the etiology to demons, witchcraft, child rearing practice, to an as yet undetected brain lesion, etc. In the recent past, Schizophrenia has been thought to be due to hereditary factors or the way the mother raised the child; this was called the nature-nurture controversy.

Nowadays scientists are seeking a brain malfunction at the neurochemical level to account for the symptoms manifested in Schizophrenia.

If there are neurochemical imbalances in the brains of schizophrenics which play a causative role in manifestations of Schizophrenia, chances are that they are genetically predetermined since the genes operate through biochemical mechanisms. Indeed, a genetic link between low platelet monoamine oxidase (MAO) activity and chronic Schizophrenia has been recently suggested and confirmed by some, although not all investigators. This is an important potential bridge between genetic and neurotransmitter studies because MAO plays a principal role in the degradation of brain monoamines, including dopamine and serotonin.

Among monozygotic twins with diseases such as Huntington's Chorea and phenylpyruvic oligophrenia, the concordance rate, or chances that both twins will be affected, is very close to 100%. Concordance among monozygotic twins for Schizophrenia is about 50%. This is a figure remarkably above that encountered among the general population in which the lifetime risk of Schizophrenia is about 1%, but quite below that found in Huntington's Chorea (100%).

These figures suggest that there are grossly about equal endogenous and exogenous forces (nature and nurture, respectively) working toward the development of Schizophrenia. Thus, the relative contributions of genetic and environmental factors is no longer a highly controversial issue. The concordance rates in fraternal (dizygotic) twins is much lower (10%) than in identical (monozygotic) and not significantly different from that found in non-twin siblings. This difference is therefore nowadays largely attributed to the identity of genetic endowment shared by monozygotic twins. The genetic loading for Schizophrenia increases with the closeness of biological relatedness and varies with the type of Schizophrenia. These two factors interplay in the quantitative but empirical determination of an individual at risk. Chronic Schizophrenia carries great genetic loading and risk for the development of this syndrome among first-degree relatives, while schizo-phreniform reactions carry little or none. With the above premise in mind, one can estimate approximate risks of Schizophrenia in the relatives of a chronic schizophrenic. These are: 1) 10% in full siblings and children not yet born; the risk past age 40 will be roughly half of the risk he had at birth - therefore only 5%; the remaining risk beyond the age of 50 will be practically negligible. 2) The offspring of a chronic schizophrenic couple has a risk close to 40% of becoming schizophrenic during his lifetime; such risk is second only to that of the identical twin of a chronic schizophrenic. 3) The risk for Schizophrenia increases directly with the number of relatives with definite Schizophrenia and with the closeness of the biological relation to him and somewhat inversely with the number of years beyond the age of maximum risk.

What you need to remember from all this are the principles involved. Some examinations might require you to select a certain percentage from a list, but you can usually do this if you recall the principal ideas.

Two main genetic models, the polygenic and the monogenic theories, have emerged largely to accommodate the conviction that there is a rather marked genetic variability in the predisposition or morbidity risk for Schizophrenia. The polygenic concept allows for the causation of a Schizophrenic Syndrome by a threshold multiadditive effect. In a monogenic view, however, the single autosomal gene assumed to be primarily responsible for the appearance of the syndrome would express itself in all homozygotes of sufficiently long survival and in about 25% of the heterozygotes. If a polygenic model were to prevail, it is very unlikely that a single biochemical abnormality would be found. The monogenic concept implies that there may be a single mutant gene leading to an error in metabolism. In the current search for such a metabolic abnormality the two most assiduously scrutinized problems are the disposition of dopamine (DA) and serotonin (5-HT). Most investigators of the role of these two neurotransmitters in the biochemistry of the mind and behavior think that they are intricately interrelated with each other and with other neurotransmitters as well, such as norepinephrine, gamma-aminobutyric acid and acetylcholine. But we will focus on DA and 5-HT in this discussion.

Dopamine will be considered first. Figure 7-1 gives an overview of possible approaches to studying dopamine.

Figure 7-1

APPROACHES TO STUDYING DOPAMINE

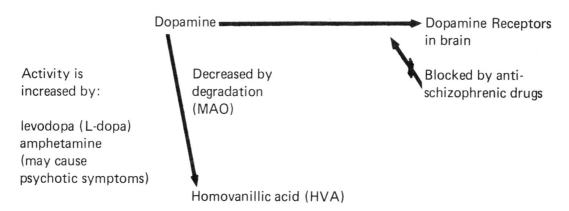

The dopamine theory of Schizophrenia originated on the basis of indirect evidence provided by the understanding gained of the mechanisms of action of antipsychotic drugs. Drugs such as phenothiazines and haloperidol cause a decided blocking effect on dopamine receptors. Of the various pharmacological actions of antipsychotics demonstrable in in vitro models, the relative dopamine receptor blocking potency of the various drugs correlates best with their antischizophrenic potency on a mg per mg basis. Clinical support for a dopamine receptor blocking effect by neuroleptics can also be gleaned from the marked increase in the levels of homovanillic acid (HVA) in the cerebrospinal fluid of patients treated with neuroleptics. HVA is the principal metabolite of dopamine. It has been demonstrated that antipsychotics cause an increased turnover of DA - both the synthesis and degradation of DA are accelerated - leading to increased HVA formation. It is thought that the increased dopamine turnover represents an effort by the neurochemical circuit involved to compensate for the receptor blockade caused by the antipsychotic.

Additional evidence for the DA theory has to do with the actions of some dopamine analogs or substances that mimic the action of dopamine. Dopamine itself cannot be studied directly because it does not pass the blood-brain barrier. But levodopa (L-dopa) which is the precursor of DA does pass the blood-brain barrier. L-dopa acts indirectly by producing DA. L-dopa produces a state of hypervigilance in both man and animals. In humans it may aggravate symptoms of Schizophrenia or may induce a Schizophreniform Psychosis in nonschizophrenics. Amphetamines also act indirectly by causing a massive extrusion of dopamine from nerve terminals. Amphetamines may cause paranoid psychoses which are quite indistinguishable from Paranoid Schizophrenia. Amphetamines release norepinephrine as well as dopamine from nerve terminals. It is thought that the release of norepinephrine is responsible for increased motor activity, while the release of dopamine determines the behavioral stereotypes and aberrations associated with amphetamines.

There are three dopaminergic pathways with fairly well-identified and localized sites of origin and termination of their neuronal elements. These are the nigro-neostriatial, the mesolimbic, and tuberohypophyseal systems. The nigrostriatal contains about 75% of the dopaminergic neurons. This is the most thoroughly investigated of the DA systems and is important in understanding the neuroleptic-induced extrapyramidal symptomatology. Dopamine receptor blockage of the tuberohypophyseal system is thought to be responsible for the endocrine constellation of neuroleptic-induced side effects. The mesolimbic system originates in neurons of the nuclear interpeduncularis in the ventral tegmentum of the brain stem and terminates in the nucleus accumbens, the tuberculum olfactorium and the cerebral cortex. Understanding of the mesolimbic system lags behind that of the other two systems, and this presents a severe impediment to a more precise understanding of our topic because the mesolimbic system is suspected, almost entirely by default, of being the most directly involved with Schizophrenia.

The belief that the mesolimbic system is involved in Schizophrenia has been fostered by the theory that the limbic system is the visceral or emotional brain. It was once thought that the extrapyramidal side effects were inseparable from the antischizophrenic effects of neuroleptic drugs. However, the fact that thioridazine causes hardly any extrapyramidal side effects and yet is a good antipsychotic is taken to suggest that thioridazine acts preferentially on the dopamine receptors in the mesolimbic system. The low incidence of extrapyramidal symptoms with thioridazine may also be due to its anticholinergic potential. Thioridazine is the most potent anticholinergic of the neuroleptics.

Serotonin (5-HT) has also been implicated in Schizophrenia. The idea that there may be a malfunction in serotonin neurons underlies much research, both in endogenous depression and in Schizophrenia. As for Schizophrenia, this view began to grow with the observation that lysergic acid diethylamide (LSD) and other hallucinogens are inhibitors of serotonin effects. The hallucinogenic effects of LSD are potentiated by reserpine. Reserpine deletes brain monoamines including serotonin. Other agents can prevent the hallucinogenic effects of LSD.

The hallucinogenic effects of LSD are not prevented by drugs that raise brain serotonin levels either by preventing its deamination such as the monoamine oxidase inhibitors (MAOI) or by fostering its synthesis such as 5-hydroxytryptophane (5-HTP), the serotonin precursor.

The methylation theory of Schizophrenia presupposes that serotonin or a closely related compound is methylated, and this would yield a psychotogenic derivative. LSD is not a suspected candidate since tolerance develops to LSD. If tolerance were to develop, increasing amounts of the psychotoxin would have to be generated or accumulated to sustain the psychosis. Dimethyltryptamine (DMT) is a hallucinogen of short action to which tolerance does not develop. DMT can conceivably be synthesized in vitro, being a methylated compound otherwise identical to tryptamine or serotonin. However, DMT has not been discovered (in a satisfactorily verifiable manner) in human body fluids.

Experiments involving administration of DMT to human subjects in doses sufficient to cause a model psychosis have shown that it is possible to detect the unchanged DMT excreted in the urine, as well as determinations of levels in circulating blood. It has therefore been concluded that if DMT were formed endogenously in schizophrenics, currently available methods of detection would have succeeded in detecting it in a less ambiguous fashion than has so far been possible. However, other lines of reasoning tend to support the methylation theory. One such approach is as follows: If a psychotogenic methylated derivative of tryptamine or serotonin accumulates in the brain of schizophrenics, this might be due to accumulation of tryptamine or serotonin. Some studies have shown that the serotonin content of platelets in chronic schizophrenics is about twice that found in schizophreniform patients or normals. Possible explanations for the elevated levels of serotonin in chronic schizophrenics may be that synthesis in this population is accelerated, or degradation is slowed up, or both. If degradation is impaired, the deaminating enzyme MAO may be low. Support for this last possibility is available. MAO activity has been found decreased in platelets of chronic schizophrenics, but again not in schizophreniform patients.

Nicotinic acid has been used in treatment of Schizophrenia because it is a methyl-receptor. The assumption was that if Schizophrenia is a state due to an excess of methylated derivatives of serotonin or tryptamine, perhaps nicotinic acid would demethylate the psychotogenic compounds. There is more claim than proof, however, for this therapeutic approach to Schizophrenia.

The polygenic theory of Schizophrenia implies a threshold effect and the possibility that two or more biochemical aberrations may be operative in Schizophrenia. It is conceivable, therefore, that some symptoms of Schizophrenia more likely may be related to an abnormality of serotonin, while other signs may be more dependent on an alteration in dopaminergic activity or sensitivity of dopaminergic receptors, or that each of the subtypes of Schizophrenia may be differentially and more selectively attributable to one of the various neurochemical abnormalities.

The psychoses caused by amphetamines more closely resemble some forms of Schizophrenia than any other psychotogen or hallucinogen, including LSD. Schizophrenics can distinguish the effects of LSD better than those of amphetamines from their endogenous symptoms. Amphetamines release norepinephrine and dopamine from nerve terminals.

It is likely that the arousal or hypervigilance characteristic of the schizophrenic state may be partly due to an alteration of the central noradrenergic system similar to that caused by amphetamines.

It is likely that alterations in other aminergic systems such as the cholinergic and the gabaminergic may be more involved in Schizophrenia than it would appear from the currently available evidence. Many lines of evidence indicate that the balance and interdependence of all the neurotransmitters are very intricate and delicate. Acetylcholine and GABA alterations may not be directly responsible for schizophrenic symptomatology, but they may directly influence the vicissitudes of dopamine and serotonin.

QUIZ, Section VI.

Circle the letter corresponding to the one correct response.

1. The high concordance among monozygotic twins for Schizophrenia suggests that

    a. Schizophrenia is not a genetic disease.
    b. genetic as well as other factors contribute to the development of Schizophrenia.

2. Chronic Schizophrenia carries a _____ _____ for monozygotic twins.

    a. high risk.
    b. low risk.

3. With increasing numbers of relatives with definite Schizophrenia and with increasing closeness of biological relatedness, risk

    a. increases.
    b. decreases.

4. With increasing age, risk

    a. increases.
    b. decreases.

Use the following diagram to answer questions 5-6.

$$\text{Dopamine} \xrightarrow{\text{MAO}} \text{Homovanillic acid (HVA)}$$

5. Low MAO activity would be expected to be associated with (check one)

    a. high levels of dopamine.
    b. low levels of dopamine.

6. Increased levels of urinary HVA would be expected to be associated with (check one)

   a. increased dopamine degradation.
   b. decreased dopamine degradation.

Circle the correct answer(s). <u>One</u> or <u>more than one</u> answer may be correct.

7. Figure 7-1 shows two reasons why increased DA activity is thought to be associated with Schizophrenia. The reasons are:

   a. L-dopa and amphetamines can precipitate schizophrenia-like symptoms.
   b. Antischizophrenic drugs are powerful dopamine receptor blockers.
   c. MAOI are powerful antischizophrenic drugs.
   d. Increased excretion of HVA is very often found in patients with Schizophrenia.

8. Two factors suggesting the involvement of DA in Schizophrenia are related to antipsychotic drug effects:

   a. antipsychotic drugs block dopamine receptors.
   b. antischizophrenic potency of drugs correlates best with their anticholinergic effect.
   c. antipsychotic drugs cause increased DA turnover.
   d. antipsychotic drugs lead to decreased formation of homovanillic acid.

9. Two drugs that support the DA theory of Schizophrenia are _____ and _____ which indirectly increase DA and can be associated with a schizophreniform psychosis.

   a. amphetamines
   b. L-dopa
   c. homovanillic acid
   d. monoamine oxidase

10. Two drugs that can raise brain serotonin levels are

    a. BAL.
    b. L-dopa.
    c. MAOI.
    d. 5-HTP.

11. If an endogenous hallucinogen were found to be the cause of Schizophrenia, it would have to meet several criteria.

    a. Tolerance does not develop.
    b. It would have to be a compound that could be synthesized by the body.
    c. It should be possible to discover the compound in body fluids.
    d. The compound should chemically resemble amphetamines.

12. Experimental findings that support the methylation of serotonin theory of Schizophrenia are:

    a. Serotonin content of platelets in chronic schizophrenics is high.
    b. MAO activity of platelets in chronic schizophrenics is low.
    c. Good therapeutic results with nicotinic acid in treatment of Schizophrenia.

TRUE or FALSE: Circle the correct answer.

T   F   13. MAOI and 5-HTP prevent hallucinogenic effects of LSD.

Match the following risks for Schizophrenia. Lettered items may be used once or more than once.

_____14. risk for monozygotic twin of   a.   1%
         chronic schizophrenic   b.   10%
_____15. risk in general population   c.   3%
_____16. risk for fraternal twin of   d.   90%
         chronic schizophrenic   e.   50%
_____17. risk for other sibling of   f.   40%
         chronic schizophrenic   g.   25%
_____18. risk if both parents schizophrenic

Dopamine receptor blockage of the following systems is thought to account for which effects of antipsychotic drugs? Match the following.

_____19. tuberohypophyseal   a.   extrapyramidal side effects
_____20. mesolimbic   b.   endocrine side effects
_____21. nigrostriatal   c.   reduction of schizophrenic symptoms

VII. PSYCHOSES NOT ELSEWHERE CLASSIFIED

This classification contains three specific categories, Schizophreniform Disorder, Brief Reactive Psychosis, and Schizoaffective Disorder and a residual category, Atypical Psychosis, for all psychotic disorders that do not meet the criteria for any specific disorder.

The diagnostic criteria for a Schizophreniform Disorder are:

    A. Meets all the criteria for Schizophrenia except for duration.

    B. The duration of illness is more than one week but less than six months. The duration includes prodromal, active, and residual phases.

The Brief Reactive Psychosis is of even shorter duration: from a few hours to less than one week. Another distinguishing feature of this disorder is that the onset immediately follows an identifiable stressor, hence the name "reactive."

The diagnostic criteria for a Brief Reactive Psychosis are:

A. The symptoms in B appear immediately following a recognizable stressor. The stressor is of a magnitude that symptoms of distress would be expected from almost all individuals. Such stresses would be loss of a loved one, combat.

B. The clinical picture involves emotional turmoil and at least one of the following:
    1. Looseness of associations or marked illogicality
    2. Delusions
    3. Hallucinations
    4. Behavior that is grossly disorganized or catatonic

C. The duration is from a few hours to less than a week.

D. This diagnosis should not be made if the symptoms in B are preceded by a period of increasing psychopathology.

E. Does not meet the criteria for an Organic Mental Disorder, manic episode, or factitious illness with psychological symptoms.

The category of Schizoaffective Disorder has been retained by DSM-III, but no diagnostic criteria are included. Schizoaffective implies a combination of schizophrenic and affective symptoms. DSM-III suggests that this occurrence is probably best categorized under Major Affective Disorder with Psychotic Features.

QUIZ, Section VII.

Circle the letter corresponding to the one correct answer.

1. You will recall from the discussion on Schizophrenia that Schizophrenic Disorders and Schizophreniform Disorders are distinguished from each other only on the basis of

    a. type of symptoms.
    b. manner of onset.
    c. duration of symptoms.
    d. degree of disorientation.

2. A Brief Reactive Psychosis differs from Schizophrenia and Schizophreniform Disorders in that in a brief psychotic reaction

    a. the duration is shorter.
    b. there are no prodromal symptoms.
    c. a recognizable stressor is always present.
    d. all of the above.

TRUE or FALSE: Circle the correct letter.

T   F   3. Stressors may or may not be identifiable before the onset of Schizophreniform or Schizophrenic Disorders.

VIII. TREATMENT OF SCHIZOPHRENIC DISORDERS

There are four major approaches to treatment of Schizophrenia: milieu, psychotherapy, drugs, and behavior modification. Only antipsychotic drug therapy has been demonstrated to be of unequivocal benefit in reducing psychotic symptoms, but results in removing residual (negative) symptoms of Schizophrenia are often disappointing.

Electroconvulsive therapy (ECT) was widely used in treatment of all types of Schizophrenia in the past, but its efficacy was rarely evaluated and it has not been compared with drug therapy in controlled studies. ECT is occassionally used nowadays to treat agitated and excited patients with Catatonic Schizophrenia. Psychosurgery was also used in the past, but is no longer an accepted method of treatment of Schizophrenia (or any other psychiatric disorder). Renal dialysis has been reported to improve a few patients with Schizophrenic Disorder; this is still an experimental approach.

A.   MILIEU THERAPY

The milieu or environment in which an individual is placed has a profound effect on behavior; most people respond to the expectations and constraints of the environment. Active psychotic symptoms will often diminish shortly after the patient is admitted to the hospital, presumably because the hospital provides a less stressful environment than the one from which the patient has just come.

Institutions are more or less authoritarian and custodial so that patients admitted to hospitals are expected to behave in a dependent and compliant manner. Long-term treatment in mental hospitals tends to promote failure to take responsibility for one's self and de-culturation. The use of a "Therapeutic Community" as a means of countering the effects of chronic hospitalization was originated in England by Maxwell Jones. He also wrote a book with that title. This model is widely used in U.S. hospitals. Its key points are:

1.	b	8.	a,c,	15.	a
2.	a	9.	a,b	16.	b
3.	a	10.	c,d	17.	b
4.	b	11.	a,b,c	18.	f
5.	a	12.	a,b	19.	b
6.	a	13.		20.	c
7.	a,b	14.	e	21.	a

(1) open wards whenever possible

(2) participation of patients and staff in group activity and patient government

(3) control of disturbed behavior by psychotherapy, chemotherapy, social, occupational, and work therapy, and rehabilitation programs (rather than by physical restraints)

(4) efforts to increase the contact between the patient in the hospital and the outside community: visiting is encouraged; home visits whenever possible.

Hospitals usually provide a variety of programs such as occupational therapy, work therapy, education, remotivation, resocialization, and patient government in order to present a better therapeutic environment. Most of these programs have been developed for use with chronically hospitalized patients, and are believed to be beneficial for this group, although the value of milieu therapy has not been conclusively demonstrated. Whatever the type of milieu, improvement does occur if drugs are a part of the treatment.

What should be remembered is that an appropriate hospital milieu should be provided--appropriate to the schizophrenic's impaired perceptual and cognitive abilities--and optimal drug therapy achieved.

In order to prevent the dependency and de-culturation associated with chronic hospitalizations, the trend today is to treat patients with Schizophrenic Disorder as outpatients or keep hospitalization time as brief as possible, and in some states efforts have been made to abolish mental hospitals altogether. Unfortunately the rehabilitation and support systems available in hospitals are usually not present in the community, so that many discharged patients are now as neglected as they were formerly in mental hospital.

Ludwig (1971) describes three major phases of treatment:

(1) modification of behavior in the hospital

(2) preparation for discharge

(3) maintenance of rehabilitation in the community.

The community mental health movement in the U.S. has had disastrous effects on many individuals because of failure to take into account the necessity of the 2nd and 3rd phases.

There are many treatment-resistant patients for whom long-term hospitalization is indicated, but for most patients with Schizophrenia brief hospitalization is preferable and adequate.

B. PSYCHOTHERAPY

A number of psychotherapy approaches have been developed for treating Schizophrenia. These include psychoanalysis and modified psychoanalytic techniques, direct analysis, and existential approaches, as well as group and family therapy. In the treatment of Schizophrenia, there appears to be little place for the use of dynamic interpretation or therapy that promotes insight. Whether treatment is individual, group, or family based, positive results are more likely if the treatment focuses on current, real-life issues and relationships, work, or other practical issues. This approach is generally termed supportive psychotherapy.

Few believe that psychotherapy should be conducted without the concurrent use of drugs. Drugs plus supportive psychotherapy produce better results in the treatment of Schizophrenia than drugs alone.

C. ANTIPSYCHOTIC DRUGS

The use of antipsychotic drugs is discussed in Chapter 16. Drugs are used in the treatment of Schizophrenic Disorders to reduce psychotic and residual symptoms and to enable the patient to participate in other forms of therapy. Maintenance drug therapy helps to prevent relapses but also may lead to the development of tardive dyskinesia. There is no hard evidence that total dosage of antipsychotic drugs increases the likelihood of tardive dyskinesia, but this is thought to be so. Thus, most authorities advocate using the lowest possible maintenance dosage and drug holidays.

D. BEHAVIOR THERAPY

Behavior therapy is based on the theory of operant conditioning first described by Skinner and employs rewards and punishment to reinforce or eliminate behaviors. Carefully designed and consistent behavior modification programs can improve functioning in some chronic patients. The critical principle involved is that receiving a reward is contingent on the patient's showing a specified improvement, geared to the patient's level of functioning in social, personal, or work behavior. Behavior modification can not be expected to cure Schizophrenia, in the sense of reversing the assumed biological or psychological causes. But altering behavior and improving social skills will help rehabilitate many patients.

E. TREATMENT-RESISTANT PATIENTS

Some individuals with Schizophrenic Disorder do recover; many others have residual symptoms but nevertheless function adequately at work and fulfill family reponsibilities. Some become treatment failures and spend a large part of their lives in hospitals. A large number are partial treatment failures who never return to a normal level of functioning, but who nevertheless are able

ANSWERS, Section VII._____

1. c
2. d
3. T

_____

to remain in the community. For these there are usually inadequate support systems. To think of a cure for this large group in the sense of being able to do without continued supportive services, is unrealistic. Schizophrenic Disorder is defined as being chronic; it doesn't usually go away. Ludwig's three phases of treatment are useful to remember and are here repeated:

  (1) modifications of behavior in the hospital
  (2) preparation for discharge
  (3) maintenance of rehabilitations in the community.

_____

QUIZ, Section VIII.

Circle the letter corresponding to the one correct answer.

1. Unequivocally useful in reducing psychotic symptoms in Schizophrenic Disorders is

    a. milieu therapy.
    b. psychotherapy.
    c. antipsychotic drug therapy.
    d. ECT.
    e. psychosurgery.

2. All the following are true regarding the Therapeutic Community approach to treatment except

    a. the forerunner of the modern U.S. mental hospital milieu therapy.
    b. thought to decrease dependency of the patient.
    c. of unequivocal value in treatment of Schizophrenia.
    d. is less authoritarian than mental hospitals of the past.

3. The best results in the treatment of Schizophrenia occur with

    a. antipsychotic drugs.
    b. a therapeutic milieu.
    c. psychoanalytically oriented psychotherapy plus antipsychotic drugs.
    d. supportive psychotherapy.
    e. supportive psychotherapy plus antipsychotic drugs.

4. The only method demonstrated to reverse the biological or social cause of Schizophrenia is

    a. milieu therapy.
    b. psychological treatments.
    c. antipsychotic drugs.
    d. supportive psychotherapy.
    e. none of the above.

5. Which of the following is useful in modifying behavior in individuals with Schizophrenic Disorder:

    a. selection of an appropriate milieu
    b. antipsychotic drugs
    c. supportive psychotherapy
    d. behavior modification programs
    e. all of the above

TRUE or FALSE: Circle the correct letter.

Prevention of institutionalization (dependency, loss of initiative, de-culturation) can be accomplished by

T F 6. discharging all patients from long-term institutions.

T F 7. brief periods of hospitalization.

IX. PARANOID DISORDERS

A. INTRODUCTION

The term "paranoia" comes from the Greek, meaning beside or beyond reason. This definition captures the main behavior involved in the Paranoid Disorders, namely, a false belief (delusion) which is not subject to logical argument. Behaviors likely to be viewed as paranoid range from suspiciousness, sensitiveness to slights, rigid adherence to rules, overcriticism of others, and self-righteousness all the way to full-blown delusions of persecution. Only in those instances in which the behavior reaches delusional proportions (i.e., delusions of persecution or delusional jealousy) do we consider the diagnosis of Paranoid Disorder. The Paranoid Disorders are divided into four categories: Paranoia, Shared Paranoid Disorder, Acute Paranoid Disorder, and Atypical Paranoid Disorder.

Along with delusions of persecution and delusional jealousy, the other essential features of the Paranoid Disorders are that: (1) the delusions are not due to any other psychiatric or organic disorder, (2) the emotional response to these delusions is appropriate, and (3) the daily functioning (e.g., intellectual and occupational skills) of the individual remains intact or deteriorates minimally over a prolonged period of time. In the purest cases, the delusions are not bizarre or disorganized but generally involve a systemized theme or series of connected themes, such as being spied upon, cheated, followed, or poisoned. The theme may be simple or elaborate. In other instances there may be only delusional jealousy (conjugal paranoia) in which the delusion revolves around a spouse's believed infidelity.

B. ASSOCIATED FEATURES

Other features commonly associated with the Paranoid Disorders include suspiciousness, anger and hostility which may lead to violence, seclusiveness, and eccentricity. Litigious activities and letter writing are also common. Other symptoms which are frequently noted in conjunction with paranoid delusions are delusions of reference in which the individual assigns a personal meaning to fortuitous events and grandiose delusions in which the person believes he is particularly important and hence may see himself as a talented scientist, inventor, politician, or prophet.

C. DIFFERENTIAL DIAGNOSIS

Paranoid behaviors frequently occur in several other clinical syndromes including Organic Mental Disorders, Affective Disorders, Schizophrenia, and Personality Disorders. In order to differentiate between one of these syndromes and the Paranoid Disorders, one must look for clinical features which are associated with the other syndromes but are not found with the Paranoid Disorders. For example, an individual suffering from a Major Depressive Episode may have delusions of persecution, but the presence of a prominent dysphoric mood and neurovegetative signs consistent wth depression would argue in favor of the diagnosis of depression. Individuals who have organically based mental disorders have symptoms of memory impairment and/or disorientation which are not found in the Paranoid Disorders. Along these same lines, in Schizophrenia, Paranoid Type, or Schizophreniform Disorder, the delusions are more apt to be fragmented and bizarre (as in the case of being controlled by alien forces) than is the case with the Paranoid Disorders. The presence of other symptoms such as thought derailment, prominent hallucinations, and a deteriorating course over time also indicates that diagnosis of a Schizophrenic Disorder is appropriate.

D. ETIOLOGY

Regarding the etiology of paranoia, neither genetic nor biochemical alterations have been emphasized. Rather, available evidence indicates that psychosocial factors are of primary importance in the development of paranoid disturbances. Two contributions made by Freud have received considerable attention from authors attempting to understand paranoia. Freud postulated that projection (i.e., the attribution of one's own unacceptable traits to another person) is the main defense mechanism employed by paranoiacs. He also hypothesized that paranoid projection involved unacceptable and unconscious homosexual impulses. That is, the male paranoiac's true belief of "I love him" is denied and changed by the defense mechanism of reaction formation into "I hate him." This belief is further distorted by projection into "I do not hate him; he hates me." (Kaplan,

Freedman, & Sadock, 1980). Clinical evidence, however, has failed to consistently support Freud's thesis, and while some paranoid patients may
harbor unconscious homosexual impulses, this etiological factor does not
pertain to the majority of paranoiacs.

Faulty learning and development have also been postulated to be of etiological importance in the development of paranoid disturbances. Often the
family background of paranoiacs was authoritarian, excessively dominating,
suppressive, and critical. Thus the person fails to develop "basic trust" in
others and relationships and comes to view the environment as hostile and
rejecting of him. As a defense against expected rejection he develops
attitudes of superiority, staunch independence and hostility, as well as
a tendency to blame others for his difficulties and to project onto them the
weaknesses he cannot acknowledge in himself.

Two other authors, Cameron (1959) and Lemert (1962), argued that there is
a reasonable and, if you will, logical progression in the development of the
paranoiac's behavior. The self-important, blaming individual, such as we
described, may, indeed, be viewed as "strange" or be disliked by others
and hence become isolated. As people often do when they are in isolated
situations, he may become anxious, watchful, or hypersensitive which may
cause others to reject him further. The person may realize something is
wrong but not be able to explain it. These circumstances lead the person to
develop a delusional belief which helps assimilate many heretofore unexplained
experiences and feelings. Given the organizing, albeit delusional, belief, the
individual then reinterprets environmental events and develops a "pseudocommunity." The "pseudocommunity" encapsulates his delusional beliefs and
becomes the target of his fears, thus allowing him to interact fairly appropriately with those outside his delusional system.

E.   DIAGNOSTIC CRITERIA

As noted earlier, the Paranoid Disorders are subdivided into Paranoia,
Shared Paranoid Disorder, Acute Paranoid Disorder, and Atypical Paranoid
Disorder. In order for any of these diagnoses to be made, the individual
must first meet the criteria of Paranoid Disorder. The criteria for the
Paranoid Disorders, as delineated in the DSM-III are as follows:

Paranoid Disorder

A.   Persistent persecutory delusions or delusional jealousy.

B.   Emotion and behavior appropriate to the content of the delusional system.

C.   Duration of illness of at least one week.

D.   None of the symptoms of criterion A of Schizophrenia, such
as bizarre delusions, incoherence, or marked loosening of
associations.

ANSWERS, Section VIII.

1. c
2. c
3. e
4. e
5. e
6. F
7. T

E. No prominent hallucinations.

F. The full depressive or manic syndrome (criteria A and B of major depressive or manic episode) is either not present, developed after any psychotic symptoms, or was brief in duration relative to the duration of the psychotic symptoms.

G. Not due to an Organic Mental Disorder.

1. Paranoia (DSM-III 297.10).

    According to DSM-III, the central feature of this disorder is the insidious development of a Paranoid Disorder with a permanent and unshakable delusional system. Despite the delusional belief, the individual maintains his ability to think in a clear and orderly fashion, and typically the delusion is so well-encapsulated that the remainder of the personality is able to operate relatively normally. Often the delusional system is elaborated from a false interpretation of an actual occurrence. With time, more and more of the environment is integrated into the delusional system. Although the evidence the paranoiac advances to justify his claims may be very tenuous, he is unwilling to accept any other possible explanation, and logic and argument to the contrary are futile. Cases of "conjugal paranoia" in which an individual believes without due cause that his mate has been unfaithful are diagnosed in this category. Also diagnosed here are instances of what were heretofore referred to as involutional paranoid states - i.e., paranoid disturbances occurring in the elderly in which signs of dementia or affective illnesses cannot account for the paranoid symptoms. The DSM-III criteria for Paranoia are:

    A. Meets the criteria for Paranoid Disorder.

    B. A chronic and stable persecutory delusional system of at least six months duration.

    C. Does not meet the criteria for Shared Paranoid Disorder.

    Two cases reported in the literature demonstrate the clinical features commonly seen in Paranoia. Milner (1949) reported a case of a thirty-three-year-old paranoiac who murdered his wife with a hammer. Prior to the murder, he had become convinced his wife was infected by a "cancer consumption germ" and that she was trying to kill him by infecting him with the germ. He based his conclusion on several pieces of "evidence" - that his wife had insured him for a small sum shortly after their marriage, that a man who had been a friend of his wife's before their marriage had died suddenly, and that for a few weeks before the murder he had suffered from a pain in his chest and an unusual taste in his mouth.

In a case of conjugal paranoia (Kaplan, Freedman, & Sadock, 1980) the patient had been reared by a dominant mother and ineffectual father. At age 41 and after 10 years of marriage, his wife became very active in civic meetings and frequently left him alone in the evenings to care for the children. One evening he was unable to reach her by phone at the supposed meeting place. Shortly thereafter, when he was requested by his company to work evenings, he saw a colleague who worked with his wife at the civic meetings leave at the regular time. He became convinced he was being plotted against and began spying on his wife and his colleague. Although he found no evidence of a plot, he began to feel more angry and anxious and came to believe his wife and associate were attempting to kill him. He was hospitalized when he flew into a rage because he believed his wife was trying to poison him one evening when she served him an after-dinner drink, but did not have one herself.

2.   Shared Paranoid Disorder (DSM-III 297.30).

In the past this syndrome was referred to as "Folie à deux," but in rare instances more than two people may be involved. DSM-III defines the essential feature of Shared Paranoid Disorder as a persecutory delusional system that develops as a result of a close relationship with another person who already has a disorder with persecutory delusions. One of the two persons has fixed delusions and is usually the dominant member of the pair. The other person is typically a dependent and suggestible person who incorporates the dominant one's delusions while they are together, but relinquishes them fairly quickly once they are separated and he is given therapy. The two people have generally lived a very close existence for a long time in relative isolation from outside influences. Women more frequently than men develop this exceedingly rare disorder. Among the 103 cases reported in the literature, 40 consisted of sisters, 26 were husband and wife, 24 were mother and child, 11 were brothers, six were brother and sister, and two were father and child (Gralnick, 1942).

The DSM-III criteria for Shared Paranoid Disorder are:

A.   Meets the criteria for Paranoid Disorder.

B.   Delusional system develops as a result of a close friendship with another person or persons who have an established paranoid psychotic disorder.

The following case illustrates the essential features of Shared Paranoid Disorder (Gregory, 1968). The Folie à deux involved a mother and her 28-year-old daughter. Both they and the father immigrated from Poland when the daughter was eight years old. They were poor and the daughter quit school in the seventh grade for financial reasons. For many years the daughter and mother slept together, were constant companions, and thus were isolated from outside forces. The daughter's problems seemed to have begun when she was involved in an auto accident shortly after having had surgery for the repair of a nasal obstruction. Following the accident, she complained of constant facial pain and difficulty with her nose and consequently attempted to sue the plastic surgeon for a half million dollars. When this attempt was unsuccessful, the daughter and mother occupied the doctor's home and refused to leave until he had paid them. They were arrested and subsequently deported to Canada. After five occasions on which the pair entered the U.S. and attempted to sue the physician, the U.S. immigration officer in Canada refused to issue them a visa. The daughter became convinced there was a plot to keep them from the U.S. and that the physician was paying the immigration officer. She also believed they were being persecuted by persons in their rooming house who were after their money. The mother came to believe her daughter's beliefs were well-founded. Consequently, they both attempted to get the half million dollars from the immigration officer by occupying his office every day for several weeks prior to being taken to a mental hospital. Throughout the hospitalization and treatment, the daughter's beliefs remained unshakable. The mother, however, after being separated from her daughter, began to lose her conviction in the daughter's delusional system.

3. Acute Paranoid Disorder (DSM-III 298.30).

As described by DSM-III, the essential feature of Acute Paranoid Disorder is that the Paranoid Disorder is acutely precipitated and clears within a six-month period. The disorder is most commonly seen in persons who experience dramatic changes in their environments, such as immigrants, prisoners, refugees, prisoners of war, and inductees into military service. The disturbance rarely becomes chronic.

The DSM-III diagnostic criteria for Acute Paranoid Disorder are:

A. Meets the criteria for Paranoid Disorder.

B. Duration of less than six months.

C. Does not meet the criteria for Shared Paranoid Disorder.

The following case illustrates the essential features of an Acute Paranoid Disorder (Kaplan, Freedman, & Sadock, 1980). The patient was a 28-year-old surgical resident from Central America who was reared in a wealthy family by a domineering mother. Upon coming to the U.S. for his residency, he became completely overwhelmed and puzzled by the adjustments facing him. His understanding of English was minimal, and he did not know how to go about meeting his basic needs, such as getting his laundry done. He was acutely embarrassed in a restaurant when his poor English led to others laughing at him. He began to suspect other residents were plotting to give him the most difficult patients and then developed an elaborate delusional system in which the hospital personnel were conspiring with the immigration office to have him deported. One day during a surgical procedure he decompensated and attacked an anesthesiologist because he thought the anesthesiologist had deliberately caused his patient to develop a hypotensive crisis. With a three-month hospitalization and an improved understanding of the English language, the patient was able to successfully complete the residency program.

4. Atypical Paranoid Disorder (DSM-III 297.90).

This is a residual category for Paranoid Disorders which are not classified elsewhere. Included in this category are the esoteric paranoid states such as the Capgras syndrome in which a person falsely believes his or her spouse has been replaced by an imposter. Also included here are the Amok syndrome and voodoo deaths. In the Amok syndrome, (which occurs almost exclusively in Africa), paranoid ideations in a confused, mute man precipitate an uncontrolled rage and rampage of destruction and killing. In the voodoo death syndrome, the patient becomes convinced a death curse has been placed on him, and his delusions lead to an excess of adrenaline or vagal overstimulation which produces a fatal state of shock.

Some clinicians would also include in the Atypical category several less exotic paranoid states - i.e., hypochondriacal, grandiose, and erotic paranoid reactions. Other authors have placed these in the Paranoia category (Kaplan, Freedman, & Sadock, 1980). In hypochondriacal paranoid psychosis, the patient becomes delusional about an unfounded physical disease or complaint. Grandiose paranoid reactions consist of the person believing himself to have special abilities or to be an important person. In erotic paranoid reactions, the person has the delusion that someone loves him, but is unable to communicate the love because of extenuating circumstances. Usually the love object is a prominent person such as a political figure.

F. INCIDENCE

Efforts to measure the incidence of the Paranoid Disorders have been hindered by the considerable confusion regarding the boundaries between the various clinical syndromes which include paranoid ideation (i.e., Schizophrenia, Paranoid Type, Paranoid Personality, and the subcategories within the Paranoid Disorders). The problems in estimating the incidence are compounded by the fact that since most paranoiacs remain fairly well-compensated in most areas of their functioning, they rarely seek professional intervention themselves. They are likely to be tolerated by their associates and the community as "crackpots" or eccentric loners. Hence, they come to the attention of professional mental health workers only if their angry or litigious behavior becomes quite extreme. Despite these problems, there seems to be agreement that the Paranoid Disorders are rare - with estimates that Paranoid Disorders account for from 0.1 % to 10 % of hospitalized psychiatric patients, depending on the sample studied (Kaplan, Freedman, & Sadock, 1980). There are no consistent findings regarding the sex ratio of the disorder.

G.   COURSE

The age of onset for the Paranoid Disorders is typically during middle or late adult life. The course of Acute Paranoid Disorders is limited to six months by definition. In contrast to this, the course for Paranoia and Shared Paranoid Disorder appears to be chronic with few periods of remission or exacerbations.

QUIZ, Section IX.

Circle the correct answer(s). One or more than one answer may be correct.

1.   Which of the following are features frequently associated with the Paranoid Disorders?

    a. onset in early adult life or late teens
    b. letter writing and litigious behavior
    c. seclusiveness and hostility
    d. unsystemized and scattered delusions

2.   In conjugal paranoia

    a. a person believes his spouse has exceptional qualities and power.
    b. spouses share a belief in a delusional system.
    c. a person believes his spouse has been replaced by a substitute.
    d. a spouse falsely believes his mate has been unfaithful.

3.   If a physician believes a patient's paranoid delusions are secondary to the ingestion of amphetamines, he should diagnose

    a. Paranoia.
    b. Paranoia secondary to amphetamines.
    c. Organic Delusional Syndrome.
    d. Organic Delusional Syndrome with Paranoia.
    e. Paranoia on Axis I and Organic Delusional Syndrome on Axis II.

4. With regard to the etiology of Paranoid Disorders

    a. Freud felt projection of homosexual impulses was a primary etiological factor.
    b. Freud's theory about this has been consistently supported by clinical cases and empirical research.
    c. failure to develop "basic trust" due to authoritarian parenting has been postulated as an etiological factor.
    d. genetic and biochemical factors appear to be of primary importance.

5. In order to diagnose Paranoid Disorder, which of the following must be present?

    a. emotions and behavior appropriate to the content of the delusional system
    b. persistent delusions of persecution or delusional jealousy
    c. the delusions must not be due to Organic Mental Disorder, Affective Syndrome, or Schizophrenia
    d. there may be no prominent hallucinations

6. In Paranoia

    a. the onset is usually gradual.
    b. the delusional system is often elaborated from a false interpretation of an actual event.
    c. the duration is longer than six months.
    d. with appropriate therapy the patient will almost always give up the delusional belief.

7. Shared Paranoid Disorder

    a. in the past has been referred to as Deux à Capgras.
    b. involves two people who are quite dominant and equally share in the delusion.
    c. entails the development of a persecutory delusional system as the result of close association with a person who already has the delusions.
    d. occurs fairly commonly, especially in males.

8. Which of the following is true regarding the treatment and course of the Paranoid Disorders?

    a. Most paranoiacs do not seek treatment on their own volition.
    b. Many paranoiacs do not receive professional help because they are tolerated as eccentrics by the community.
    c. The success rate for treating paranoiacs is high.
    d. The condition is commonly seen.

9. Which of the following is/are DSM-III Diagnostic Criteria for Acute Paranoid Disorder?

    a. duration of greater than six months.
    b. acute onset.
    c. first appearance of a paranoid episode for patient.
    d. meets the criteria for Paranoid Disorder.

ANSWERS, Section IX. _____

1. b,c
2. d
3. c
4. a,c
5. a,b,c,d
6. a,b,c
7. c
8. a,b
9. d

POST-TEST

For the following questions, circle the letter corresponding to the one correct response.

1. Prognostic factors in Schizophrenia include all except

    a. type of clinical symptom.
    b. age at onset.
    c. mode of onset.
    d. premorbid adjustment.
    e. cultural background.

2. All of the following are useful in the treatment of Schizophrenic Disorders except

    a. psychoanalysis.
    b. antipsychotic drugs.
    c. milieu therapy.
    d. behavioral modification.
    e. supportive psychotherapy.

Use the following case study to answer questions 3-4.

A 27-year-old single, white female who had been employed as a clerk-typist until 10 days ago was brought to the hospital by her parents who reported progressive withdrawal until she became mute, negative, and refused to eat. There was no history of previous mental illness.

The patient appeared as a withdrawn, immobile person who did not gesture or move her body and who was difficult to understand because she would only whisper a few words. She did state that she felt thoughts were being put into her mind which she could not decode, and as a result she could not talk. She laughed after she said this.

3. The patient exhibited all of the following symptoms except

    a. hallucinations.
    b. delusions.
    c. autism.
    d. motor disturbance.
    e. inappropriate affect.

4. The most likely diagnosis would be

    a. Briquet's syndrome.
    b. Catatonic Schizophrenia.
    c. Paranoid Schizophrenia.
    d. Schizophreniform Disorder.
    e. amphetamine psychosis.

Use the following case study to answer questions 5-6.

A 28-year-old man states that he has invented a device that could be used to monitor the thoughts of world leaders. Because of the sensitive nature of this invention, the Patent Office has tried to steal it and the FBI has scrutinized his activities, including wire tapping his telephone. The FBI has also developed subtle ways of brain washing which it has employed on the patient for the past two years.

5. Here we have an example of

    a. thought insertion.
    b. grandiose and persecutory delusions.
    c. thought withdrawal.
    d. superstitiousness.
    e. religiosity.

6. According to DSM-III, symptoms of this nature are highly suggestive of

    a. manic depressive illness.
    b. Paranoid Schizophrenia.
    c. Schizoid Personality.
    d. amphetamine psychosis.
    e. none of the above.

7. All the following are among Bleuler's 4 A's except

    a. anhedonia.
    b. ambivalence.
    c. looseness of associations.
    d. affect.
    e. autism.

For the following questions, one or more than one answer may be correct. Circle the correct answer(s).

8. If an endogenous hallucinogen were found to be the cause of Schizophrenia, it would have to meet which of the following criteria?

    a. Tolerance to it does not develop.
    b. It would have to be a compound that could be synthesized by the body.
    c. It should be possible to discover the compound in body fluids.
    d. The compound should chemically resemble amphetamines.

9. Factor(s) that suggest the involvement of dopamine in Schizophrenia are related to which of the following antipsychotic drug effects?

    a. Antipsychotic drugs block dopamine receptor blockade.
    b. Antipsychotic drugs may cause extrapyramidal side effects.
    c. Antipsychotic drugs cause increased dopamine turnover.
    d. Antipsychotic drugs produce a sedative effect.

10. Argument(s) in support of the serotonin or methylation theory of Schizophrenia include:

    a. LSD and other hallucinogens include EEG patterns typical of arousal.
    b. Serotonin content of platelets in chronic schizophrenics is high.
    c. MAO activity of platelets in chronic schizophrenics is low.
    d. Good therapeutic results with nicotinic acid (a methyl receptor) are seen in treatment of Schizophrenia.

11. Which of the following symptoms commonly occur(s) in Schizophrenia?

    a. impaired intelligence
    b. impaired orientation
    c. impaired memory
    d. autism

12. Which of the following is/are true?

    a. Schizophrenia can be reliably diagnosed if catatonic symptoms are present.
    b. Schizophrenia can be reliably diagnosed if looseness of associations is present.
    c. Schizophrenia can be reliably diagnosed if autism is present.
    d. A diagnosis of Schizophrenia based on signs and symptoms is unreliable.

13. Drug(s) that support(s) the dopamine theory of Schizophrenia, because they indirectly increase dopamine and can be associated with schizophreniform psychoses, is/are

    a. nicotinic acid.
    b. levodopa.
    c. lysergic acid diethylamide.
    d. amphetamines.

14. Which of the following is/are essential criteria for a diagnosis of Schizophrenia?

    a. characteristic symptoms.
    b. disorganization of a previous level of functioning.
    c. duration of at least six months.
    d. early age of onset.

15. Which of the following clinical features is/are consistent with a diagnosis of Paranoid Disorder?

    a. Persecutory delusions or delusional jealousy is present.
    b. Daily functioning of the individual is severely disrupted.
    c. The delusions are not due to another psychiatric or organic syndrome.
    d. The emotional response to the delusions is inappropriate.

16. In Acute Paranoid Disorder

    a. the onset is usually gradual.
    b. the duration of the illness is less than six months.
    c. there are prominent hallucinations.
    d. changes in the person's environment such as immigration or prison are often precipitating factors.

17. The DSM-III diagnostic criteria for Paranoid Disorders include

    a. persistent persecutory delusions or delusional jealousy.
    b. not due to organic mental disorder.
    c. duration at least one week.
    d. prominent hallucinations.

18. The Paranoid Disorders are divided into

    a. Paranoia.
    b. Shared Paranoid Disorder.
    c. Acute Paranoid Disorder.
    d. Conjugal Paranoid Disorder.

19. With regard to Paranoia

    a. the onset is usually gradual.
    b. it is a rare disorder.
    c. the course is usually chronic with few cures.
    d. few patients with this disorder seek treatment on their initiative.

Matching: Lettered items may be used once, more than once, or not at all.

Match the following risks for Schizophrenia with the corresponding percentages.

___20.	risk for other sibling	a.	1%
___21.	risk for monozygotic twin	b.	3%
___22.	risk if both parents schizophrenic	c.	10%
___23.	risk in general population	d.	25%
___24.	risk for fraternal twins	e.	40%
		f.	50%
		g.	90%

Match the following terms and definitions.

___25. derailment

___26. hallucination
___27. poverty of content
        of speech
___28. autism
___29. concreteness
___30. neologism
___31. vagueness

a. perceptual experience without a stim-
    ulus
b. an undefined, made-up word
c. ideas do not proceed logically

d. preference for fantasy over reality
e. responses that are literal rather
    than abstract
f. failure to convey much information,
    although there is an adequate amount
    of speech
g. obscure or unclear responses

Match the following terms with the corresponding examples.

___32. neologism
___33. delusion of grandeur
___34. superstition
___35. delusion of influence
___36. somatic delusion

a. "I am the Virgin Mary."
b. The brakish-brack waters scalidify
    the snails.
c. A postmenopausal woman believes
    she is pregnant.
d. "My horoscope says I am under the
    influence of Mars and Pluto today."
e. A woman believes that her every
    move is controlled by unseen agents.

PRE-TEST ANSWERS

1.	a,b,c	13.	a
2.	a,b,c	14.	b
3.	b,d	15.	b
4.	a,b,c	16.	a
5.	a,b,c	17.	d
6.	d	18.	a
7.	d	19.	a
8.	a,c	20.	f
9.	b,d	21.	a
10.	a,b,c	22.	c
11.	a,b,c	23.	c
12.	a,b,c,d	24.	e

25. a
26. b
27. c
28. e
29. d
30. b
31. a
32. e
33. c
34. f
35. g
36. d

POST-TEST ANSWERS

1.	a	13.	b,d	25.	c
2.	a	14.	a,b,c	26.	a
3.	a	15.	a,c	27.	f
4.	d	16.	b,d	28.	d
5.	b	17.	a,b,c	29.	e
6.	b	18.	a,b,c	30.	b
7.	a	19.	a,b,c,d	31.	g
8.	a,b,c	20.	c	32.	b
9.	a,b,c	21.	f	33.	a
10.	a,b,c	22.	e	34.	d
11.	d	23.	a	35.	e
12.	d	24.	c	36.	c

REFERENCES

Bleuler, E. Dementia praecox or the group of schizophrenias. Translated by Zinkin, J. New York: International Universities Press, 1950.

Cameron, N. Paranoid conditions and paranoia. In S. Arieti (Ed.), American handbook of psychiatry. New York: Basic Books, 1959, 508-539.

Crow T. J. Molecular pathology of schizophrenia: More than one disease process? British Medical Journal, 1980, 280, 66-68.

Gralnick, A. Folie à deux: The psychosis of association. Psychiatric Quarterly, 1942, 16, 230-260.

Gregory, I. Fundamentals of psychiatry. Toronto: W.B. Saunders Company, 1968.

Johnstone, E.C., Crow, T.J., Frith, C.D., Carney, M.W.P., & Price, J.S. Mechanism of the antipsychotic effect in the treatment of acute Schizophrenia: Lancet, 1978, i, 848-851.

Kaplan, H. I., Freedman, A. M., & Sadock, B. J. Comprehensive textbook of psychiatry, III. London: Williams & Wilkins, 1980.

Langfeldt, G. Schizophrenia: Diagnosis and prognosis in the schizophrenic syndrome: An annual review. K. Cancro, (Ed.) New York: Brummer/Mazel, 1971.

Lemert, E. M. Paranoia and the dynamics of exclusion. Sociometry, 1962, 25, 2-25.

Ludwig, A. M. Treating the treatment failures. New York: Grune and Stratton, 1971.

Mackay A. V. P. Positive and negative schizophrenic symptoms and the role of dopamine. British Journal of Psychiatry, 1980, 137, 379-386.

Milner, K. O. The environment as a factor in the aetiology of criminal paranoia. Journal of Mental Science, 1949, 95, 124-132.

Sartorius, N., Jablensky, A., Stromgren, E., & Shapiro, R. Validity of diagnostic concepts across cultures: A preliminary report from the international pilot study of schizophrenia. In L. C. Wynn, R. L. Cromwell, & S. Matthysse, (Eds.), The nature of schizophrenia. New York: John Wiley and Sons, 1978.

Wing, J. K. Clinical concepts of schizophrenia. In J.K. Wing (Ed.), Schizophrenia: Towards a new synthesis. London: Academic Press, 1978.

CHAPTER 8

Affective Disorders

Thomas E. Steele, M.D.

CHAPTER OUTLINE

LEARNING OBJECTIVES

After completing this chapter, you will be able to:

1. Define affect and Affective Disorder.

2. Distinguish depression from age- or situation-appropriate worry, from sadness, and from grief.

3. Define depression, hypomania, and mania.

4. Describe disturbances in cognition, perception, neurovegetative function, and behavior that accompany Affective Disorders.

5. Describe influences of the patient's age upon the symptoms of depression.

6. Describe influences of the stage in the life cycle upon the psychological symptoms or concerns of the depressed patient.

7. Describe possible relationships between life events and depression.

8. Describe differences in history and symptoms between patients who experience both depression and mania, and patients who experience depression only.

9. List factors that suggest an increased risk of suicide in depressed patients.

10. List symptoms and signs that are common to Affective and Schizophrenic Disorders, and factors that help distinguish Affective from Schizophrenic disorders.

11. Describe biogenic amine hypotheses of Affective Disorders, including examples of evidence upon which these hypotheses are based.

12. Describe the indications for, and limitations of, somatic treatment (drugs or electroconvulsive therapy) and psychosocial treatment in patients with Affective Disorders.

PRE-TEST

For the following questions, <u>one</u> or <u>more</u> <u>than</u> <u>one</u> answer may be correct. Circle the correct answer(s).

1. DSM-III provides both inclusion and exclusion criteria for diagnosing Affective Disorders. In addition to the presence or absence of specific symptoms, disorders are classified according to

    a. severity.
    b. presence or absence of precipitating stresses.
    c. duration of disturbance.
    d. etiology.

2. The sleep disorder of depression

    a. may consist of excessive sleep rather than decreased sleep.
    b. can be appropriately treated with benzodiazepines.
    c. provides a sensitive index to pharmacologic treatment.
    d. is usually restricted to prolonged sleep latency (difficulty falling asleep).

3. Depression and Dementia may be difficult to distinguish. Which of the following is(are) more characteristic of depression than Dementia?

    a. recent memory more impaired than remote memory
    b. objective signs of cognitive deficit are greater than subjective complaints
    c. family members are unlikely to be aware of the severity of the patient's difficulties
    d. symptoms are worse in the morning, and improve as the day progresses

4. Which of the following might represent typical delusions as seen in depressed patients?

    a. A 25-year-old man believes he is an agent of the C.I.A., and has a powerful radio transmitter implanted in his teeth.
    b. A 46-year-old woman believes that her heart has stopped beating.
    c. A 30-year-old woman believes that God has summoned her to Saudi Arabia to take over the OPEC Cartel.
    d. A 44-year-old man knows that he emits a horrible body odor, even though he bathes several times a day.

5. Choose the correct statement(s).

    a. Depressed patients who also have histories of mania tend to have become depressed at a younger age than depressed patients without histories of mania.
    b. Patients with little or no sleep disturbance are unlikely to be severely depressed.
    c. Patients who talk about suicide are more likely to commit suicide than are patients who don't talk about it.
    d. The presence of hallucinations and/or delusions in a patient favors a diagnosis of Schizophrenia over a diagnosis of depression.

6. Choose the correct statement(s).

    a. The presence of paranoid delusions in a patient tends to rule out an Affective Disorder.
    b. Patients with Affective Disorders may exhibit catatonic excitement, or catatonic stupor.
    c. In acutely psychotic patients, a detailed mental status examination is the most reliable way to distinguish Schizophrenia from Affective Disorder.
    d. Patients with mania may exhibit bizarre behavior and formal thought disorders.

7. Choose the correct statement(s).
    a. The suicide rate generally increases as age increases.
    b. Ingestion of benzodiazepines is unlikely to be lethal unless other drugs or alcohol are ingested concomitantly.
    c. A majority of people who commit suicide have seen a physician during the months prior to their death.
    d. If a physician brings up the topic of suicide with a depressed patient, the risk of suicide increases.

8. A 55-year-old man, with no previous history of depression or mania, presents with typical symptoms of profound depression, including the belief that his "insides have rotted away" and that all of his relatives have died because of his sins. The best treatment(s) would be

    a. ECT.
    b. amitriptyline.
    c. amitriptyline plus haloperidol.
    d. phenelzine plus perphenazine.

9. Choose the correct statement(s).

    a. Intensive psychotherapeutic treatment is best begun at the height of a patient's depression, when he is most motivated to relieve his suffering.
    b. Most patients with severe Affective Disorders will need extensive psychotherapeutic treatment after their acute symptoms are in remission.
    c. Long-standing problems in relating comfortably to others--based on the patient's lack of adequate role models--are likely to be helped by the appropriate psychotropic medication.
    d. Psychotherapy is unlikely to be effective in relieving the neuro-vegetative symptoms that accompany a depressive episode.

10. Regarding depression and grief, choose the correct statement(s).

    a. Low self-esteem is common in depression but not in grief.
    b. A major loss may precede both depression and grief.
    c. Freud believed that ambivalence toward the lost object was present in depression but not in grief.
    d. Sleep disturbance is common in depression but not in grief.

11. The biogenic amine permissive hypothesis

    a. states that low levels of serotonin and high levels of norepinephrine lead to mania.
    b. states that high levels of serotonin and low levels of norepinephrine lead to depression.
    c. is consistent with clinically observed effects of reserpine.
    d. implies that psychological factors play little or no role in Affective Disorders.

12. The primary determinant(s) of a patient's thought content when depressed is(are)

    a. the severity of the sleep disorder.
    b. the quality of the marital relationship (in married patients).
    c. the duration of the depressive episode.
    d. the patient's age and place in the life cycle.

13. Which of the following provide(s) strong evidence for a genetic factor in Affective Disorders?

    a. greater concordance in monozygotic than dizygotic twins
    b. increased incidence of depression in families of depressed probands
    c. similar patterns of antidepressant drug response in depressed relatives of depressed patients
    d. increasing incidence of depression with advancing age

14. In a patient with an acute psychosis, the diagnosis of Schizophrenia is more likely to be correct than the diagnosis of mania if

    a. the patient is less than 25 years old.
    b. delusions and hallucinations are present.
    c. treatment with haloperidol brings about improvement in symptoms.
    d. the patient shows marked blunting or flattening of affect.

15. Depressive delusions are congruent with

    a. depressive affect.
    b. impaired concentration.
    c. lowered self-esteem.
    d. early-morning awakening.

16. A 17-year-old boy has been expelled from school because of persistent fighting with peers, and an assault upon a teacher. He has been arrested several times in the last two years for petty offenses, he frequently becomes intoxicated with alcohol, and he has wrecked his car several times. He has no close friends, although he "hangs around" with several other boys who have been expelled. In grade school, he had seemed well-adjusted and free of problems. His distraught parents consult you:

a. They should be reassured that he will "grow out of it" if his external circumstances change--e.g., if he joins the Army.

b. The possibility that he is suffering from an Affective Disorder should be considered.

c. He should be sent to reform school as probably incorrigible.

Circle the letter corresponding to the one correct response.

17. A middle-aged man complains of abdominal pain and weight loss, and notes that he has recently become constipated. Sigmoidoscopy and barium enema are negative. He reports no disturbance of sleep.

    The most likely diagnosis at this point is

    a. depression.
    b. hysteria.
    c. unknown.
    d. adenocarcinoma of the colon.

18. Patients with "classical" depressive syndromes tend to be between ages

    a. 15-30.
    b. 30-40.
    c. 40-60.
    d. 60-75.

19. Depressed patients beyond the age of 60 will generally show _____ confusion than younger depressives.

    a. more
    b. less

I. INTRODUCTION

Affects are feelings, as distinct from thoughts or actions. Examples of affects include sadness, euphoria, anger, and fearfulness. If a relative or close friend died, you would initially miss them and find yourself preoccupied with thoughts about them--and, in addition to experiencing these thoughts, you would probably also experience the feeling, or affect, of sadness. If a careless driver backed into your parked car, you might think, "That jerk!", but your affect would probably be one of anger.

The term mood is also used to describe feeling states, with the connotation that a mood is a more enduring state of feeling than an affect which may be transient; the comparison has been drawn that mood is to affect as climate is to weather. In practice, the terms mood and affect are often used synonymously, and the psychiatric illnesses characterized by disturbance in mood are known as Affective Disorders. Furthermore, the Affective Disorders do not include disorders involving the entire range of feeling states, but rather only those disorders characterized by pathological lowering or pathological elevation of mood. A mood is pathological when it is disproportionate--either in severity or duration--to the feeling state the average person would be expected to experience in similar circumstances. For example, if an elderly woman feels sad, cries easily, and talks only of her husband--and you learn that her husband of 40 years died two days ago--you would not consider her sadness pathological; it is an expected, typical reaction to a major loss. However, if she feels exactly the same way six months later, you should suspect that a disorder of mood, or an Affective Disorder, has supervened. Similarly, if a man is excited and bubbling over with joy, and you learn that he has just won $100,000 in the sweepstakes, you are not surprised at his expansive and elated mood. By contrast, if a man is filled with enthusiasm for schemes to save the world and spends day after day (and most of each night) telephoning friends, casual acquaintances, and Congressmen to harangue them about his wondrous gifts, one suspects that his elation is pathological.

Implicit in the concept of disorder, when referring to Affective Disorder, are discomfort and disturbed social function. For example, if a person suffers from a significant degree of depression (to be defined below), he would experience discomfort--not only from the emotionally painful affect itself (sadness, "blues," down-in-the-dumps), but also from associated physical symptoms such as lack of energy and disturbed sleep. Such a person would also show a decreased capacity to work (whether as an employee or as a homemaker) and decreased skill and comfort in interpersonal relationships. While a mildly depressed person might be able to continue to work (although less efficiently, and with less enjoyment, than previously) and might be able to maintain, with effort, satisfactory relationships with friends and family, a more severely depressed person would show significant impairment in these areas.

The presence of psychic discomfort (e.g., prolonged sadness), plus evidence of associated "biological" dysfunction (e.g., sleep disorder, lack of energy, anorexia), plus psychosocial dysfunction (e.g., declining work performance, or increased marital friction) would be evidence that a person was suffering from an Affective Disorder, rather than from the transient fluctuations in mood that are part and parcel of the human condition.

QUIZ, Section I.

Circle the correct answer(s). One or more than one answer may be correct.

1. Affects are

    a. thoughts.
    b. feelings.
    c. perceptions.

2. The presence of a significant Affective Disorder implies not only discomfort, but also psychosocial dysfunction. Psychosocial dysfunction is defined as impairment in

    a. energy level.
    b. interpersonal relationships and work function.

3. A pathological mood is one that is _____ to the circumstances.

    a. proportionate
    b. disproportionate

An Affective Disorder serious enough to warrant treatment is likely to be characterized by three types of disturbance: pathological mood, biologic dysfunction, and social dysfunction. Match the numbered disturbance with the appropriate lettered classification; each lettered classification may be used once, more than once, or not at all.

___4.   decreased sleep   a. altered mood
___5.   excessive arguments with spouse   b. biologic dysfunction
___6.   excessive sadness   c. social dysfunction
___7.   lack of energy
___8.   anorexia
___9.   making stupid mistakes at work

II. DEPRESSION

Depression is the most common Affective Disorder, and indeed is probably the most common psychiatric illness. Because significant degrees of depression are accompanied by physical symptoms, primary care physicians see many patients with depression, especially when--as is common--the physical symptoms are more prominent (or more readily volunteered by the patient) than the disturbance in affect per se. Perhaps one-third of all patients seen in a general practice of medicine will complain of physical symptoms for which no organic cause can be found, and many of these patients are depressed. Approximately 5% of all men and 10% of all women will experience at least one serious depressive episode in their lives. Correctly diagnosing depression can prevent exhaustive but unnecessary work-ups for nonexistent physical disorders, can reduce patient suffering, and can reduce "doctor shopping" and "specialist hopping." Once diagnosed, many depressions can be successfully treated by the nonpsychiatric physician. Failure to diagnose depression not only needlessly prolongs the patient's distress, but can also, as Detre and Jarecki (1971) emphasize, lead to the one step--suicide--that ensures that the patient will not recover.

The word "depression" is commonly used in several ways. Synonyms for depressive affect per se include sadness, feeling "low" or "blue," or being "down-in-the-dumps." In typical depressions, depressive affect is prominent and is accompanied by changes in thinking and physical symptoms to be described below. These physical symptoms, changes in thinking, and associated behavioral changes, in combination with depressive affect, define the typical syndrome of depression. However, depressive affect can appear as a symptom in other psychiatric and nonpsychiatric illnesses. For example, patients with Organic Brain Syndromes (see Chapter 5) may experience sadness and tearfulness, but may not be suffering primarily from depression: their cognitive dysfunction--e.g., impaired memory--may impair their psychosocial functioning, but this is not a direct result of depression because the dysfunction reflects impairment of memory rather than impairment of mood. Patients with chronic physical illnesses may also experience depressive affect--i.e., feel sad--but not all chronically ill patients experience the enduring change in mood, plus the associated physical symptoms, plus an associated social dysfunction that is a result of the mood disturbance that would indicate that a concomitant syndrome of depression is present. The picture is further complicated by the existence of atypical depressive syndromes, in which depressive affect is not prominent but is overshadowed by other psychological symptoms such as panic attacks, anxiety, or obsessional thoughts.

A. TYPICAL, OR "CLASSIC," DEPRESSION

The patient with a classic depression experiences depressive affect or profound sadness. The patient will also experience anhedonia, or the inability to experience pleasure. This anhedonia not only influences the present, but also memories of the past: the patient derives little or no pleasure from previously enjoyable activities (work, playing cards, watching TV, visiting friends, sexual intercourse, etc.), and furthermore has difficulty recalling or anticipating pleasure. This may color the history you obtain: a previously satisfactory marriage is now described as "a mistake"; a previously competent housewife may say, "I've always been a slob"; your inquiry about general health may be met by a barrage of past and present ailments. In severe depressions, the future holds no promise: "It's hopeless--what's the use--I'll never get well."

Depressed patients also experience a lack of energy and a lack of motivation. This lack of energy, or anergia, coupled with a reduced capacity to experience pleasure, usually results in impaired social functioning. Patients no longer engage in purposeful, pleasurable activity--they feel weak and depleted, and also "know" that such pursuits are futile and unrewarding. Their withdrawal from family and friends, plus their cessation of pleasure-seeking behavior, may accentuate their distress and create a vicious cycle of depression-promoting behavior. Depressed people are often irritable and short-tempered as well, which further strains relationships with others.

A hallmark of significant depression is neurovegetative dysfunction--that is, disorders of sleep, appetite, and libido (sexual drive). The most typical depressive sleep disorders are middle-of-the-night awakening (MNA) and early-morning awakening (EMA). Even if the sleep loss is relatively mild, the patient will find sleep unsatisfactory and will not awaken refreshed. Sleep disorder is an especially important symptom because: the severity of sleep disorder is an index of the severity of the depression; sleep disorder is a guide to drug treatment in that the dose of medication needed to normalize sleep is usually the dose needed to treat the depression; and the sleep disorder may be more prominent than other depressive symptoms, thus offering a clue to otherwise obscure complaints. Sleep is a relatively quantifiable phenomenon and a relatively conflict-free area: patients are willing to describe their sleep pattern in detail despite reticence in discussing other areas such as sexual function.

The presence of MNA and/or EMA is helpful in distinguishing depression from syndromes primarily involving anxiety. The characteristic sleep disorder in syndromes characterized by anxiety is prolonged sleep latency-- that is, difficulty falling asleep (DFA). Many, if not most, depressed patients are also anxious, but if MNA or EMA is prominent, the anxiety present is most likely a concomitant of depression, and it will resolve as the depression improves. Because anxiety often accompanies depression, many depressed patients are incorrectly diagnosed as primarily anxious, and are treated with sedatives such as benzodiazepines. This is unfortunate on at least three counts: benzodiazepines can be habituating; they may, over prolonged periods, heighten the severity of depression; and they may mask the sleep disorder of depression which leads to the erroneous conclusion that the problem causing the sleep disorder has been appropriately treated. Primary anxiety--as an enduring disorder, rather than transient state--is far less common than depression, and vast amounts of sedatives prescribed annually are "treating" large numbers of misdiagnosed patients. The routine nightly use of sedatives in hospitals is also to be deplored, since a sleep disturbance lasting more than a few nights may represent a significant--and treatable--depression.

A severely depressed patient may experience DFA as well as MNA and EMA, and may even have total insomnia. However, the history in depression will usually reveal that the initial disturbance was MNA or EMA which only later progressed to include DFA. Self-medication with alcohol can also confuse the picture: a patient may mask his sleep disorder by becoming intoxicated, or, alternatively, a patient's MNA may represent rebound hyperexcitability of the central nervous system as a modest dose of alcohol wears off, rather than autonomous MNA.

1.	b	6.	a
2.	b	7.	b
3.	b	8.	b
4.	b	9.	c
5.	c		

Anorexia, usually with weight loss, is a common symptom of depression. Patients may report that food has "lost its taste," or "isn't cooked right anymore." Because anorexia is a symptom of many physical illnesses as well, a patient with anorexia must be carefully questioned about other symptoms of depression such as depressed mood and depressive sleep disorders; if these symptoms are absent, the physician should hesitate to ascribe anorexia, lack of energy, or other physical symptoms to depression.

The sexual appetite also suffers in depression. While some patients, in a vain attempt to seek pleasure, may increase their sexual activity early in the course of a depression, sexual drive is usually markedly decreased later in the course of the illness. Male patients commonly complain of impotence and females of orgasmic dysfunction when they are depressed.

Psychomotor activity is commonly altered with significant depressions. The pattern of altered activity may be <u>agitation</u> (restless, purposeless movements such as handwringing or pacing the floor) or <u>retardation</u> (a slowing or decrease in motor activity, speech, and thoughts). Patients with agitation may be misdiagnosed as suffering primarily from anxiety; however, concomitant findings of a depressed mood and a depressive sleep disorder will usually lead to the correct diagnosis. Patients with severe psychomotor retardation may be virtually immobile and mute and may be unable to provide any history beyond one or two words expressing hopelessness.

The sadness and anhedonia of depression--augmented perhaps by the patient's reaction to neurovegetative dysfunction and motor abnormality--lead to certain patterns of depressive thinking. Patients experience guilt and lowered self-esteem--"I've done some terrible things"--"I'm a worthless person"--"I deserve to die"--which are quite disproportionate to the facts of their lives. Patients feel worthless and hopeless; both feelings reflect the effect of anhedonia upon their self-concept and upon their view of their future. Most depressive thoughts, or depressive cognition, can be seen to be related to depressive affect and anhedonia: a patient who is profoundly sad and who cannot experience, recall, or imagine pleasure, views himself and the world around him as evil, painful, nonrewarding, and lacking in hope. The patient may feel that the physical and psychic discomforts of depression are justified punishment for exaggerated misdeeds.

The thought processes of the depressed patient are often impaired: the patient may complain of an inability to concentrate and will have trouble becoming immersed in a TV show or will not be able to finish reading an article in a magazine. A great effort of will is required to attend to any but the most mundane tasks, since sad thoughts and depressive ruminations persistently intrude. The patient may complain of impaired memory, although objective tests of memory functions often show that the patient's deficits are less severe than one would expect from the patient's description.

While patients with Dementia--impairment of memory as a result of actual neuronal deficits--may also complain of memory loss, their objective deficits are usually equal to, or greater than, their subjective complaints. Also, in Dementia recent memory is more impaired than remote memory. By contrast, depressed patients who complain of problems with memory generally do not show a clear distinction between the ability to remember recent and remote events.

The disturbance in the patient's thoughts may be so severe that a disorder of thought content--delusions--is present. Delusions are beliefs that are false, are fixed (i.e., they are not changed by logical arguments that would be persuasive to non-delusional people), and are not consistent with beliefs of others in the patient's sociocultural matrix (thus, a belief in demon possession may be nondelusional in certain religious groups). These delusions, as with other depressive thoughts, are consistent with or congruent with the affective disturbance. Thus, a severely depressed person with a delusion would not believe that he was an exalted or important person; rather, he would believe that he was a terrible sinner, that no decent person could love him, or that he was experiencing justified punishment for his grave personal failings.

The delusional depressed patient will not simply <u>feel</u> evil or impoverished; he will <u>believe</u> that many have died because of his sins of omission or commission, that he suffers from an unspeakable or fatal disease, or that all his worldly possessions have been taken away forever. The physician is especially likely to hear about somatic delusions. While the nonpsychotically depressed patient <u>wonders</u> if some physical ailment is causing his distress, the patient with somatic delusions <u>knows</u>, despite all evidence to the contrary, that his bowels have rotted away, that he is riddled with cancer, or that his misguided physician is concealing from him the awful truth about his loathsome illness. These examples of somatic delusions illustrate again the congruence between the disordered thoughts and other symptoms (worthlessness, hopelessness, anhedonia) in depression: depressive somatic delusions convey a sense of dissolution, decay, and emptiness.

Depressed patients may also exhibit paranoid ideation that may or may not be severe enough to warrant classification as delusional. The patient's anhedonia and low self-esteem may lead to a feeling that he is worthless and unlovable, and thus that his spouse has sought extramarital affairs, or that his family and friends are planning to abandon him, or that people are scheming to acquire his few remaining possessions. Ideas of reference that are congruent with depressive thinking may be seen. The patient will attach a special and unwarranted meaning to innocuous events: an overcooked meal is punishment for some imagined misdeed; an overheard fragment of conversation seems to be a discussion of how everyone would be better off if he were dead. Although the later age of onset and history of adequate premorbid social functioning should leave little question about the diagnosis, depressed patients with ideas of reference and paranoid delusions are sometimes misdiagnosed as schizophrenic.

Hallucinations--perceptual experiences occurring in the absence of an external stimulus--may occasionally occur in severe depressions. As with depressive delusions, depressive hallucinations are consonant with the disturbances of thought and affect. Thus, depressive auditory hallucinations might consist of a voice commanding the patient to commit suicide or might comment on how evil or worthless the patient is. Although hallucinations in depression may involve any of the sensory modalities, auditory hallucinations are most common.

If a depressed patient experiences hallucinations or delusions, the patient is said to be psychotic. "Psychotic" means that the individual has defective reality testing--i.e., experiences hallucinations and/or delusions--but because psychotic thinking or perceiving can occur in a variety of mental states-- e.g., Schizophrenia and Organic Brain Syndromes, as well as Affective Disorders--the term "psychotic" lacks diagnostic specificity. Rather, it connotes a high degree of disturbance and a qualitative departure from normal mental functioning.

Additional physical symptoms in depression may include dry mouth, constipation, and a variety of pains--headache, backache, abdominal pain, joint pains--in addition to the physical symptoms already mentioned. Obviously, these physical symptoms may arise from a number of physical illnesses as well as from depression, and such physical symptoms are sometimes the most prominent aspect of the patient's presentation to the physician. The physician would suspect depression as a possible cause if the physical symptoms did not have a readily identifiable physical cause, and if the patient experienced additional symptoms that are more clearly indicative of depression such as a typical sleep disorder, a depressed mood, or psychomotor agitation or retardation. While unexplained pains are common in depression, the physician should hesitate to make this diagnosis unless concomitant signs or symptoms of depression are present; depression is not diagnosed by exclusion.

In addition, patients with "classic" depression look depressed--they appear sad, may cry easily, and may neglect their grooming. They may sigh frequently. They may reveal that their mood, and other symptoms as well, undergo diurnal variation: they feel worse in the morning, somewhat better as the day progresses, and then worse again the next morning. When complaints of slowed thinking and impaired memory are prominent in elderly patients the presence of diurnal variation may help distinguish a primarily depressive illness from a Dementia accompanied by a certain degree of sadness. While the depressed patient typically feels worse in the morning, the patient with a dementiform process may show a decline in cognitive function as the day progresses. A patient with Dementia may seem reasonably intact in the morning, but quite confused at night.

The patient's age exerts a significant effect upon the pattern of symptoms that will occur when that individual is depressed. The picture of depression described above is most typically seen in patients in midlife--the 40's and 50's. Because this age group is at a relatively high risk for depression, the constellation of symptoms that occurs in patients in their 40's and 50's constitutes typical or "classic" depression. The symptom complex seen in younger and older depressed patients is more variable, but does not represent separate disease entities. The classical depression seen in midlife reflects the same basic process that occurs in younger or older patients, but each age group manifests this process in different ways.

B. LESS-TYPICAL PATTERNS OF DEPRESSION

Age exerts a major effect upon two aspects of depression. It influences the symptoms of depression, and also influences the psychological concerns, or particular worries, of the depressed patient. Detre and Jarecki (1971) summarize these two areas in their timetable of depressive symptoms and a parallel timetable of depressive life concerns.

The diagnosis of depression in children can be quite difficult. They exhibit a protean symptom pattern, and although a sad mood is sometimes seen, often other symptoms--temper tantrums, nightmares, phobias, or school refusal--may predominate. Because children are unusually sensitive to the vicissitudes of the family environment, it is difficult to distinguish distress that is reactive to external events--e.g., disharmony in the parents' relationship--from distress that may represent a more autonomous depressive process in the child; the diagnosis and treatment of depression in children is best left to the specialist.

Adolescents who are depressed may show a distinctly depressed mood, but, as with younger children, other symptoms and behaviors may overshadow purely affective symptoms. Depressed adolescents may demonstrate impulsive and self-destructive behavior, rebelliousness, a sullen negativism, irritability, conversion symptoms (see page 487), or sexual promiscuity. Episodes of anxiety and depersonalization (see page 494) may be prominent in older adolescents. It is important to distinguish transient reactions to difficult situations from symptoms that are prodromal to major disorders that will become more distinct as the patient ages. In general, an adolescent who experiences prolonged difficulty as a result of the symptoms mentioned above is more likely to develop one or more episodes of a typical Affective Disorder later in life than to be merely "going through a phase."

Depressed patients in their early 20's may exhibit phobias, severe anxiety attacks, or episodes of depersonalization as symptoms of an Affective Disorder. While these symptoms may dominate the clinical picture, the diagnosis of depression is suggested by concomitant neurovegetative symptoms such as anorexia or sleep disturbance and a diurnal fluctuation in symptoms. Many of these patients with atypical depressions will develop episodes with more classic depressive symptoms later in life and will have family histories of Affective Disorder.

From the mid-20's through the 30's a distinct depressive mood is more often seen, although vague and undiagnosable physical complaints may still predominate. As patients approach midlife, the somatic complaints and pains become more persistent and more localized (although still without demonstrable physical cause), and symptoms of anxiety become less prominent.

As patients age beyond the midlife period in which the "classical" pattern of depressive symptoms appears the physical and mental concomitants of the aging process become prominent. While some elderly patients may exhibit a clear depressive syndrome, many others appear confused and agitated. The elderly patient may perform poorly on tests of concentration and immediate recall (e.g., digit span forward and backward, serial subtraction of seven from 100) and recent memory may be impaired. The question arises: is a dementia-like process present, or is the patient too apathetic, unmotivated, and preoccupied with depressive thoughts to care about performing the doctor's silly tasks? The term pseudodementia is applied to patients who exhibit symptoms of Dementia (such as poor memory or apathy) that are actually caused by psychiatric illness (most commonly depression) rather than reflecting a structural or metabolic abnormality of brain function. If the patient appears sad and apathetic throughout the entire interview, then the cognitive deficits may reflect depression. By contrast, the patient who appears relatively normal when discussing neutral matters, but who becomes more confused, angry, agitated, or tearful when asked to perform simple calculations, is more likely to have an organic deficit. It can be difficult to distinguish the labile mood that occurs in patients whose cerebral function is compromised from the frequent crying spells of the depressive. It is certain, however, that depression may lead to decompensation in an elderly patient whose minimal Dementia might otherwise go unrecognized.

Both depression and Dementia are clinical diagnoses. Patients with definite Dementia may show no cerebral changes on computerized tomographic scans, and patients with significant cortical atrophy and/or ventricular enlargement may show no significant deficits on cognitive testing and may function quite normally. Because the prognosis and treatment in depression and Dementia are so different, correctly distinguishing the two conditions is vital. The difficulty is compounded by the tendency for older patients to exhibit some confusion when depressed--which may at times represent the unmasking of a dementiform process in a patient whose cognitive reserve is adequate only so long as the patient is neither depressed nor subjected to other stresses such as a physical illness or an abrupt change in life circumstances.

The particular diurnal pattern of symptoms and the mental status findings that may help distinguish depression from Dementia are listed in Table 8-1. Wells (1979) suggests several guidelines for diagnosing pseudodementia; they are summarized in the table on the next page.

C. DEPRESSIVE CONCERNS AND THE LIFE CYCLE

Because humans dislike uncertainty and ambiguity and have a propensity to codify their life experiences, depressed patients will often advance various reasons to "explain" their depressive symptoms. The depressed adolescent blames his failure to qualify for the football team, the depressed housewife attributes her dysphoria to her husband's apparently-waning affection, the depressed executive believes that falling profits caused his depression, the depressed septuagenarian blames his arthritis. While there is little doubt that unhappy life events can precede or aggravate a depressive episode, the major determinant of the particular thought content of the depressive is not the fact that he is depressed, but rather his place in the life cycle. People

TABLE 8-1

FEATURES DISTINGUISHING DEPRESSION
FROM DEMENTIA

Depression	Dementia
A. Clinical course and history.	
1. Fairly precise onset-- can be accurately dated.	1. Time of onset usually more vaguely recalled.
2. Rapid progression of symptoms after onset.	2. Slow progression of symptoms throughout course.
3. Family quite aware of dysfunction and its severity.	3. Family often unaware of severity of dysfunction.
B. Patient complaints and interview behavior.	
1. Complaints of cognitive loss are severe and detailed.	1. Complaints of cognitive difficulty minimal and, if present, vague.
2. Patients emphasize disability, and highlight their performance failures.	2. Patients conceal disability, and take pleasure in retained abilities.
3. Patients make little effort to perform even simple tasks, and do not try to "keep up."	3. Patients struggle to perform tasks, and use memory aids such as notes or calendars.
4. Patients communicate a strong sense of distress, particularly at early stages.	4. Patients often seem unconcerned, particularly at later stages.
5. Loss of social skills prominent.	5. Social skills often retained.
6. Frequently answers "I don't know" to tests of cognitive function.	6. Attempts to answer questions, but often scores a "near-miss."

at a given stage in their life cycle will be concerned with, or worried about, more-or-less the same tasks and problems--but when they are depressed, their worries are colored and intensified by anhedonia, guilt, and hopelessness, all of which will, in concert with the additional symptom of depression, diminish their ability to cope. The nondepressed person will worry but not feel hopeless, will be concerned but not overwhelmed, will be able to seek and experience comfort and support from friends and family, and will have the motivation and energy to try to change those aspects of life's problems that can be changed.

Detre and Jarecki (1971) present a <u>timetable of depressive life concerns</u>, emphasizing that the age-related changes in the individual's social role and responsibilities, rather than the presence or absence of depression per se, are the critical factors determining the areas of concern. For example, the depressed child feels unloved by his parents, the depressed adolescent worries about dating and feels alienated from friends and family, the depressed young married person questions his or her choice of mate and questions readiness for parenthood or career choice, the depressed woman in her thirties is devastated by her children's growing independence or her husband's preoccupation with work or feels unfulfilled in her own career, the depressed executive in his forties feels he will never advance further in his company's hierarchy; the depressed truck driver in his mid-fifties is increasingly preoccupied with physical complaints that seem trivial to others and worries about premature retirement; and as people enter their sixties and seventies and beyond, they will, if depressed, worry inordinately about their declining health, the loneliness and infirmities of old age, the deaths of friends, and their own eventual demise. All of these concerns are shared by others at a similar stage in life, but in the person with depression the concerns are pervasive, are colored by anhedonia, low self-esteem and guilt, and seem insurmountable.

Failure to appreciate the relationship between stage in the life cycle and depressive concerns leads to confusion between cause and effect in depressed patients. Thus, if a depressed patient is married, one would expect concerns over the marital relationship to be included in the patient's complaints; if a depressed patient has a concomitant physical illness, one might expect concerns about the illness to be prominent. This does not mean that in the former instance marital problems caused the depression, nor in the latter that physical illness caused the depression; one must avoid confusing why a patient feels worried or sad with why he has developed a depressive syndrome.

For example, a physician seeing a depressed man who lost his job several months ago is likely to conclude that the man is depressed because he lost his job and because he now experiences financial pressures, etc. Actually, depression may have caused the job loss rather than vice-versa. The man developed a depression, began to perform more poorly at work, then stopped caring and began to miss work, and was fired. His depression continued unabated or may have gotten worse, and in addition he now has more worries --finances, for example, plus his wife's withdrawal of affection as a result of her resentment at his drinking (which has increased as he tries to self-medicate his depression). That he worries about these problems is a realistic response to his current life circumstances; that he feels hopeless about them, and currently lacks the energy and motivation to make matters better, is a result of his depression.

Depression versus Grief. Profound sadness--often accompanied by many of the other symptoms of depressive syndromes--usually occurs when a person has suffered a major loss. In grief, the loss is significant (i.e., most people would agree that the loss was of major proportions); the degree of disturbance is proportionate to the loss, and the distress is self-limited--that is, it will gradually begin to improve over the next few days to few weeks. A major loss may or may not precede a depressive episode, but in depression the distress is more enduring--social functioning is impaired for a longer period, and the syndrome may not remit for weeks, months, or even years unless treated. Furthermore, self-esteem is commonly lowered in depression; lowered self-esteem is not a part of normal bereavement. A pattern of distress that begins as grief but which continues beyond the "normal" period for the bereaved individual's cultural matrix is indistinguishable from a depression that arises for no known reason and should be treated as a depression.

QUIZ, Section II.

Circle the letter corresponding to the <u>one</u> correct response.

1. Depressed patients complain of somatic symptoms

    a. rarely.
    b. commonly.

2. Patients with little or no sleep disturbance are _____ to be severely depressed.

    a. likely
    b. unlikely

3. Since many depressed patients are also anxious, antianxiety agents such as benzodiazepines usually _____ be given to depressed patients.

    a. should
    b. should not

4. When anxiety is primary rather than secondary to depression, the characteristic sleep disturbance is

    a. DFA.
    b. MNA.
    c. EMA.
    d. MNA and EMA.

5. In depression, complaints of poor memory may be _____ than any demonstrable deficit.

    a. greater
    b. less

6. In Dementia, objective signs of disturbed memory are often _____ than subjective complaints would indicate.

    a. greater
    b. less

7. A patient with Dementia is likely to show _____ in cognitive functioning as the day progresses.

    a. decline
    b. improvement

8. In grief, the degree of distress is _____ to the severity of the loss.

    a. proportionate
    b. out of proportion

Circle the correct answer(s). <u>One</u> or <u>more</u> <u>than</u> <u>one</u> answer may be correct.

9. Neurovegetative symptoms in depression include

   a. crying spells.
   b. sleep disorder.
   c. increased libido.
   d. anorexia.
   e. anergia.
   f. suicidal ideas.

10. Which of the following somatic delusions might be seen in severely depressed patients?

   a. A 46-year-old woman believes that her heart has stopped beating.
   b. A 25-year-old man believes he is an agent of the CIA, and has a radio transmitter implanted in his teeth.
   c. A 50-year-old man believes that his bowels have stopped working and his entire abdomen is filled with excrement.
   d. A 38-year-old woman believes, erroneously, that her skin rash is a sign that her body is consumed by syphilis.
   e. A 44-year-old man knows that he emits a horrible body odor, even though he bathes several times a day.
   f. A 22-year-old woman believes that Christ has a special plan for her patella.

11. Which of the following hallucinations might be experienced by severely depressed patients (assume no external or actual stimulus in each instance)?

   a. A 60-year-old man hears a voice ask him for his telephone number.
   b. A 43-year-old woman hears an angel condemning her sexual indiscretions.
   c. A 34-year-old man feels worms gnawing away at his vital organs.
   d. An 81-year-old man sees three dogs walking on the ceiling.
   e. A 32-year-old woman sees herself swinging from the gallows.
   f. A 51-year-old man hears his uncle castigating him for his faults.

Match the lettered manifestation of depressive thinking with the most appropriate numbered classification. Lettered items may be used once, more than once, or not at all.

___12.	thinking that one's discomfort is deserved	a. hopelessness
___13.	effect of anhedonia upon one's view of the future	b. anergia
___14.	feeling worthless	c. low self-esteem
___15.	believing one's self to be a terrible sinner	d. guilt

III.　BIPOLAR DISORDER--MANIA AND MANIC-DEPRESSIVE ILLNESS

A.　GENERAL DESCRIPTION

It is no small wonder that some persons who at times experience the profound lowering of mood that accompanies severe depression will at other times in their lives experience the profound and pathological elevation of mood known as <u>mania</u>.　Bipolar Disorder, or manic-depressive illness, is characterized by a history of one or more episodes of depression, plus one or more episodes of mania.　The particular pattern of the illness varies from person to person:　some patients with manic-depressive illness will experience several depressive episodes but only one manic episode over a lifetime; in others, manic episodes may predominate; and in still others, episodes of pathologically elevated and lowered mood occur with roughly equal frequency. To encompass patients experiencing these mood fluctuations, the term manic-depressive illness is preferable to manic-depressive psychosis, because the symptoms and social dysfunction, although severe, are not invariably of psychotic proportions.

The patient who is manic is not merely happy; he is <u>euphoric</u> or <u>elated</u> and filled with boundless <u>energy</u>.　His sleep may decrease significantly, but unlike the person with depression, he tolerates sleep loss without complaint. He may rationalize that he is too busy to sleep and that sleep would be an unnecessary interference with his plans and schemes which seem grandiose to a trained observer.　His exaggerated sense of self-importance leads him to try to involve others in his plans to solve the energy crisis, save the world, or make a million dollars overnight in real estate, and he may indiscriminately write, telephone, or attempt to visit important people such as corporation executives, Congressmen, and even the President.　The manic is <u>impulsive</u> and spends money indiscriminately; he may make excessive long-distance telephone calls, day or night, to friends or strangers.　He may impulsively buy an entire new wardrobe, decide to fly to Europe on the spur of the moment, or buy an expensive new car even though his present vehicle may be barely broken in.　Believing that he is possessed of great wealth as well as unusual intellectual, social, and sexual prowess, he may rapidly overdraw his bank account.　He may even forge checks or borrow someone else's credit card since he "knows" that unlimited funds are within his grasp (for differential diagnosis involving impulsive behaviors, see also Chapter 12, Impulse Disorders).

The manic may be so <u>hyperactive</u> that he cannot sit still for even a moment. Too busy to eat, too busy to sleep, he may become exhausted, and persons with severe mania have in the past, when untreated, died of starvation, metabolic derangements, or myocardial infarction.

The speech of the manic is <u>pressured</u>; he can be interrupted with difficulty or not at all, and he also exhibits a marked <u>flight</u> <u>of</u> <u>ideas</u>, shifting from topic to topic at a pace that leaves the interviewer far behind.　He is hyperalert and easily distractible, however, and will notice and rapidly comment upon almost anything that enters his field of vision.

1.	b	9.	b,d,e
2.	b	10.	a,c,d,e
3.	b	11.	b,c,e,f
4.	a	12.	d
5.	a	13.	a
6.	a	14.	c
7.	a	15.	d
8.	a		

With two exceptions, age has much less influence on the clinical presentation of mania than on depression; manics do not show the marked differences in signs and symptoms at various ages that characterize depression. The first exception is adolescence: impulsivity, substance abuse, and other deviant behaviors may be more obvious than an altered mood. The other exception is the elderly patient whose manic episode may show prominent elements of confusion --perhaps because the manic's sleep deprivation unmasks the hitherto-hidden cognitive deficits of the aging brain.

One subclass of manics, rather than being elated, will become markedly irritable. The hyperactivity, greatly decreased need for sleep, and pressured speech will be present, but instead of laughter, puns, and jokes, the patient will be short-tempered, nasty, and if provoked or his requests thwarted, possibly assaultive. Although the more typical euphoric manic may become irritable when someone attempts to interfere with his expansive plans, the persistently irritable manic does not show periods of expansive good fellowship or gregariousness. Such irritable manics are often quite paranoid as well; if the irritable manic is so severely ill as to be delusional, his hostility and suspiciousness may cause him to be misdiagnosed as having Paranoid Schizophrenia. The true diagnosis emerges when longitudinal data reveal that the manic: has not had the marked premorbid social deficits of the schizophrenic; has not shown the blunted or flattened affect of the schizophrenic; may have, unlike the schizophrenic, experienced symptom-free intervals between episodes of illness; and, finally, has relatives with more typical manic or depressive episodes.

The distinction between Schizophrenia and manic-depressive illness may be impossible to make on the grounds of current signs and symptoms alone, (Pope & Lipinski, 1978). Features common to Schizophrenia and Bipolar Affective Disorder include hallucinations, delusions, Schneiderian first-rank symptoms (see Chapter 7, Schizophrenic Disorders), bizarre behavior, catatonic excitement, catatonic immobility or stupor, paranoid ideation, and severe sleep disorder. Consequently, it may be impossible to make the correct diagnosis without longitudinal data, including the family history. Often only the passage of time--during which more clearly affective symptoms may emerge--will reveal the true nature of the illness.

Family history will often contribute to the correct diagnosis. If the acutely psychotic young woman has a brother who was always isolated, withdrawn, and "peculiar," who was hospitalized for several months at age 20 and who now, despite intensive and appropriate treatment, continues to show severe deficits in psychosocial functioning, then one feels some confidence in assuming that the young woman's own symptoms may represent Schizophrenia. This would be especially true if the woman herself had had a marginal premorbid adjustment and an insidious onset of more flagrant symptoms. By contrast, the acutely psychotic young woman whose mother and uncle suffered "nervous breakdowns" in midlife with complete recovery is more likely to have an Affective Disorder--even if she seems just as "crazy" and bizarre as the young woman in the preceding example.

Because the modal age of onset of Bipolar Affective Disorder is late adolescence and young adulthood, affective illness warrants careful consideration in the differential diagnosis of mental disorders in young people. Schizophrenic symptoms also become prominent in late adolescence and young adulthood, thus heightening the diagnostic dilemma. There is scant justification for preferring a diagnosis of Schizophrenia over Affective Disorder on the basis of early age of onset alone.

As mentioned in the section on Depression, patients and clinicians are all-too-ready to "explain" depression exclusively on the basis of life circumstances and to advance a multitude of plausible reasons for the patient's having become depressed. This phenomenon does not seem to occur in mania; people view the grandiosity, hyperactivity, and impulsiveness of the manic more as an autonomous morbid process than as a "reaction" to a current situation. Perhaps the persistence in America of the Protestant/Puritan ethic allows us to identify more easily with the self-flagellation of the depressive than with the pathological ebullience of the manic.

B. MANIA WITHOUT DEPRESSION

Although manic-depressive illness typically involves attacks of depression and mania, a few patients experience recurrent episodes of mania without ever developing significant depression; because these patients' manic symptoms do not seem different from the manic episodes of patients who also experience depressions, patients with mania only, have also traditionally been included under manic-depressive illness.

C. UNIPOLAR AND BIPOLAR ILLNESS

While systematic differences between manic episodes in patients with mania only and those with histories of depression as well are not apparent, differences do exist between depressions in patients who have histories of mania and those who do not. Patients with depression only are said to be unipolar, while patients with a history of depression and mania are classified as bipolar; thus, Bipolar Affective Disorder is essentially synonymous with manic-depressive illness, although the latter term sometimes implies a greater severity of mood disturbance. Bipolar patients generally have an earlier age of onset of serious affective symptoms than unipolar patients; the modal age of onset of manic-depressive illness is in the 20's, whereas the onset of unipolar illness tends to be in the 40's. These tendencies are by no means ironclad--some patients who first become depressed in their 40's or 50's will have their first manic episode a decade or more later and thus be late-onset bipolars; and some patients will develop a single serious depression in their 20's without ever in their lives developing mania. Patients with a unipolar pattern of depression are less likely to experience recurrences of depression than bipolar patients; many unipolar patients may have only one serious depressive episode in their lives, while bipolar patients commonly have several depressive episodes, as well as one or more episodes of pathological elevation of mood. Bipolar patients tend to be <u>hypersomnic</u> when depressed, while decreased sleep is typical in unipolar patients. Furthermore, many bipolar patients tend, between episodes of illness, to be cheerful and outgoing, while unipolar patients tend to be somewhat anxious and overconscientious throughout their lives. The unipolar-bipolar distinction is valuable in that it provides a guide to treatment (e.g., bipolar patients are more likely to respond to lithium carbonate as discussed in a later section), and to prognosis (e.g., unipolar patients are less likely to experience a recurrence of depression).

A pathological alteration in mood--elevation, expansiveness, or irritability--that is less severe than that needed to diagnose mania is termed <u>hypomanic</u>. Like the manic, the hypomanic will show symptoms--such as a decreased need for sleep, increased energy, overtalkativeness, or impulsive behaviors such as foolish spending of money or reckless driving--that result in some impairment in social or occupational functioning. In essence, hypomania is simply an attenuated form of mania. (Note that "hypomania" means "a little less than mania.")

The importance of recognizing hypomanic symptoms is that persons who have hypomanic episodes are at an increased risk for developing depression or frank mania. As one might expect, a person with a history of hypomania is more likely to have a family history of bipolar than unipolar illness; also, the depressions of persons who have been hypomanic tend to resemble bipolar depressions rather than unipolar depressions. Patients with recurrent periods of elevated and lowered mood are diagnosed as <u>cyclothymic</u> when the mood alterations are not severe enough to meet criteria for manic and depressive episodes; cyclothymia in fact probably represents mild Bipolar Disorder rather than a separate illness (Akiskal et al., 1977).

A certain subjectivity is involved in distinguishing the person who is "normally" energetic and ebullient from one who is mildly hypomanic, and in borderline cases the discrimination may seem more a matter of personal taste than of diagnostic precision: one clinician's hard-driving executive dynamo is another's hypomanic. However, if one remembers that psychosocial dysfunction and disruption are necessary concomitants of psychopathology, such ambiguities will be minimized or eliminated.

QUIZ, Section III.

Circle the letter corresponding to the <u>one</u> correct answer.

1. In contrast to depressed patients, who suffer because of their insomnia, the manic experiences a greatly _____ need for sleep.

    a. increased
    b. decreased

2. In contrast with depressive delusions which may involve poverty and a sense of worthlessness, a manic who is delusional may have _____ beliefs.

   a. grandiose
   b. nihilistic

3. Although the typical manic shows an elated mood, some manics are not elated but rather extremely _____.

   a. irritable
   b. passive

4. This group of manics (question 5) is also prone to develop

   a. paranoid ideation.
   b. flamboyant ideation.

5. Although exceptions exist, Bipolar Affective Disorder generally appears at a(n) _____age than Unipolar Disorder.

   a. earlier
   b. later

6. A patient who first becomes significantly depressed at age 45 is more likely to be

   a. bipolar.
   b. unipolar.

7. That is, he is _____likely ever to experience a manic episode than a patient who becomes depressed at age 25.

   a. more
   b. less

8. Unipolar depression is _____ likely to recur than bipolar depression.

   a. more
   b. less

9. Age has _____ influence upon manic symptoms than upon depressive symptoms.

   a. more
   b. less

Complete the following.

10. Two exceptions to the statement in question nine are adolescence, where deviant _____ may overshadow an abnormality of mood, and old age, in which manic patients are likely to become _____.

11. Mania represents a pathological _____ of mood; patients experiencing both mania and depression have _____ - _____ illness.

12. The speech of the manic is _____; his rapidly jumping from one subject to another is known as _____ .

13. Because the manic is so distractible, one would expect poor performance on tests of _____ such as repeating a series of digits.

14. The irritable, paranoid manic may be, erroneously, thought to be suffering from _____ . Despite the presence of grandiose or paranoid delusions, the diagnosis is more likely mania if there is a family history of _____ , if the age of onset is _____ , and if the patient has had symptom-free intervals between episodes of illness.

15. Patients with depression only are classified as _____ , whereas a patient with both mania and depression would be termed _____ .

16. The unipolar-bipolar distinction is based, not on inference, but on _____ phenomena. The unipolar-bipolar distinction also provides guidelines for _____ , as well as some estimate of _____ .

17. Symptoms and behaviors that are similar to, but less severe or disruptive than those seen in mania are called _____ .

Match the following phenomena with their corresponding moods.

___18. A 45-year-old man believes that he is going to Hell for his (nonexistent) sins.

___19. A 22-year-old woman hears, when no one is around, two male voices describing her undergarments.

___20. A 46-year-old man, while running across the street, hears the the Secretary of State inviting him to address the United Nations.

___21. A 38-year-old woman believes she is pregnant with the Messiah.

___22. A 24-year-old man believes that a recording device has secretly been implanted in his antecubital fossa.

___23. A 53-year-old man believes that he has invented a perpetual motion machine.

___24. A fundamentalist preacher is convinced that God speaks to him in his dreams.

a. consistent with depression
b. consistent with mania
c. neither

Match the following features with the lettered items.

___ 25. delusions of persecution
___ 26. flattened or blunted affect
___ 27. marked increase in psychomotor activity
___ 28. good premorbid adjustment
___ 29. prolonged psychosocial disability even
         when acute symptoms in remission
___ 30. auditory hallucinations
___ 31. catatonic behavior (either excitement
         or immobility)
___ 32. family history of Affective Disorder
___ 33. recurrences, with symptom-free intervals
         between episodes
___ 34. impulsive money-spending and grandiose
         delusions

a. more characteristic
    of Schizophrenia
b. more characteristic
    of manic-depressive
    illness
c. compatible with either
    diagnosis

TRUE or FALSE: Circle the correct letter.

T   F   35. While the border between certain character traits (such as
             cheerfulness, extroversion, and high energy level) and hypo-
             mania may be indistinct, a person without impairment in work
             or interpersonal relationships could correctly be labeled hypo-
             manic.

IV. DSM-III CLASSIFICATION OF AFFECTIVE DISORDERS

The following represents a condensation of pages 117-130 of the <u>Quick reference to the diagnostic criteria from DSM-III</u>   (American   Psychiatric Association, Washington, D.C., 1980).

Diagnostic criteria are first presented for manic episodes and for major depressive episodes; when one of these episodes is present then a major Affective Disorder can be diagnosed.

The formal criteria for a <u>manic episode</u> are:

A. One or more distinct periods with a persistently and pre-
    dominantly elevated, expansive, or irritable mood. This
    mood must be prominent and relatively persistent, although
    it may alternate with a depressive mood.

B. Duration of at least <u>one week</u> (or any duration if hospitali-
    zation is necessary), during which at least <u>three</u> of the fol-
    lowing symptoms <u>(four</u> if the predominant mood is irritable
    rather than elevated) have been prominent:

(1) More active (socially, physically, sexually, or at work) than usual.
(2) More talkative than usual.
(3) Flight of ideas, or subjective experience that thoughts are racing.
(4) Inflated self-esteem (grandiosity, which may be delusional).
(5) Decreased need for sleep.
(6) Distractibility (i.e., attention too easily drawn to unimportant external stimuli).
(7) Excessive involvement in activities (such as buying sprees, sexual indiscretions, foolish business investments, or reckless driving) without recognizing the high potential for painful consequences.

C. The following may be present only in the presence of clear affective symptoms (a and b, above): preoccupation with a mood-incongruent delusion or hallucination or bizarre behavior. If clear affective symptoms are not present, then mood-incongruent psychotic features such as thought insertion, delusions of control, or hallucinations that lack a grandiose theme would preclude the diagnosis of a manic episode.

D. Not superimposed on Schizophrenia, Schizophreniform Disorder, or a Paranoid Disorder.

E. Not due to any Organic Mental Disorder.

The formal criteria for a major depressive episode are:

A. Dysphoric mood--sad, blue, hopeless, low, down in the dumps, irritable, worried--or loss of interest or pleasure in all or almost all usual activities and pastimes. The dysphoric mood or anhedonia must be prominent and relatively persistent, but not necessarily the most predominant symptom.

B. At least four of the following symptoms, present for at least two weeks:

(1) Poor appetite or significant weight loss, or increased appetite or weight gain.
(2) Sleep difficulty or sleeping too much.
(3) Loss of energy, fatigability, or tiredness.
(4) Objective evidence of psychomotor agitation or retardation.
(5) Loss of interest or pleasure in usual activities, or decrease in sexual desire.
(6) Feelings of self-reproach, or excessive or inappropriate guilt (either may be delusional).

(7) Complaints or evidence of diminished ability to think or concentrate--such as slowed thinking or indecisiveness.

(8) Recurrent thoughts of death or suicide, or thoughts of wishing to be dead, or any suicidal behavior.

C. The following may be present only in the presence of clear affective symptoms (a and b above): preoccupation with a mood-incongruent delusion or hallucination (i.e., a delusion or hallucination that is not clearly related to guilt, personal inadequacy, disease, etc.); or bizarre behavior. Lacking a clear affective syndrome, such mood-incongruent psychotic features preclude diagnosis of a depressive episode.

D. Not superimposed on Schizophrenia, Schizophreniform Disorder or a Paranoid Disorder.

E. Not due to any Organic Mental Disorder, or uncomplicated bereavement.

The preceding criteria are used in making the following formal diagnoses of the Major Affective Disorders:

Bipolar Disorder, Mixed:
A. Current (or most recent) episode involves the full symptomatic picture of both manic and major depressive episodes, intermixed or rapidly alternating every few days.

B. Depressive symptoms are prominent, and last at least a full day.

Bipolar Disorder, Manic:
A. Currently (or most recently) in a manic episode. (If there has been a previous manic episode, the current episode need not meet the full criteria for a manic episode.)

Bipolar Disorder, Depressed:
A. Has had one or more manic episodes.
B. Currently (or most recently) in a major depressive episode.

Major Depression (single episode, or recurrent):
A. One or more depressive episodes.
B. Has never had a manic episode.

The subclassification melancholia is applied to major depression when the following features are present: prominent anhedonia, and lack of reactivity to usually pleasurable stimuli, plus at least three of the following:

(1) distinct quality to the depressed mood (i.e., it is quite different from the dysphoria experienced following the death of a loved one)

ANSWERS, Section III.

1.	b	18.	a
2.	a	19.	c
3.	a	20.	b
4.	a	21.	b
5.	a	22.	c
6.	b	23.	b
7.	b	24.	c
8.	b	25.	c
9.	b	26.	a
10.	behavior, confused	27.	b
11.	elevation, manic-depressive	28.	b
12.	pressured, flight of ideas	29.	a
13.	concentration	30.	c
14.	Paranoid Schizophrenia, Affective Disorder, later (or older)	31.	c
		32.	b
15.	unipolar, bipolar	33.	b
16.	observable, treatment, prognosis	34.	b
17.	hypomanic	35.	F

(2) prominent diurnal variation, with symptoms worse in the morning
(3) EMA of at least two hours
(4) marked psychomotor agitation or retardation
(5) significant anorexia or weight loss
(6) excessive or inappropriate guilt

DSM-III also presents criteria for two other specific affective disorders: Cyclothymic Disorder, and Dysthymic Disorder.

Cyclothymic Disorder:
   A. During the preceding <u>two</u> <u>years</u>, there have been numerous periods in which there were some symptoms characteristic of both depressive and manic syndromes. However, symptoms were not of sufficient severity or duration to meet the criteria for a major depressive or manic episode.

   B. Periods of normal mood lasting as long as several months may separate depressive and hypomanic periods; the depressive and hypomanic periods themselves may alternate, or symptoms of elevated and lowered mood may be intermixed.

   C. During periods of altered mood, there are, in addition to the mood change per se, at least three associated symptoms. For example, during a depressive period there must be a depressed mood or anhedonia, plus three depressive symptoms (e.g., sleep disorder, decreased energy, and social withdrawal); during a hypomanic period, both altered mood (elevated, expansive, or irritable) and three additional symptoms (e.g., decreased need for sleep, extreme gregariousness, and impulsive activities) must be present.

For the depressive periods, three of the following 12 symptoms must be present:

    (1) insomnia or hypersomnia
    (2) low energy or chronic fatigue
    (3) feelings of inadequacy
    (4) decreased effectiveness or productivity at school, work, or home
    (5) decreased attention, concentration, or ability to think clearly
    (6) social withdrawal
    (7) loss of interest in or enjoyment of sex
    (8) restriction of involvement in pleasurable activities, guilt over past activities
    (9) feeling slowed down
    (10) less talkative than usual
    (11) pessimistic attitude toward the future or brooding about past events
    (12) tearfulness or crying

For hypomanic periods three of the following 12 symptoms must be present:

    (1) decreased need for sleep
    (2) more energy than usual
    (3) inflated self-esteem
    (4) increased productivity, often associated with unusual, self-imposed working hours
    (5) sharpened and unusually creative thinking
    (6) uninhibited people-seeking (extreme gregariousness)
    (7) hypersexuality without recognition of possibility of painful consequences
    (8) excessive involvement in pleasurable activities with lack of concern for the high potential for painful consequences, e.g. buying sprees, foolish business investments, reckless driving
    (9) physical restlessness
    (10) more talkative than usual
    (11) over-optimism or exaggeration of past achievements
    (12) inappropriate laughing, joking, punning

    D. Absence of psychotic features.

    E. Not due to any other mental disorder.

Dysthymic Disorder:
    A. During the past two years (or one year for children and adolescents), the patient has experienced characteristics of the depressive syndrome for most or all of the time; however, symptoms are not of sufficient severity or duration to warrant the diagnosis of depressive episode.

B.   Periods of normal mood may be present during the two year period, but do not last more than a few months.

C.   During the depressive periods one of the following is prominent: either a depressed mood per se (i.e., sad, down in the dumps) or anhedonia.

D.   During the depressive period, at least <u>three</u> of the following 13 symptoms are present.

(1) insomnia or hypersomnia
(2) low energy level or chronic tiredness
(3) feelings of inadequacy, loss of self-esteem, or self-deprecation
(4) decreased effectiveness or productivity at school, work, or home
(5) decreased attention, concentration, or ability to think clearly
(6) social withdrawal
(7) loss of interest in, or enjoyment of, pleasurable activities
(8) irritability or excessive anger (in children, expressed toward parents or caretakers)
(9) inability to respond with apparent pleasure to praise or rewards
(10) less active or talkative than usual, or feels slowed down or restless
(11) pessimistic attitude toward the future, brooding about past events, or feeling sorry for self
(12) tearfulness or crying
(13) recurrent thoughts of death or suicide

E.   Absence of psychotic features.

F.   If the depressive syndrome is superimposed on another mental disorder, the depressed mood is sufficiently intense or disruptive of functioning so that it can be clearly distinguished from the individual's usual mood.

Finally, there are two Atypical Affective Disorders: <u>Atypical Depression</u> and <u>Atypical Bipolar Disorder</u>.   These are atypical only in that they fail to meet <u>all</u> of the necessary formal criteria for the "typical" disorders.   For example, a depression that fulfills the criteria for Dysthymic Disorder, except for having periods of normal mood lasting more than a few months, would be diagnosed as Atypical Depression; or, an illness that has many features of a Bipolar Disorder but lacks the required number of associated symptoms would be diagnosed as Atypical Bipolar Disorder; or, an illness with a distinct depressive episode plus some manic features--but not enough to meet the criteria for a manic episode--would be diagnosed as Atypical Bipolar Disorder.

QUIZ, Section IV.

TRUE or FALSE: Circle the correct letter.

T   F   1.   "Atypical" Affective Disorders are so-called because their symptom patterns are unusual or bizarre.

Complete the following.

2.   The principal difference between Typical and Atypical Affective Disorders is that the Atypical Disorders do not meet the formal criteria in terms of the required _____ of specified symptoms, or the required degree of _____, or the _____of disturbance.

V.   ASSESSMENT OF SUICIDAL RISK

While any patient who is confused or impulsive may be at risk for self-harm, patients who commit suicide are often depressed.   Thus, recognition of depression becomes a major step in the assessment of suicidal risk, and any patient who is significantly depressed must be considered a potential suicide. The physician is in an especially strategic position to prevent suicide since at least half of the people who kill themselves have seen a physician (not necessarily a psychiatrist) within six months of their death, and a majority of these patients have entertained suicidal thoughts during the months preceding their death.   Thus, if the physician is willing to inquire about suicide, he or she is in an excellent position to identify many potential suicides.

Some physicians are reluctant to ask about suicide; this probably reflects their own discomfort with a painful and frightening subject, although they may rationalize their avoidance by believing that asking might "upset the patient," or "give him ideas."   Actually, most patients are relieved to be able to discuss their suicidal thoughts and discussing them with the physician may reduce the painful isolation and shame about suicide that the patient experiences.   While you would not begin the interview with "Hello. Are you thinking of killing yourself?," the physician can, if depression is present, gently but quickly elicit the presence and severity of suicidal concerns.   In the course of assessing the severity of the depressed patient's mood, one might ask questions like the following:
   "Have you been feeling sad, or down in the dumps?"
   "Do you sometimes feel hopeless?"
   "Does it seem like life isn't worth living?"
   "Have you felt that you (or others) would be better off if you were dead?"
   "Have you thought about harming yourself?"
   "How did you think you would do it?"

Within six questions you will have ascertained not only the presence of suicidal thoughts, but also whether or not there is a plan. The presence of suicidal plans is an especially ominous sign--for while occasional suicidal thoughts are probably universal, plans are not. The suicidal plan provides the bridge between thought and action. Many "sudden" or seemingly impulsive suicides probably represent the impulsive decision to implement a more long-standing plan--a plan that could have been discovered if the physician had asked about suicide.

The dimensions of suicidal plans include: whether or not a plan is present, how lethal is the contemplated method, and how detailed is the plan. The more lethal the method and the more detailed the plan, the greater the risk. For example, a depressed young woman who acknowledges suicidal thoughts might, when asked about method, say "I don't know--maybe take some aspirin." This situation is of relatively low risk compared to the middle-aged man who says, "I'm going to blow my brains out with my shotgun. I can rest it on the floor, put the muzzle in my mouth, and pull the trigger with my foot."; this is obviously a very high-risk situation.

Usually, when a person says he will not kill himself he can be believed (for the moment, at least). An exception would be a person who has recently made a serious suicide attempt that was somehow interrupted, whose degree of depression and other circumstances have not changed, and who is merely trying to avoid interference with a repeat attempt.

A history of a prior attempt is a high-risk sign; a substantial number of people who kill themselves have made previous attempts. Suicidal communications are also a sign of risk; it is a myth that "people who talk about suicide aren't really serious about it." Two-thirds of those who succeed at suicide have talked about it to someone--usually a family member--which emphasizes the importance of obtaining information from others when the possibility of suicide is suspected.

Although some self-damaging acts seem clearly to be attention-seeking behaviors without lethal intent and thus are called suicide "gestures," they nevertheless represent a risk factor. They suggest a poverty of strategies for coping with distress as well as poor judgment, and many patients who make "gestures" will at some point in the future succeed in killing themselves. Also, many people are poor pharmacologists; they may intend a "gesture," but ingest a lethal quantity of pills.

Suicidal communications may be quite direct--"I'm going to kill myself"--or somewhat more indirect: "You won't have to worry about me anymore," "Things would be better if I were dead," "It will be all over soon." Giving away prized possessions or suddenly putting one's affairs in order for no known reason is a high-risk sign. A depressed person's increased preoccupation with the afterlife can be a sign of impending suicide, and people who write suicide notes are at high risk for successfully completing the act.

The risk of suicide generally parallels the depth of the depression; one exception is the patient who is intensely preoccupied with suicide, but who is too anergic and retarded to carry out the act. Such a patient may improve enough to implement his plan before he improves still further and abandons it.

Recent major changes in life circumstances--especially recent loss--increase the risk of suicide. Common stressful losses include death of a loved one, marital separation or divorce, financial reverses, and loss of health. While some losses might seem relatively trivial to the physician--e.g., the death of a nephew or the death of a pet--the loss may be especially meaningful to the patient in some idiosyncratic or personal way. For example, a depressed elderly widower's 18-year-old dog may be the only "significant other" in his life, and if this pet were to die it might be a major blow--"the last straw."

Certain demographic factors are helpful in assessing suicidal risk: the risk is higher in men than in women; increases with advancing age (although suicide is the second leading cause of death in college students); and is higher in persons who are separated, widowed, or divorced than in married persons. The rate is also higher in people who abuse alcohol or drugs and higher in persons with chronic or debilitating physical illness. Combining these factors with the severity of the patient's depression, the presence or absence of prior attempts, the presence of suicidal communications--and most important of all, the presence or absence of a suicidal plan--allows the physician to identify those patients who are at high risk for suicide.

The weighting of the various factors is not, in the individual instance, a precise science. You should pay attention to your intuition in assessing suicidal risk; if, despite a patient's seeming to be at low risk on the basis of the preceding factors, you have an uncanny feeling that he or she is seriously suicidal, you are probably right.

Doctors sometimes feel fatalistic about preventing suicide: "If someone really wants to kill himself, he will." While not all suicides can be prevented, such an attitude ignores three facts:

(1) Suicidal intent may be intense but transient. If the immediate attempt is prevented, the suicidal risk may decrease, especially if effective treatment is offered.
(2) Most suicidal people are ambivalent about dying, and a fatalistic attitude ignores the positive side of this ambivalence. Suicidal behavior represents not only a wish to die, but also an attempt to solve a problem and often a "cry for help."
(3) A person may be quite willing to use one method but not another. Thus, removing pills or guns may be lifesaving, even though an electric cord could still be used for hanging. In addition, removing a readily available method may introduce the delay necessary for intervention to occur.

Another way in which you can contribute to suicide prevention is through limiting the prescribing of certain especially dangerous drugs. At typical daily doses, a 7-10 day supply of barbiturates, meprobamate, or glutethimide can, if ingested all at once, lead to serious medical complications (e.g., severe respiratory depression, hypotension, coma and death). Unfortunately, antidepressants, which depressed patients are likely to receive, can

ANSWERS, Section IV._____

1. F
2. numbers, severity, duration
_____

also be life-threatening when a 7-10 day supply is ingested. The risks of overdose with any drug are compounded when multiple drugs or alcohol are also ingested. The risks from benzodiazepines (such as diazepam or chlordiazepoxide) overdosage are significantly less, unless alcohol or other drugs are also taken--in which case benzodiazepine ingestion can be fatal. The implications of all of this for prescribing habits are obvious: depressed patients should not be given sedatives in the first place (they are mistakenly prescribed to treat depressive sleep disorder), and it would be most imprudent to give a depressed patient with suicidal ideation more than a one-week's supply of antidepressant medication.

_____

QUIZ, Section V.

Circle the letter corresponding to the <u>one</u> correct response.

1. A history of prior suicidal behavior indicates _____risk.

    a. increased
    b. decreased

2. As a general rule, the risk of suicide is _____ with patients who are more severely depressed.

    a. greater
    b. less

3. Overdosage of antidepressants is a _____ risk situation from a purely medical standpoint.

    a. high
    b. low

TRUE or FALSE: Circle the correct letter.

T F 4. Most people who commit suicide have given the matter little prior thought.

T F 5. If the physician asks a depressed patient about suicide, the risk of suicide increases.

T F 6. Patients who threaten suicide, or who make seemingly half-hearted attempts, are at low risk for suicide compared to the general population.

Complete the following.

7. Among the many factors contributing to the risk of suicide, the presence of a _____ is probably the indicator of greatest risk.

8. The more _____ the plan, and the more _____ the method, the greater the risk of suicide.

9. One should try to remove whatever means of suicide--such as a gun, or pills--that the patient is contemplating using because most suicidal patients are _____ about dying; suicidal impulses may be _____, and the patient might not use other _____ of suicide even though they are potentially available.

10. Because depressed patients are especially likely to attempt suicide, a patient with suicidal ideation should receive no more than a _____ week(s) supply of antidepressants at any one time.

Match the following factors or situations with their relative risk for suicide. Lettered items may be used more than once.

____11. increasing age
____12. female
____13. teetotaler
____14. detailed suicidal plan
____15. talks about suicide
____16. divorced
____17. history of alcohol abuse
____18. physically ill
____19. no previous attempt
____20. suicide note
____21. widowed alcoholic male gun-collector
____22. apprehended trying to leap off bridge but says, "I didn't mean it--let me go home now."
____23. 28-year-old married woman
____24. your "gut feeling" that risk is high
____25. lives alone
____26. no history of impulsive behavior

a. relatively high risk for suicide
b. relatively lower risk for suicide

Match the following drugs with their corresponding risk factor with regard to lethality when used in suicide attempts.

____27. diazepam
____28. antidepressants
____29. secobarbital
____30. chlordiazepoxide plus alcohol

a. relatively high risk
b. relatively lower risk

VI. CAUSES OF AFFECTIVE DISORDERS

The most accurate statement summarizing the causes of the Affective Disorders would be "unknown." Factors at sociocultural, psychological (mind), and biological (brain) levels interact with one another in all forms of behavior; thus, one would expect causal explanations in the Affective Disorders to be multifactorial, complex, and intertwined. Much of the confusion in understanding Affective Disorders reflects a dualistic and reductionistic adherence to the mind-body dichotomy which states that certain events are essentially "psychological" and free from physiological (e.g., neurochemical) influence, while other events are "physical" or "organic," and essentially free from psychic influences. In the real world, these various frames of reference--the sociocultural, the psychological, and the neural--are simply different perspectives (each with its own questions and methods of inquiry) for looking at complex phenomena that are occurring simultaneously at all three levels. A human is at once an organism with a brain, a person with a mind, and a member of a sociocultural matrix. While a given perspective may be more useful for a given question (e.g., the perspective of the organism is the primary focus during a neurosurgical operation), no one perspective is inherently superior to any other. Consequently, various aspects of the Affective Disorders have been explained at each of the three levels.

A. SOCIOLOGICAL FACTORS

From a sociocultural standpoint, some have explained the increased incidence of depression in women as the outcome of a social structure that deprives women of the full range of choices or opportunities that are available to men. Similarly, a depression occurring in a man whose educational and occupational opportunities are limited because of his race could be said to be determined, in part, by the values and beliefs held by a particular society at a particular time and place. Durkheim, in his classic monograph on suicide, examined the influence of religious affiliation, marital status, and several other sociological variables upon suicide rate. Thus, for some people--career military officers, in one of his examples--suicide was less the deviant act of a "sick" individual than a behavior that conformed to a set of social values. The hara-kiri of the Japanese soldier, the self-immolation of the Buddhist monks during the Vietnam War, and the immolation of widows in India are acts that accord with a well-developed tradition of beliefs; although one may need to examine individual psychological factors to understand why a particular military officer kills himself at a particular time, the fact of a high suicide rate is a sociological phenomenon.

B. PSYCHOLOGICAL FACTORS

At the individual or psychological level, loss is the most prominent explanation for depression. Freud's 1917 monograph Mourning and melancholia postulated that the loss of an ambivalently valued love object was the major cause of depression. If a husband's feelings for his wife were primarily positive and the wife died, the husband would mourn. However, if the husband harbored strong negative feelings as well (even if these were at an unconscious level) and his wife died, he would develop melancholia (depression). According to Freud, the husband's anger--which might be accentuated by his wife's "deserting" him through death--could not be consciously expressed, but rather would be turned inward against the self, or introjected. The widower would then experience self-hatred and self-reproach, as well as guilt arising from his unacceptable feelings toward his wife. Such a metapsychological model is notoriously resistant to systematic empirical study, depending as it does upon specialized techniques (such as psychoanalysis) for probing the unconscious aspects of the individual's psyche. While by no means a comprehensive theory, it may contribute to understanding why some losses lead to transient dysphoria while others are followed by depression.

Beck's cognitive theory, in which depressive thinking precedes depressive affect, offers another psychological model of depression (Beck et al., 1979): the patient has a negative view of himself or herself, interprets ongoing experiences in a negative way, and has negative expectations of the future. This cognitive triad influences behavior as well as mood: the depressed person fails to engage in behaviors that might lead to pleasure, thus maintaining the depressive cycle.

C. BIOLOGICAL FACTORS

Investigation of the biochemical aspects of the Affective Disorders is one of the most active areas of psychiatric research; the success of anti-depressant and antimanic drugs in relieving the symptoms of severe affective disturbances has provided a major impetus to pursuing a neurochemical understanding of behavior.

The biogenic amine hypothesis has been a major theme in biological psychiatric research. Simply stated, depression results from a relative deficiency of norepinephrine at certain critical sites in the brain, while mania results from a relative excess of norepinephrine at critical brain sites. A variant of this hypothesis, the biogenic amine permissive hypothesis, states that a deficiency of the indoleamine serotonin creates the necessary vulnerability to Affective Disorder, which then will become manifest as mania if norepinephrine becomes excessive, or as depression if norepinephrine becomes deficient.

Much of the early evidence for these hypotheses was indirect, such as the observation that some patients treated with reserpine, which depletes monoamines, develop a syndrome which closely resembles naturally-occurring depression. Also, certain drugs used to treat depression (some tricyclic antidepressants and the monamine oxidase inhibitors) cause an increase in available norepinephrine in the brain. In addition, these noradrenergic drugs may precipitate mania in certain individuals.

Somewhat more direct evidence for biogenic amine hypotheses comes from measurement of neurotransmitter metabolism. Maas (1975) and other investigators have found a decrease in the urinary excretion of 3-methoxy-4-hydroxyphenethylene glycol (MHPG) in certain depressed patients. MHPG is believed to provide a reasonably good index of norepinephrine metabolism in the brain, and a decrease in MHPG excretion in some depressives is consistent with a relationship between a relative deficiency of norepinephrine and depression. Furthermore, imipramine, which in vivo has primarily noradrenergic action, seems effective in treating depressed patients who have decreased MHPG excretion; this includes depressed manic-depressives, and some unipolar depressives. Preliminary evidence suggests increased MHPG levels in manics which is consistent with biogenic amine theories.

ANSWERS, Section V.

1. a	10. one	20. a
2. a	11. a	21. a
3. a	12. b	22. a
4. F	13. b	23. b
5. F	14. a	24. a
6. F	15. a	25. a
7. plan	16. a	26. b
8. detailed, lethal	17. a	27. b
9. ambivalent, transient,	18. a	28. a
methods	19. b	29. a
		30. a

MHPG has been used to select the proper antidepressant drug: while some patients have decreased MHPG levels, other depressives show normal or increased MHPG excretion; the latter patients tend not to respond to imipramine. Some studies have shown that these high-MHPG, imipramine non-responders excrete below-normal levels of 5-hydroxyindole acetic acid (5-HIAA), which is a serotonin metabolite, and these patients tend to respond to amitriptyline. These results are consistent with bits and pieces of biogenic amine theories: patients with decreased MHPG, suggesting norepinephrine deficiency, respond to the imipramine but not the amitriptyline. Patients with normal or increased MHPG excretion which suggests that norepinephrine is not deficient, do not respond to imipramine, but do respond to amitriptyline. According to some investigators, the high-MHPG, low 5-HIAA, amitriptyline responders are, phenomenologically, unipolar depressives who are unlikely ever to develop mania.

The results of studies of hypothalamic-pituitary-adrenal activity in depression are consistent with a role for biogenic amines in Affective Disorders, and may eventually contribute to an improved classification of these illnesses. The dexamethasone suppression test (Carroll et al., 1981) gives abnormal results in a subgroup of severely depressed patients whose mood state is relatively autonomous (i.e., uninfluenced by environmental events) and who are likely to require treatment with drugs or ECT (see section VII, below). The test consists of administering l mg of dexamethasone orally at 11:30 p.m., then measuring plasma cortisol at 4:00 p.m. the next day. Plasma cortisol values above 5µg/dL are abnormal and represent escape from suppression by dexamethasone. Although the test is not sensitive (that is, false-negative results are common), it is highly specific, with few false positives. The yield of positive results improves somewhat, if in addition to the 4:00 p.m. sample, 8:00 a.m. and 11:00 p.m. samples are collected as well.

Studies of the hypothalamic-pituitary-thyroid axis are also relevant to Affective Disorder. Biogenic amines modulate release of the hypothalamic peptide thyrotropin-releasing hormone (TRH). Some manic patients show a blunted thyroid-stimulating hormone (TSH) response to TRH, and there is evidence that this could help distinguish between acute mania and acute Schizophrenia (Extein et al., 1982).

Despite their utility, there are many loose ends to biogenic amine theories and many observations that are unexplained by, or frankly inconsistent with, the theory in its simplest form (Baldessarini, 1975). For example, treatment of depression with large doses of precursors of the supposedly-deficient neurotransmitters has yielded inconsistent and generally unpromising results. Also, while several laboratories have reproduced the previously-cited MHPG results, others have failed to do so or have found contradictory results. Furthermore, the metabolic effects (such as reuptake block) that have been proposed to explain the efficacy of antidepressants occur rapidly--yet improvement in depressed mood usually does not occur for several weeks. Although deficient production, increased destruction, increased excretion, or competition with other neurohumors could contribute to a neurotransmitter deficiency, the most promising candidate for altered function in depression now seems to be the postsynaptic receptor (Charney, Menkes, & Heninger, 1981). Despite variable or divergent presynaptic effects, a variety of effective treatments--tricyclic antidepressants, monoamine oxidase inhibitors, and ECT--share postsynaptic effects: after long-term administration they reduce β-adrenergic and enhance serotonergic and α-adrenergic postsynaptic receptor sensitivity. The effects of thyroid hormone upon affective symptoms--e.g., deficient thyroid hormone may predispose to depression, and administering small doses of thyroid may enhance responsiveness to tricyclic antidepressants--may also be mediated by catecholamine-β-receptor interactions (Whybrow & Prange, 1981).

Genetic factors presumably underlie many of the biochemical aspects of the Affective Disorders, such as responsiveness to particular drugs or particular patterns of neurohumoral metabolism such as MHPG excretion. However, the exact mechanisms of genetic influence and the particular modes of inheritance (i.e., monogenic vs. polygenic) are unknown.

Similarities in illness patterns shared by biologic relatives do not, in themselves, constitute evidence of genetic factors--children acquire a psychological and cultural, as well as genetic, endowment from their parents--but striking differences in concordance between monozygotic and dizygotic twins, increased incidence of affective disorder in adopted-out children of parents with affective illness, and the tendency for affectively-ill biologic relatives to show similar patterns of drug response do support a strong genetic influence upon the Major Affective Disorders.

Akiskal and McKinney (1975) have presented an intriguing hypothesis that is consistent with much of what is known about depression. They suggest that a fundamental disruption in the neurochemistry of the diencephalon--which seems intimately involved in the experiencing of pleasure or reward--represents the final common pathway for depression. The model integrates chemical, experiential, and behavioral variables and outlines pathways and mechanisms whereby each set of variables can influence the other. For example, an alteration in the neurochemistry of critical diencephalic areas would interfere with the ability to experience pleasure (i.e., would be felt as anhedonia), which would in turn reduce pleasure-seeking behavior. Both catecholamines and indoleamines are known to play significant roles in modulating the function of the diencephalic areas that serve as the neuroanatomical substrates of "reward" and "punishment." Genetic factors might alter enzymes involved in neurotransmitter synthesis, destruction, or transport. A history of deprivation in early life (such as loss of a parent or parental coldness and indifference) could be reflected by subtle alteration in the diencephalic pleasure-regulating mechanisms, which would in turn sensitize the individual to the effects of frustration in adult life. Stresses could include purely physiologic stressors (e.g., reserpine), as well as psychologically-defined stressors whose meaning derives from the individual's unique experience. In their model, dysphorias such as reactive sadness or mild depression represent a readily-reversible alteration of function of diencephalic reinforcement mechanisms, whereas the anhedonia of significant depression reflects a more severe and enduring dysfunction of diencephalic homeostasis. The diencephalic final common pathway is responsible for the shared features of depressive disorders, while the multiplicity of pathogenic factors (genetic, psychological, environmental, etc.) explains their heterogeneity. A major virtue of their model is its inclusion of variables from the three levels--social, psychological, organismic--that must be taken into account when explaining complex behavioral phenomena.

We must add that the mechanisms whereby the brain transduces experience into alterations in the chemical and electrical activities of neurons, or whereby neuronal states are transduced into thoughts and feelings, remain an utter mystery.

QUIZ, Section VI.

Circle the correct answer(s). <u>One</u> or <u>more</u> <u>than</u> <u>one</u> answer may be correct.

1. Which of the following provide(s) strong evidence of genetic factors in Affective Disorders?

    a. much higher concordance in monozygotic than dizygotic twins
    b. increased incidence of depression in families of depressed probands
    c. similar patterns of antidepressant drug response in depressed relatives of depressed patients
    d. increased incidence of depression with advancing age

Circle the letter corresponding to the <u>one</u> correct response.

2. An abnormal, or positive, result of the dexamethasone suppression test (DST) would be
    a. 3μg/dL.
    b. 9μg/dL.

3. While the results of neurochemical studies of depression and its treatment often seem quite variable, studies of _____ are yielding consistent results.

    a. presynaptic receptor function
    b. MHPG excretion
    c. norepinephrine turnover
    d. postsynaptic receptor function

Complete the following.

4. Freud postulated that turning anger inward, by a process known as
    _____, resulted in depression. This occurred fol-
    lowing the loss of a love object toward whom one had mixed, or
    _____, feelings.

5. Drugs which _____ the availability of norepinephrine,
    such as reserpine, seem to cause depression in certain individuals.
    Drugs which _____ the level of _____ are
    used to treat depression, and, in addition, may provoke _____
    in certain patients. These findings are (direct/indirect) support for
    biogenic _____ hypotheses of Affective Disorders.

6. Of the various norepinephrine metabolites, _____ provides
    the best index of CNS norepinephrine metabolism. Depressed patients
    with _____ levels of this metabolite in the urine are
    likely to respond to imipramine, which in vivo has _____
    effects.

7. Low MHPG tends to predict a positive response to _____,
    which has primarily noradrenergic action, while high MHPG tends to
    predict positive response to _____, whose action is
    _____.

8. According to Akiskal and McKinney, the area of the brain known as the
    _____ serves as the final common pathway for
    depression.

9. Deficient thyroid hormone predisposes to

    a. depression.
    b. mania.
    c. both.
    d. neither.

Assuming the correctness of the indoleamine permissive hypothesis, complete
the following chart:

Relative level of: Mood State

Serotonin	Norepinephrine	
Normal	Normal	10. _____
Decreased	Increased	11. _____
Normal	Decreased	12. _____
Decreased	Normal	13. _____
Normal	Increased	14. _____
Decreased	Decreased	15. _____

TRUE or FALSE: Circle the correct letter.

T   F   16. A positive DST strongly suggests the diagnosis of significant
            depression.

T   F   17. A negative DST is strong evidence against the diagnosis of significant depression.

Match the following descriptions with the corresponding types of phenomena. Lettered items may be used once or more than once.

___18.   The suicide rate among Catholics is lower than among Protestants.

___19.   A boy becomes depressed after his parents are killed in an auto accident.

___20.   A woman in India, whose husband has just died, throws herself on his funeral pyre as prescribed by the Hindu ritual of Suttee.

a. primarily socially-influenced phenomena

b. primarily psychologically-influenced phenomena

VII.   TREATMENT OF AFFECTIVE DISORDERS

The nonpsychiatric physician needs to be knowledgeable in the diagnosis of Affective Disorder since he or she will probably see more patients with depression than all other psychiatric disorders combined, and should be familiar with their treatment since many can be successfully managed without extensive help from a psychiatrist.

Treatments fall into two broad categories: somatic (e.g., drugs, ECT) and psychosocial (e.g., the various forms of psychotherapy). Somatic treatments are the mainstay of therapy for the symptoms of the Major Affective Disorders. By contrast, psychosocial treatments are more effective in improving areas of overall life-adjustment, such as having appropriate and realistic expectations of self and others, and the ability to form and maintain gratifying relationships with others. Such problems may be present in patients whose Major Affective Disorders are in remission and in patients with more long-standing, experientially-based "characterologic" problems that are not primarily symptoms of biologically-based Affective Disorder.

A.   TREATMENT OF DEPRESSION

The presence of significant neurovegetative symptoms and a relative autonomy of mood are the major indications for somatic treatment of depression; thus, patients meeting criteria for melancholia epitomize the need for somatic treatment. Patients whose sleep, appetite, sexual drive, and energy level are relatively normal, and who can be easily "cheered up," are unlikely to have a severe degree of depressive affect and are unlikely to respond to somatic treatments. The presence of a severely depressed mood accompanied by a normal pattern of sleep should prompt an inquiry about the use of sedatives or alcohol, or should lead to questioning the diagnosis.

Patients with significant neurovegetative symptoms and a significantly depressed mood are also likely to have significant impairment of psychosocial functioning (e.g., at work, at school, or with interpersonal relationships), and this provides another index of the need for treatment. A patient who feels a little "down," who occasionally sleeps restlessly, and whose social functioning is neither a great strain nor impaired is either in the earliest stages of depression or else has a disturbance that is likely to be transient; in either case, drug treatment would be premature (unless history reveals that these symptoms were previously prodromal to a serious depression). In essence, depression should be treated on the same basis as any other illness: when the discomfort is severe enough, and/or the disability severe enough--and the treatment effective enough--so that the risks of inaction outweigh the risks of treatment.

Significant depression should be treated regardless of whether or not you think the depression has a "cause." A patient with a chronic physical illness has reason to worry, or feel sad, but he does not have "a reason" to have MNA and EMA, persistent crying spells, psychomotor agitation, and diurnal mood fluctuation. Because patients with severe physical illness usually cling to hope, even when this is unrealistic, the presence of hopelessness should raise suspicion that a pathological depression has supervened. While physical illness, like other life stress, may precede or accompany significant depressive episodes, a depression with significant neuro-vegetative dysfunction that follows life changes is, phenomenologically and therapeutically, indistinguishable from one that arises out of the blue. Again, remember to distinguish age-appropriate worry from depression, and do not forget that a patient's explanation of the cause of his depression ("my wife left me") may, in fact, be the result of the depression. Obviously, efforts to reduce life stresses can be helpful, but a fully-developed depression will generally run its course, little influenced by environmental contingencies, without somatic treatment.

In considering treatment of depression, it is useful to know the natural history of the illness. Most depressions last six to 18 months. Thus, if you saw a patient who first came to you after he had been developing depression of moderate severity for the better part of a year, but in the last two months had gradually but significantly improved, you would probably want to observe the patient closely over a several week period to see if the depression continued to improve before offering specific treatment.

Antidepressant drugs are generally the first line of defense in treating significant depression. Although ECT is faster, usually safer, and often more efficacious, the stigma attached to its use, and its overuse and abuse in the past, have led doctors and patients to relegate it to the status of a last resort. Certainly, prescribing and taking pills is more in keeping with what doctors and patients expect of one another than is the induction of electrically-induced convulsions. See Chapter 16, Psychopharmacology, for a detailed discussion of the use of antidepressant medication.

B.   TREATMENT OF MANIA

Lithium carbonate has become the treatment of choice for acute episodes. It is little short of miraculous that this simple action can reverse the myriad affective, cognitive, perceptual, and behavioral manifestations of mania, and such an action lends credence to the notion of a unitary neurochemical imbalance at the core of at least some Affective Disorders. While lithium's currently approved indications are the treatment of mania and prophylaxis

ANSWERS, SECTION VI.

1. a,c
2. b
3. d
4. introjection, ambivalent
5. decrease, increase, norepinephrine, mania, indirect, amine
6. MHPG, decreased, noradrenergic
7. imipramine, amitriptyline, serotonergic
8. diencephalon
9. a
10. normal
11. mania
12. normal
13. normal
14. normal
15. depression
16. T
17. F
18. a
19. b
20. a

against recurrent manic episodes, it also reduces the severity and frequency of depressive episodes in bipolar patients and, in some bipolar patients, it is an effective antidepressant. Many depressed bipolar patients will, however, require combined treatment: lithium plus imipramine (or desipramine), or, less commonly, lithium plus an MAOI. In general, the more "classic" the manic and depressive episodes, the better the response to lithium.

Because cyclothymia and manic-depressive illness are quantitatively differing points on a continuum, just as are hypomania and mania, lithium should be considered in patients whose comfort or social functioning is impaired by recurrent mood swings. Thus, lithium has been useful in treating recurrent depressions when these depressions resemble those of depressed manic-depressives and in treating recurrent hypomanic or Cyclothymic Disorders, even when they do not attain the severity of a manic or depressive episode. As with any form of psychiatric drug treatment, a decision whether to treat or not depends upon the risks (including adverse psychosocial consequences) and discomfort of the illness versus the risks of the treatment itself.

See Chapter 16 for a description of the drug treatment of mania.

Although bipolar illness is typically an episodic disorder characterized by relative freedom from symptoms between attacks, some patients have chronic, non-remitting forms of manic-depressive illness. While Kraepelin was well-aware of such variants in the earlier part of the 20th century, his observations seem to have lain fallow until recent years. With the advent of lithium treatment, some chronic, apparently hopeless patients thought to be suffering from chronic Schizophrenia or some other severe but undiagnosable psychosis have responded dramatically to lithium. The difficulty in deciding whether an acute psychosis represents Schizophrenia or manic-depressive illness has already been discussed, and this difficulty is, of course, compounded when the mania or depression assumes a chronic or otherwise quite atypical course. Van Putten and Sanders (1975) describe several such patients; that their illness was, in fact, Bipolar Affective Disorder was shown not only by their favorable response to lithium, but also by more careful history-taking which revealed mood swings earlier in life and, in some patients, the disappearance of atypical symptoms and the emergence of more obvious affective symptoms during lithium treatment. They suggest that a lithium trial may be worthwhile in patients who have failed to respond to other treatments, especially when one considers the previously mentioned practice in this country of overdiagnosing Schizophrenia and underdiagnosing manic-depressive illness. Comparison of Kraepelin's and Van Putten and Sanders' clinical observations with many textbooks' descriptions of "schizophrenic" patients is sobering.

C. ECT

Electroconvulsive therapy, because of the rapidity of its beneficial effects and its relative safety, may be the treatment of choice in patients who are severely depressed and suicidal, and for whom the two-or-more week wait for antidepressants to become effective is unacceptable. It may also be indicated in manic patients who are extremely excited, hyperactive, or assaultive, and at risk of harming others or exhausting themselves. Some patients with catatonic excitement or stupor who may have been misdiagnosed as schizophrenic, respond rapidly to ECT; for such patients ECT is often safer than the very high doses of drugs needed to bring them under a modicum of control. In addition to the manic episode which is too dangerous or too severe to be controlled with drugs, severe depressions with prominent neurovegetative symptoms occurring in older patients may be especially amenable to ECT. As with a given psychotropic drug, a previous response to ECT is the best predictor of its future success.

ECT is generally safer than psychotropic drugs since it is given under closely supervised conditions, and, unlike drugs which exert their potentially noxious effects 24 hours a day, the duration of each treatment is very brief. Convulsive therapy may be the first choice when a medical condition such as cardiovascular disease is sufficiently severe to preclude antidepressant drugs. ECT is discussed in more detail in Chapter 19, Other Treatment Modalities.

D. PSYCHOSOCIAL TREATMENT OF AFFECTIVE DISORDERS

Symbolic interventions--such as the various forms of psychotherapy--are generally acknowledged to be ineffective in treating the symptoms of Major Affective Disorders. That is, when a mood disorder is manifest by significant neurovegetative symptoms which, in concert with the disordered mood itself, significantly impair social functioning, the underlying biologic derangement seems to be autonomous and is insensitive to purely verbal input; the derangement will either remit spontaneously at some future point and for no known reason, or else must be treated with somatic modalities (drugs, or ECT). Trying to "help" a severely depressed (not sad, but depressed) patient understand how his own unconscious thoughts or wishes have caused his distress is painful as well as useless, and his inability to profit from intensive psychotherapy adds one more failure experience to a patient who already feels demoralized.

That traditional insight-oriented psychotherapy has little role in the treatment of severe affective symptoms does not mean that psychotherapeutic skills are unnecessary for the clinician who treats patients with Affective Disorders. In the acute phase of treatment, when symptoms are severe, considerable psychological and psychodynamic sophistication may be needed to: engage patients in treatment; explain their illness to them in a way that they are likely to understand and accept; foster the trust and confidence necessary for compliance with the regimen of treatment; and understand and cope with whatever factors (in the patient or patient's family) arise that might interfere with, or undermine, successful treatment. Furthermore, when neurovegetative symptoms have subsided, various forms of psychotherapy may be quite useful: in understanding why particular people or events are unusually stressful to the patient and in helping him do something about it, in helping patient and family "pick up the pieces" after a period of severe disruption of normal function, and in educating patient and family about the chances for recurrence of the illness and what symptoms or behaviors should serve as warning signals. While it is true that psychotherapy is ineffective in treating the symptoms that accompany major disorders of mood, it is equally true that drugs are ineffective in improving personal adjustment or social functioning, except to the degree that they treat symptoms which are directly interfering with psychosocial functioning.

A possible exception to the general ineffectiveness of psychosocial therapy as a definitive treatment of depression is Beck's Cognitive therapy (Beck et al., 1979). Beck's approach involves a systematic attack on the depressive cognitive triad, mentioned in Section VI, and shows promise in treating depressions of less-than-melancholic proportion.

When considering the role of somatic and psychosocial treatments for patients with Affective Disorders, it is most important to remember the scope and limitations of each: studies have shown that while drugs (or ECT) effectively relieve the Affective Disorder per se, many patients' overall level of functioning is significantly enhanced when appropriate psychotherapy is included. Philip May has coined the term "psychotherapeutic management" to describe a form of doctor-patient interaction that is quite distinct from the sort of psychotherapy that intends to alter long-standing, psychologically influenced patterns of behavior. Psychotherapeutic management deals with those issues, described in the preceding paragraph, necessary to engage and successfully treat the patient's episode of illness. While psychotherapeutic management is certainly enhanced by a knowledge of personality development and dynamic psychology, the psychotherapeutic management of many patients with acute Affective Disorders can be successfully undertaken by the well-informed nonpsychiatric physician.

Because it may be impossible accurately to determine the acutely ill patient's premorbid adjustment (the pillar of the community may, when depressed, say "I've always been a failure, and I always will be."), decisions about the need for more extensive psychotherapy should be deferred until the acute episode is in remission. You will then find that some patients, once they are no longer manic or depressed, are essentially free from significant problems. Others, however, will exhibit patterns of behavior or discuss feelings that are relatively independent of the Affective Disorder--problems in forming lasting or gratifying relationships with others, low self-esteem that is a result of early experience and long-standing intrapsychic conflict rather than a reflection of an acute lowering of mood, difficulties in relating to authority figures, etc.--and these patients would be candidates for psychosocial treatment at the hands of a specialist. See Chapter 17 for further discussion of psychosocial treatment modalities.

QUIZ, Section VII.

Circle the letter corresponding to the <u>one</u> correct answer.

1.   An atypical depressive episode would be _____ likely to respond to lithium than an episode characterized by hypersomnia, anergia, and psychomotor retardation.

      a. more
      b. less

2.   A patient whose mood is easily changed in response to environmental events is _____ to respond well to somatic treatment.

      a. likely
      b. unlikely

Complete the following.

3.   Although lithium's primary indications are the treatment of _____ and the prevention of recurrence of _____ episodes, it is often effective in preventing episodes of _____ as well, and in some bipolar patients it effectively treats acute _____ episodes.

4.   _____ works more rapidly than do drugs used to treat mood disorders; it is also _____. It may be especially useful when a patient's illness is so _____ that the risk of harm to himself or others is great, and one cannot wait for drugs to become effective. It is relatively little-used today-- not because it is a poor treatment in properly-selected patients, but rather because of the _____ attached to its use.

5.   The presence of significant _____ indicates that antidepressant medication is likely to be helpful.

6.   In addition to neurovegetative disturbance, the presence of a significantly _____ mood and impairment of _____ function suggests that somatic treatment is warranted.

Use the following case study to answer questions 7-10.

A 39-year-old housewife is slowly dying of breast cancer and is expected to live six to nine months. Until recently, she managed to keep up with a modicum of housework and relate well to her husband and children, despite occasional crying spells and episodes of anger at her oncologist. For the past month, she has been awakening at 3:00 or 4:00 a.m., unable to return to sleep, and feels "horrible" until 10:00 or 11:00 a.m. She has anorexia (which has been attributed to her chemotherapy). She frequently flies into a rage at her children, then is filled with remorse. She has begun to feel hopeless.

TRUE or FALSE: Circle the correct letter.

T   F   7. She is experiencing a normal reaction to a serious illness.

T   F   8. Even though she has ample reason to feel distressed, antide-pressant treatment should be considered.

Complete the following.

9. Her feeling "horrible" until late morning probably represents a
    _____ mood fluctuation.

10. A diagnosis of depression should be considered because she has sig-nificant _____ disorder, accompanied by impaired
    _____ function, and a feeling of ___,_____ .

TRUE or FALSE: Circle the correct letter.

T   F   11. Psychotherapy is unlikely to be effective in relieving the ano-rexia and decreased sleep that accompany a depressive epi-sode, or the pressured speech and hyperactivity that accompany a manic episode.

T   F   12. Long-standing problems in relating comfortably with others--based on the patient's lack of adequate role models--are likely to be helped by the appropriate psychotropic medication.

T   F   13. The clinician should avoid mixing psychosocial and somatic treatments in the overall management of a patient with a sig-nificant Affective Disorder.

T   F   14. Intensive psychotherapeutic treatment is best begun at the height of a patient's depression, when he is most motivated to relieve his suffering.

T   F   15. Antidepressant medication is unlikely to improve depression if stressful environmental circumstances--"reasons to be de-pressed"--are present.

T   F   16. Lithium may be indicated in mood disturbances that are too mild to be classified accurately as manic or depressive episodes.

T   F   17. When a patient is significantly depressed, it may be impossible to determine the need for longer-term psychosocial treatment.

T   F   18. Many patients with severe Affective Disorders do not need exten-sive psychotherapeutic treatment aimed at fundamental alteration of personality patterns.

T   F   19. "Psychotherapeutic management" (Philip May's term) is a special-ized technique restricted to mental health professionals.

ANSWERS,   Section   VII._____

1.   b
2.   b
3.   mania, manic, depression, depressive
4.   ECT, safer, severe, stigma
5.   neurovegetative symptoms
6.   depressed, psychosocial
7.   F
8.   T
9.   diurnal
10.   sleep, psychosocial, hopelessness

11.   T
12.   F
13.   F
14.   F
15.   F
16.   T
17.   T
18.   T
19.   F

POST-TEST

For the following questions, <u>one</u> or <u>more</u> <u>than</u> <u>one</u> answer may be correct. Circle the correct answer(s).

1. Which of the following might represent typical delusions as seen in depressed patients?

    a. A 25-year-old man believes he is an agent of the C.I.A., and has a powerful radio transmitter implanted in his teeth.
    b. A 46-year-old woman believes that her heart has stopped beating.
    c. A 30-year-old woman believes that God has summoned her to Saudi Arabia to take over the OPEC Cartel.
    d. A 44-year-old man knows that he emits a horrible body odor, even though he bathes several times a day.

2. Choose the correct statement(s).

    a. Intensive psychotherapeutic treatment is best begun at the height of a patient's depression, when he is most motivated to relieve his suffering.
    b. Most patients with severe Affective Disorders will need extensive psychotherapeutic treatment after their acute symptoms are in remission.
    c. Long-standing problems in relating comfortably to others--based on the patient's lack of adequate role models--are likely to be helped by the appropriate psychotropic medication.
    d. Psychotherapy is unlikely to be effective in relieving the neuro-vegetative symptoms that accompany a depressive episode.

3. Regarding depression and grief, choose the correct statement(s).

    a. Low self-esteem is common in depression but not in grief.
    b. A major loss may precede both depression and grief.
    c. Freud believed that ambivalence toward the lost object was present in depression but not in grief.
    d. Sleep disturbance is common in depression but not in grief.

4. DSM-III provides both inclusion and exclusion criteria for diagnosing Affective Disorders. In addition to the presence or absence of specific symptoms, disorders are classified according to

    a. severity.
    b. presence or absence of precipitating stresses.
    c. duration of disturbance.
    d. etiology.

5. Choose the correct statement(s).

    a. The presence of paranoid delusions in a patient tends to rule out an Affective Disorder.

b. Patients with Affective Disorders may exhibit catatonic excitement or catatonic stupor.

c. In acutely psychotic patients, a detailed mental status examination is the most reliable way to distinguish Schizophrenia from Affective Disorder.

d. Patients with mania may exhibit bizarre behavior and formal thought disorders.

6. Which of the following provide(s) strong evidence for a genetic factor in Affective Disorders?

a. greater concordance in monozygotic than dizygotic twins
b. increased incidence of depression in families of depressed probands
c. similar patterns of antidepressant drug response in depressed relatives of depressed patients
d. increasing incidence of depression with advancing age

7. Depression and Dementia may be difficult to distinguish. Which of the following are more characteristic of depression than Dementia?

a. recent memory more impaired than remote memory
b. objective signs of cognitive deficit are greater than subjective complaints
c. family members are unlikely to be aware of the severity of the patient's difficulties
d. symptoms are worse in the morning, and improve as the day progresses

8. In a patient with an acute psychosis, the diagnosis of Schizophrenia is more likely to be correct than the diagnosis of mania if

a. the patient is less than 25 years old.
b. delusions and hallucinations are present.
c. treatment with haloperidol brings about improvement in symptoms.
d. the patient shows marked blunting or flattening of affect.

9. Choose the correct statement(s).

a. Depressed patients who also have histories of mania tend to have become depressed at a younger age than depressed patients without histories of mania.
b. Patients with little or no sleep disturbance are unlikely to be severely depressed.
c. Patients who talk about suicide are more likely to commit suicide than are patients who don't talk about it.
d. The presence of hallucinations and/or delusions in a patient favors a diagnosis of Schizophrenia over a diagnosis of depression.

10. A 55-year-old man with no previous history of depression or mania presents with typical symptoms of profound depression, including the belief that his "insides have rotted away" and that all of his relatives have died because of his sins. The best treatment(s) would be

    a. ECT.
    b. amitriptyline.
    c. amitriptyline plus haloperidol.
    d. phenelzine plus perphenazine.

11. The primary determinant(s) of a patient's thought content when depressed is(are)

    a. the severity of the sleep disorder.
    b. the quality of the marital relationship (in married patients).
    c. the duration of the depressive episode.
    d. the patient's age and place in the life cycle.

12. Choose the correct statement(s).

    a. The suicide rate generally increases as age increases.
    b. Ingestion of benzodiazepines is unlikely to be lethal unless other drugs or alcohol are ingested concomitantly.
    c. A majority of people who commit suicide have seen a physician during the months prior to their death.
    d. If a physician brings up the topic of suicide with a depressed patient, the risk of suicide increases.

13. The sleep disorder of depression

    a. may consist of excessive sleep rather than decreased sleep.
    b. can be appropriately treated with benzodiazepines.
    c. provides a sensitive index to pharmacologic treatment.
    d. is usually restricted to prolonged sleep latency (difficulty falling asleep).

14. The biogenic amine permissive hypothesis

    a. states that low levels of serotonin and high levels of norepinephrine lead to mania.
    b. states that high levels of serotonin and low levels of norepinephrine lead to depression.
    c. is consistent with clinically observed effects of reserpine.
    d. implies that psychological factors play little or no role in Affective Disorders.

Use the following case study to answer questions 15-16.

A 48-year-old man feels hopeless, cries easily, and believes that he has always been a sinner. Although he functioned well at home and at work until six months ago, he is now convinced that he has always been a terrible husband and father. His food has "lost its taste" and he has lost 10 pounds in the last three months. He sleeps eight hours per night with the aid of Dalmane® (flurazepam) 30 mg h.s. prescribed by his family doctor. He has recently begun to doubt his wife's fidelity and believes she is having an affair with their minister, whom she has frequently consulted in recent months as she has become more worried about her husband. He also thinks she may be poisoning his food.

15. Which of the following are quite <u>inconsistent</u> with a diagnosis of Schizophrenia?

    a. belief that his wife may be unfaithful
    b. relatively late age of onset
    c. good premorbid psychosocial functioning
    d. believing his food may be poisoned

Complete the following.

16. Reconcile the diagnosis of severe depression with a normal sleep pattern in this patient. _____

_____

Circle the letter corresponding to the <u>one</u> correct response.

Use the following case study to answer questions 17-25.

A 42-year-old married woman physician has developed, over several weeks, a sleep pattern characterized by brief awakenings throughout the night, finally awakening at 3:00 or 4:00 a.m. and being unable to return to sleep. She has also noticed increasing nightmares, a loss of appetite, and a diminished interest in and enjoyment of sexual relations with her husband. Previously, sex was quite pleasurable. She is more irritable with her colleagues and was recently passed over for the chairmanship of an important medical school committee. Her husband seems less affectionate and solicitous than previously and she has begun to wonder if he is seeing another woman. She no longer enjoys caring for patients and must force herself to struggle through each clinical encounter. She notices that she has made several errors in caring for patients and wonders whether her becoming a physician was a mistake as her parents always seemed to think. She has developed a mild but persistent lower backache, although an orthopedic colleague reassured her that "nothing is wrong" after careful physical and neurologic examination.

17. The most likely diagnosis is

    a. marital maladjustment.
    b. depression.
    c. paranoid personality, manifested by unrealistic fantasies about her husband's infidelity.
    d. hypochondriasis.

18. Since this patient is 42 years old, a finding of a severe deficit of recent memory would raise what diagnostic possibility?

    a. psychotic depression
    b. hysteria
    c. Organic Mental Disorder

19. Her current distaste for medical practice probably means

    a. her parents were correct in their judgment of her career choice.
    b. that she is anhedonic.
    c. that she has an Organic Brain Syndrome.

20. Which is more likely?

    a. Her depression caused her to miss an important career opportunity (committee chairmanship).
    b. Being passed over for the committee chairmanship has caused her depression.

21. Anxiety and phobias are prominent symptoms in depressed patients who are, compared to this patient

    a. significantly younger.
    b. around the same age.
    c. significantly older.

22. Her sexual difficulties are likely to respond to

    a. sexual therapy à la Masters and Johnson (see Chapter 11).
    b. marital counseling.
    c. her being considered for committee chairman.
    d. treatment of her depression.

Circle the correct answer(s). One or more than one answer may be correct.

23. This patient's marital problems

    a. may aggravate her depression.
    b. probably result from her depression.
    c. are the primary cause of her depression.

24. Dalmane® (flurazepam) 30 mg h.s. might

    a. improve her sleep pattern, at least temporarily.
    b. lead to habituation.
    c. mask a symptom that is useful in monitoring response to antidepressant treatment.
    d. all in all, be a bad choice.

25. This patient is worried about her marriage and career because

    a. they are central issues in her life at this point.
    b. problems in these areas have caused her to become depressed.
    c. her ability to cope with these difficulties is impaired.

PRE-TEST ANSWERS

1.	a,c	8.	a,c	14.	d
2.	a,c	9.	d	15.	a,c
3.	d	10.	a,b,c	16.	b
4.	b,d	11.	a,c	17.	c
5.	a,b,c	12.	d	18.	c
6.	b,d	13.	a,c	19.	a
7.	a,b,c				

POST-TEST ANSWERS

1.	b,d	10.	a,c	17.	b
2.	d	11.	d	18.	c
3.	a,b,c	12.	a,b,c	19.	b
4.	a,c	13.	a,c	20.	a
5.	b,d	14.	a,c	21.	a
6.	a,c	15.	b,c	22.	d
7.	d	16.	his sedative medication is probably masking a sleep disorder	23.	a,b
8.	d			24.	a,b,c,d
9.	a,b,c			25.	a,c

REFERENCES

Akiskal, H. S., Djenderedjian, A. H., Rosenthal, R. H., & Khani, M. K. Cyclothymic disorder: Validating criteria for inclusion in the bipolar affective group. American Journal of Psychiatry, 1977, 134, 1227-1233.

Akiskal, H. S., & McKinney, W. T. Jr. Overview of recent research in depression. Integration of ten conceptual models into a comprehensive clinical frame. Archives of General Psychiatry, 1975, 32, 285-305.

Baldessarini, R. The basis for amine hypotheses in affective disorders. A critical evaluation. Archives of General Psychiatry, 1975, 32, 1087-1093.

Beck, A. T., Rush, A. J., Shaw, B. F., & Emery, G. Cognitive therapy of depression. New York: The Guilford Press, 1979.

Carroll, B. J., Feinberg, M., Greden, J. F., Tarika, J., Albala, A. A., Haskett, R. F., James, N. McI., Kronfol, Z., Lohr, N., Steiner, M., de Vigne, J. P., & Young, E. A specific laboratory test for the diagnosis of melancholia. Archives of General Psychiatry, 1981, 38, 15-22.

Charney, D. S., Menkes, D. B., & Heninger, G. R. Receptor sensitivity and the mechanism of action of antidepressant treatment. Archives of General Psychiatry, 1981, 38, 1160-1180.

Detre, T. P., & Jarecki, H. G. Modern psychiatric treatment. Philadelphia: J.B. Lippincott, 1971.

Diagnostic and statistical manual of mental disorders (3rd Edition). Washington, D.C.: American Psychiatric Association, 1980.

Extein, I., Pottash, A. L. C., Gold, M. S., & Cowdry, R. W. Using the protirelin test to distinguish mania from schizophrenia. Archives of General Psychiatry, 1982, 39, 77-81.

Loranger, A. W., & Levine, P. M. Age at onset of bipolar affective illness. Archives of General Psychiatry, 1978, 35, 1345-1348.

Maas, J. W. Biogenic amines and depression. Archives of General Psychiatry, 1975, 32, 1357-1361.

Pope, H. G. Jr., & Lipinski, J. F. Jr. Diagnosis in schizophrenia and manic-depressive illness. Archives of General Psychiatry, 1978, 35, 811-828.

Van Putten, T., & Sanders, D. G. Lithium in treatment failures. Journal of Nervous and Mental Disease, 1975, 161, 255-264.

Wells, C. E. Pseudodementia. American Journal of Psychiatry, 1979, 136, 895-900.

Whybrow, P. C., & Prange, A. J. Jr. A hypothesis of thyroid-catecholamine-receptor interaction. Archives of General Psychiatry, 1981, 38, 106-113.

SUGGESTIONS FOR FURTHER READING

Detre and Jarecki's excellent book, listed under <u>REFERENCES</u>, contains, in addition to a chapter on "Affective Disorders," two chapters on "The Assessment of the Patient," and "Examination, Disposition, and Management." These chapters are useful for approaching a broad spectrum of psychiatric illnesses in addition to the affective disorders.

Barchas, J. D., Berger, P. A., Ciaranello, R. D., & Elliott, G. R. <u>Psychopharmacology: From theory to practice</u>. New York: Oxford University Press, 1977.

This broad-ranging book is another source of further details of drug treatment.

Tighe, P. (Ed.) <u>Depression today: Confident clinical office management</u>. New York: C.M.E. Communications, Inc., 1978.

Part One: Recognizing and Diagnosing Depression.
Part Two: Managing the Acute Episode and Follow-Up Phase.
Part Three: Special Cases in the Pharmacologic Management
               of Depression.

These pamphlets, written for the nonpsychiatric physician, are well-written, authoritative, and reasonably concise.

CHAPTER 9

ANXIETY DISORDERS

Miriam DeAntonio, M.D.
Lorenz Villeponteaux, Ph.D.

CHAPTER OUTLINE

LEARNING OBJECTIVES

After completing this chapter you will be able to:

1. Describe the concept of anxiety.

2. Differentiate between normal and abnormal anxiety.

3. Differentiate between fear and anxiety.

4. Name ten physiological responses to anxiety which are aroused by the autonomic nervous system.

5. Name and define three types of Phobic Disorders.

6. Define and differentiate between the concepts of primary and secondary gain.

7. List the characteristic features of panic attacks.

8. List the diagnostic criteria for Generalized Panic Disorder.

9. List the diagnostic criteria for Generalized Anxiety Disorder.

10. Define obsession and compulsion.

11. List the diagnostic criteria for Obsessive Compulsive Disorder.

12. Name and define five ego defense mechanisms often found in persons with Obsessive Compulsive Disorder.

13. List the diagnostic criteria for Post-Traumatic Stress Disorder.

14. Describe Atypical Anxiety Disorder; specify when this diagnosis is used.

PRE-TEST

For the following questions one or more than one answer may be correct. Circle the correct answer(s).

1. Anxiety

    a. plays an important, positive role in our lives.
    b. promotes action toward homeostasis.
    c. may be protective.
    d. is ego-syntonic.

2. A number of organ systems may be affected by anxiety. These include

    a. cardiovascular system.
    b. genitourinary system.
    c. gastrointestinal system.
    d. musculoskeletal system.

3. People who experience anxiety include

    a. medical students.
    b. schizophrenics.
    c. infants and children.
    d. depressed patients.

4. Phobic Disorders include

    a. Simple Phobia.
    b. Social Phobia.
    c. Agoraphobia.
    d. Compulsive Phobia.

5. Agoraphobia

    a. has anxiety as a prominent feature.
    b. is more commonly seen in males.
    c. is often associated with recurrent panic attacks.
    d. is associated with a specific, circumscribed feared object.

6. Panic attacks have which of the following characteristics?

    a. sudden, overwhelming anxiety
    b. physiological responses such as dyspnea
    c. feelings of apprehension, helplessness, impending doom
    d. brief duration of the symptoms

7. Free-floating anxiety is characterized by signs and symptoms of

    a. apprehensive expectation.
    b. vigilance and scanning.
    c. motor tension.
    d. autonomic hyperactivity.

8. Characteristics of obsessions and compulsions are that they

    a. persistently intrude into one's consciousness.
    b. are ego-syntonic.
    c. are recognized by the patient as irrational.
    d. have a relatively easily identifiable source.

9. Post-Traumatic Stress Disorders

    a. frequently involve "flashbacks."
    b. are usually time-limited.
    c. may be confused with Organic Mental Disorders.
    d. are always associated with the death of one or more persons.

10. Physiological responses expressed via the autonomic nervous system
    and associated with both fear and anxiety include

    a. dyspnea.
    b. chest pain.
    c. pounding heartbeat.
    d. excessive salivation.

11. A young, single woman has a fear of thunderstorms. She adamantly
    refuses to leave her house whenever there is even the slightest chance
    of rain. Her mother "understands" and will literally sit with her
    daughter under these circumstances. This example illustrates

    a. primary gain.
    b. Simple Phobia.
    c. secondary gain.
    d. Social Phobia.

12. A middle-aged man reports that whenever he opens a door he thinks,
    "Someone will die." He then unfailingly returns to the door, touches
    the doorknob, and says, "I take that back." This example involves

    a. obsession.
    b. compulsion.
    c. undoing.
    d. phobia.

13. A Vietnam combat veteran reports "flashbacks" of war experiences, depression, withdrawal, difficulty sleeping, guilt over his own survival, trouble concentrating, and inability to hold a job. He also becomes panicky if he hears firecrackers going off in his neighborhood. On the basis of this information alone the diagnosis is likely to be

   a. Panic Disorder.
   b. Phobic Disorder.
   c. Generalized Anxiety Disorder.
   d. Post-Traumatic Stress Disorder.

14. Anxiety is the most prominent feature of

   a. Phobic Disorders.
   b. Schizophrenias.
   c. Post-Traumatic Stress Disorders.
   d. Impulse Disorders.

15. Anxiety results if the individual resists giving in to the symptoms which he has developed for relieving anxiety in

   a. Generalized Anxiety Disorders.
   b. Phobic Disorders.
   c. Panic Disorders.
   d. Obsessive Compulsive Disorders.

Match the following numbered items with the proper symptoms.

____16. apprehensive expectation
____17. vigilance and scanning
____18. motor tension
____19. autonomic hyperactivity

a. sweating, palpitations, clammy hands, dizziness, parathesias, dry mouth

b. anxious, frightened, scared feeling that something bad will happen to oneself or loved ones, constant worrying and ruminating about this

c. difficulty sleeping, distractibility, irritability, cautious guarded behavior, impatience, on edge

d. restlessness, trembling, keyed up, fatigued, tense, muscle twitches, frowning, strained faces, easily startled

I. INTRODUCTION

A basic belief in our society is that every person is unique. Genetic endowment, human interaction, internal and external physiological-biological influences, and all manner of nonorganic forces contribute to the production of this uniqueness. Certain structural and functional characteristics are shared by virtually all human organisms. The structural features are generally more visible and, therefore, more readily identifiable; the functional features, on the other hand, are more difficult to measure and therefore it is more difficult to compare one person to another. We know that we share, for example, a wide range of emotions with other humans; everyone, from time to time, feels sad, happy, frightened, angry, loving, or worried.

There are ranges of these emotions which are considered normal, but the lines defining the limits are not precisely drawn. When an individual moves far enough outside the normal range, he comes or is brought for care to the attention of psychiatry.

Of all the emotions, anxiety probably occupies the most prominent place in psychiatry. If there is a thread that runs through nearly all the psychiatric disorders it probably is anxiety, even though such a thread would vary a great deal in thickness and in hue. Furthermore, since the apparent absence of anxiety may be a diagnostic criterion, such a thread would also vary in its visibility.

Within the range of normal human emotions anxiety also plays a very prominent role. There are many nontechnical words which convey the notion of anxiety. We talk about people as being nervous or uptight. We recognize in ourselves, at times, that we are uneasy about something even though we may not know specifically what it is that we are uneasy* about. We speak of discomfort, of worry, jitters, of having butterflies in the stomach. We respond to a wide variety of circumstances with anxiety: taking tests, speaking in public, hearing scary noises, being sick, having bad things happen to our loved ones, to name but a few.

Anything which makes us uncomfortable, such as anxiety, has a negative connotation. However, anxiety plays an important positive role in our lives. Without any discomfort or anxiety, for example, we would probably be devoid of motivation. Why act or change anything if we are perfectly comfortable, anxiety-free, in our current situation? If we feel no anxiety about the neuroanatomy examination, why study?

Complicating matters even more is the fact that a bridge exists between the emotional or affective response and the physiological response to anxiety. Furthermore, the physiological response to fear is the same as the physiological response to anxiety.

---

*It is interesting to note that the words disease and uneasiness derive from the same Anglo-Norman and Old French words.

Although somewhat oversimplified, a useful way of differentiating fear from anxiety has to do with the concept of <u>threat</u> as perceived by the individual. Fear results from a real threat or danger to the individual. Being confronted by a large, vicious dog will usually produce a fear response. Anxiety, on the other hand, usually results from a threat or danger which is internal. Going for an admissions interview for medical school normally will produce anxiety. The internal threat in this situation usually has to do with a threat or danger to one's well-being or self-esteem. In addition, anxiety may have as a stimulus an external object (as in fear), but the response to the object is out of proportion to the reality of the object, i.e., it is a kind of overreaction to the threat.

Anxiety, then, is a common human experience which may reach abnormal proportions. It has an affective component which is unpleasant or uncomfortable. It also has a physiological component expressed through the autonomic nervous system. Some of these physiological responses to anxiety are: rapid, pounding heartbeat; tightness in the chest; perspiration; headache; dry mouth; shortness of breath; sudden urge to urinate; tremor; flushing or pallor; cold, clammy hands. Fear produces these same responses in an individual and is differentiated from anxiety only by the source of the threat or danger to the person's well-being. In addition, the overreaction or unrealistic response to an external threat produces anxiety which is abnormal. You will learn later in this chapter that this kind of overreaction is the essence of the phobic response.

One of the basic drives of all human beings is toward homeostasis, both physiologically and psychologically. When something goes wrong we act to regain a kind of balance-in-motion. This is relatively easy to see anatomically, as in the case of the body's autoimmune system. It is in this drive to maintain psychological homeostasis that anxiety plays a very useful role, that of warning us of threats, either internal or external ones. We talk about this type of anxiety as signal anxiety. It signals us to prepare to take action to cope with a threat of some type.

Obviously, then, we do not simply accept fear or anxiety without trying to return to a homeostatic state. Usually we begin by making conscious maneuvers to cope with the anxiety or the fear. If we see a car coming toward us we quickly try to move out of its path. If we are facing an examination we try to reduce the anxiety by studying. It is when these conscious coping mechanisms have failed that we call upon unconscious means to deal with the anxiety, the ego defense mechanisms.

[If you do not understand the role or concept of ego defense mechanisms, you should review Chapter 2.]

In this chapter you will learn about some abnormal, psychopathological aspects of anxiety. While some types of anxiety occur in the vast majority of psychiatric disorders, it is the most prominent feature in what the DSM-III refers to as the Anxiety Disorders. These disorders include: 1) Phobic Disorders; 2) Anxiety Disorders; 3) Post-Traumatic Stress Disorders; and 4) Obsessive Compulsive Disorders.

A great deal has been written about anxiety, and interest in this phenomenon has not been limited to psychology or psychiatry. Theologians, philosophers, writers, anthropologists, sociologists and others have paid a great deal of attention to anxiety. If you are interested in reading more globally about anxiety see Stein, Vidich, and White (1960). A more recent view of anxiety is in the area of state versus trait anxiety (Spielberger, 1966). In this conceptualization trait anxiety refers to a person's tendency to be anxious over time. State anxiety, on the other hand, refers to anxiety which is experienced just at a given moment. The individual who ranks high on the scale of anxiety as a personality trait is one who tends to "perceive a wide range of objectively nondangerous circumstances as threatening, and to respond to these with A-state reactions disproportionate in intensity to the magnitude of the objective danger" (Spielberger, 1966, pp. 16-17).

But why is there such variation on the scale of trait anxiety? Why is it that some individuals seem to be more susceptible than others to anxiety when confronted with the same stimuli? At this time there are no clear, simple answers to such questions. At least one thing is certain, and that is that anxiety is a highly complex phenomenon involving a wide variety of components which interact with one another. These components include genetic, instinctual, cognitive, CNS, and peripheral nervous system factors. One would have to include unconscious factors as well, like an individual's unique set of ego defense mechanisms, developed in large measure to cope with anxiety.

It should be clear at this point that anxiety is indeed an emotion which is shared by human beings, but which in some individuals moves quantitatively into levels which are functionally disabling. The associated perception, in general terms, is that the organism is being threatened in some way by some stimulus, and the stimulus may be an external one or an internal one. Lader (1978) points out that the external stimulus may be physical, social, or psychological; and the internal stimulus may be thoughts, needs, aspirations, or drives. If a stimulus is perceived as a threat, then central nervous system arousal occurs and interacts with peripheral nervous system activity, leading to additional stimuli for anxiety. For example, an anxiety-producing stimulus may lead to, among other things, a rapid and pounding heartbeat, which, in turn, may produce a higher level of anxiety in the individual.

Now consider the Anxiety Disorders. In DSM-III these disorders are classified on the basis of: 1) anxiety which is experienced as the predominant feature of the disorder, as in generalized anxiety and panic; and 2) anxiety which results if the individual resists giving in to the symptoms which he has developed to relieve anxiety, as in Phobic and Obsessive Compulsive Disorders.

QUIZ, Section I.

Circle the letter corresponding to the <u>one</u> correct response.

1. Physiological responses to either fear or anxiety may include all of the following <u>except</u>

    a. shortness of breath.
    b. rapid heartbeat.
    c. tightness of chest.
    d. excessive salivation.
    e. tremor.

TRUE or FALSE: Indicate which of the following questions are true (T) and which are false (F) by circling the appropriate letter.

T   F   2. We usually make conscious efforts to reduce anxiety or fear.

T   F   3. Ego defenses may be either conscious or unconscious.

T   F   4. The perception of anxiety by an individual may be a signal to prepare for a threat of some sort.

T   F   5. Of all the emotions, anxiety probably occupies the most prominent place in psychiatry.

T   F   6. The range of limits of normalcy regarding human emotions is precisely drawn.

T   F   7. Anxiety may often play a role in National Board Scores in that anxiety may increase motivation to study.

Match the following types of threats with the response they produce. Lettered items may be used once or more than once.

___8.	internal threat	a.	anxiety
___9.	external, real threat	b.	fear
__10.	overreaction to a real external threat		

Match the following definitions with the corresponding types of anxiety.

__11.	a person's tendency to be anxious over time	a.	state
__12.	anxiety experienced at a given moment in time	b.	trait

II. PHOBIC DISORDERS (Phobic Neurosis)

Phobia is defined as an irrational fear of an object or a situation which leads to persistent avoidance of that object or situation. Furthermore, for such a fear to be diagnosed as a phobia the avoidance behavior must interfere with the person's ability to function or must cause the individual significant distress. A person may go through life in a metropolitan area in a reasonably functional way even though he is deathly afraid of zebras.

Psychoanalytic theory contends that the object of the fear is a symbolic and unconscious one. According to this view, the conflict surrounding an unconscious object is displaced onto a real object about which it is "safe" to express a fear. In this way a person, on an unconscious level, may be afraid of giving in to an impulse to be very exhibitionistic, and the phobic reaction may be in the form of fear of appearing in front of an audience, or a fear of the theater itself, or a fear of crowded places.

Learning theory, on the other hand, suggests that phobic reactions are the result of a very aversive stimulus being paired with the feared object. The classical example of this was the case of Watson and Rayner (1920), who conditioned Albert, a child of nearly one year of age, to be afraid of furry objects by pairing a very loud noise with the child's approach to a white rat. While this was an experimentally induced phobia (one which no ethics committee would approve today), learning theorists maintain that phobias develop in a similar manner, with the pairing of the aversive stimulus and the feared object occurring more or less accidentally.

At any rate, the DSM-III provides four categories of Phobic Disorders: 1) Agoraphobia with Panic Attacks, 2) Agoraphobia without Panic Attacks, 3) Social Phobia, and 4) Simple Phobia.

A. AGORAPHOBIA WITH PANIC ATTACKS (DSM-III 300.21) AND AGORA-
    PHOBIA WITHOUT PANIC ATTACKS (DSM-III 300.2)

The word Agoraphobia is taken from the Greek, meaning a fear of the market place (or agora), with the implication of any public place. In psychiatry, it refers to a fear of leaving the house, of being left alone, or going out or being in any unfamiliar place alone. There are varying degrees of disability within this disorder including, in its extreme form, literally being unable to leave the home.

Just as with all Phobic Disorders, Agoraphobia has anxiety as an important component, and, in fact, Marks (1978) refers to it as a "phobic anxiety state" (p. 77). The anxiety is most prominent when the individual is confronted with leaving the familiar setting of the home, particularly if the excursion must be made alone. Even in the home the individual may experience anxiety if left alone. The fear, then, is also related to the notion that help may be needed but inaccessible if the individual is either alone or outside the familiar setting.

Onset of Agoraphobia is usually in late adolescence or young adulthood (18 to 35 years of age), and the incidence is more prevalent among women (2/3).

ANSWERS, Section I. _____

1.	d	7.	T
2.	T	8.	a
3.	F	9.	b
4.	T	10.	a
5.	T	11.	b
6.	F	12.	a

The disorder is unusual in children, although there may well be a history in the adolescent agoraphobic of some type of separation anxiety in childhood, e.g., School Phobia.

There is a wide variation in both the disability and the duration of Agoraphobia. The onset may be sudden or very insidious, developing over a period of years. According to Marks (1978), some people develop the symptoms of Agoraphobia and then, without specific treatment, the symptoms disappear over a period of weeks or months. Others are able to hide their symptoms for long periods of time in spite of the accompanying anxiety.

The DSM-III differentiates between two types of Agoraphobia, one with panic attacks and the other without. Since a history of panic attacks is the usual case, the latter diagnosis is not often used except when one is not able to elicit such a history. (For a summary of the specific features of panic attacks see p. 460).

Agoraphobia is diagnosed when an individual develops an irrational fear of leaving the familiar setting of the home and subsequently resists or avoids leaving the house. Recurrent episodes of panic almost always precede the phobic symptoms and lead to feelings of anticipatory anxiety, helplessness, and impending doom. The individual then avoids situations that would leave him alone or without access to help. He tenaciously avoids being alone under any circumstances, even in the home, and is typically reluctant to be in closed or open spaces, crowds, buses, planes, cars, trains, churches, stores, and the like. The individual may be so dominated by his fears that he becomes incapacitated and housebound.

What is gained by this elaborate psychological maneuvering is relief from anxiety. Displacement binds the anxiety associated with the patient's conflict and keeps the conflict out of awareness. This is known as primary gain. Not only displacement, but any mental mechanism can accomplish primary gain, or relief of anxiety.

Secondary gain occurs as a result of being sick. What is gained may range from extra care and attention, to "leave of absence" from work and responsibilities, to monetary compensation and other such "gains." The gain may even be enough to cause some patients (unconsciously) to remain "sick." This can be seen in both physical and psychiatric illnesses.

Diagnostic criteria for Agoraphobia
(DSM-III 300.2x)

A. The individual has marked fear of and thus avoids being alone
    or in public places from which escape might be difficult or
    help not available in case of sudden incapacitation, e.g.,
    crowds, tunnels, bridges, public transportation.

B. There is increasing constriction of normal activities until
    the fears or avoidance behaviors dominate the individual's
    life.

C. Not due to a major depressive episode, Obsessive Compulsive
    Disorder, Paranoid Personality Disorder, or Schizophrenia.

Agoraphobia must also be differentiated from other disorders or clinical
states that have paranoid features which in turn can lead to isolation,
withdrawal, incapacitation, and refusal to leave the setting of the home.

****

GO TO VIDEOTAPE

****

B. SOCIAL PHOBIA (DSM-III 300.23)

It is quite common for any person to feel mildly anxious when entering a
novel social situation, such as a party or a dance, especially if the other
people present are not close friends of that person. In fact, any new
situation normally will generate a certain amount of anxiety in most of us.
In other words, an unfamiliar situation poses at least a mild threat to a
person since he does not know what to expect. You will recall, for
example, that your first test in anatomy or biochemistry produced a
certain amount of anxiety.

In the case of Social Phobia, the individual seems to focus on the fear that
people are watching him (not in a paranoid sense) and will see that his
hand shakes, that he blushes, that he will not be able to eat because his
throat will constrict. As Marks (1978) says, the fear is of the people
themselves and of what they will think of him. This is in contrast to the
agoraphobic who fears what the crowd itself might do to him. These
anonymous people may somehow suffocate or crush the individual or may
keep him from reaching help if he suddenly becomes ill.

The predominant feature of the Social Phobia, then, is a fear of any
social situation which leaves the individual open to possible criticism and
embarrassment. When the possibility of being faced with such a situation
exists then two things typically occur. First, the individual experiences
what is called anticipatory anxiety, i.e., the person begins to feel anxious about not only the feared situation, but about the anxiety he knows is

coming. He is anxious about anxiety. Second, he typically begins using avoidance behavior. Somehow he must avoid being thrust into the social situation he fears. After all, if one does not eat in public no one can see--and be critical of--the manifestations of anxiety, like trembling hands or profuse sweating.

As with all phobias, there is a wide range of disability associated with Social Phobias. While a Social Phobia is always quite restricting, it may not always be significantly disabling for the individual. In people whose livelihood depends on interacting with others (entertaining clients, speaking in public, etc.) the development of a Social Phobia obviously can be severely disabling.

Another dimension of the Social Phobia is related to how generalized the disorder is. Some people may be unable to eat in a crowded restaurant, but may do very well at home. Others, however, may be so disabled that they must always eat alone even though they have spouses and children. The disability may become so generalized that the individual finds himself unable to be looked at by others, unable to talk with others, or even unable to have intercourse with the spouse.

The age at onset for the Social Phobia is usually the teen years through young adulthood. This type of phobia commonly develops insidiously over a period of some months. In some instances, however, a specific event may be identified as the source of the phobic reaction. For example, a person who has a particularly embarrassing thing happen to him in a social situation may immediately develop a Social Phobia.

Social Phobia must not be confused with other disorders that have social withdrawal and generalized anxiety as part of their clinical picture. It is to be differentiated from Obsessive Compulsive Disorder, Major Depressive Disorder, Schizophrenia, Paranoid State, Avoidant Personality Disorder, Simple Phobia, and Agoraphobia.

Diagnostic criteria for Social Phobia

A. A persistent irrational fear of, and compelling desire to avoid, a situation in which the individual is exposed to possible scrutiny by others and fears that he or she may act in a way that will be humiliating or embarrassing.

B. Significant distress because of the disturbance, and recognition by the individual that his or her fear is excessive or unreasonable.

C. Not due to another mental disorder, such as Major Depression or Avoidant Personality Disorder.

C. SIMPLE PHOBIA (DSM-III 300.29)

Simple Phobia is probably the Phobic Disorder most familiar in the general population. It refers to fear and avoidance of specific situations and objects not included in Agoraphobia and Social Phobia. Therefore, an individual who develops an irrational fear and avoidance of an object or situation other than that of leaving the home and of social situations is said to have a Simple Phobia.

The fears involved in Simple Phobia are much more discreet and circumscribed than in Agoraphobia, in which case the fear is more generalized. Fear of thunderstorms, elevators, and heights is common. Fear of animals, especially reptiles, insects, and rodents is even more common.

It is important to bear in mind that many of these simple fears are realistic to some degree. Most individuals would normally avoid snakes, thunderstorms, and dangerous heights. These fears become disordered when the reaction or avoidance behavior secondary to the phobic stimulus exceeds normal proportions and interferes with normal functioning.

While spontaneous panic attacks without a specific stimulus do not occur in Simple Phobia, a person may experience overwhelming anxiety and symptoms of panic if suddenly exposed to the feared object or situation. Some individuals have been surprised to find that they have become nonphobic after incidental exposure to the dreaded stimulus and apparent elimination of the anticipatory anxiety associated with it.

Obviously, Simple Phobias may lead to impaired functioning from a very mild to severe degree. It is quite easy to avoid poisonous snakes, especially if one lives in a city. On the other hand, a business executive with fear of elevators may be incapacitated if his business is in New York City's mid-Manhattan.

Diagnostic criteria for Simple Phobia

A. A persistent, irrational fear of, and compelling desire to avoid, an object or a situation other than being alone, or in public places away from home (Agoraphobia), or of humiliation or embarrassment in certain social situations (Social Phobia). Phobic objects are often animals, and phobic situations frequently involve heights or closed spaces.

B. Significant distress from the disturbance and recognition by the individual that his or her fear is excessive or unreasonable.

C. Not due to another mental disorder, such as Schizophrenia or Obsessive Compulsive Disorder.

QUIZ, Section II.

Circle the correct answer(s). One or more than one answer may be correct.

1. Which of the following is not true regarding Phobic Disorders?

    a. Persistent avoidance behavior of a feared object or situation must be present in an individual in order to diagnose a Phobic Disorder.
    b. The fear must be an irrational one in order to diagnose a Phobic Disorder.
    c. Learning theory contends that a phobia originates when an aversive stimulus is paired, usually accidentally, with the object which becomes the feared one.
    d. A person may consciously express a fear of one object in order to avoid revealing the real or "unsafe" object he fears.

2. Which of the following is (are) true regarding Agoraphobia?

    a. The onset of the disorder is usually in young adulthood.
    b. The onset is usually quite sudden.
    c. Anxiety may or may not be a component of the disorder.
    d. Without any treatment the symptom may disappear in a few weeks or months.
    e. Usually the history reveals the presence of panic attacks.

3. Agoraphobia must be differentiated from

    a. Major Depressive Disorders.
    b. Schizophrenia.
    c. Somatoform Disorders.
    d. various paranoid states.

4. When faced with a social situation a person suffering from a Social Phobia typically will experience

    a. trait anxiety.
    b. anticipatory anxiety.
    c. avoidance behavior.
    d. depressed behavior.

5. Which of the following statements is (are) true regarding Social Phobias?

    a. Onset is usually in teen or young adult years.
    b. In most instances the onset is acute and is associated with a specific embarrassing situation.
    c. Disability from the disorder may vary from very mild to severe.
    d. Social withdrawal usually is symptomatic of a Social Phobia.
    e. A predominant feature is a fear of crowds.

Match the following symptoms with the corresponding disorders.

___6.　　a person becomes anxious about and　　　a.　Agoraphobia
　　　　　avoids eating in public　　　　　　　　b.　Social Phobia
___7.　　a person becomes anxious about and　　　c.　Simple Phobia
　　　　　avoids leaving home
___8.　　a person becomes anxious about and
　　　　　avoids flying in airplanes

III.　ANXIETY STATES (Anxiety Neuroses)

The disorders in this group are, like the Phobic Disorders, characterized by anxiety. Unlike the Phobic Disorders, however, there may be no specific object, of which the patient is aware, that triggers the anxiety (i.e., the source is internal); or, if the source is external the threat posed is out of proportion to the real danger. As Lader (1972) writes, ". . . there is either no discernible danger or the danger is by common sense standards disproportionate to the emotion produced (p. 484)."

A.　PANIC DISORDER (DSM-III 300.01)

Just as with anxiety in general, panic may be judged to be normal or abnormal, depending on the stimulus or source of threat and upon the individual's reaction to that threat. Panic in the midst of a natural disaster, like an earthquake, is understandable, expected, and considered a normal response. The same type of response, when there is no apparent stimulus for it, is confounding and usually considered abnormal. It is this latter type of panic response to which the term Panic Disorder is applied.

Panic refers to sudden, overwhelming anxiety. It may be associated with an object, a thought, a person, a situation, or with no discernible stimulus at all. The most prominent feature of the Panic Disorder is recurrent attacks of panic. Such attacks are defined by the following features:

(1) Sudden onset of anxiety
(2) The psychological feeling of severe apprehension, helplessness, and impending doom
(3) Physiological responses associated with autonomic nervous system arousal
(4) Cessation of symptoms usually after a brief period of time (although the attack may last for hours)

The individual who suffers from a Panic Disorder experiences the physiological responses associated with acute stimulation of the autonomic nervous system and with increases in production of epinephrine and norepinephrine. Klein, Zitrin, and Woerner (1978) indicate that the most frequently described symptoms of autonomic nervous system arousal seen in panic attacks are:

(1) Dyspnea
(2) Palpitations
(3) Chest pains or discomfort
(4) Choking or smothering sensation
(5) Dizziness
(6) Paresthesias

Recurrent panic attacks, then, are an important feature of Panic Disorder. In addition, the patient with this disorder may also develop what is called free-floating anxiety which occurs between episodes of panic.

Free-floating anxiety refers to a general sense of anxiety which is not attached to a specific object or situation. The characteristics of free-floating anxiety are: 1) apprehensive expectation, 2) vigilance and scanning, 3) motor tension, and 4) autonomic hyperactivity (Klein, Zitrin, & Woerner, 1978). These will be explained in more detail in a later section of this chapter on Generalized Anxiety Disorder. For the present time, remember that the more severe the Panic Disorder becomes the more likely the patient will suffer from a general kind of anxiety between the episodes of panic.

The notion is that when the individual suffers panic attacks, it is not uncommon for him to become anxious about the possibility of experiencing another of these attacks which are unexpected and unpredictable. The psychological experience associated with panic attacks can be so intensely terrifying that the person may become disorganized, disoriented, and/or depersonalized. These attacks may be described as anxiety in its most extreme form. They usually occur when the individual feels that access to help is too restricted. This may lead to avoidance of such situations to the point that the patient resists leaving his home and develops Agoraphobia (with panic attacks).

Panic Disorder most often begins in adolescence or young adulthood. It is relatively common to find a history of Separation Anxiety (see p. 717) in childhood. This does not mean that all children who suffer from Separation Anxiety Disorders will later develop Panic Disorders, but the presence of the former may well be a predisposing factor for the latter.

The signs and symptoms of Panic Disorder may be present in such mental disorders as Schizophrenia, Major Depressive Disorder, or Somatization Disorder. If other mental disorders can be diagnosed, this will rule out the diagnosis of Panic Disorder. Certain physical disorders may produce symptoms similar to those of Panic Disorder. Some of these disorders are withdrawal from sedatives, hypoglycemia, pheochromocytoma, and hyper-thyroidism.

Diagnostic criteria for Panic Disorder

A.   At least three panic attacks within a three-week period in circumstances other than during marked physical exertion or in a life-threatening situation. The attacks are not precipitated only by exposure to a circumscribed phobic stimulus.

B. Panic attacks are manifested by discrete periods of apprehension or fear, and at least four of the following symptoms appear during each attack:

   (1) Dyspnea
   (2) Palpitations
   (3) Chest pain or discomfort
   (4) Choking or smothering sensations
   (5) Dizziness, vertigo or unsteady feelings
   (6) Feelings of unreality
   (7) Paresthesias (tingling in hands or feet)
   (8) Hot and cold flashes
   (9) Sweating
 (10) Faintness
 (11) Trembling or shaking
 (12) Fear of dying, going crazy, or doing something uncontrolled during an attack

C. Not due to a physical disorder or another mental disorder, such as Major Depression, Somatization Disorder, or Schizophrenia.

D. This disorder is not associated with Agoraphobia.

B. GENERALIZED ANXIETY DISORDER (DSM-III 300.02)

Remember that earlier in this chapter the concept of <u>state</u> versus <u>trait</u> anxiety was discussed. In a sense the Generalized Anxiety Disorder is similar to a high level of trait anxiety in that it represents an ongoing, relatively high level of arousal. This is different from anxiety seen in such things as Phobic or Panic Disorders in which the anxiety rapidly increases to very high levels. In the Generalized Anxiety Disorder, there is some day-to-day variation in anxiety levels, but over time the levels remain high. Put another way, the individual remains almost constantly aware that he is anxious, although unaware of the source or stimulus for his persistent anxiety. Put yet another way, the anxiety seen in this disorder is analogous to <u>free-floating</u> anxiety which was briefly described in the section on Panic Disorder.

The persistent type of anxiety seen in the Generalized Anxiety Disorder must have been present for at least six (6) months in order to make this diagnosis. If it has been present for less than six months, the diagnosis of Atypical Anxiety Disorder (DSM-III 300.00) is used. Furthermore, if the onset of the persistent anxiety is associated with some psychosocial stressor (birth of a child, divorce, illness, etc.) then the diagnosis of Adjustment Disorder with Anxious Mood is used (DSM-III 309.24). The assumption is that in the last diagnosis the anxiety will cease when the source of the anxiety ceases and therefore the prognosis is less serious.

Most prominent in the Generalized Anxiety Disorder is the presence of chronic autonomic hyperactivity. Klein, Zitrin, and Woerner (1978) have delineated four categories of features seen in general anxiety. These are used in DSM-III as a major method of assessing anxiety of the generalized or the free-floating type. These four are:

(1) Apprehensive expectation: The patient behaves in a guarded and cautious manner. He may seem distracted, irritable, unable to concentrate, impatient, and defensive. Sleep is often disturbed--(DFA), middle of the night awakening (MNA), early morning awakening (EMA), restless unsatisfying sleep, and fatigue on awakening have been described.

(2) Vigilance and scanning: This is seen in the frightened and anxious person who constantly fears that some fate will befall him or someone close to him. He worries, ruminates, watches, checks, and anticipates that he or a loved one will die or be stricken with something bad.

(3) Motor tension: This is both felt by the individual as well as observed by others. People report feeling jumpy, jittery, shaky, trembling, tense, keyed up, tight, unable to relax, easily fatigued, achiness. One may observe muscular twitching, jumpiness, restlessness, frowning, strained face, trembling, shaking, sighing respirations, and easy startle, all of which are secondary to increased striated muscle tone.

All of the above must not be confused with agitation in which there is manifest gross motor activity.

(4) Autonomic hyperactivity: This results from stimulation of the sympathetic and parasympathetic nervous systems.

In addition to the symptoms described above, people often report dry mouth, cold clammy hands, lump in the throat, diarrhea, nausea, and frequent urination.

Clearly, anxiety and panic are unpleasant, distressing, and debilitating.

The Diagnostic criteria for Generalized Anxiety Disorder are:

A. Generalized, persistent anxiety is manifested by symptoms from three of the following four categories:

(1) Motor tension: Shakiness, jitteriness, jumpiness, trembling, tension, muscle aches, fatigability, inability to relax, eyelid twitch, furrowed brow, strained face, fidgeting, restlessness, easy startle

(2) Autonomic hyperactivity: Sweating, heart pounding or racing, cold clammy hands, dry mouth, dizziness, light-headedness, paresthesias (tingling in hands or feet), upset stomach, hot or cold spells, frequent urination, diarrhea, discomfort in the pit of the stomach, lump in the throat, flushing, pallor, high resting pulse and respiration rate

(3) Apprehensive expectation: Anxiety, worry, fear, rumination, and anticipation of misfortune to self or others

(4) Vigilance and scanning: Hyperattentiveness resulting in distractibility, difficulty in concentrating, insomnia, feeling "on edge," irritability, impatience

B. The anxious mood has been continuous for at least one month.

C. Not due to another mental disorder, such as a Depressive Disorder or Schizophrenia.

D. At least 18 years of age.

It is important to be fully aware that a number of physical disorders can present with signs and symptoms that mimic or are very similar to psychiatric disorders. In the case of the Generalized Anxiety Disorder, the chronic autonomic hyperactivity and motor tension may cause symptoms which require that you consider a number of physical conditions, including:

(1) Normal fear
(2) Intoxication - amphetamines, alcohol, aspirin, caffeine, cannabis, cocaine, PCP
(3) Withdrawal - barbiturates, hypnotics, sedatives
(4) Medication side-effects
(5) Allergies
(6) Coronary artery disease - angina pectoris, MI
(7) Paroxysmal rapid arrhythmias
(8) Hypertension, hypotension

(9) Bronchial asthma, COPD, hyperventilation, pulmonary embolism
(10) Peptic ulcer, esophagitis, irritable colon
(11) Hyperthyroidism
(12) Pheochromocytoma
(13) Hypoglycemia
(14) Endocrine variations associated with puberty, menstrual cycle, menopause
(15) Brain tumor
(16) Seizures (psychomotor)
(17) Benign familial tremor
(18) Mitral valve prolapse

****

GO TO VIDEOTAPE

****

C.   OBSESSIVE COMPULSIVE DISORDER (DSM-III 300.30) (Obsessive Compulsive Neurosis)

To adequately understand Obsessive Compulsive Disorders it is very important that you first understand the concept of ego-alien or ego-dystonic impulses. If you do not understand this concept you should review Chapter 2, Psychodynamic Considerations and Defense Mechanisms.

An obsession is a recurrent, persistent, ego-alien idea, or impulse. The thought, idea, or impulse enters the conscious mind uninvited, so to speak, and the patient faces the virtually impossible task of removing it from conscious awareness. In an effort to deal with the obsession a compulsion often develops.

A compulsion is a recurrent, persistent, ego-alien urge or impulse to behave in what is recognized by the patient as well as others as an unreasonable way. It is one way of dealing with the obsession. The classic example in literature of the compulsive ritual is Lady Macbeth's handwashing compulsion. However, unlike the case of Lady Macbeth, the compulsive behavior usually is not so clearly connected with the impetus of the behavior. (As you may recall, Lady Macbeth participated in the murder of Duncan and persisted in trying to wash away the nonexistent blood from her hands.) Compulsive behaviors or rituals most often take the form of a more obscure kind of symbolism. Checking and rechecking doors and windows, counting objects repeatedly, touching things in a ritualized kind of order or sequence, repetitive handwashing, are all fairly common compulsions. It is not unusual to see someone suffering from this disorder use a whole cake of soap in a day.

While one diagnostic criterion of this disorder is that it produces significant distress in the individual, it is important to recognize that the neat, orderly qualities which are a part of the obsessive compulsive personality are also highly regarded traits in our society. Being neat, orderly, clean, and paying attention to details are generally considered virtues and are often rewarded. Consider for example, accountants, housekeepers, dentists, physicians, secretaries, bankers, and engineers. You could add a great many others to this list, of course. When the generally desirable traits become ritualized and also begin to cause a person distress, however, a psychiatric disorder ensues.

The patient recognizes the irrational nature of his behavior and very often will attempt to resist performing the ritual. With the resistance to performing the compulsive behavior comes heightened tension and anxiety which can only be diminished by performing the irrational ritual. Repeated failures to resist the behavior often lead to giving up the resistance. It is thought that anxiety also is heightened by a fear on the part of the individual that he will give in to the obsessional thought which is most often of an aggressive or dangerous sexual nature (Weintraub, 1974). As far as the patient is concerned the source of the anxiety is not conscious, but rather is of a nonspecific nature. He is aware, however, that when he resists the compulsion, anxiety increases.

Psychodynamically, attempts to repress ego-alien impulses (thoughts or behaviors) have failed and these impulses begin to intrude into the conscious mind. Other defenses are then called into play to control anxiety and restore homeostasis. The most common ones used by persons with Obsessive Compulsive Disorders are:

(1) Isolation of affect: Conflict over control and associated aggressive and hostile feelings lead to the need to control one's affect to the point that underlying feelings remain hidden or isolated. This leads to aloofness.

(2) Undoing: The individual with Obsessive Compulsive Disorder magically thinks that he can prevent or undo or counteract his unwanted thought or urge by performing a certain act. Undoing leads to rituals.

For example, a patient reported that whenever he turned off a light he obsessively thought, "My father will die," and he was always compelled to return to the light switch, touch it, and say, "I take back that thought." It is as if the thought itself effects the action, with no intervening physical activity.

(3) Reaction formation: Efforts to control aggressive, hostile, or unacceptable feelings may lead to development of behaviors and attitudes which are exactly opposite to the underlying impulses. Overprotectiveness may "cover" a mother's rejecting feelings toward her infant. This leads to overdoing.

(4) Displacement: Unable to tolerate the anxiety associated with murderous feelings towards one's parent, an individual with Obsessive Compulsive Disorder may transfer these feelings to passers-by on the street. A patient reports having to check with the transport

authority periodically to ascertain whether anyone he brushed by was thrown into the path of a subway train and killed.

(5) Symbolization: The compulsive acts associated with Obsessive Compulsive Disorder represent and symbolically replace the real, underlying, unwanted, or unacceptable thoughts and impulses.

****

GO TO VIDEOTAPE

****

D.   POST-TRAUMATIC STRESS DISORDER (DSM-III 308.30) or (DSM-III 309.81)

If you do not have firsthand experience with severe trauma, and most people do not, you have certainly read about and seen television accounts of natural disasters, such as hurricanes, floods, and earthquakes, and of "man-made" disasters, such as fires, airplane crashes, wars, and the like. This category applies to many of the survivors of such traumatic events. The individual does not in fact have to be involved in a mass disaster, one which becomes a front page headline. The automobile wreck in which one person is killed or maimed and another person survives may produce a Post-Traumatic Stress Disorder in the survivor. A major part of the dynamics of such a disorder usually is the fact that one person survived while another, or others, did not.

The traumatic event associated with the disorder is not necessarily one which is associated with death of others, although this is frequently the case. The threat of death, however, often seems to be a component of the trauma, as, for example, in cases of torture. Rape is another such event which frequently produces this syndrome in the victim. In this instance, most victims are more traumatized by the threat of death or bodily harm than from the sexual act.* In any case, the stressor which is associated with the traumatic event may occur to an individual or to a group of persons.

One of the first major disasters to be studied and reported in the psychiatric literature was the Coconut Grove Fire, a nightclub fire in which a great many people were killed. Lindemann (1944) wrote about grief reaction of survivors of this fire, and his work became the basis for modern crisis intervention work. One basic principle elaborated on was that the affective response to loss is typically, normally, one of grief.

More recently, a great deal has been written about the post-disaster effect -- psychic trauma -- on the survivors of the Buffalo Creek flood in

---

*Clinical interviews by Villeponteaux with approximately 75 rape victims consistently found that the major fear during a rape was related to the life threatening aspect of the event.

West Virginia. Lifton and Olson (1976) concluded that all persons exposed to the flood at Buffalo Creek experienced some or all of the following symptoms of the survivor:

(1) Death Imprint (and its effect on death anxiety). A number of persons were observed as long as 2½ years later to exhibit symptoms of fear and anxiety associated with such things as rain, thunder, crowds of people.

(2) Death Guilt. The frequent, painful self-recrimination for having survived while others died was present 2½ years after the disaster. At the same time there is also a feeling among survivors of being thankful that they did survive, which enhances the guilt.

(3) Psychic Numbing. This is an apparent decrease in the affective ability of the survivor and looks like apathy, sadness, depression, withdrawal from social contact. This is thought to be a defensive process in which protection against the memories, the guilt, the grief, and the loss is sustained.

(4) Impaired Human Relationships. This takes the form, primarily, of a need for nurturance, a need to be cared for, on the one hand, and a distrust of others on the other. Close relationships often dissolve under a pall of distrust of the world as being counterfeit. Often associated with this is a smoldering anger directed at someone who was responsible for the disaster.

(5) Struggle for Significance. The survivors search for some meaning or significance, some explanation for the disaster in the sense of an internal resolution. It is only after such an internal conflict can be resolved that the survivor can go on with his life.

Frequently the individual re-experiences the traumatic event. This may be in the form of recalling the painful experience, having the experience intrude with dreams, or even in the form of a kind of "flashback" in which the individual seems actually to re-live the experience. In this latter case the individual may seem to be in a dissociative state as he or she re-lives the traumatic event.

Other symptoms commonly associated with this disorder are directly related to anxiety, like autonomic hyperarousal, and to phobias in which various stimuli to remembering the event are avoided. Frequently found are various symptoms of depression, particularly in the form of sleep disturbances. If the patient meets the criteria for Anxiety or Depressive Disorder the diagnosis should be made in addition to the Post-Traumatic Stress Disorder.

Furthermore, some individuals exhibit symptoms of Organic Mental Disorder, such as difficulty with concentration, memory failures, headache, and so forth. Whether or not the person suffered physical trauma which could account for the organicity, if the symptoms meet the criteria for Organic Mental Disorder, this should be an additional diagnosis.

A disorder of impulse control sometimes must be differentiated from Post-traumatic Stress Disorder, since sometimes patients in the latter category will explode aggressively, will suddenly leave town, change jobs, or change homes without planning or discussion.

DSM-III lists four diagnostic criteria for the
Post-Traumatic Stress Disorder:

A. Existence of a recognizable stressor that would evoke significant symptoms of distress in almost anyone.

B. Re-experiencing the trauma as evidenced by at least one of the following:

   (1) recurrent and intrusive recollections of the event
   (2) recurrent dreams of the event
   (3) sudden acting or feeling as if the traumatic event were reoccurring, because of an association with an environmental or ideational stimulus

C. Numbing of responsiveness to or reduced involvement with the external world, beginning some time after the trauma, as shown by at least one of the following:

   (1) markedly diminished interest in one or more significant activities
   (2) feelings of detachment or estrangement from others
   (3) constricted affect

D. At least two of the following symptoms that were not present before the trauma:

   (1) hyperalertness or exaggerated startle response
   (2) sleep disturbance
   (3) guilt about surviving when others have not, or about behavior required for survival
   (4) memory impairment or trouble concentrating
   (5) avoidance of activities that arouse recollection of the traumatic event
   (6) intensification of symptoms by exposure to events that symbolize or resemble the traumatic event

There are really three subtypes of this disorder: acute, chronic, and delayed. In the case of the acute type the symptoms began within six months of the event. In the chronic type the symptoms have persisted for more than six months, obviously making it possible for an acute form to become chronic. In the delayed type the symptoms did not appear until at least six months after the traumatic event.

Prognostically, the chronic and the delayed types are more persistent and more difficult to treat. When symptoms develop within six months the prognosis is much better for remission of the symptoms.

```
***************************************************************************

                            GO TO VIDEOTAPE

***************************************************************************
```

E.   ATYPICAL ANXIETY DISORDER (DSM-III 300.00)

This category is provided primarily for those individuals who do not meet all of the diagnostic criteria for one of the Anxiety Disorders but who still seem to be suffering from an anxiety. For example, a person who meets all of the criteria for a Generalized Anxiety Disorder except that the disability is of less than six months duration might fall into this category.

The category may also be used for a much more difficult diagnostic problem, that of the person who presents with a morbid fear of disease, usually cancer. Although the terms, "cancer phobia" or "disease phobia" are often used, these people usually do not represent a true phobic reaction since their anxiety continues even when they are able to avoid the stimuli, the reminders of the disease. Remember that the phobic person is generally comfortable when he is not confronted with the stimulus to his phobic reaction.

There is a similarity between "disease phobia" and an obsessive compulsive reaction. The difference, as DSM-III points out, is that the thinking about the feared illness has more the quality of rumination than of obsessional thinking.

Perhaps the most difficult diagnostic differentiation here is between "illness phobia" and the Atypical Somatoform Disorder (which you will learn about in Chapter 10). The differentiation is not a really clear-cut one and is based on the predominance of physical symptoms and complaints in the Somatoform Disorder, which do not fit with the physical findings. Put another way, the patient suffering from the Somatoform Disorder reports physical symptoms, whereas the patient with an "illness phobia" focuses more on the fear that he might have a disease, even though actual symptoms of one kind or another are not present.

QUIZ, Section III.

Circle the correct answer(s). <u>One</u> or <u>more</u> <u>than</u> <u>one</u> answer may be correct.

1.   Panic attacks have which of the following features?

     a.   subjective feelings of apprehension
     b.   stimulation of autonomic nervous system responses
     c.   insidious increase in anxiety leading to panic
     d.   relatively brief (minutes to hours) duration of the panic

2. The patient is a 23-year-old female who is seen by you in the emergency room. She has been brought to the E.R. by her boyfriend who was with her in a movie theater when she suddenly became quite upset. She was breathing rapidly, felt lightheaded, and reported feeling a tightness in her chest. She has never experienced anything like this in the past and has no idea of what caused her to suddenly become so frightened and apprehensive. It has been two hours since the event in the theater and she is now only mildly anxious. You would be justified in

    a. doing a complete mental status examination.
    b. diagnosing a Panic Disorder.
    c. ordering blood and urine work on the patient.
    d. referring her for psychiatric consultation immediately.

3. Regarding Panic Disorders, which of the following is (are) true?

    a. Onset is usually in teen or early adult years.
    b. A history of separation anxiety is not uncommon.
    c. The presence of free-floating anxiety between attacks rules out the diagnosis of Panic Disorder.
    d. A variety of endocrine disorders may produce symptoms of Panic Disorder.

4. A person with an Obsessive Compulsive Disorder

    a. decreases anxiety by performance of the compulsive behavior.
    b. increases anxiety when he resists performing the compulsive behavior.
    c. is conscious of the source of his anxiety.
    d. recognizes the irrational nature of his behavior.

5. An individual with a Post-Traumatic Stress Disorder may experience which of the following?

    a. difficulty with concentration and memory
    b. rapid, pounding heartbeat
    c. increase in number and intensity of close relationships
    d. sleep disturbances
    e. flashback of the traumatic event

6. The patient is a 48-year-old male. He tells you that for the past four months he has been having difficulty sleeping at night, has been having trouble remembering things, at times feels like his heart is going to pound through his chest, has lost his appetite, has chronic headaches, and often feels like he wants to be alone. These symptoms have gotten worse in the last six weeks. Upon further discussion he reveals that about seven months ago he and a fellow worker at the local

shipyard were involved in an accident in which the other man was killed. The patient is now at the point where he feels he cannot continue to work.

On the basis of this information you could rule out

a. Somatoform Disorder.
b. Chronic Post-Traumatic Stress Disorder.
c. Organic Mental Disorder.
d. Depressive Disorder.

Match the following symptoms with the corresponding categories of anxiety.

___7.   patient behaves in a guarded   a. motor tension
        cautious manner   b. apprehensive
___8.   patient almost constantly looks   expectation
        around, worries   c. autonomic hyper-
___9.   patient frequently moves, jumps,   activity
        startles easily   d. vigilance and
__10.   patient has difficulty swallowing,   scanning
        feels cold, urinates frequently

Match the following descriptions with the corresponding lettered items. Lettered items may be used once or more than once.

___11. recurrent, persistent, ego-alien urge or   a. obsession
        impulse to act in a way that the patient   b. compulsion
        himself recognizes as unreasonable
___12. recurrent, persistent, ego-alien thoughts
___13. enters the conscious mind uninvited
___14. touching objects in a ritualized order

Match the following descriptions with the corresponding lettered items.

___15. need for nurturance by others along with   a. death imprint
        distrust of others   b. death guilt
___16. search for some meaning or explanation for c. psychic numbing
        the disaster   d. impaired human
___17. anxiety associated with stimuli associated   relationships
        with the disaster   e. struggle for
___18. decreased emotional lability in favor of   significance
        sadness or apathy
___19. self-recrimination and gratitude for one's
        own survival

TRUE or FALSE: Circle the correct letter.

Anxiety in a Generalized Anxiety Disorder is

T   F   20. similar to state anxiety.
T   F   21. similar to trait anxiety.

T   F   22. different from anxiety in Phobic and Panic Disorders in terms of onset.
T   F   23. similar to free-floating anxiety.
T   F   24. out of the awareness of the patient.

IV. TREATMENT OF ANXIETY DISORDERS

The question of which treatment approach is most efficacious for the various Anxiety Disorders is one which has not been clearly answered at this time. It is likely that combinations of therapies often are more effective than a single approach.

Since anxiety is the common thread running through these disorders, and to the patients this is usually the most distressing aspect of the disorders, there is a tendency for many physicians to write prescriptions for antianxiety drugs (anxiolytics). The most popular of these are the benzodiazepines, of course, and with good reason. You should remember, however, that anxiety may have a very useful purpose, and the chemical removal of anxiety at times may be contraindicated. Moreover, the long term use of anxiolytics, as you will learn in Chapter 16, may have serious consequences.

This is not to say that the benzodiazepines are never to be used with Anxiety Disorders, but only that they should be used primarily for the management of acute, anxiety-related symptoms. Put another way, these drugs are best used as an adjunct to other treatment modalities, not as the treatment of choice for the Anxiety Disorders.

[For a more thorough understanding of the uses of antianxiety medications see Chapter 16, Psychopharmacology.]

Behavioral Therapy may be quite useful in the treatment of Anxiety Disorders. For example, a patient may be taught progressive relaxation techniques to help deal with the anxiety. Progressive relaxation is a method of controlling muscle tension by having the patient go through a process of tensing and then relaxing muscle groups. The initial goal is to help the patient become aware of the difference between tensed and relaxed muscles since many are not conscious of the fact that muscles are tightly contracted. The theoretical - and logical - idea is that it is impossible to be simultaneously tense and relaxed. Remember that a frequent concomitant of anxiety is the autonomic nervous system response of tightened muscles. Once the patient has learned to relax, even in the face of the anxiety-producing stimulus, he is able to assume more control over his response to anxiety.

[For further elaboration of behavioral techniques, see Chapter 18, Behavioral Treatment.]

Many argue that the mere control of symptoms of anxiety is not sufficient to adequately deal with the disorder; that uncovering or insight-oriented

ANSWERS, Section III._____

1.	a,b,d	9.	a	17.	a
2.	a,c	10.	c	18.	c
3.	a,b,d	11.	b	19.	b
4.	a,b,d	12.	a	20.	F
5.	a,b,d,e	13.	a	21.	T
6.	b	14.	b	22.	T
7.	b	15.	d	23.	T
8.	d	16.	e	24.	F

techniques are often necessary, i.e., one should use a therapeutic approach based on psychodynamic theory. Anxiety, in short, is rooted in conflict and exacerbated by some threat to the integrity of the individual's ego.

[See Chapter 17, Psychosocial Treatments, for further elaboration of the psychodynamic approach.]

The judgment about which approach to take with a specific patient is based on a variety of factors, not the least of which is a carefully administered mental status examination, history, physical examination, and a clear diagnosis. Situational anxiety <u>may</u> best be treated with anxiolytics. Chronic anxiety may best be treated by some combination of techniques. Anxiety as a feature of a psychotic process may require hospitalization and ongoing management by a psychiatrist. By the same token, Obsessive Compulsive Disorders and phobias may require a variety of techniques, depending on severity of the disorder and the extent to which the patient is disabled by the disorder.

POST-TEST

Circle the correct answer(s). One or more than one answer may be correct.

1. Agoraphobia

    a. has anxiety as a prominent feature.
    b. is more commonly seen in males.
    c. is often associated with recurrent panic attacks.
    d. is associated with a specific, circumscribed feared object.

2. Free-floating anxiety is characterized by signs and symptoms of

    a. apprehensive expectation.
    b. vigilance and scanning.
    c. motor tension.
    d. autonomic hyperactivity.

3. Anxiety results if the individual resists giving in to the symptoms which he has developed for relieving anxiety in

    a. Generalized Anxiety Disorders.
    b. Phobic Disorders.
    c. Panic Disorders.
    d. Obsessive Compulsive Disorders.

4. Anxiety

    a. plays an important, positive role in our lives.
    b. promotes action toward homeostasis.
    c. may be protective.
    d. is ego-syntonic.

5. Physiological responses expressed via the autonomic nervous system and associated with both fear and anxiety include

    a. dyspnea.
    b. chest pain.
    c. pounding heartbeat.
    d. excessive salivation.

6. People who experience anxiety include

    a. medical students.
    b. schizophrenics.
    c. infants and children.
    d. depressed patients.

7. A Vietnam combat veteran reports "flashbacks" of war experiences, depression, withdrawal, difficulty sleeping, guilt over his own survival, trouble concentrating, and inability to hold a job. He also becomes panicky if he hears firecrackers going off in his neighborhood. On the basis of this information alone the diagnosis is likely to be

   a. Panic Disorder.
   b. Phobic Disorder.
   c. Generalized Anxiety Disorder.
   d. Post-Traumatic Stress Disorder.

8. Phobic disorders include

   a. Simple Phobia.
   b. Social Phobia.
   c. Agoraphobia.
   d. Compulsive Phobia.

9. Anxiety is the most prominent feature of

   a. Phobic Disorders.
   b. Schizophrenia.
   c. Post-Traumatic Stress Disorders.
   d. Impulse Disorders.

10. Panic attacks have which of the following characteristics?

   a. sudden, overwhelming anxiety
   b. physiological responses such as dyspnea
   c. feelings of apprehension, helplessness, impending doom
   d. brief duration of the symptoms

11. Characteristics of obsessions and compulsions are that they

   a. persistently intrude into one's consciousness.
   b. are ego-syntonic.
   c. are recognized by the patient as irrational.
   d. have a relatively easily identifiable source.

12. A young, single woman has a fear of thunderstorms. She adamantly refuses to leave her house whenever there is even the slightest chance of rain. Her mother "understands" and will literally sit with her daughter under these circumstances. This example illustrates

   a. primary gain.
   b. Simple Phobia.
   c. secondary gain.
   d. Social Phobia.

13. A number of organ systems may be affected by anxiety. These include

    a. cardiovascular system.
    b. genitourinary system.
    c. gastrointestinal system.
    d. musculoskeletal system.

14. Post-Traumatic Stress Disorders

    a. frequently involve "flashbacks."
    b. are usually time-limited.
    c. may be confused with Organic Mental Disorders.
    d. are always associated with the death of one or more persons.

15. A middle-aged man reports that whenever he opens a door he thinks, "Someone will die." He then unfailingly returns to the door, touches the doorknob, and says, "I take that back." This example involves

    a. obsession.
    b. compulsion.
    c. undoing.
    d. phobia.

Match the following with the proper symptoms.

____16. autonomic hyperactivity
____17. motor tension
____18. apprehensive expectation
____19. vigilance and scanning

a. restlessness, trembling, keyed up, fatigued, tense, muscle twitches, frowning, strained faces, easily startled

b. sweating, palpitations, clammy hands, dizziness, parathesias, dry mouth

c. anxious, frightened, scared feeling that something bad will happen to oneself or loved one, constant worrying and ruminating about this

d. difficulty sleeping, distractibility, irritability, cautious guarded behavior, impatience, on edge

PRE-TEST ANSWERS

1. a,b,c
2. a,b,c,d
3. a,b,c,d
4. a,b,c
5. a,c
6. a,b,c,d
7. a,b,c,d
8. a,c
9. a,c
10. a,b,c

11. a,b,c
12. a,b,c
13. d
14. a,c
15. b,d
16. b
17. c
18. d
19. a

POST-TEST ANSWERS

1. a,c
2. a,b,c,d
3. b,d
4. a,b,c
5. a,b,c
6. a,b,c,d
7. d
8. a,b,c
9. a,c
10. a,b,c,d

11. a,c
12. a,b,c
13. a,b,c,d
14. a,c
15. a,b,c
16. b
17. a
18. c
19. d

REFERENCES

Diagnostic and statistical manual of mental disorders (3rd Ed.). Washington: American Psychiatric Association, 1979.

Klein, D. F., Zitrin, C. M., & Woerner, M. Antidepressants, anxiety, panic and phobia. In M. A. Lipton, A. Dimascio, & K. F. Killam (Eds.), Psychopharmacology: A generation of progress. New York: Raven Press, 1978.

Lader, M. The nature of anxiety. British Journal of Psychiatry, 1972, 121, 481-491.

Lader, M. Current psychophysiological theories of anxiety. In M. A. Lipton, A. Dimascio, & K. F. Killam (Eds.), Psychopharmacology: A generation of progress. New York: Raven Press, 1978.

Lifton, R., & Olson, E. The human meaning of total disaster. Psychiatry, 1976, 39, 1-18.

Lindemann, E. The symptomatology and management of acute grief. American Journal of Psychiatry, 1944, 101, 141-148.

Marks, I. Living with fear. New York: McGraw-Hill, 1978.

Spielberger, C. D. Theory and research in anxiety. In C. D. Spielberger (Ed.), Anxiety and behavior. New York: Academic Press, 1966, p. 3-20.

Stein, M. R., Vidich, A. J., & White, D. M. (Eds.) Identity and anxiety. Glencoe: The Free Press, 1960.

Watson, J. B. & Rayner, R. Conditioned emotional reactions. Journal of Experimental Psychology, 1920, 3, 1-14.

Weintraub, W. Obsessive-compulsive and paranoid personalities. In J. Lion (Ed.), Personality disorders: Diagnosis and management. Baltimore: The Williams and Wilkins Co., 1974.

CHAPTER 10
Somatoform and Dissociative Disorders
Donald E. Manning, M.D.

CHAPTER OUTLINE

LEARNING OBJECTIVES

After completing this chapter, you will be able to:

1. Recognize the elements of the psychoanalytic theory of the neuroses as related to the etiology of the Somatoform and Dissociative Disorders.

2. Recognize the definitions of the following mental mechanisms:

    Conversion
    Displacement
    Symbolization
    Somatization
    Dissociation

3. Recall descriptions and categorizations of the following disorders:

    Somatization Disorder
    Conversion Disorder
    Psychogenic Pain Disorder
    Hypochondriasis
    Psychogenic Amnesia
    Psychogenic Fugue
    Multiple Personality
    Depersonalization Disorder

4. Recall treatment approaches for each of the disorders above.

5. Recall the kinds of Psychogenic Amnesia, including:

    localized
    selective
    generalized
    continuous

6. Recognize definitions of the following terms:

    "la belle indifference"
    Secondary Gain
    Primary Gain
    Pseudocyesis

PRE-TEST

For the following questions, circle the letter corresponding to the one correct answer.

1. Which of the following statements is not correct?

    a. Current stresses can trigger the release of previously repressed psychic material.
    b. Neurotic defenses aid in keeping conflicts in the unconscious.
    c. Anxiety is often associated with unconscious conflicts.
    d. Failure of repression can lead to the use of new, abnormal, or neurotic mental mechanisms.
    e. Hypochondriasis is often responsive to drug therapy.

2. All of the following may be the presenting symptom of a Conversion Disorder, except

    a. seizures.
    b. vomiting.
    c. unconscious episodes.
    d. sterility.

3. Psychogenic Pain Disorder is not associated with which of the following?

    a. psychogenic pain without physical findings
    b. pain temporally related to meaningful environmental stimuli
    c. associated with primary and secondary gain
    d. may become chronic
    e. should be treated with analgesics

For the following questions, one or more than one answer may be correct. Circle the correct answer(s).

4. Somatization Disorder

    a. is one of several Somatoform Disorders.
    b. is also known as Briquet's syndrome.
    c. has symptoms in many organ systems.
    d. uses the mental mechanism of somatization.

5. Briquet's syndrome is characterized by

    a. multiple-organ physical complaints.
    b. onset before age 30.
    c. frequent pseudoneurologic symptoms.
    d. use of the mental mechanisms of conversion.

6. Complications of the Somatization Disorder include

   a. addiction to amphetamines.
   b. abuse of prescribed drugs.
   c. sexual sterility.
   d. frequent surgical procedures.

7. In Conversion Disorder the patient

   a. uses conversion as a mental mechanism.
   b. may use displacement and symbolization as mental mechanisms.
   c. usually gives primary and secondary gains.
   d. frequently exhibits "la belle indifference."

8. Patients with Hypochondriasis

   a. are chronic complainers.
   b. are preoccupied with worries about the presence of undetected physical illness.
   c. have frequent physical symptoms.
   d. are preoccupied with bodily functions.

9. Dissociation

   a. is a mental mechanism that includes a loss of part of consciousness, behavior, or identity.
   b. aids repression.
   c. is a way of binding anxiety.
   d. is a mental representation of previous psychic conflicts.

10. Psychogenic Amnesia is

    a. sudden in onset and gradually clears.
    b. frequently disabling.
    c. the least common Dissociative Disorder.
    d. a dissociation of consciousness.

11. The Multiple Personality Disorder

    a. is characterized by two or more <u>partial</u> personalities.
    b. is characterized by sudden shifts between personalities.
    c. usually remits spontaneously.
    d. is characterized by personality shifts in response to suggestion.

12. Symptoms of Depersonalization Disorder include

    a. loss of sense of one's own reality.
    b. loss of sense of time.
    c. dizziness.
    d. gradual onset and remission.

Match each mental mechanism with the appropriate description.

13. shifting affect from
    conflict to physical symptom
14. changing psychic conflict
    into physical symptom
15. "special" meaning of
    physical symptom
16. focusing on physical
    symptoms or concerns

a. somatization

b. conversion

c. displacement

d. symbolization

Match the following disorders with the corresponding terms.

___17.   disorder of identity
___18.   disorder of consciousness
___19.   disorder of behavior
___20.   disorder of sense of reality

a. fugue
b. amnesia
c. depersonalization
d. multiple personality

Match the following disorders with the corresponding therapy.

___21.   Somatization Disorder
___22.   Conversion Disorder
___23.   Psychogenic Amnesia
___24.   Psychogenic Pain Disorder

a. surgery
b. medication
c. psychotherapy

Match the following types of amnesia with their corresponding definitions.

___25.   localized amnesia
___26.   generalized amnesia
___27.   continuous amnesia
___28.   selective amnesia

a. total memory loss for entire life
b. total memory loss for events for a fixed time interval
c. total memory loss from event to present
d. partial memory loss for a fixed time period

I. SOMATOFORM DISORDERS

The Somatoform Disorders were once called hysterical neuroses, conversion type. They are now divided into four distinct entities:

    A. Somatization Disorder (Briquet's syndrome)
    B. Conversion Disorder (conversion hysteria)
    C. Psychogenic Pain Disorder
    D. Atypical Somatoform Disorder (Hypochondriasis)

According to the DSM-III, the hallmark of the Somatoform Disorders is the presence of or concern with physical symptoms suggesting a physical disorder for which there are no demonstrable organic findings to explain the symptoms. Thus, the symptoms result from psychological conflicts, not from physical disorder. To explain the etiology of these disorders, this text will utilize the psychoanalytic theory of the neuroses. According to this theory a current situation or life stress causes the mobilization (or making conscious) of an old conflict. The old conflict, a psychic trauma from early development, had been repressed utilizing any of several mental mechanisms. The new stress causes the failure of previously adequate repressive mechanisms, and the old conflict surfaces as anxiety. In order to cope with or "bind" this anxiety, new and abnormal (neurotic) mental mechanisms are called upon. These keep both the conflict and much of the anxiety in the unconscious. This was discussed in greater detail in the chapter on "Defense Mechanisms."

These new, neurotic, or abnormal mental mechanisms which arise differ with different syndromes. For example, if the psychic symptom is changed into a discrete physical symptom isolated to a specific function of the voluntary nervous system or special nervous sensory system, then the mental mechanism is called conversion. Conversion frequently has other mental mechanisms associated with it. Included among these are symbolization, in which the physical disorder symbolically represents the psychic conflict and displacement, in which the affect is displaced from the original conflict to the physical symptom. Somatization is another defense, wherein anxiety is bound by the focusing on multiple somatic complaints or concerns.

A.   SOMATIZATION DISORDER (DSM-III 300.81)

There are four Somatoform Disorders. The most common of these is the Somatization Disorder, which is also known as Briquet's syndrome. There are three essential elements to this disorder: 1) there must be the onset of vague, dramatic, or complicated medical history prior to age 30; 2) there must be significant symptoms in many organ systems; 3) the individual usually consults many physicians without defining any apparent physical illness.

According to the DSM-III, individuals with a Somatization Disorder must have many symptoms (14 in women, 12 in men) in the following six symptom groups:

1) he must believe he has been sickly most of his life
2) pseudoneurologic symptoms (paralysis, blindness, difficulty swallow-ing, loss of voice, blurred vision, muscle weakness, urinary problems, convulsions, deafness, diplopia, etc.) or dissociative symptoms (amnesia, syncopal episodes)
3) abdominal pain, vomiting spells, bloating, diarrhea, food intoler-ance
4) in women, complaints of dysmenorrhea or menstrual irregularity
5) chronic sexual difficulties, including indifference, disinterest, lack of sexual pleasure, or dyspareunia
6) musculoskeletal pain or frequent headaches

Individuals with a Somatization Disorder frequently have symptoms of de-pression in addition to their physical symptoms. In fact, the DSM-III reports that the reason they usually come to psychiatric attention is because of symptoms related to depression, including suicidal thoughts or gestures. Other disorders are commonly associated, including substance abuse, anti-social behavior or personality disorder, and Histrionic Personality Disorder. The first of these associated disorders, substance abuse, is not uncommonly iatrogenic - an outgrowth of the patient's incessant seeking of treatment from multiple physicians. Included among these abused substances are minor tranquilizers, amphetamines, barbiturates, opiates, and synthetic analgesics. In addition, people with this disorder frequently have had multiple surgical procedures.

The disorder is probably more common in women; some studies estimate an incidence as high as one percent of the general population.

****

GO TO VIDEOTAPE

****

B.   CONVERSION DISORDER (DSM-III 300.11)

A second Somatoform Disorder is the Conversion Disorder. This disorder was originally described as presenting with symptoms which mimicked neur-ologic disease such as paralysis, anesthesia, blindness, or seizures. Other possible presentations are now recognized, such as vomiting or pseudocyesis. The diagnosis of a Conversion Disorder implies a specific mechanism to account for the disorder. As referred to earlier, due to current stresses, the individual has experienced a reduced ability to repress a previously unconscious conflict. This psychic conflict is "converted" to a physical symptom. This conversion provides the individual with a primary gain and a secondary gain. The primary gain is the maintenance of the psychic conflict in the unconscious. The secondary gain is the support the indi-vidual receives from others or the avoidance of something which is unpleas-ant to him. These two gains, primary and secondary, frequently allow the individual to accept an obviously disabling symptom with an air of quiet unconcern. This acceptance is referred to by its original French term "la belle indifference."

Case Study: M.G., a 26-year-old female, is brought to the emergency room by her husband after the sudden onset of total paralysis of both legs. A neurologist has seen the patient and describes a total flaccid paralysis of both lower extremities with an associated total anesthesia and moderately brisk, symmetrical reflexes.

The patient is examined while lying calmly on a stretcher. She can offer no clues as to what has produced these symptoms, relating that everything was fine until shortly after dinner when, while watching television, she noticed she was unable to move her legs. During the interview, the patient was conversant and appropriate, although it was noted that she did not seem very concerned about her paralysis. Her mental status exam was otherwise unremarkable.

In order to diagnose Conversion Disorder, additional information is necessary. Review the diagnostic criteria below:

Diagnostic criteria for Conversion Disorder:

A.   The predominant disturbance is a loss of or alteration in physical functioning suggesting a physical disorder.

B.   Psychological factors are judged to be etiologically involved in the symptom, as evidenced by either:

(1) there is a temporal relationship between an environmental stimulus that is apparently related to a psychological conflict or need and the initiation or exacerbation of the symptom
(2) the symptom enables the individual to avoid some activity that is noxious to him or her
(3) the symptom enables the individual to get support from the environment that otherwise might not be forthcoming

C.   It has been determined that the symptom is <u>not</u> under voluntary control.

D.   The symptom cannot, after appropriate investigation, be explained by a known physical disorder or pathophysiological mechanism.

E.   The symptom is not limited to pain or to a disturbance in sexual functioning.

F.   Not due to Somatization Disorder or Schizophrenia.

The chief differences between a Somatization Disorder and a Conversion Disorder lie in three areas:

1.   Whereas both involve physical symptoms in the absence of demonstrable organic illness, the Somatization Disorder is chronic and

involves multiple organ systems. The Conversion Disorder is usually of sudden onset in the face of marked stress, is short-lived, and remits completely.

2. Treatment of a Conversion Disorder is usually short-term and usually involves psychotherapy. Both hypnosis and the sodium amytal interview have also been used in the diagnosis of Conversion Disorder and in exploring the preconscious dynamics leading to the symptom. Frequently, the symptom will remit completely during one of these procedures. On the other hand, the Somatization Disorder is not responsive to these procedures, and in fact, Somatization Disorders rarely respond well to medication and frequently require long-term psychotherapy with poor or mixed results.

3. Conversion Disorders are relatively rare; Somatization Disorders are fairly common.

****

GO TO VIDEOTAPE

****

C. PSYCHOGENIC PAIN DISORDER (DSM-III 307.80) AND HYPOCHONDRI-ASIS (DSM-III 300.70)

Two special categories of Somatoform Disorders can be regarded as closely related to the Somatization and Conversion Disorders. In Psychogenic Pain Disorder, there is the presence of nonorganic pain instead of specific physical symptoms. In contrast to Conversion Disorders, psychogenic pain is usually chronic, unrelenting, and unresponsive to treatment. Early in the course, the pain may be temporally related to meaningful environmental stimuli and may remit if it is not reinforced and the secondary gains are insufficient. Treatment with analgesics is contraindicated because of the abuse potential and surgical ablation frequently leads to the transference of the pain to another location.

A second syndrome is that of Hypochondriasis. Individuals with this disorder are preoccupied with bodily function or fear of various diseases. They do not, however, have the physical symptoms or complaints of Somatization Disorders nor the specific physical symptom of the Conversion Disorder. Hypochondriasis is typically also unresponsive to treatment, although mixed results have been reported with psychotropic medication and long-term psychotherapy.

QUIZ, Section I.

Circle the correct answer(s). <u>One</u> or <u>more</u> <u>than</u> <u>one</u> answer may be correct.

1. Somatization Disorder

    a. is one of several Somatoform Disorders.
    b. is also known as Briquet's syndrome.
    c. has symptoms in many organ systems.
    d. uses the mental mechanism of somatization.

2. Briquet's syndrome is characterized by

    a. multiple-organ physical complaints.
    b. onset before age 30.
    c. frequent pseudoneurologic symptoms.
    d. use of the mental mechanism of conversion.

3. Complications of the Somatization Disorder include

    a. addiction to amphetamines.
    b. abuse of prescribed drugs.
    c. sexual sterility.
    d. frequent surgical procedures.

Use the following case study to answer question 4.

H.K., a 42-year-old female, was seen in consultation on the request of her internist. She had been hospitalized for the evaluation and treatment of severe episodic epigastric pains. However, an extensive evaluation has provided no possible cause for the patient's pains, which she describes as unrelated to food intake, time of day, or external stress. The patient has experienced similar pains in the past and has been treated with anticholinergics/antispasmodics with some relief. Although these symptoms have only been present for 1-2 years, the patient has had other abdominal symptoms in the past, and has had an appendectomy and a cholecystectomy. Her only other surgery has been an ovarian wedge biopsy for dyspareunia thought to be secondary to an ovarian cyst and a dilatation and curettage to evaluate dysmenorrhea. In addition to this, a review of systems is positive for bursitis, recurrent in both shoulders, partially remitting following steroid injection. The patient takes no regular medications other than the antispasmodics mentioned above. She does take phenacetin with codeine 4-6 times a week for recurrent bifrontal headache.

Her mental status examination is remarkable in that she focuses almost exclusively on her physical symptoms and is resentful that a psychiatrist has been consulted.

4. In this case, which of the following information would be <u>necessary</u>?

    a. age of patient when symptoms first appeared
    b. the pathology reports from the patient's appendectomy and chole-
        cystectomy
    c. the medical history before the patient was 25
    d. the number of prior physicians consulted

5. In Conversion Disorder the patient

    a. uses conversion as a mental mechanism.
    b. may use displacement and symbolization as mental mechanisms.
    c. usually gives primary and secondary gains.
    d. frequently exhibits "la belle indifference."

6. The diagnosis of Conversion Disorder (case study on page 488) can now
    be confirmed by a positive response to which of the following questions?

    a. Has there been an event recently that was psychologically stressful?
    b. Is there something the patient is supposed to do, but that she
        strongly did not want to do?
    c. Was one of the patient's parents a paraplegic during the time she
        was growing up?
    d. Is the husband being supportive now when he was not before?

7. Psychogenic Pain Disorder is associated with which of the following?

    a. psychogenic pain without physical findings
    b. pain temporally related to meaningful environmental stimuli
    c. associated with primary and secondary gain
    d. may become chronic

8. Patients with Hypochondriasis

    a. are chronic complainers.
    b. are preoccupied with worries about the presence of undetected
        physical illness.
    c. have frequent physical symptoms.
    d. are preoccupied with bodily functions.

Circle the letter corresponding to the <u>one</u> correct response.

9. The following statements are true <u>except</u>:

    a. Current stresses can trigger the release of previously repressed
        psychic material.
    b. Neurotic defenses aid in keeping conflicts in the unconscious.
    c. Anxiety is associated with unconscious conflicts.
    d. Failure of repression can lead to the use of new, abnormal, or
        neurotic mental mechanisms.
    e. Secondary gain is the maintenance of the psychic conflict in the
        unconscious.

10. All of the following may be the presenting symptom of a Conversion Disorder except

    a. seizures.
    b. vomiting.
    c. unconscious episodes.
    d. dyspareunia.

TRUE or FALSE: Indicate which of the following statements are true (T) and which are false (F) by circling the appropriate letter.

T   F   11. Somatization Disorders should be treated with appropriate medication for symptom relief.

T   F   12. Secondary gain is seen in both Somatization and Conversion Disorders.

T   F   13. "La belle indifference" is seen in Somatization Disorders.

T   F   14. Conversion is the symbolic physical representation of an unconscious physical stress.

T   F   15. Conversion Disorders are short-lived.

T   F   16. Conversion Disorders are temporally related to psychologically meaningful and stressful stimuli.

Match the following descriptions with their corresponding terms.

___17. shifting affect from conflict   a. somatization
        to physical symptom
___18. changing psychic conflict into   b. conversion
        physical symptom
___19. "special" meaning of physical   c. displacement
        symptom
___20. focusing on physical symptoms   d. symbolization
        or concerns

II. DISSOCIATIVE DISORDERS

The Dissociative Disorders have also been called hysterical neuroses, dissociative type. There are four categories of Dissociative Disorders:

    A. Psychogenic Amnesia
    B. Psychogenic Fugue
    C. Multiple Personality
    D. Depersonalization Disorder

Each of these conditions will be considered separately below, but there are some general comments concerning the etiology and treatment of these disorders.

Dissociation is a mental mechanism, as are conversion, somatization, displacement, and symbolization, which were discussed in the earlier part of this chapter. Dissociation occurs when stress, which is psychologically meaningful, threatens repression of previously traumatic, conflicted issues. This leads to an increase in anxiety. In order to deal with the anxiety and aid repression, the mental mechanism of dissociation is employed. In dissociation, a part of consciousness, identity, or motor behavior is separated from the remainder of the conscious ego. This separation of part of the ego leads to symptoms of the different disorders in this class. In all these disorders, however, there is a primary gain of repression of the conflicted material; there may frequently be a secondary gain of avoiding unpleasantness in the environment or gaining support from the environment. There may also be "la belle indifference" in regard to the symptoms (Nemiah, 1975).

As mentioned in the DSM-III, dissociation may involve:

1) The separation of a part of consciousness
2) The separation of a part of motor behavior
3) The separation of a part of identity

In the first case, the resultant disorder is Psychogenic Amnesia. In the second case, the separation of a part of motor behavior, the wanderings of the Psychogenic Fugue result. In the last case, there are two resultant disorders: 1) the Multiple Personality, wherein the individual's customary identity is forgotten and a new identity or identities take over the individual's behavior; and 2) the Depersonalization Disorder, wherein the individual loses the sense of his own reality (an important part of identity).

In all Dissociative Disorders, when psychiatric treatment is indicated, psychotherapy is the treatment of choice.

A.   PSYCHOGENIC AMNESIA (DSM-III 300.12)

Psychogenic Amnesia is the most common Dissociative Disorder. According to the DSM-III, it is the sudden onset of an inability to recall important personal information registered and stored in memory. The amnesia begins suddenly, usually following severe psychological stress. During the episode, the patient is typically disoriented, perplexed, and indifferent. The episode is usually self-limiting and ends abruptly. There are four types of amnesia that may be seen in this condition:

1.   Localized amnesia, the most frequent form, is a failure to recall all events related to a fixed period of time.
2.   Selective amnesia is a failure to recall some important events during a fixed period of time.
3.   Generalized amnesia is a failure to recall all events of one's life.
4.   Continuous amnesia is a failure to recall all events from a specific period up to the present.

****

GO TO VIDEOTAPE

****

B.　PSYCHOGENIC FUGUE (DSM-III 300.13)

Psychogenic Fugue is an exceedingly rare condition characterized by the sudden onset of travel away from home with loss of memory for one's identity, and following recovery there is memory loss for the fugue. Fugues frequently occur while the individual is using alcohol and follow psychological stresses. The travel may be limited or extensive and may include the assumption of a new identity. This new identity is usually incomplete and not elaborate, but may be quite complex. The fugue usually lasts hours to days, but may extend for months. Recovery is usually rapid and complete.

Although the course for both Psychogenic Fugue and Psychogenic Amnesia is usually rapid and recovery is complete, both conditions are if protracted, amenable to psychotherapy. Also, in both cases, hypnosis or a sodium amytal interview may be helpful diagnostically, may uncover the preconscious dynamics of the symptom, or may actually be curative.

C.　MULTIPLE PERSONALITY (DSM-III 300.14)

This disorder is an exceedingly rare condition in which an individual has two or more complex, distinct, frequently opposite personalities. At any given time, one of these personalities dominates the individual. Transition between personalities is abrupt and may be triggered by psychological stress or suggestion. The condition usually appears initially in young females and runs a chronic course. The treatment of choice is psychotherapy; therapeutic intervention consists of attempting to achieve a synthesis between the personalities, but this is rarely more than partially successful.

****

GO TO VIDEOTAPE

****

D.　DEPERSONALIZATION DISORDER (DSM-III 300.60)

According to the DSM-III, the hallmark of the Depersonalization Disorder is the sudden onset of a sense of loss of one's own reality. This may be described as a feeling of unreality, seeing oneself from a distance, perceiving a distortion of one's extremities, or feeling as if one is dreaming. These episodes are usually prolonged, remit gradually over minutes to hours, and recur frequently, at least weekly. (Isolated episodes are thought to occur normally in young adults.) Associated complaints with the disorder are distortions in perception of the environment, dizziness, loss of subjective sense of time, and feeling of derealization. The onset of the disorder is invariably in adolescence or young adulthood and the occurrence of episodes

1.	a,b,c,d	8.	b,d	15.	T
2.	a,b,c	9.	e	16.	T
3.	a,b,d	10.	d	17.	c
4.	a,c	11.	F	18.	b
5.	a,b,c,d	12.	T	19.	d
6.	a,b,d	13.	F	20.	a
7.	a,b,c,d	14.	F		

usually follows a psychological stress. The course is chronic, the individual is asymptomatic between episodes, and treatment is rarely successful, although supportive psychotherapy is probably beneficial during the acute episodes.

In summary, the Somatoform and Dissociative Disorders can be viewed in one other way. One group contains disorders that are relatively rare, including Multiple Personality, Psychogenic Fugue, Psychogenic Amnesia, Depersonalization Disorder, and Conversion Disorder. Although treatment results are mixed, most of these conditions are at least somewhat responsive to psychotherapy, amytal interviews, hypnosis, and/or psychotropic medication. The second group of disorders includes Somatization Disorder and Psychogenic Pain Disorder. These two conditions are relatively common, resistant to treatment, and carry a high risk of nonpalliative surgery and iatrogenic substance abuse.

QUIZ, Section II.

Circle the correct answer(s). One or more than one answer may be correct.

1. Dissociation

   a. is a mental mechanism that includes a loss of part of consciousness, motor behavior, or identity.
   b. aids repression.
   c. is a way of binding anxiety.
   d. is a mental representation of previous psychic conflicts.

2. Psychogenic Amnesia is

   a. sudden in onset and rapidly clears.
   b. frequently disabling.
   c. the least common Dissociative Disorder.
   d. a dissociation of consciousness.

3. Hypnosis and sodium amytal interview may be indicated in which of the following?

   a. Psychogenic Fugue
   b. Psychogenic Amnesia
   c. Somatization Disorder
   d. Conversion Disorder

4.   The Multiple Personality Disorder

   a.   is characterized by two or more <u>partial</u> personalities.
   b.   is characterized by sudden shifts between personalities.
   c.   usually remits spontaneously.
   d.   is characterized by personality shifts in response to suggestion.

5.   Symptoms of Depersonalization Disorder include

   a.   depersonalization - loss of sense of one's own reality.
   b.   loss of sense of time.
   c.   dizziness.
   d.   gradual onset and remission.

Use the following case study to answer questions 6-7.

P. W., a 26-year-old female, was doing well until the evening before admission. Shortly after dinner she began arguing with her husband about his staying out late the night before. She then began crying and pounding on the walls and her husband with her fist. She suddenly became limp and fell to the floor sobbing. She finally stopped crying and remained limp, unresponsive to verbal or physical stimuli. After about 30 minutes, she regained consciousness but was disoriented to time, place, and person, and didn't know that their two children had been born. She slept erratically through the night. When she remained disoriented the next morning, she was taken to the hospital and was admitted. During the day she gradually began remembering more and more. There was no history of seizure activity or prior episodes similar to this.

On examination at admission she was an attractive, crying, white female who appeared her stated age, wearing neat jeans and a shirt. She was cooperative but became agitated when she could not remember something she thought she should know. She maintained no eye contact; alternately she was calm and then would begin crying and sobbing. She was occasionally shaky and obviously confused. Her speech was logical and coherent though she would stop when she could not remember and would state that, "Yes, I believe that's so because Johnny told me so." Her affect was depressed and anxious. She knew that she knew the answers to questions but could not find them. She stated that her thoughts were very confused, just "floating around in my head, but they are all my own thoughts." She denied any delusions, homicidal thoughts, but has thought at times that things would be better if she were dead. She denied any hallucinations except the day before, when shortly after regaining consciousness she thought she saw and heard her father who had been dead for two years. She was oriented to place, but did not know how old she was, nor the month and year. Her immediate memory was fair; she remembered two out of three objects at five minutes; she didn't know her children's names or ages; Kennedy was the only president she could remember. Concentration was decreased. She was able to abstract proverbs well. Insight and judgment were impaired.

Circle the letter corresponding to the <u>one</u> correct answer.

6.   This patient exhibits which type of amnesia?

      a. generalized
      b. localized
      c. continuous
      d. selective

7.   In order to diagnose Psychogenic Amnesia in this patient all of the
      following are important <u>except</u>

      a. sudden onset.
      b. precipitating stress of husband's night-out drinking.
      c. father's death.
      d. negative history for seizures or previous episodes.
      e. avoidance of stress of child rearing.

TRUE or FALSE: Circle the correct answer.

T   F   8. Psychogenic Fugue is the dissociation of part of identity.

T   F   9. After recovery, the individual remembers what he did during
            the fugue.

T   F   10. Psychogenic Fugue is rare.

T   F   11. Psychogenic Fugue is often related to the heavy use of alcohol.

Match the following symptoms with the corresponding disorders.   Lettered
items may be used once, more than once, or not at all.

___12.   a separation of a part of identity   a. fugue
___13.   a separation of a part of consciousness   b. amnesia
___14.   a separation of a part of motor behavior   c. depersonalization
___15.   loss of sense of own reality   d. multiple personality

Match the following disorders with the corresponding treatments.   Lettered
items may be used once, more than once, or not at all.

___16.   Somatization Disorder   a. surgery
___17.   Conversion Disorder   b. medication
___18.   Psychogenic Amnesia   c. psychotherapy
___19.   Psychogenic Pain Disorder

Match the following types of Psychogenic Amnesia with the appropriate description.

___ 20. localized amnesia
___ 21. generalized amnesia
___ 22. continuous amnesia
___ 23. selective amnesia

a. total memory loss for entire life
b. total memory loss for events for a fixed time interval
c. total memory loss from event to present
d. partial memory loss for a fixed time period

ANSWERS, Section II.

1.	a,b,c	9.	F	17.	c
2.	a,b,d	10.	T	18.	c
3.	a,b,d	11.	T	19.	c
4.	b,d	12.	c,d	20.	b
5.	a,b,c	13.	b	21.	a
6.	b	14.	a	22.	c
7.	c	15.	c	23.	d
8.	F	16.	c		

POST-TEST

For the following questions, one or more than one answer may be correct. Circle the correct answer(s).

1. Briquet's syndrome is characterized by

   a. multiple-organ physical complaints.
   b. onset before age 30.
   c. frequent pseudoneurologic symptoms.
   d. use of the mental mechanisms of conversion.

2. The Multiple Personality Disorder

   a. is characterized by two or more partial personalities.
   b. is characterized by sudden shifts between personalities.
   c. usually remits spontaneously.
   d. is characterized by personality shifts in response to suggestion.

3. Symptoms of Depersonalization Disorder include

   a. loss of sense of one's own reality.
   b. loss of sense of time.
   c. dizziness.
   d. gradual onset and remission.

4. Complications of the Somatization Disorder include

   a. addiction to amphetamines.
   b. abuse of prescribed drugs.
   c. sexual sterility.
   d. frequent surgical procedures.

5. Patients with Hypochondriasis

   a. are chronic complainers.
   b. are preoccupied with worries about the presence of undetected physical illness.
   c. have frequent physical symptoms.
   d. are preoccupied with bodily functions.

6. Somatization Disorder

   a. is one of several Somatoform Disorders.
   b. is also known as Briquet's syndrome.
   c. has symptoms in many organ systems.
   d. uses the mental mechanism of somatization.

7. Dissociation

    a. is a mental mechanism that includes a loss of part of consciousness, behavior, or identity.
    b. aids repression.
    c. is a way of binding anxiety.
    d. is a mental representation of previous psychic conflicts.

8. In Conversion Disorder the patient

    a. uses conversion as a mental mechanism.
    b. may use displacement and symbolization as mental mechanisms.
    c. usually gives primary and secondary gains.
    d. frequently exhibits "la belle indifference."

9. Psychogenic Amnesia is

    a. sudden in onset and gradually clears.
    b. frequently disabling.
    c. the least common Dissociative Disorder.
    d. a dissociation of consciousness.

For the following questions, circle the letter corresponding to the one correct answer.

10. Psychogenic Pain Disorder is not associated with which of the following?

    a. psychogenic pain without physical findings
    b. pain temporally related to meaningful environmental stimuli
    c. associated with primary and secondary gain
    d. may become chronic
    e. should be treated with analgesics

11. Which of the following statements is not correct?

    a. Current stresses can trigger the release of previously repressed psychic material.
    b. Neurotic defenses aid in keeping conflicts in the unconscious.
    c. Anxiety is often associated with unconscious conflicts.
    d. Failure of repression can lead to the use of new, abnormal, or neurotic mental mechanisms.
    e. Hypochondriasis is often responsive to drug therapy.

12. All of the following may be the presenting symptom of a Conversion Disorder except

    a. seizures.
    b. vomiting.
    c. unconscious episodes.
    d. sterility.

Match the following disorders with the corresponding terms.

___ 13. Somatization Disorder
___ 14. Conversion Disorder
___ 15. Psychogenic Amnesia
___ 16. Psychogenic Pain Disorder

a. medication
b. surgery
c. psychotherapy
d. all of the above
e. none of the above

Match the following types of amnesia with their corresponding definitions.

___ 17. generalized amnesia
___ 18. continuous amnesia
___ 19. selective amnesia
___ 20. localized amnesia

a. total memory loss from event to present
b. partial memory loss for a fixed time period
c. total memory loss for entire life
d. total memory loss for events for a fixed time interval

Match each mental mechanism with the appropriate description

___ 21. changing psychic conflict into physical symptom
___ 22. focusing on physical symptoms or concerns
___ 23. "Special" meaning of physical symptom
___ 24. shifting affect from conflict to physical symptom

a. symbolization
b. displacement
c. conversion
d. somatization

Match the following disorders with corresponding terms.

___ 25. disorder of identity
___ 26. disorder of behavior
___ 27. disorder of consciousness
___ 28. disorder of sense of reality

a. multiple personality
b. depersonalization
c. fugue
d. amnesia

PRE-TEST ANSWERS

1. e	11. b,d	20. c
2. d	12. a,b,c	21. c
3. e	13. c	22. c
4. a,b,c,d	14. b	23. c
5. a,b,c	15. d	24. c
6. a,b,d	16. a	25. b
7. a,b,c,d	17. d	26. a
8. b,d	18. b	27. c
9. a,b,c	19. a	28. d
10. d		

POST-TEST ANSWERS

1. a,b,c	11. e	20. d
2. b,d	12. d	21. c
3. a,b,c	13. c	22. d
4. a,b,d	14. c	23. a
5. b,d	15. c	24. b
6. a,b,c,d	16. c	25. a
7. a,b,c	17. c	26. c
8. a,b,c,d	18. a	27. d
9. d	19. b	28. b
10. e		

REFERENCES

Diagnostic and statistical manual of mental disorders (3rd Ed.). Washington: American Psychiatric Association, 1980.

Nemiah, J. Hysterical neurosis, conversion type, and hysterical neurosis, dissociative type. In Freedman, A. M., Kaplan, H. I., & Sadock B. J. (Eds.), Comprehensive textbook of psychiatry II. Baltimore: Williams & Wilkins, 1975.

CHAPTER 11

Psychosexual Disorders
Darlene L. Shaw, Ph.D.
Dean G. Kilpatrick, Ph.D.

CHAPTER OUTLINE

Learning Objectives

Pre-Test

I. Myths Concerning Human Sexuality

II. Psychosexual Disorders

   A. Gender Identity Disorders

      1. Transsexualism
      2. Gender Identity Disorder of Childhood
      3. Atypical Gender Identity Disorder

   B. Paraphilias

      1. Fetishism
      2. Transvestism
      3. Zoophilia
      4. Pedophilia
      5. Exhibitionism
      6. Voyeurism
      7. Sexual Masochism
      8. Sexual Sadism
      9. Atypical Paraphilias

   C. Psychosexual Dysfunctions

      1. Inhibited Sexual Desire
      2. Inhibited Sexual Excitement
      3. Inhibited Female Orgasm
      4. Inhibited Male Orgasm
      5. Premature Ejaculation
      6. Functional Dyspareunia
      7. Functional Vaginismus
      8. Atypical Psychosexual Dysfunctions

   D. Other Psychosexual Disorders

      1. Ego-Dystonic Homosexuality
      2. Psychosexual Disorders Not Elsewhere Classified

III.   Treatment of Psychosexual Disorders

Post-Test

Pre-Test/Post-Test Answers

References

LEARNING OBJECTIVES

After completing this chapter you will be able to:

1. Recognize common myths concerning human sexuality and recall the correct information which dispels these myths.

2. Recognize the DSM-III diagnostic criteria which define each of the Gender Identity Disorders, Paraphilias, and Psychosexual Dysfunctions.

3. Assign correct diagnostic labels to written case descriptions which characterize the Gender Identity Disorders, the Paraphilias, and the Psychosexual Dysfunctions.

4. Identify each of the four phases constituting the normal sexual response cycle.

5. Recognize general treatment considerations and approaches for dealing with Psychosexual Disorders.

PRE-TEST

For each of the following questions, one or more than one answer may be correct. Circle the correct answer(s).

1. Which of the following is (are) considered Psychosexual Disorders by DSM-III?

    a. Gender Identity Disorders
    b. Paraphilias
    c. Psychosexual Dysfunctions
    d. Heterophilia

2.. Which of the following would not be classified as a Paraphilia?

    a. Homosexuality
    b. Voyeurism
    c. Pedophilia
    d. Sexual Sadism
    e. Zenophilia

For the following questions, circle the letter corresponding to the one correct response.

3. Which of the following is not characteristic of Paraphilias?

    a. preference for nonhuman object for sexual arousal
    b. sexual activity with humans involving real or simulated suffering or humiliation
    c. sexual activity with consenting adults
    d. sexual activity with nonconsenting adults

4. The most dangerous Paraphilia is

    a. Fetishism.
    b. Exhibitionism.
    c. Sexual Masochism.
    d. Sexual Sadism.
    e. Zoophilia.

5. Which of the following is not a part of the sexual response cycle?

    a. appetitive
    b. excitement
    c. repetitive
    d. orgasm
    e. resolution

6. Which of the following is <u>not</u> classified as a Psychosexual Dysfunction?

    a. Inhibited Sexual Desire
    b. Inhibited Sexual Arousal
    c. Inhibited Female Orgasm
    d. Multiple Orgasmic Failure in Females
    e. Premature Ejaculation
    f. Functional Vaginismus

TRUE or FALSE: Indicate which of the following questions are true (T) and which are false (F) by circling the appropriate letter.

T   F   7. Our culture encourages children to explore their sexuality.

T   F   8. Penis size varies more in the flaccid than in the erect state.

T   F   9. There are two types of orgasms among women - clitoral and vaginal.

T   F   10. Anatomical sexual characteristics and gender identity must be different for an individual to be diagnosed as having a Gender Identity Disorder.

T   F   11. Transsexuals are individuals who dress up in the clothes of the opposite sex.

T   F   12. A child whose gender identity and anatomical sexual characteristics are different would be diagnosed as having Gender Disorder of Childhood.

T   F   13. Transvestites generally prefer sex with those of their same gender.

T   F   14. Most fetishists are males.

T   F   15. Zoophilia is defined as an insatiable desire to make love in the public zoo.

T   F   16. Most exhibitionists are dangerous.

T   F   17. Masochists and sadists together make good bedfellows.

T   F   18. Psychosexual dysfunction can occur in all but the appetitive portion of the sexual response cycle.

T   F   19. It is permissible to diagnose relatively minor disturbances and/or those which result from organic factors as Psychosexual Disorders according to DSM-III.

T   F   20. During the excitement phase of the sexual response cycle, physiological changes are mediated primarily by the parasympathetic nervous system.

T   F   21. During the orgasmic phase, sympathetic nervous system activity predominates.

T   F   22. Homosexuality should always be classified as a Psychosexual Disorder.

T   F   23. Psychoanalytic therapy is the treatment of choice for most cases of Psychosexual Dysfunction.

T   F   24. Unfortunately, most Psychosexual Disorders do not respond well to treatment.

I. MYTHS CONCERNING HUMAN SEXUALITY

Sexuality plays a major part in all of our lives, and most persons consider physicians to be experts on human sexuality. Individuals who wish to obtain accurate information about sexual matters or who wish to receive help with sexual problems often contact their physician. Therefore, you should become knowledgeable about human sexuality. In particular, you should be familiar with several commonly held myths, or false beliefs, about human sexuality since many patients will believe these myths.

The first myth is that children are not sexual beings. Children are sexual beings and during childhood explore both their own bodies and the bodies of others. Male and female children experience similar sexual drives, and, if left unimpeded, they can stimulate themselves to orgasm. No damage results from childhood masturbation. Furthermore, while children are capable of sexual intercourse, in our society most childhood sexual experiences are solitary stimulation or mutual stimulation with occasional oral-genital contact. Children in our culture are frequently and unnecessarily punished for sexual play.

There are numerous sexual myths concerning adults which are widely believed in our society. For instance, men are particularly concerned with the belief that there is great variation in penis size. While this may be true when the penis is in the flaccid state, there exists minimal variation in the size of the erect penis. Another myth along these lines is that there is a relationship between penis size and body size and that the man with a large penis is more sexually potent than the man with a small penis. In fact, there is little correlation between body and penis size, and penis size in no way affects sexual potency. Similarly, there is no correlation between race and the size of the erect penis (McCary, 1967).

Another myth is that females experience two kinds of orgasm. In the past, largely due to an essay on the subject by Freud, it was believed that females experience two types of orgasm, one clitoral (and immature), the other vaginal (and adult). This belief is erroneous and contrary to research findings. Only one type of female orgasm exists, and that comes from adequate stimulation of the clitoris or other erotogenic zones or by erotic thoughts.

Other myths surround the topic of masturbation. Contrary to popular belief, both men and women masturbate. The incidence of masturbation to orgasm among men is commonly estimated to be 95% of the total male population (McCary, 1967). Among women, depending upon the group, from 50% to 80% masturbate at some time, and the incidence increases with higher educational level (McCary, 1967). Both sexes begin this activity at an early age, with 13% of boys and girls having masturbated by 10 years of age (McCary, 1967). Adolescent boys masturbate an average of 2.5 times a week, and the frequency of this practice declines after the teens. Among women, the frequency increases until middle age and remains fairly unchanged thereafter (Kinsey, Pomeroy, Martin, & Gebhard, 1953). Among both sexes, masturbation often continues throughout life and well into old age. While the frequency of masturbation usually depends upon the availability of other sexual outlets, it is an acceptable sexual activity which many individuals continue to engage in, although they have enjoyable sexual partnerships. Of all sexual activities, masturbation is the most successful way of reaching orgasm for women. It is also a myth that masturbation is a cause of poor eyesight, hairy palms, softening of the spinal cord, acne, or physical damage.

Another myth is that individuals lose interest in sex as they get older. With availability of a sexual partner, many individuals maintain sexual potency until 70, 80, or 90 years of age.

The populace largely believes that lower socioeconomic and minority groups do not wish to limit family size and that they engage in more varied and frequent sexual behavior. In addition, many people think incest occurs more frequently in lower socioeconomic groups. These assumptions are false. Lower socioeconomic groups usually have less varied sexual activity than middle and high socioeconomic groups, and incest is as common in high socioeconomic groups as in low socioeconomic groups.

Many myths surround the event of pregnancy. Although it is widely believed that females can become pregnant at menarche, pregnancy usually cannot occur until one or two years after menarche. Also, while menopause is believed to end fertility, conception is possible as long as menstrual periods occur, however sporadically. Intercourse is often thought to be dangerous during the last trimester of pregnancy. This is incorrect. Except when the membrane has ruptured, intercourse during the third trimester is not dangerous.

Sexual offenders are often thought to be oversexed, lecherous people. In fact, the typical convicted sex offender is severely sexually inhibited, rather than oversexed. Furthermore, despite the popularity of books and movies about fictional "sex-crazed killers," homicide seldom occurs in conjunction with sexual offenses. Indeed, the likelihood of being murdered by a "sex fiend" is far less than that of being killed by a family member or close friend (Falk, 1965).

A final myth about human sexuality is that there are few, if any, social or cultural influences on sexual behavior or mores. Nothing could be further from the truth. An examination of different cultures reveals considerable variation in the types of sexual behaviors which are permitted or condoned. For example, some cultures, such as ancient Greece or modern San Francisco, condone homosexual behavior, while other cultures strongly condemn such behavior.

QUIZ, Section I.

TRUE or FALSE: Circle the correct letter.

T   F   1. Freud's tenet that women experience two types of orgasm, clitoral and vaginal, is one of only a few of his beliefs which has been borne out by present day research.

T   F   2. The frequency with which incest occurs shows little variability across socioeconomic groups.

T   F   3. There are minimal differences in penis size when the penis is in the erect state.

T   F   4. Normal children have almost no interest in sexual play.

T   F   5. Only lecherous, dirty old men continue to have an interest in sex past the age of 65.

T   F   6. For normal men and women the frequency of masturbation peaks around age 28 and gradually declines until it stops at either age 50 or when the person marries--whichever comes first.

T   F   7. Penis size and body size are highly correlated.

T   F   8. The erect penis of black men is generally larger than the erect penis of white males.

II. PSYCHOSEXUAL DISORDERS

The DSM-III divides Psychosexual Disorders into four major groups: 1) Gender Identity Disorders, 2) Paraphilias, 3) Psychosexual Dysfunctions, and 4) Other Psychosexual Disorders. Psychosexual Disorders are defined on the basis of an assumption that psychological factors play a major part in the acquisition and/or maintenance of these disorders. Thus, disorders in sexual functioning which are caused by organic factors are not designated as Psychosexual Disorders even though there may be psychological reactions to the organically caused dysfunction. For example, impotence occurring following a spinal cord injury or diabetes would be coded on Axis III as a physical disorder, and the resulting adjustment reaction would be coded on Axis I.

A. GENDER IDENTITY DISORDERS

The first group of Psychosexual Disorders is the Gender Identity Disorders. The common element in all Gender Identity Disorders is that there is a discrepancy between an individual's anatomic sex and gender identity.

Anatomical sexual characteristics are determined by chromosomal makeup. Thus, an individual with an X-Y chromosomal makeup and female genitalia is anatomically female. In contrast, gender identity can be defined as one's perceptions of oneself as male, female, or ambivalent. The DSM-III states that gender identity is the private experience of gender role and that gender role is defined as everything a person says and does to indicate to others that one is female, male, or ambivalent. Thus, gender role and identity refer to a wide variety of thoughts, feelings, and behaviors regarding whether one is "male," "female," or "ambivalent" about it. The key point to remember is that it is possible for one's anatomical sex and gender identity to be discrepant.

In normal children, gender identity or the sense of oneself as male or female is fixed during early childhood, most often by two years of age. Current opinion favors the view that environmental factors override genetic and biological ones in determining an individual's gender identity. Disordered gender identity almost always develops in the context of a pathological parent-child relationship, often times one in which the parent was rejecting of the child's anatomical sex.

There are three subgroups within the Gender Identity Disorders: 1) Transsexualism, 2) Gender Identity Disorder of Childhood, and 3) Atypical Gender Identity Disorders of Adolescence or Adult Life. It should be noted that all of these disorders are quite rare.

1.   Transsexualism (DSM-III 302.5).
     Transsexualism is a chronic disorder which is characterized by: 1) a persistent sense of discomfort and inappropriateness about one's anatomic sex, 2) a persistent wish to be rid of one's genitals, and 3) a persistent desire to live as a member of the opposite anatomic sex. These feelings must persist for at least two years before a diagnosis of Transsexualism can be made. Additionally, this diagnosis should not be made if these feelings are symptomatic of another mental disorder (e.g., Schizophrenia) or are associated with a genetic abnormality or physical intersex disorder. According to DSM-III, these characteristics form the basis for the diagnosis of Transsexualism:

     A.   Sense of discomfort and inappropriateness about one's anatomic sex.
     B.   Wish to be rid of one's own genitals and to live as a member of the other sex.
     C.   The disturbance has been continuous (not limited to periods of stress) for at least two years.
     D.   Absence of physical intersex or genetic abnormality.
     E.   Not due to another mental disorder, such as Schizophrenia.

ANSWERS, Section I.

1. F	5. F
2. T	6. F
3. T	7. F
4. F	8. F

Transsexuals usually exhibit several characteristic behaviors. They often complain that they feel uncomfortable wearing the clothes of their anatomical sex and frequently cross-dress in the clothes of the other sex. They also frequently engage in activities which they believe to be stereotypic of the opposite sex. Thus, a transsexual man may pursue "feminine" activities while a transsexual woman may seek out stereotypic "masculine" activities. Transsexuals generally find their genitals so repugnant that they make frequent requests for sex reassignments.

With respect to the course of Transsexualism, there are three major types of history: 1) asexual, 2) homosexual, and 3) heterosexual. As you might guess, transsexuals with an asexual history deny ever having had strong sexual feelings. They also report histories of never or rarely experiencing sexual activity or pleasure from the genitals. In contrast, some transsexuals have a history of primarily homosexual behavior prior to the onset of Transsexualism; that is, they are attracted to members of their same anatomical sex. A third group of transsexuals claims to have had an active heterosexual life. Occasionally, a transsexual's history may not neatly fit into any of these three types, in which case they should be classified as unspecified.

Transsexuality is a rare disorder which develops most frequently in individuals who have experienced gender identity problems as children. The onset for those with an asexual or homosexual history usually occurs during late adolescence or early adult life, while the onset may be somewhat later for those with a heterosexual history. Additionally, males present with this disorder much more frequently than females.

****

GO TO VIDEOTAPE

****

2. Gender Identity Disorder of Childhood (DSM-III, 302.60).
The essential features of this disorder are persistent feelings of discomfort and inappropriateness in a child about his or her anatomical sex and a desire to be, or a conviction that he or she actually is, a member of the opposite sex. These feelings must be more than a rejection of stereotypical sex role behavior and often include a persistent desire to be a member of the opposite sex and

a repudiation of their own genitalia. In order to diagnose Gender Identity Disorder of Childhood the individual may not have reached adolescence and must meet the following criteria:

For Females:

A. Strongly and persistently stated desire to be a boy, or insistence that she is a boy (not merely a desire for any perceived cultural advantages from being a boy).

B. Persistent repudiation of female anatomic structures, as manifested by at least one of the following repeated assertions:

(1) that she will grow up to become a man (not merely in role)
(2) that she is biologically unable to become pregnant
(3) that she will not develop breasts
(4) that she has no vagina
(5) that she has, or will grow, a penis

C. Onset of the disturbance before puberty. (For adults and adolescents, see Atypical Gender Identity Disorder.)

For Males:

A. Strongly and persistently stated desire to be a girl, or insistence that he is a girl.

B. Either (1) or (2):

(1) Persistent repudiation of male anatomic structures, as manifested by at least one of the following repeated assertions:

(a) that he will grow up to become a woman (not merely in role)
(b) that his penis or testes are disgusting or will disappear
(c) that it would be better not to have a penis or testes

(2) Preoccupation with female stereotypical activities as manifested by a preference for either cross-dressing or simulating female attire, or by a compelling desire to participate in the games and pastimes of girls.

C. Onset of the disturbance before puberty. (For adults and adolescents, see Atypical Gender Identity Disorder.)

With respect to associated features, children with the Gender Identity Disorder do not report being disturbed by it except as it causes them difficulty with family and friends. As in the case with other Gender Identity Disorders, Gender Identity Disorder of Childhood is quite rare. Moreover, not all children who experience a gender identity problem develop the complete syndrome, nor do the majority of these children develop Gender Identity Disorders as adults. Approximately three-fourths of boys who cross-dress begin to do so prior to their fourth birthday. Later, during the early years of school, the child is subjected to a considerable amount of social ostracism from peers, and a significant proportion of children respond to this social pressure by giving up their exaggerated insistence on the activities and attire of the opposite sex. Among those who do not, some develop a homosexual orientation and a smaller number may develop Transsexualism. There is no information about whether the disorder occurs more frequently among males or females.

3. Atypical Gender Identity Disorder (DSM-III 302.85).
As stated in the DSM-III: This is a residual category for coding gender identity problems that are not classifiable as a specific Gender Identity Disorder. In most instances, this category will be used for adolescents or adults, who, as children, met the criteria for Gender Identity Disorder of Childhood and who still have significant signs of that disorder.

B. PARAPHILIAS

The term Paraphilia is defined as a deviation in what one is attracted to sexually. Hence, Paraphilias are sometimes called sexual deviations. Paraphilias are a group of disorders which are characterized by persistent and repetitive sexually arousing fantasies or acts which are associated with: 1) preference for use of nonhuman objects for sexual arousal, 2) sexual activity with humans involving real or simulated suffering or humiliation, or 3) sexual activity with nonconsenting partners. These disorders are considerably more common in males than in females. Individuals with this disorder often have an impairment in their capacity to engage in affectionate sexual activity with an adult human partner of either sex. Psychosexual dysfunctions are also frequent in this group.

Individuals with a Paraphilia seldom experience erotic arousal without the use of paraphiliac fantasies. These fantasies are frequently present during masturbation or coitus and make sex partners feel that they are superfluous. The content of paraphiliac fantasy is not, in and of itself, unusual. For example, many men are sexually excited by women's underclothing, but a fantasy is considered paraphiliac if an individual becomes sexually excited only by the undergarments or by thinking about them.

The following Paraphilias will be defined:

1.   Fetishism
2.   Transvestism
3.   Zoophilia
4.   Pedophilia

5.   Exhibitionism
6.   Voyeurism
7.   Sexual Masochism
8.   Sexual Sadism
9.   Atypical Paraphilias

1.   Fetishism (DSM-III 302.81).
     This is a Paraphilia which is characterized by the use of nonliving objects as the preferred or exclusive method of producing sexual excitement. Common fetishes include female undergarments, shoes, boots, and parts of the human body such as hair or nails. The disorder usually begins during adolescence and tends to be chronic. Almost all reported cases have been males.

     DSM-III Diagnostic criteria for Fetishism:

     A.   The use of nonliving objects (fetishes) is a repeatedly preferred or exclusive method of achieving sexual excitement.

     B.   The fetishes are not limited to articles of female clothing used in cross-dressing (Transvestism) or to objects designed to be used for the purpose of sexual stimulation (e.g., vibrator).

2.   Transvestism (DSM-III 302.30).
     Transvestism is defined as recurrent and persistent cross-dressing for the purpose of sexual arousal by a heterosexual male. If the cross-dressing is interfered with, intense frustration results. The transvestite usually wears more than one article of women's clothing and may dress entirely as a woman. The cross-dressing usually begins in early adolescence or childhood. This disorder is rare, and, as defined, only occurs in males. These are the diagnostic criteria for Transvestism:

     A.   Recurrent and persistent cross-dressing by a heterosexual male.

     B.   Use of cross-dressing for the purpose of sexual excitement, at least initially, in the course of the disorder.

     C.   Intense frustration when the cross-dressing is interfered with.

     D.   Does not meet the criteria for Transsexualism.

3.   Zoophilia (DSM-III 302.10).
     Zoophilia is defined as the use of animals (zoo) as the preferred (philos) or exclusive method of producing sexual excitement. The animal may be used in intercourse or may be trained to excite the

human partner by licking or rubbing erotogenic zones. Additionally, the fantasy of sexual activity with animals is sexually arousing to individuals with Zoophilia. This is an extremely rare disorder which is seen almost exclusively in males and is more frequent among rural or farm boys. While there is little information regarding the age of onset, the disorder usually occurs by early adulthood and the course is chronic. Keep in mind the diagnostic criterion for Zoophilia:

> The act or fantasy of engaging in sexual activity with animals is a repeatedly preferred or exclusive method of achieving sexual excitement.

4. Pedophilia (DSM-III 302.20).
Pedophilia is the preference for repetitive sexual activity with prepubertal children. Adults must be at least 10 years older than the children, but for late adolescents, no precise age difference has been officially selected. Male adults who are heterosexually oriented prefer 8- to 10-year-old girls and usually desire looking or touching rather than intercourse. They often occupy some position of authority in the girl's environment and are usually well-known to the girl, such as her step-father, uncle, or a close family friend. Homosexually oriented male pedophiles prefer slightly older boys than the heterosexually oriented. Adults with no particular preference for either boys or girls tend to select younger children than adults who are exclusively homo- or heterosexual. Most pedophiles are male, and about twice as many pedophiles are heterosexually oriented as are homosexually oriented.

With regard to the course of the disorder little is known, but homosexual pedophiles have a relatively high recidivism rate, ranging from 13% to 28% of those apprehended, a rate which is approximately twice that of their heterosexual counterparts (DSM-III). No good information exists about the prevalence of sexual offenses against children, but pedophiles are thought to constitute approximately 30% of all apprehended sexual offenders (McCary, 1967).

The following criteria are needed to diagnose Pedophilia:

A. The act or fantasy of engaging in sexual activity with prepubertal children is a repeatedly preferred or exclusive method of achieving sexual excitement.

B. If the individual is an adult, the prepubertal children are at least ten years younger than the individual. If the individual is a late adolescent, no precise age difference is required, and clinical judgment must take into account the age difference as well as the sexual maturity of the child .

5. Exhibitionism (DSM-III 302.40).
To use a phrase made popular in the '60s, Exhibitionism is "letting

it all hang out" or a repetitive pattern of exposing the genitals to an unsuspecting stranger for the purpose of producing sexual excitement. Exhibitionists obtain sexual gratification by exposing themselves and do not attempt other sexual acts with their victims. Almost all exhibitionists, who are sometimes called "flashers," are males, and many are married. They are also not usually dangerous to their victims and often will scurry away if their behavior does not elicit the desired response from the victim. Exhibitionists have the highest recidivism rate of any sexual offenders, with about 20% being rearrested. They constitute about a third of all apprehended sexual offenders, but the prevalence of the disorder among the general population is unknown.

The important diagnostic criterion for Exhibitionism is:

> Repetitive acts of exposing the genitals to an unsuspecting stranger for the purpose of achieving sexual excitement, with no attempt at further sexual activity with the stranger.

Remember, to classify as Exhibitionism, exposure of the genitals must be for the purpose of producing sexual gratification. The "dirty old man" who exhibits his genitals in the middle of the street or hospital corridor may be delirious or demented rather than exhibitionistic.

There are several approaches to dealing with the exhibitionist's problem behavior, and the following story illustrates one novel approach. When an exhibitionist exposed himself to two women who were walking down the street, the first woman turned to the second and calmly stated, "That looks like a penis, only smaller!"

6. Voyeurism (DSM-III 302.82).
    Voyeurism is defined as a repetitive seeking out of situations in which the voyeur looks at an unsuspecting woman who is naked, disrobing, or engaging in sexual activity. He obtains sexual excitement by doing so, and this is the preferred or exclusive method of obtaining sexual excitement. Looking is the only sexual contact, and the voyeur frequently achieves orgasm by masturbation, either during the voyeuristic episode itself or in response to memories of prior voyeuristic episodes. Reported cases of voyeurs, sometimes called "peeping Toms," have all been males.

In general, voyeurs are not dangerous, although being observed by a strange man is frequently upsetting to his victim. Data on the prevalence of this disorder is lacking. Obviously, normal sexual activity includes obtaining sexual excitement from observing one's partner, and this type of behavior, which is generally a precursor to other sexual activity, should not be considered voyeuristic.

The DSM-III diagnostic criteria for Voyeurism are:

A. The individual repeatedly observes unsuspecting people who are either naked, in the act of disrobing, or engaging in sexual activity and no sexual activity with the observed people is sought.

B. The observing is the repeatedly preferred or exclusive method of achieving sexual excitement.

7. Sexual Masochism (DSM-III 302.83).
This disorder is characterized by an individual's obtaining sexual excitement through his own suffering. If either of the following criteria is present, the diagnosis of Sexual Masochism may be made:

(1) A preferred or exclusive mode of producing sexual excitement is to be humiliated, bound, beaten, or otherwise made to suffer.

(2) The individual has intentionally participated in an activity in which he or she was physically harmed or his or her life was threatened, in order to produce sexual excitement.

Masochistic fantasies are not sufficient to diagnose Sexual Masochism; the diagnosis is made only if the individual engages in masochistic sexual acts. In instances in which the individual's life is threatened or physical harm is inflicted, a single well-documented episode is sufficient to make the diagnosis. Individuals with Sexual Masochism vary considerably as to the severity and intensity of the disorder, ranging from occasional acting out of bondage and/or humiliation fantasies to cases in which serious injury or death occurs as the result of intentional acts on the part of the masochist.

No good data exist regarding the prevalence of Sexual Masochism. While it is thought to be a relatively rare disorder, since it is hidden, it may be more prevalent than is generally recognized. The disorder occurs more frequently in males than in females and the disorder tends to be chronic as well. As you might imagine, sexual masochists and sexual sadists make complementary, if somewhat unusual, bedfellows.

8. Sexual Sadism (DSM-III, 302.84).
In contrast to Sexual Masochism, the key feature in Sexual Sadism is obtaining sexual excitement and/or orgasm by inflicting physical or psychological suffering upon another individual. These DSM-III criteria will earmark the diagnosis:

Either A, B, or C:

A. On a nonconsenting partner, the individual has repeatedly intentionally inflicted psychological or physical suffering in order to produce sexual excitement.

B. With a consenting partner, the preferred or exclusive mode of achieving sexual excitement combines humiliation with simulated or mildly injurious bodily suffering.

C. On a consenting partner, bodily injury that is extensive, permanent, or possibly mortal is inflicted in order to achieve sexual excitement.

The severity of Sexual Sadism ranges from individuals who occasionally feel excited by torture fantasies but who do not act them out except in simulated forms to lust murderers who obtain sexual excitement by the death of their partners. Other sexual sadists may brutally torture or rape their victims.

Unlike most of the other Paraphilias we have discussed, Sexual Sadism is a potentially dangerous disorder which poses a major hazard to the safety and well-being of society. It occurs far more frequently in males and, in its more severe forms, occurs almost exclusively in males. In its more extreme forms, Sexual Sadism is generally a chronic disorder.

It is interesting to note that rape is not included as a diagnostic category in DSM-III. While Sexual Sadism may include rape, certainly not all, or even many, rapists are sexual sadists. Current discussions of rape suggest that in most instances rape should not be viewed as a sexual act, but rather, as an act of pure aggression. In making the differential diagnosis the important thing to determine is whether the rapist obtained sexual gratification from the sadistic elements of the act. If this is not the case (a distinction which would be admittedly difficult to make in some cases), Sexual Sadism should not be diagnosed.

9. Atypical Paraphilias (DSM-III 302.90).
    This category is used to classify individuals who do not fit into one of the other types of Paraphilias. The mind boggles at the wide variety of peculiar objects and situations from which certain individuals obtain sexual excitation, and a comprehensive presentation of these other Paraphilias is impossible. However, a partial listing would include: 1) coprophilia (obtaining sexual gratification from feces), 2) frotteurism (obtaining sexual gratification from rubbing one's penis against women in crowded public places), 3) klismaphilia (obtaining sexual gratification from enemas), 4) necrophilia (having sexual intercourse with a corpse), 5) telephone scatologia (obscene phone calls), and 6) urophilia (obtaining gratification from urine).

The Paraphilias are not disorders which come frequently to the attention of primary care physicians. One videotaped example is used for this section. It is of a voyeur. This does not imply that Voyeurism is the most frequently seen or the most serious disorder of the Paraphilias.

****

GO TO VIDEOTAPE

****

C. PSYCHOSEXUAL DYSFUNCTIONS

The characteristic feature in all Psychosexual Dysfunctions is a significant inhibition in the appetitive or psychophysiological changes which characterize the complete sexual response cycle. Sporadic or occasional failures in sexual functioning (e.g., impotence or failure to reach orgasm) are common and do not qualify for diagnosis as Psychosexual Dysfunctions. To be diagnosed, a disturbance should be relatively major and should not be entirely attributable to organic factors or symptomatic of another clinical psychiatric syndrome. Loss of sexual desire is a frequent outcome of Recurrent Major Depressive Disorders, for example, and hence would not be diagnosed as a Psychosexual Dysfunction if the symptom was secondary to the Depressive Disorder.

In order to diagnose Psychosexual Dysfunctions, it is necessary to understand the complete sexual response cycle. Typically, the sexual response cycle has been conceptualized as having four phases: 1) appetitive, 2) excitement, 3) orgasm, and 4) resolution. The appetitive phase consists of fantasies about sexual activity and psychological interest in or desire to engage in sexual activity. · The parasympathetic nervous system tends to predominate during the appetitive phase.

The excitement phase consists of a subjective sense of sexual pleasure, as well as a repertoire of physiological changes which are predominantly mediated by the parasympathetic nervous system. Among males, major changes are penile tumescence leading to erection and secretion of the Cowper's gland. Among females, major changes are vasocongestion in the pelvis, vaginal lubrication, swelling of the external genitalia, development of the orgasmic platform (a narrowing of the outer third of the vagina by increased pubococcygeal muscle tension and vasocongestion), vasocongestion of the labia minora, breast tumescence, and lengthening and widening of the inner two-thirds of the vagina.

The orgasmic phase consists of a peaking of sexual pleasure with release of sexual tension. While men have only one orgasm, women may experience multiple orgasms during the orgasmic phase. In men, the orgasmic reflex is divided into two components -- emission and ejaculation. The first, emission, consists of contractions of the internal reproductive organs (the vas deferens, the prostate, the seminal vesicles, and the internal part of the urethra) and signals the sensation of "ejaculatory inevitability." This visceral response is under the control of the sympathetic branch of the autonomic nervous system. The second component, ejaculation, is experienced as the pleasurable orgasm proper and consists of rhythmic contractions of the bulbar muscles which serve to force semen from the penis. In contrast, the female orgasm is comprised of only one component which is analogous to ejaculation and consists of a series of reflex rhythmic contractions of the circumvaginal and perineal muscles and of the swollen tissues of the orgasmic platform. These contractions may or may not be subjectively experienced by the woman's partner during coitus. Frequently in both genders, orgasm is accompanied by generalized muscular tension or contractions such as involuntary pelvic thrusting.

The resolution phase consists of a sense of relaxation and well-being with a reversal back to parasympathetic predominance. For both sexes the general somatic components of the sexual response diminish rapidly. Increased blood pressure, heart rate, and respiration return to their basal state minutes after orgasm. Men are physiologically refractory to further erection and orgasm during this phase. The duration of the refractory period varies directly with age, growing longer as the man grows older. A decrease in the male's frequency of ejaculation also occurs with increasing age. The elderly man will remain refractory to orgasm longer than to erection and may achieve good erections during subsequent sexual activity, but not be able to feel the urge to ejaculate. The refractory phenomenon is absent in women who may be responsive to further stimulation immediately following the orgasm.

Inhibition may occur during any or all of these four phases of the sexual response cycle. Additionally, the inhibition may be in actual performance, in subjective pleasure or desire, or both. The DSM-III leaves a fair amount of latitude to the clinician in the diagnosis of these disorders, encouraging the clinician to take into account such factors as frequency, chronicity, and effect on other areas of functioning prior to making a diagnosis of Psychosexual Dysfunction. It is imperative to note that a Psychosexual Dysfunction may be diagnosed only after the clinician has determined the disturbance is not caused exclusively by organic factors and that it is not symptomatic of another clinical psychiatric syndrome. Several specific Psychosexual Dysfunctions are listed in the DSM-III, and the diagnostic criteria for each will be listed.

1. Inhibited Sexual Desire (DSM-III 302.71).

    A. Persistent and pervasive inhibition of sexual desire. The judgment of inhibition is made by the clinician's taking into account factors that affect sexual desire such as age, sex, health, intensity and frequency of sexual desire, and the context of this individual's life. In actual practice this diagnosis will rarely be made unless the lack of desire is a source of distress to either the individual or his or her partner. Frequently this category will be used in conjunction with one or more of the other Psychosexual Dysfunction categories.

B. The disturbance is not caused exclusively by organic factors (e.g., physical disorder or medication) and is not due to another Axis I disorder.

****

GO TO VIDEOTAPE

****

2. Inhibited Sexual Excitement (Frigidity, Impotence) (DSM-III 302.72).
This disorder has the following criteria for diagnosis:

A. Recurrent and persistent inhibition of sexual
excitement during sexual activity, manifested by:
In males, partial or complete failure to attain or
maintain erection until the completion of the sexual
act, or

In females, partial or complete failure to attain or
maintain the lubrication-swelling response of sexual
excitement until completion of the sexual act.

B. A clinical judgment that the individual engages in
sexual activity that is adequate in focus,
intensity, and duration.

C. The disturbance is not caused exclusively by organic factors (e.g., physical disorder or medication) and is not due to another Axis I disorder.

****

GO TO VIDEOTAPE

****

3. Inhibited Female Orgasm (DSM-III 302.73).

A. Recurrent and persistent inhibition of the female orgasm as manifested by a delay in or absence of orgasm
following a normal sexual excitement phase during
sexual activity that is judged by the clinician to be
adequate in focus, intensity, and duration. The same
individual may also meet the criteria for Inhibited Sexual Excitement if at other times there is a problem with
the excitement phase of sexual activity. In such cases
both categories of Psychosexual Dysfunction should be
noted.

Some women are able to experience orgasm during non-
coital clitoral stimulation, but are unable to experience

it during coitus in the absence of manual clitoral stimulation. There is evidence to suggest that in some
instances this represents a pathological inhibition that
justifies this diagnosis whereas in other instances it
represents a normal variation of the female sexual
response. This difficult judgment is assisted by a
thorough sexual evaluation, which may even require a
trial of treatment.

    B.   The disturbance is not caused exclusively by organic
factors (e.g., physical disorder or medication) and is
not due to another Axis I disorder.

4.   Inhibited Male Orgasm (DSM-III 302.74).
The following DSM-III diagnostic criteria exist for this disorder:

    A.   Recurrent and persistent inhibition of the male or-
gasm as manifested by a delay in or absence of
ejaculation following an adequate phase of sexual
excitement. The same individual may also meet
the criteria for Inhibited Sexual Excitement if at
other times there is a problem with the excitement
phase of sexual activity. In such cases both categories of Psychosexual Dysfunction should be
noted.

    B.   The disturbance is not caused exclusively by or-
ganic factors (e.g., physical disorder or medication) and is not due to another Axis I disorder.

****

GO TO VIDEOTAPE

****

5.   Premature Ejaculation (DSM-III 302.75).
The following DMS-III diagnostic criteria exist for this disorder:

    A.   Ejaculation occurs before the individual wishes it,
because of recurrent and persistent absence of
reasonable voluntary control of ejaculation and orgasm during sexual activity. The judgment of
"reasonable control" is made by the clinician's taking into account factors that affect duration of the
excitement phase, such as age, novelty of the
sexual partner, and the frequency and duration of
coitus.

    B.   The disturbance is not due to another Axis I dis-
order.

```
***********************************************************************

                         GO TO VIDEOTAPE

***********************************************************************
```

6. Functional Dyspareunia (DSM-III 302.76).
   The following DSM-III diagnostic criteria exist for this disorder:

   A. Coitus is associated with recurrent and persistent genital pain, in either the male or the female.

   B. The disturbance is not caused exclusively by a physical disorder, and is not due to lack of lubrication, Functional Vaginismus, or another Axis I disorder.

7. Functional Vaginismus (DSM-III 302.51).
   The following DSM-III diagnostic criteria exist for this disorder:

   A. There is a history of recurrent and persistent involuntary spasm of the musculature of the outer third of the vagina that interferes with coitus.
   B. The disturbance is not caused exclusively by a physical disorder, and is not due to another Axis I disorder.

8. Atypical Psychosexual Dysfunctions(DSM-III 302.70).
   The DSM-III describes this as a residual category to be used for Psychosexual Dysfunctions which are not easily classifiable elsewhere.

D. OTHER PSYCHOSEXUAL DISORDERS

1. Ego-Dystonic Homosexuality (DSM-III 302.00).
   The key features in this disorder are: 1) a desire to acquire or increase heterosexual arousal to initiate or maintain heterosexual relationships and 2) a sustained pattern of overt homosexual arousal that the individual explicitly complains is unwanted and is a source of distress. Frequently, the individual has a history of unsuccessful attempts at initiating heterosexual relationships. Often in adults, there is a strong desire to have a family life and children. Such individuals have often had homosexual relationships but experience little satisfaction because of strong negative feelings about homosexuality. There is little information regarding prevalence of the disorder or about whether it occurs more frequently among males or females. It is important to note that the DSM-III does not classify homosexuality per se as a mental disorder. The DSM-III diagnostic criteria for Ego-Dystonic Homosexuality are the following:

A. The individual complains that heterosexual arousal is persistently absent or weak and significantly interferes with initiating or maintaining wanted heterosexual relationships.

B. There is a sustained pattern of homosexual arousal that the individual explicitly states has been unwanted and a persistent source of distress.

There has been and continues to be, a tremendous controversy regarding the status of homosexuality per se as a mental disorder. Some clinicians, not to mention some extremely self-righteous private citizens, believe that homosexuality is always the result of some mental disorder and/or moral defect. Other clinicians and investigators cite evidence that many homosexuals lead well-adjusted, happy, productive lives and experience no distress over their sexual preference, and state that there is no reason to call homosexuality a disorder under these conditions. Those who state that homosexuality is not a disorder note that parts of this society still have heavy sanctions against homosexuality, while other parts are indifferent to it or are even supportive. These differences of opinion illustrate quite nicely the fact that the DSM-III is a classification system which reflects political as well as medical/diagnostic considerations. The issue was resolved by a vote of the members of the American Psychiatric Association, which voted that homosexuality was not a mental disorder. The DSM-III classification reflects the outcome of this vote. Irrespective of this political process, it is fair to say that there is little definitive scientific information about the etiology of homosexuality or about the psychological adjustment of homosexuals as a group.

2. Psychosexual Disorders Not Elsewhere Classified.
This DSM-III category is a residual category for coding mental disorders with a disturbance in sexuality which have not been covered by other diagnostic categories. The following are a few examples of disturbances which would fall in this category: 1) Marked feelings of inadequacy related to self-imposed standards of masculinity or femininity, such as body habitus, or size and shape of sex organs; 2) impaired pleasure during the normal physiological pelvic responses of orgasm; 3) distress over a pattern of repeated sexual conquests with a succession of individuals who exist only as things to be used (Don Juanism and Nymphomania).

QUIZ, Section II.

Circle the correct answer(s). <u>One</u> or <u>more</u> <u>than</u> <u>one</u> answer may be correct.

1. Psychosexual Disorders are subdivided into

   a. Gender Identity Disorders.
   b. Paraphilias.
   c. Psychosexual Disorders occurring secondary to medical disorders.
   d. Psychosexual Dysfunctions.
   e. Other Psychosexual Disorders.

2. According to DSM-III, to be classified as a Psychosexual Disorder, the etiology of the disorder

   a. must be primarily physical or organic.
   b. must be primarily psychological.
   c. may be physical <u>or</u> psychological, depending on the specific Psychosexual Disorder you are diagnosing.
   d. may be mixed, involving both primary organic and psychological factors.

3. The important feature(s) in all Gender Identity Disorders is (are)

   a. there is a discrepancy between gender identity and anatomical sex.
   b. there is a discrepancy between gender role and gender identity.
   c. there is a discrepancy between anatomical sex and chromosomal makeup.

4. Which of the following is (are) included among the diagnostic criteria for males and females for Gender Identity Disorder of Childhood?

   a. persistent rejection of stereotypical sex role behavior
   b. persistent repudiation of anatomic sexual attributes
   c. persistently stated desire to be or assertion that he is a member of the opposite sex
   d. the disturbance has been continuous for two years

5. Paraphilias are characterized by repetitive sexually arousing fantasies associated with repetitive

   a. sexual activity with a nonconsenting person.
   b. desire to live as a member of the opposite sex.
   c. sexual activity involving real or simulated suffering or humiliation.
   d. preference for use of a nonhuman object for sexual arousal.
   e. seeking of adult partners of the same sex for affectional sexual gratification.

6. In the sexual response cycle the appetitive phase consists of

    a. subjective sense of sexual pleasure with accompanying physiological change.
    b. fantasies about sex.
    c. interest in or desire to engage in sex.
    d. ejaculatory inevitability.

7. Inhibition in the sexual response cycle may occur

    a. in all four of the phases.
    b. in the excitement and orgasmic phases, only.
    c. in the performance of all Paraphilias.
    d. in the subjective pleasure received from sexual acts.

Use the following case history to answer questions 8-11.

Mr. and Mrs. T. came to their family physician complaining of marital discord. They are both in their early thirties, college-educated, and aspiring in their respective careers--he as a certified accountant with a large corporation and she as an attorney with a prestigious law firm. They have been married nine years and have no children. Mrs. T. complains that her husband has no interest in her sexually; she is feeling angry at him for not initiating sex more frequently and wonders if her career threatens his masculinity. In response to his wife's comments, Mr. T. states, "Of course I find my wife sexually attractive, and I feel like we should have sex more often. I'm just tired when I get home from work; I've been under a lot of pressure lately." A sexual history reveals that although the couple used to enjoy sexual relations approximately two times weekly, for the past eight months they have been attempting to have sex only once or twice a month, and on almost all of these occasions Mrs. T. is the initiator. Furthermore, Mr. T. has been unable to maintain an erection sufficient for penetration on over half of the occasions on which they attempted sex in the past eight months. On those occasions on which Mr. T. maintains an erection he experiences orgasm and ejaculation without difficulty.

8. When considering Mr. T.'s sexual problem the physician should

    a. rule out the presence of another psychiatric syndrome.
    b. rule out the presence of organic or medical factors which may be leading to his sexual disinterest and his performance problem.
    c. determine the presence of Ego-Syntonic Homosexuality.
    d. determine whether the attempts at sexual intercourse are adequate in focus and duration to produce erection.

9. Providing the physician determines Mr. T. is clinically depressed, the appropriate diagnosis would

    a. be Episodic Depression with a Secondary Psychosexual Dysfunction of Inhibited Sexual Excitement.
    b. be Episodic Depression with a Secondary Psychosexual Dysfunction of Inhibited Sexual Desire.

    c.   not include a Psychosexual Dysfunction.
    d.   require that both a and b be included in the diagnosis.

10.   Providing the physician can find no evidence of a psychiatric syndrome or of organic factors which are leading to Mr. T.'s sexual difficulties the appropriate diagnosis would be

    a.   Inhibited Sexual Desire.
    b.   Inhibited Sexual Excitement.
    c.   Inhibited Male Orgasm.

11.   Providing the physician can find no evidence of another psychiatric syndrome or of organic factors which are leading to Mrs. T.'s sexual difficulties, the appropriate diagnosis for her would be

    a.   Psychosexual Dysfunction with Inhibited Sexual Desire.
    b.   Psychosexual Dysfunction with Inhibited Sexual Excitement.
    c.   Psychosexual Disorder not Elsewhere Classified (Nymphomania).
    d.   None of the above.

Use the following case history to answer questions 12-14.

Ms. M. has contacted her OB-GYN specialist because of sexual problems arising with her boyfriend. Interview reveals that Ms. M. feels sexually attracted to her boyfriend and desires to have intercourse with him. However, intercourse is persistently painful for Ms. M., and she has recurring inability to reach a climax during coitus. Further questioning indicates that although there is sufficient lubrication to allow comfortable insertion of the penis, as sexual activity continues the lubrication decreases markedly and penetration becomes increasingly uncomfortable.

12.   In order to diagnose Ms. M.'s problem appropriately, the clinician must

    a.   rule out Latent Ego-Dystonic Homosexuality.
    b.   investigate organic factors, including medications, which might cause her problems.
    c.   determine whether a psychiatric syndrome is present which might lead to her sexual problems.
    d.   determine whether Ms. M. and her boyfriend are engaging in sexual activity of adequate intensity and duration to produce orgasm for Ms. M.

13.   Providing it is determined that no organic or psychiatric syndromes are causing Ms. M.'s sexual problems, and that her sexual activity is of adequate intensity and duration, which of the following diagnoses is (are) appropriate?

    a.   Functional Vaginismus
    b.   Functional Dyspareunia
    c.   Inhibited Female Orgasm
    d.   Inhibited Sexual Excitement

14. Providing Ms. M.'s sexual problems are not caused exclusively by organic factors or another psychiatric syndrome and that she can reach an orgasm when coitus is accompanied by manual clitoral stimulation, the correct diagnosis

     a. continues to include Inhibited Sexual Excitement.
     b. continues to include Functional Dyspareunia.
     c. continues to include Inhibited Female Orgasm.
     d. may or may not include Psychosexual Dysfunction with Inhibited Female Orgasm as more information is needed to make this determination.

15. Mr. A., a 28-year-old white male, was self-referred to an outpatient psychiatric clinic. Mr. A. expressed a desire to have sexual relations with his girlfriend of two weeks, but reported that he was unable to maintain his arousal long enough to achieve penetration. The client's history reveals prior unsuccessful attempts at establishing sexual relationships with women. Furthermore, he reports that although he is able to perform sexually with other men, he does not want to engage in this type of sexual activity. In fact, he feels intensely remorseful following sex with men. When speaking of his feelings of remorse the patient begins to cry and states that he feels totally confused about why he continues to engage in sex with men when he really doesn't want to be identified as a homosexual. The most likely diagnosis for the fellow is

     a. Inhibited Sexual Excitement.
     b. Ego-Dystonic Homosexuality.
     c. Gender Identity Disorder.
     d. Transsexualism.
     e. Ego-Syntonic Homosexuality.

Use the following case history to answer questions 16-18 only.

Mr. J. is a 32-year-old white male who presented at an outpatient psychiatric clinic stating he desired counseling in preparation for a sex-change operation. Interview revealed that Mr. J. had been married for 12 years, and was currently employed as a hair stylist. History revealed that the patient had been cross-dressing as a female off and on since the age of 13. Until the past year the cross-dressing had been confined to his home, and he had enjoyed infrequent, though satisfactory, sex with his wife. Approximately a year ago, however, his sexual relationship with his wife had deteriorated and he had begun to experience increasingly frequent urges to go out in public dressed as a woman. At that time he also began to feel that he was "not meant to be a man" but, rather, a woman, and he began hating his male genitalia and wishing to change them. This persistent and intense wish had prompted his current request for a sexual reassignment.

TRUE or FALSE: Circle the correct letter.

T   F   16. Given that Mr. J. has no genetic abnormality or another mental disorder, his symptoms fulfill the DSM-III diagnostic criteria for Transsexualism.

T   F   17. Mr. J. exhibits several behavioral characteristics of trans-sexuals in that he sought a stereotypically feminine occupation and had gender identity problems in adolescence as evidenced by his cross-dressing.

T   F   18. Mr. J.'s sexual history may best be classified as asexual.

T   F   19. Paraphilias represent a severe impairment in the ability to engage in affectionate sexual activity with an adult partner.

T   F   20. Paraphiliacs are overwhelmingly predominately males.

T   F   21. By definition, Transvestism, Voyeurism, and Pedophilia occur only in men.

T   F   22. Pedophilia occurs more frequently among homosexuals.

T   F   23. Exhibitionists and voyeurs are usually not dangerous to their victims.

T   F   24. In both Exhibitionism and Voyeurism, the diagnostic criteria include the elements of: 1) repetitiveness, 2) the act of exposure or looking is accompanied by sexual excitement, and 3) no further contact occurs with the victim.

T   F   25. In Sexual Masochism, the individual must intentionally submit to harm, while in Sexual Sadism harm is inflicted on a nonconsenting partner.

Match the following Paraphilias with the phrase which best summarizes the core feature of the syndrome.

_____26. use of animals as the preferred method of obtaining sexual excitement

_____27. looking at unsuspecting women is the only sexual contact

_____28. use of nonliving objects as the preferred method for securing sexual excitement

_____29. repetitive sexual activity with prepubertal children

_____30. obtaining sexual excitement through submitting to physical harm or humiliation

_____31. persistent cross-dressing by heterosexual males

a. Sexual Sadism
b. Exhibitionism
c. Transvestism
d. Voyeurism
e. Zoophilia
f. Sexual Masochism
g. Fetishism
h. Pedophilia

_____32. repetitive exposure of genitals to unsuspecting
strangers for obtaining sexual excitement
_____33. obtaining sexual excitement by inflicting physical
or psychological harm

Match the following sexual response cycles with the corresponding nervous system.

34. predominates in the appetitive phase of the sexual response cycle
35. mediates the excitement phase of the sexual response cycle
36. mediates the emission component of the orgasmic phase of the sexual response cycle
37. controls the resolution phase of the sexual response cycle

a. sympathetic nervous system
b. parasympathetic nervous system

III. TREATMENT OF PSYCHOSEXUAL DISORDERS

Having first discussed common myths about human sexuality and then presented the DSM-III diagnostic categories for the Psychosexual Disorders, we will devote the remainder of this chapter to treatment of Psychosexual Disorders. Obviously, a comprehensive discussion of treatment approaches is beyond the scope of this chapter, but we would like to present some basic information on this topic. The reader interested in a more detailed discussion of treatment approaches should consult one of several excellent references on the topic (e.g., Kaplan, 1974; LoPiccolo & LoPiccolo, 1978; Masters & Johnson, 1970). After completion of this chapter, you will not know how to treat Psychosexual Disorders. However, it is quite important that you know that many Psychosexual Disorders are treatable.

Prior to presentation of specific treatment information, some general aspects of treatment intervention will be considered. One important consideration is whether or not a treatment intervention is warranted. The sexual behavior of some individuals may differ from usual cultural or social rules and mores. These variations in sexual behavior may be at either extreme, involving nonparticipation in any form of sexual activity or participation in activities condemned by the general society such as group sex, mate swapping, homosexuality, or casual sex. While these deviations from the norm may systematically alienate individuals from general society, variant sexual behaviors are not necessarily pathological or abnormal and do not always require change. An attempt by the physician to change the sexual behavior of a patient should usually not be undertaken unless the patient expresses a desire to change, excepting situations in which the behavior is clearly injurious to the patient or to others. Variant types of sexual activity which are not harmful to the participants, if carried out by consenting adults who are free of any coercion and if done privately, should be considered acceptable behavior, even if others choose not to participate in similar activities. Sexual behavior should be deemed acceptable if it meets three criteria:

1) It is not harmful to the participants.
2) Participants in the behavior are consenting adults who are free of any coercion.
3) The activity takes place away from unwilling observers.

Gender Identity Disorders are quite difficult to treat if the treatment goal is to change the gender identity to match the patient's anatomical sex. Particularly with transsexuals, treatment often focuses upon changing the patient's anatomical sexual characteristics to be congruent with his or her gender identity. Generally such treatment begins with a thorough evaluation to insure that the patient is truly a transsexual and really understands the consequences of sex change procedures. Treatment should include a considerable amount of psychological counseling as well as administration of hormones appropriate to the gender identity the patient wishes to adopt. After a period of time (at least one year) during which the patient cross-dresses and takes appropriate hormones, surgical procedures may be initiated which change the patient's external genitalia to match his or her gender identity. Obviously, sexual reassignment surgery is a serious procedure which should not be done without careful assessment and counseling.

With respect to paraphiliacs, the chief problems in treatment are the following. First, the paraphiliac is sexually aroused by an inappropriate object or person and is not sufficiently aroused by "normal" sexual activity. Second, the paraphiliac is often rather satisfied with this state of affairs and is not particularly motivated to change his or her behavior. Thus, the paraphiliac's behavior is more frequently disturbing to other people than it is to himself, a state of affairs which leads to reduced motivation for treatment.

Many approaches for treating Paraphilias exist, but behavior therapists have been particularly active in developing treatment approaches for these conditions. Behaviorists generally assume that the deviant sexual arousal patterns exhibited by paraphiliacs have been learned and that more appropriate arousal patterns can be learned and substituted for the deviant ones. Behavioral treatment approaches often involve direct measurement of sexual arousal to both deviant and "normal" sexual stimuli and/or fantasies. Penile tumescence and vaginal blood flow changes in response to sexual stimuli are measured to produce information on arousal patterns. Treatment approaches then focus on reducing sexual arousal to deviant stimuli and increasing sexual arousal to "normal" stimuli. Frequently, paraphiliacs are found to have poor social skills as well; that is, they have difficulty dealing with members of the opposite sex in an effective, appropriate manner. Therefore, treatment may also include social skills training in which they are taught how to make conversation, ask for dates, etc. Paraphiliacs are difficult to treat, but these approaches have been used with some success.

Sexual dysfunction is a problem for many patients, and the physician will see many such patients. Indeed, Masters and Johnson (1970) concluded from their research that 50% of American marriages suffer from sexual inadequacies. The sexual dysfunction syndromes differ to some degree with regard to prognosis. In general, however, the results of therapy outcome studies are encouraging in that the majority of patients with these disorders respond favorably to a variety of treatment modalities.

With the sexual dysfunctions of males, Premature Ejaculation is the most responsive to sex therapy. Kaplan's (1974) results indicate Premature Ejaculation is virtually always amenable to brief treatment techniques, and Masters and Johnson (1970) reported a 98% cure rate.

Inhibited Sexual Excitement (Impotence) also shows a good prognosis for rapid remission, particularly in males who have previously functioned well but subsequently developed difficulties. Masters and Johnson (1970) reported an initial cure rate of 74%. Relapse of the impotent patient is usually related to stress and life situations or environmental changes.

While Inhibited Male Orgasm has the poorest prognosis among the sexual dysfunctions of males, the consensus seems to be that 50 to 60% of males with this disorder respond to brief treatment procedures (Kaplan, 1974; Masters & Johnson, 1970). Moreover, the cure achieved appears to be quite stable and relatively resistant to changes occurring in the individual's life circumstances.

With regard to sexual dysfunctions in women, treatment of Functional Vaginismus has met with excellent and permanent results using brief treatment techniques. Masters and Johnson (1970) reported a 100% cure rate, using progressive dilation of the vagina during heterosexual encounters. In addition, 100% cure rates have been reported by gynecologists who used gradual dilation of the spastic vagina and concurrent education (Kaplan, 1974).

Inhibited Sexual Excitement in women shows a lesser, though still "good," prognosis for improvement with brief therapy. Kaplan (1974) reported that the "great majority" of women with Inhibited Sexual Excitement achieve enhanced sexual response with treatment. She cautions, however, that response to treatment appears to be dependent, to a greater extent than is true with male dysfunctions, on the quality of the relationship the patient has with her sexual partner.

With Inhibited Female Orgasm, the cure rate is virtually 100% if the criterion for a cure is based solely on ability to achieve orgasm. Kaplan (1974) reported the "great majority" of women with orgasmic dysfunction are able to reach orgasm in heterosexual settings, given brief treatment procedures.

The woman who is highly responsive but suffers from coital orgasmic dysfunction has a less favorable prognosis.

Some patients experiencing sexual dysfunction will identify their problem to the physician and seek help. However, many patients with sexual dysfunctions will be too shy or embarrassed to discuss their problem unless they are specifically asked about potential problems in a sympathetic, supportive manner.

ANSWERS, Section II. _____

1.	a,b,d,e	13.	c,d	26.	e
2.	b	14.	a,d	27.	d
3.	a	15.	b	28.	g
4.	b,c	16.	F	29.	h
5.	a,c,d	17.	T	30.	f
6.	b,c	18.	F	31.	c
7.	a,d	19.	T	32.	b
8.	a,b,d	20.	T	33.	a
9.	c	21.	F	34.	b
10.	a,b	22.	F	35.	b
11.	d	23.	T	36.	a
12.	b,c,d	24.	T	37.	b
		25.	F		

For this reason, questions regarding sexual functioning should be routinely included in medical histories and patient evaluations. The physician should be particularly careful to evaluate sexual functioning when problems such as marital discord or depression are evident, as these problems along with many psychological disorders often have concomitant symptoms of sexual dysfunction. In addition, since sexual dysfunction is a frequent consequence of certain medical disorders such as diabetes mellitus and of certain treatment regimens such as that for chronic hypertension, when these conditions are present the physician should take a thorough sexual history and encourage the patient to discuss the sexual ramifications of his disease. A complete sexual history should include information concerning: 1) the nature, onset, and duration of the sexual problem; 2) the relationship of the partners, particularly issues concerning commitment, conflicts, and power struggles; 3) family background regarding sex education; 4) sexual development including early sexual experiences; 5) the exact pattern of sexual response for each partner; 6) evidence of "involuntary" normal sexual responses such as morning erections in an impotent man; and, of course, 7) a thorough medical history including medications taken which may contribute to the sexual problem.

QUIZ, Section III.

Circle the correct answer(s). One or more than one answer may be correct.

1. Behavioral treatment programs for paraphiliacs often involve

   a. blood flow studies to measure sexual arousal patterns.
   b. punishing sexual arousal to deviant stimuli.
   c. increasing sexual arousal to appropriate stimuli.
   d. social skills training.

2. Which of the following types of information should be elicited when taking a sexual history?

    a. the onset, duration, and nature of the sexual problem
    b. evidence of involuntary "normal" sexual responses
    c. evidence of successful resolution of the Oedipal complex
    d. the quality of the relationship between the partners

TRUE or FALSE: Circle the correct letter.

T   F   3. The clinician should follow his own instincts when attempting to change the sexual behavior of a patient, regardless of whether the patient expresses a desire to change.

T   F   4. Gender Identity Disorders are easily treated, with a good cure rate.

T   F   5. Sex change operations with transsexuals should be undertaken only <u>after</u> extensive counseling and a period of time during which the patient has cross-dressed, received hormones, and assumed the gender identity of the sex he or she wishes to be.

T   F   6. The majority of sexual dysfunction syndromes do not respond favorably to brief treatment.

T   F   7. Premature Ejaculation and Functional Vaginismus virtually always respond to treatment, with cure rates nearing 100%.

T   F   8. The cure rate in impotent males is approximately 75%, if the individual is otherwise healthy and there is no physical cause for the disorder.

T   F   9. With treatment, nearly all women who suffer from Inhibited Female Orgasm are able to reach orgasm, but the prognosis for coital orgasm is less favorable.

T   F   10. Since sexual problems rarely occur concomitantly with medical problems and other psychiatric syndromes, the clinician need not take a sexual history unless the patient mentions the subject of sex first.

T   F   11. Since numerous medications affect portions of the normal sexual response cycle, it is important to inquire about current medications when a patient complains of sexual dysfunction.

ANSWERS, Section III. _____

1. a,b,c,d
2. a,b,d
3. F
4. F
5. T
6. F
7. T
8. T
9. T
10. F
11. T

POST-TEST

For the following questions, circle the letter corresponding to the <u>one</u> correct answer.

1. The most dangerous Paraphilia is

    a. Fetishism.
    b. Exhibitionism.
    c. Sexual Masochism.
    d. Sexual Sadism.
    e. Zoophilia.

2. Which of the following is <u>not</u> characteristic of Paraphilias?

    a. preference for nonhuman object for sexual arousal
    b. sexual activity with humans involving real or simulated suffering or humiliation
    c. sexual activity with consenting adults
    d. sexual activity with nonconsenting adults

3. Which of the following is <u>not</u> classified as a Psychosexual Dysfunction?

    a. Inhibited Sexual Desire
    b. Inhibited Sexual Excitement
    c. Inhibited Female Orgasm
    d. Multiple Orgasmic Failure in Females
    e. Premature Ejaculation
    f. Functional Vaginismus

4. Which of the following is <u>not</u> a part of the sexual response cycle?

    a. appetitive
    b. excitement
    c. repetitive
    d. orgasm
    e. resolution

For each of the following questions, <u>one</u> or <u>more</u> than <u>one</u> answer may be correct. Circle the correct answer(s).

5. Which of the following would <u>not</u> be classified as a Paraphilia?

    a. Homosexuality
    b. Voyeurism
    c. Pedophilia
    d. Sexual Sadism
    e. Zoophilia

6. Which of the following is (are) considered Psychosexual Disorders by DSM-III?

    a.   Gender Identity Disorders
    b.   Paraphilias
    c.   Psychosexual Dysfunction

TRUE or FALSE: Circle the correct letter.

T   F   7. During the excitement phase of the sexual response cycle, physiological changes are mediated primarily by the parasympathetic nervous system.

T   F   8. Psychosexual Dysfunction can occur in all but the appetitive portion of the sexual response cycle.

T   F   9. Our culture encourages children to explore their sexuality.

T   F   10. It is permissible to diagnose relatively minor disturbances and/or those which result from organic factors as Psychosexual Disorders according to DSM-III.

T   F   11. Penis size varies more in the flaccid than in the erect state.

T   F   12. There are two types of orgasms among women - clitoral and vaginal.

T   F   13. Most fetishists are males.

T   F   14. During the orgasmic phase, sympathetic nervous system activity predominates.

T   F   15. Transsexuals are individuals who dress up in the clothes of the opposite sex.

T   F   16. Unfortunately, most Psychosexual Disorders do not respond well to treatment.

T   F   17. Homosexuality should always be classified as a Psychosexual Disorder.

T   F   18. Psychoanalytic therapy is the treatment of choice for most cases of Psychosexual Dysfunction.

T   F   19. Most exhibitionists are dangerous.

T   F   20. Zoophilia is defined as an insatiable desire to make love in the public zoo.

T   F   21. Masochists and sadists together make good bedfellows.

T   F   22. Transvestites generally prefer sex with those of their same gender.

T   F   23. Anatomical sexual characteristics and gender identity must be different for an individual to be diagnosed as having a Gender Identity Disorder.

T   F   24. A child whose gender identity and anatomical sexual characteristics are different would be diagnosed as having Gender Disorder of Childhood.

PRE-TEST ANSWERS

1.	a,b,c	13.	F
2.	a,e	14.	T
3.	c	15.	F
4.	d	16.	F
5.	c	17.	T
6.	d	18.	F
7.	F	19.	F
8.	T	20.	T
9.	F	21.	T
10.	T	22.	F
11.	F	23.	F
12.	T	24.	F

POST-TEST ANSWERS

1.	d	13.	T
2.	c	14.	T
3.	d	15.	F
4.	c	16.	F
5.	a	17.	F
6.	a,b,c	18.	F
7.	T	19.	F
8.	F	20.	F
9.	F	21.	T
10.	F	22.	F
11.	T	23.	T
12.	F	24.	T

REFERENCES

Diagnostic and statistical manual of mental disorders (3rd ed.) Washington, D.C.: American Psychiatric Association, 1980.

Falk, G. J. The truth about sex offenders. Sexology, 1965, 32, 271-273.

Kaplan, H. S. The new sex therapy: Active treatment of sexual dysfunctions. New York: Brunner/Mazel, 1974.

Kinsey, A. C., Pomeroy, W. B., Martin, C. E., & Gebhard, P. H. Sexual behavior in the human female. Philadelphia: W.B. Saunders, 1953.

LoPiccolo, J., & LoPiccolo, L. (Eds.) Handbook of sex therapy. New York: Plenum Press, 1978.

Masters, W. H., & Johnson, V. E. Human sexual inadequacy. Boston: Little, Brown, 1970.

McCary, J. L. Human sexuality. New York: Van Nostrand Reinhold Company, 1967.

CHAPTER 12

Impulse Control Disorders
Lorenz Villeponteaux, Ph.D.

CHAPTER OUTLINE

LEARNING OBJECTIVES

After completing this chapter you will be able to:

1. Describe the psychoanalytic and psychodynamic concept of impulsivity.

2. Describe the learning theory concept of impulsivity.

3. Describe the organic basis for impulsive behavior.

4. Differentiate between normal and pathological levels of impulsive behavior.

5. Describe the connection between hyperactive behavior in childhood and lowered levels of impulse control in adulthood.

6. Name and define the criteria for the diagnosis of Pathological Gambling.

7. Differentiate between Pathological Gambling and Manic-Depressive Illness.

8. Define the concept of "chasing" seen in Pathological Gambling.

9. Name and define the criteria for the diagnosis of Kleptomania.

10. Differentiate between Kleptomania and Antisocial Personality (Conduct Disorders in children).

11. Name and define the criteria for the diagnosis of Pyromania.

12. Name the triad of behaviors in childhood which some claim predict violent and dangerous behavior in adulthood.

13. Name three other psychiatric illnesses with which firesetting may be associated.

14. Name and define the diagnostic criteria for Intermittent Explosive Disorder and for Isolated Explosive Disorder.

15. Differentiate between Intermittent and Isolated Explosive Disorders.

16. Name three other terms used to describe the Explosive Disorders.

17. Differentiate between Explosive Disorders and Dissociative Disorder.

18. Differentiate between Explosive Disorders and Antisocial Personality (Conduct Disorder in children).

19. Name the four common features associated with poor impulse control and episodes of destructive behavior, as described by Mark and Ervin (1970).

PRE-TEST

For each of the following questions, <u>one</u> or <u>more</u> <u>than</u> <u>one</u> answer may be correct. Circle the correct answer(s).

1. Impulses are sometimes

    a. ego-syntonic.
    b. controlled by defense mechanisms.
    c. ego-dystonic.
    d. converted to words (rather than action).

2. It is thought that, neuroanatomically, aggressive, attack behaviors may be interactive with

    a. autonomic nervous system.
    b. limbic system.
    c. neocortex.
    d. pineal gland.

3. Psychodynamically, which of the following is (are) considered to be features of kleptomaniacs?

    a. tension
    b. anxiety
    c. conflict
    d. guilt

4. Which of the following pieces of information would be important for you to have in order to diagnose Kleptomania?

    a. whether or not the individual suffers from delusions or hallucinations
    b. the person experienced orgasm at the time of the theft
    c. whether the person was alone or with someone else at the time of the theft
    d. the usefulness of the object stolen

5. Which of the following disorders must be ruled out before making a diagnosis of Pyromania?

    a. Schizophrenia
    b. Antisocial Personality Disorder
    c. Conduct Disorder
    d. Klein-Levin syndrome

6. There are two types of Explosive Personality Disorders described in DSM-III, Intermittent and Isolated. These are distinguished from each other in terms of the

    a. quantity of the violent episodes.
    b. presence or absence of remorse about the violent episodes.
    c. quality of the violent episodes.
    d. object (person or thing) of the violent episode.

7. Mark and Ervin have listed certain characteristics of individuals who exhibit poor impulse control along with periods of destructive behavior. These characteristics include which of the following?

    a. physical assault
    b. pathological intoxication
    c. impulsive sexual behavior
    d. numerous traffic violations

8. Differential diagnosis of Explosive Disorders should include

    a. Schizophrenia.
    b. Antisocial Personality Disorder.
    c. Conduct Disorder.
    d. Dissociative Disorder.

9. Reading the psychiatric literature on Intermittent Explosive Disorders you will find which of the following used as synonymous for this entity?

    a. Epileptoid Personality Disorder
    b. Episodic Dyscontrol Syndrome
    c. Explosive Personality Disorder
    d. Instinct Dyscontrol

10. In the framework of learning theory, control of impulsive behavior is

    a. referred to as passive-avoidance behavior or nonbehavior.
    b. related to the conditioning of an aversive state of arousal.
    c. attained through developing ego function.
    d. usually dependent on aversive conditioning.

11. Which of the following would rule out a diagnosis of Kleptomania?

    a. an increased sense of tension prior to the act of stealing
    b. a history of six acts of stealing
    c. a concurrent diagnosis of Antisocial Personality Disorder
    d. the use of two confederates to carry out the theft

12. In psychodynamic theory the control of impulses is primarily a function of

    a. id.
    b. ego.
    c. superego.
    d. society.
    e. genetics.

13. Pathological Gambling as a disorder is determined by the amount of money

    a. risked.
    b. lost.
    c. won.
    d. none of the above.

14. Which of the following is <u>not</u> in the triad of behaviors which, when seen in children, is said to predict violent and dangerous behavior in adulthood?

    a. firesetting
    b. enuresis
    c. autism
    d. cruelty to animals

TRUE or FALSE: Circle the correct letter.

T F 15. Impulses to do things which are socially unacceptable (such as, stealing, sexual promiscuity, fighting) are pathological.

T F 16. A 25-year-old male has been diagnosed as having Intermittent Explosive Disorder. EEG reveals the likelihood of a temporal lobe lesion. You begin treating him with Dilantin and find that both the frequency and severity of the violent episodes decrease. You should include psychotherapy in his treatment regimen.

Define the following.

17. Define the concept of "chasing" as it is applied to pathological gamblers.

_____

_____

_____
_____

I. INTRODUCTION

You have already learned about <u>impulsivity</u> as a symptom of a variety of psychiatric disorders. As a symptom it figures very prominently in the antisocial personality, in Conduct Disorders in Children, in some Organic Mental Disorders, in manic episodes, and in the Paraphilias. It is also frequently seen in the Schizophrenias as well as in Dissociative Disorders.

This chapter deals with disorders of impulse control which have not been classified elsewhere in the DSM-III. These disorders have as a common thread running through them an apparent inability to control impulses, specifically impulses to act in a socially unacceptable manner.

If one accepts the notion that being subject to impulses in varying degrees of quality and quantity is a part of the human condition, and, moreover, that there is a wide range of ability to control these impulses (that is, to keep them from being converted into unacceptable action), then it is important to look at impulsivity from an etiological standpoint.

A. PSYCHODYNAMIC THEORY AND IMPULSES

Within the framework of the structural theory of the personality the id is the source of basic needs or drives, and it demands satisfaction of these needs or drives. It becomes the function of the ego to postpone gratification of id drives, to <u>control</u> them.

The uncontrolled id always demands immediate gratification of needs. For example, the hunger drive stirs the neonate to action regardless of the time or place. (The rooting reflex, even though it is genetically programmed or instinctual, might well be viewed as a primitive kind of impulsive behavior related to the hunger drive.) A delay in satisfying the hunger drive often produces in the infant a reaction which can best be described as rage. It is only after the ego begins to form and function that the young child is able to postpone gratification.

The process of what is called "socialization" of children takes place primarily through the development of the ego which exerts controls on the drives of the id. This process begins with controls being exercised externally. That is to say, parents or their substitutes control the behavior of the child from without. The process continues with the child incorporating these controls internally so that the parent no longer has to be physically present to inhibit a forbidden behavior.

[If you do not understand these concepts you should review Chapter 2. For further elaboration of the concept of the development of internal controls see Redl and Wineman (1957).]

It should be obvious that the process of learning to internalize controls is a gradual one and its development extends over a period of years. Furthermore, the concept of ego control is not subject to the "all-or-none" law. There are certain areas of control established first, and then other areas of control develop later -- or perhaps fail to develop later. The important point here is that one of the major functions of the ego is to control impulses, i.e., to keep behavior within the bounds set by society as initially represented by parents.

Grossbard (1962) suggests that normally we all learn to control our impulses by converting them into language, fantasies, or symbols. For example, we usually do not act on an impulse to take unlawful possession of a particularly attractive sports car (which just happens to have the key in the ignition). Rather, we may control the impulse by converting it to a fantasy of us driving around town in the car, or we may talk about how exciting it would be to own such a car.

There are a great many other examples of normal, healthy ways of dealing with impulses. By late adolescence or certainly by young adulthood most males have stopped acting on the impulse to be physically aggressive. They may well have converted these impulses to verbal aggressions in the form of sarcasm, arguing, or criticism, to say nothing of mildly passive aggressive behaviors. One of the most popular ways the adolescent or young adult deals with the aggressive impulse is by using sports such as football to express the impulse in a socially acceptable manner.

It is often said that aggressive impulses are symbolically expressed by many surgeons. It is theorized by some that by the use of sublimation (see Chapter 2) the surgeon has rechanneled the impulses into a behavior which is not only socially acceptable, but also highly regarded and rewarding.

Psychodynamic theory differentiates between Impulse Disorders and Anxiety Disorders (generally referred to as neuroses in other classification systems such as the DSM-II) in terms of the effect on the ego. For one suffering from an impulse disorder, the thoughts, feelings, and behaviors associated with the impulses are ego-syntonic; on the other hand the thoughts, feelings, and behaviors associated with the Anxiety Disorders are said to be ego-dystonic. That is to say, in the latter case a great deal of distress is caused, taking the form of anxiety and guilt. In fact, the apparent absence of guilt and anxiety related to a socially unacceptable behavior is one diagnostic criterion of the antisocial personality, while impulsivity is another.

A very similar differential view is provided by Leaff (1974) when he writes that, "In contrast to the neurotic whose symptomatology results primarily from intrapsychic conflict, the diagnostic psychopathology of the (impulse disorders) results from rigid, syntonic personality traits and patterns" (p. 4).

B.   LEARNING THEORY AND IMPULSES

Modern learning theory (behaviorism) is based on the premise that behavior is determined or learned by means of the consequences of the behavior. Put another way, any behavior which is rewarded or reinforced will tend to continue to occur. Behavior patterns which are defined here as pathologically impulsive, therefore, are being reinforced in some manner. The individual is getting something out of behaving the way he or she does. The diagnostic/treatment problem comes in determining the type of reinforcement the individual is getting, for what is rewarding to one person may not be rewarding to another.

Take, for example, the young child who is distracting in the classroom. He is brought to the front of the room, scolded by the teacher, and made to sit by the teacher's desk. For some children such an experience may be quite embarrassing and therefore aversive to the behavior which led to the reprimand. For others, however, the experience may be rewarding, as in the case of the boy who needs more attention than he is getting. For him the attention could be much more rewarding than aversive.

The Skinnerian model of behavior theory, Trasler (1978) points out, does not explain "socially-based behavioral inhibitions" (p. 277). These inhibitions are essentially the same as the internal controls mentioned earlier in this chapter, but learning theorists view them as developing through learning during socialization. This concept of internal controls is often referred to as "passive avoidance" types of behavior, or nonbehavior.

It has been suggested that inhibitions which develop during the socialization process are actually evolved through the conditioning of an aversive state of arousal which some call anxiety.

C.   ORGANIC THEORY AND IMPULSES

There is considerable evidence that some impulsive behaviors are associated with some types of central nervous system dysfunction. You will recall from your study of neuroanatomy that the "old" brain, phylogenetically speaking, contains the limbic system (or, as some prefer, the limbic brain). A great many studies of animals, including some with man, using ablation and direct stimulation of the brain have concluded that there exists a "definable neural system which organizes effective and directed attack behavior, and that this system is linked to structures of the limbic brain" (Mark & Ervin, 1970, p. 31).

While there is a great deal more to discover about the specific correlations between the brain and behavior, some things seem clear at this time. The limbic system, particularly the hippocampus, and the hypothalamus, seems to play an important role in the control and influence of emotional activity. From an evolutionary standpoint this makes very good sense since these structures are physiologically proximal to olfaction structures, which in turn are so important to such things as fight, flight, and fright as well as to sexual responses in lower species. It is also important to realize that there logically must be a connection between the limbic brain and the autonomic nervous system since such things as pupil dilation, increased heart rate, etc., occur in response to emotional reactions of fear, aggression, etc. (Pincus & Tucker, 1974).

Furthermore, while there are certainly connections between the limbic brain and the neocortex, there are a great many connections within the limbic system including both afferent and efferent fibers. The point here is that there is good evidence that the numerous parts of the limbic system are interconnected and may continue to discharge within the limbic system either with or without much neocortical involvement.

Figure 12-1

Limbic - Neocortical Interactions

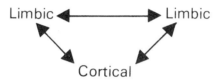

READING NOTE: For a more detailed description of the structure and function of the limbic system as known today see Pincus' and Tucker's Behavioral neurology, 1974. See also Mark and Ervin, Violence and the brain, 1970.

Probably one of the most important differential diagnoses to be made in psychiatry is, generally, between neurologically induced deviant behavior and functional psychopathology. Damage, destruction, stimulation, irritation of various limbic structures can produce alterations in behavior presenting symptoms which are remarkably like those seen in Schizophrenia, depression, mania, hysteria, and in other functional disorders.

D.   HYPERACTIVITY AND LOW IMPULSE CONTROL

There is evidence which links some hyperactive child syndromes and low impulse control. It is important to understand that all hyperactive children are not alike, nor do they all develop traits or behaviors in later life which are viewed as psychopathological.

Satterfield (1978) found that a substantial number of children who have been diagnosed as hyperactive have lowered levels of central nervous system arousal (as measured by various indicators of autonomic nervous system arousal). The model which Satterfield (1978) suggests is one of low CNS arousal coupled with low CNS inhibition. Such a model accounts for several of the major symptoms of hyperactive children: excessive motor activity, short attention span, and impulsivity. It also accounts for the reason that CNS stimulants which heighten the CNS arousal level seem to be quite effective in the treatment of many hyperactive children.

Lewis and Balla (1976) found that the hyperactive child syndrome was "one of the most common central nervous system precursors of delinquency" (p. 65) which they found in their court clinic in Hartford, Connecticut. They prefer the term "central nervous system dysfunction" to describe the children who display a combination (not all in one child at one time) of symptoms. These symptoms include: hyperactivity, impulsivity, distractibility, shortened attention span, and learning problems of one kind or another.

These symptoms, where seen together, have recently been taken as indicators of Minimal Brain Dysfunction (MBD). Obviously this is a nonspecific term with regard to the area of organic impairment, but chemical stimulation with low doses of amphetamine have been reported to be successful in many instances.

In their study Lewis and Balla (1976) carefully examined 285 delinquent children referred by the court to their clinic. Although previously undetected, many of these children were found to have clear evidence of central nervous system dysfunction, including 18 who had symptoms of temporal lobe epilepsy and psychosis.

In summary, then, poor impulse control may be viewed in psychodynamic, learning, or neurological terms. It is likely that in many instances a combination of interacting factors is involved. For example, a 12-year-old boy was placed on Ritalin® for hyperactive behavior. (Although used to treat mild depression, Ritalin® has an apparently paradoxical effect with some hyperactive children.) One of the two doses had to be taken in school, and the principal of the school brought the pill to the youngster each day at lunchtime. The implications of this for the boy were many and undoubtedly confusing to him. He began hiding the medicine, refusing to take it, even though the effect of the medicine had been to improve dramatically his hyperactivity. Now his behavior became worse than it was prior to beginning the course of treatment.

E. IMPULSIVITY AND PSYCHOPATHOLOGY

Redlich and Freedman (1966) refer to such impulsive behaviors as "irresistible acts, which are incompatible with overt social and ethical standards and do not serve a useful purpose" (p. 383). Put another way, to be considered pathological, acting on an impulse must be socially unacceptable and have no overriding or redeeming value. For example, it is generally considered socially unacceptable to assault another person physically. There are instances, however, when such behavior is not only acceptable but even desirable (as in the case of one defending oneself or a loved one).

If an impulsive act is socially unacceptable and serves no useful purpose then, it is likely that the act poses a threat of some sort to either the individual committing the act or to someone else in that individual's environment. The threat may be aimed at a person physically or emotionally, or it may be more indirect, in terms of being aimed at something which is highly valued by someone else. For instance, the individual who is suffering from a manic-depressive illness may spend a great deal of money on impulse. This behavior may well pose a threat to him and his family in regard to financial ruin, to say nothing of anxiety generated in his family.

In summary, then, to be considered pathological, acting on an impulse must: 1) be socially unacceptable, 2) not serve a useful purpose, and 3) pose a threat to the individual himself or to others.

The general criteria for impulse disorders given in the DSM-III are:

A. A failure to resist an impulse to perform some act which is harmful to the patient himself or to others. The resistance may be conscious or unconscious and the act may or may not be premeditated.

B. Prior to the act there is an increasing sense of tension.

C. At the time of the act the patient experiences pleasure or gratification or release.

It is important to realize that an impulse is not in itself pathological; indeed it is quite normal to have impulses. It is how we deal with impulses that is important. All impulses spring from internal drives which are directed at meeting needs as perceived by the person experiencing the impulse. It is the conversion of the impulse to action which gives it the potential for being pathological.

Furthermore, many persons could be described as being nonpathologically impulsive, that is, persons who do indeed act on impulse, but are able to control their impulses when these impulses lead to behaviors which would be socially unacceptable. For example, Zuckerman et al. (1964) describe "sensation seeking" individuals who seem to need more than the usual amount of excitement in their day-to-day lives. Their Sensation Seeking Scale measures this characteristic along a continuum from very low to very high. Many of the persons who are high on this dimension may meet the criteria of impulsiveness, but many stay within the bounds of socially acceptable behavior.

There is a great deal more to be learned about the causes of impulse-driven behavior in human beings, but against this background consider the following disorders which have as a cardinal symptom the apparent lack of ability to control impulses of a fairly specific nature.

QUIZ, Section I.

Circle the correct answer(s). <u>One</u> or <u>more than one</u> answer may be correct.

1. Acquiring control over one's own behavior is

   a. an instinctual process.
   b. a developmental phenomenon.
   c. normally preceded by external controls.
   d. a function of the id.
   e. either present or absent in a child by age seven years.

2. It is likely, neuroanatomically, that in "attack" behaviors the limbic brain may be interacting with

   a. the autonomic nervous system.
   b. the neocortex.

3. One model which is offered to explain hyperactivity among children is

   a. high CNS arousal with low CNS inhibition.
   b. low CNS arousal with high CNS inhibition .
   c. high CNS arousal with high CNS inhibition.
   d. low CNS arousal with low CNS inhibition.

TRUE or FALSE: Circle the correct letter.

T   F   4. Controlling impulses allows one to postpone gratification of a need or desire.

T   F   5. One of the most common ways of controlling impulses is converting the impulse into words rather than action.

T   F   6. It is usually pathological if one experiences socially unacceptable impulses after adolescence.

T   F   7. Certain ego defense mechanisms are used to control impulses.

T   F   8. If the impulse does not seem to produce anxiety, it is said to be ego-syntonic.

T   F   9. Socially undesirable behavior may be unintentionally reinforced.

T   F   10. Having an impulse to steal an automobile is considered pathological.

Complete the following.

11. Acting on an impulse is considered pathological when the behavior

     a. is socially _____.
     b. does not serve a useful _____.
     c. poses a threat to the individual himself or to_____.

===
===

II. PATHOLOGICAL GAMBLING (DSM-III 312.31)

The person who fits into this diagnostic category is one who, usually beginning in adolescence, has become chronically unable to resist the impulse to gamble. The behavior has become a distinct threat to the individual and to his or her family usually because of the financial problems arising out of the gambling behavior. It is not uncommon for the individual to become involved in behaviors which are frankly against the law (forgery, writing "bad" checks, embezzlement, etc.), or at best on the fringes of socially unacceptable behavior (borrowing from and not repaying friends, frequent loss of jobs, etc.). All of these activities are aimed at getting money in order to gamble, and the gambling will lead, so the person rationalizes, to winning enough money to pay off all debts.

The pathological gambler may look as though he is in a manic or hypomanic state, but often will show signs of anxiety and/or depression around the issue of the deep trouble in which he has become embroiled.

Differentially one must distinguish between pathological gambling and a manic episode of manic-depressive illness. In the former the elation is usually associated with winning, while in the case of manic-depressive illness the history will indicate that the mood swing to elation occurred prior to the gambling.

One must also differentiate between Pathological Gambling and Antisocial Personality. If the criteria for Antisocial Personality are met, then this should be the diagnosis used even though pathological gambling is a clear feature of the personality or character structure of the individual. In other words, the pathological gambler may commit antisocial acts, usually stealing in some form, but the goal is clearly to get money for gambling. He or she does not commit such acts when money for gambling is available.

Finally, there are features of both obsession and compulsion in terms of preoccupation with and rumination about gambling. These features do not extend, pathologically, to other areas of the person's life, however.

Lesieur (1979) describes the development of the compulsive (pathological) gambler. He or she moves from an introduction to gambling into a vicious cycle of gambling to "get even" so that he or she can gamble some more. The crucial difference Lesieur (1979) sees between the pathological and nonpathological gambler is what he refers to as "chasing." This term refers to the use of gambling to get even with gambling debts or debts related to gambling. Once the individual is committed to "chasing," the vicious cycle becomes a spiral which often leads to more and more involvement in unlawful activity.

The compulsive or pathological gambler, according to Lesieur (1979), uses rationalization and denial to deal with the unacceptable behaviors, e.g., using the family resources to gamble, "borrowing" (stealing or embezzling) money from employers, and getting further involved in the gambling culture.

It is important to understand that the pathological gambler has what is described as a craving for the "action" of gambling, that the satisfaction comes from having a bet on a game or event and being caught up in the unfolding of the final outcome. Many pathological gamblers will tell you that the amount of money involved is not the crucial factor, although they usually will bet as much as they can. If they are able to place only a small bet, however, they can still get caught up in the action.

The DSM-III gives three major criteria which must be met in order to establish a diagnosis of Pathological Gambling:

A. The individual is chronically and progressively unable to resist impulses to gamble.

B. Gambling compromises, disrupts or damages family, personal, and vocational pursuits, as indicated by at least three of the following:

(1) arrest for forgery, fraud, embezzlement, or income tax evasion due to attempts to obtain money for gambling
(2) default on debts and other financial responsibilities
(3) disrupted family or spouse relationship due to gambling
(4) borrowing of money from illegal sources (loan sharks)
(5) inability to account for loss of money or to produce evidence of winning money, if this is claimed
(6) loss of work due to absenteeism in order to pursue gambling activity
(7) necessity for another person to provide money to relieve a desperate financial situation

C. The gambling is not due to Antisocial Personality Disorder.

Probably the most effective treatment for the pathological gambler is the Gamblers Anonymous organization. The principles are essentially the same as those of Alcoholics Anonymous in that both peer pressure and support are important ingredients. Ongoing psychiatric treatment may be necessary in addition to involvement in Gamblers Anonymous.

****

GO TO VIDEOTAPE

****

ANSWERS, Section I. _____

1. b,c
2. a,b
3. d
4. T
5. T
6. F
7. T

8. T
9. T
10. F
11. a. unacceptable
    b. purpose
    c. others

_____

QUIZ, Section II

TRUE or FALSE: Circle the correct letter.

T   F   1. The behavior of the pathological gambler, as described above, meets the criteria you learned for pathologically impulsive behavior.

T   F   2. Chronic and progressive gambling in an individual is sufficient to diagnose pathological gambling.

Circle the letter corresponding to the one correct response.

3. You are seeing a 32-year-old male in a prison population. He has been serving a term for grand larceny and reports to you that he has made his living for the last six years by stealing and fencing goods of various kinds. He has maintained an apartment in a fairly exclusive subdivision with only the money he has made in his illegal activities. He estimates that he has lost between $10,000 and $12,000 per year playing blackjack and betting on sporting events over the last four years.

    Given only that information, what would be the most likely diagnosis of this man?

    a. pathological gambler
    b. Antisocial Personality
    c. manic depressive
    d. Conduct Disorder

Circle the correct answer(s). One or more than one answer may be correct.

4. The concept of "chasing" with reference to gamblers

    a. is used in connection with pathological gamblers.
    b. may be used to describe the dynamics of embezzlers.
    c. often leads to escalation of gambling behavior.
    d. refers to the gambler's defense mechanisms of denial and rationalization.

III. KLEPTOMANIA (DSM-III 312.32)

In the <u>Encyclopedia</u> <u>of</u> <u>Psychoanalysis</u> (Eidelberg, 1968), the following description of Kleptomania is given:

> Kleptomania is characterized by obsessive stealing, usually without sufficient economic motivation, traceable to profound frustrations during the oral, anal, or phallic stage. The stolen objects are substitute pleasures for those previously denied. The act is one of revenge on the images of those held responsible for the supposed malfeasance. In women, Kleptomania represents an active castration tendency directed against the penis of the male, with incorporative aims. Kleptomania represents an exhibitionistic and masochistic provocation of external punishment for both sexes (p. 213).

As the above quotation indicates, Kleptomania is thought of in more traditional psychoanalytic theory as being a highly symbolized disturbance. The symbolism is a sexual one in both males and females. The hidden, secret aspect of the behavior itself is symbolically akin to the secret, hidden masturbatory fantasy and behavior of the child or adolescent. On another level, still symbolic, the behavior is a somewhat narcissistic act which is used to obtain something which represents love. The unconscious formula is, "I am owed something. I deserve it. I have a right to take it." This kind of unconscious process might well account for the fact that the object taken by the kleptomaniac is usually of little monetary value. It is not the objective worth, but rather the symbolic value of the object which is important to the kleptomaniac.

On still another level, <u>anxiety</u>, <u>tension</u>, <u>conflict</u>, and <u>guilt</u> are important aspects of the disorder. The conflict is one among ego, id, and superego. The kleptomaniac <u>does</u> know right from wrong. His superego does contain the societal prohibition against stealing; however, the drive for gratification is not controlled effectively. The impulse to steal in order to satisfy the drive or need is rationalized on an unconscious level, and yet it also produces anxiety and guilt in the individual. The guilt and anxiety seem to be more related to the shame, humiliation, loss of status, etc. which accompany being apprehended.

The tension seems to be directly related to the conflict, increasing as the act of stealing gets closer. There also seems to be a release of tension just as or shortly after the act is completed. Description of this by persons who are kleptomanic are startlingly like descriptions of sexual tension and discharge of tension at orgasm. In fact some actually report orgasm at the time of the theft. This same phenomenon is also seen in some pyromaniacs at the time of setting a fire.

The differential diagnosis is usually relatively easy to make, although many disorders may have some type of stealing associated with them. Some schizophrenics will steal objects of relatively little value. Some individuals suffering from some types of brain dysfunction may also steal. It is

ANSWERS, Section II._____

1. T
2. F
3. b
4. a,c

_____

sometimes difficult to differentiate between Kleptomania and Antisocial Personality or Conduct Disorders in children. These individuals steal impulsively, but one major differential factor is that the latter usually steal for material gain. Another major difference is that the person with Antisocial Personality or Conduct Disorder will often, but not always, act with others, whereas the kleptomanic individual invariably acts alone.

One other differential problem arises not infrequently when a person is apprehended after stealing some object and then attempts to convince others that the act was uncontrollable. This type of malingering has the obvious goal of escaping criminal prosecution for stealing. By carefully examining the patient with respect to the diagnostic criteria for Kleptomania as well as for Antisocial Personality or Conduct Disorder, the accurate diagnosis usually can be made without too much difficulty.

DSM-III lists the following five criteria for the diagnosis of Kleptomania:

A. Recurrent failure to resist impulses to steal objects that are not for immediate use or their monetary value.

B. Increasing sense of tension before committing the act.

C. An experience of either pleasure or release at the time of committing the theft.

D. Stealing is done without long-term planning and assistance from, or collaboration with, others.

E. Not due to Conduct Disorder or Antisocial Personality Disorder.

****

GO TO VIDEOTAPE

****

QUIZ, Section III.

TRUE or FALSE: Circle the correct letter.

T   F   1.   The monetary value of the stolen object is an important diagnostic aspect of Kleptomania.

T   F   2.   A person suffering from Kleptomania almost always acts alone.

Circle the correct answer(s). <u>One</u> or <u>more</u> <u>than</u> <u>one</u> answer may be correct.

3.   Which of the following is (are) thought to be a facet(s) of Kleptomania?

    a.   tension
    b.   conflict
    c.   anxiety
    d.   guilt

4.   Name two differential diagnosis considerations regarding Kleptomania.

_____

_____

_____

IV.   PYROMANIA (DSM-III 312.33)

The <u>Encyclopedia</u> <u>of</u> <u>Psychoanalysis</u> (Eidelberg, 1968) defines Pyromania as "a compulsion to set fires, usually neither for practical reasons nor for material profit" (p. 357). This definition does differentiate between pyromaniacs and firesetters who for pay or out of anger and hostility set fires. It should be noted, though, that the dynamics of the pyromaniac may be seen in some arsonists who do not meet the criteria for diagnosis in this category.

The classic study on Pyromania was done by Lewis and Yarnell (1951), but relatively little has been written on this subject since that time. This is true in spite of the fact that in 1970 over 200 million dollars in losses of property were sustained from incendiary fires (Axberger, 1973).

Lewis and Yarnell (1951) reported over 1,100 cases of firesetters, and found that about two-fifths of the males met their criteria for Pyromania, that is, persons who acted on an irresistible impulse and without a discernible motive. While there are reported cases of females suffering from Pyromania, the overwhelming number are male, as is true in the case of firesetting in general.

The onset of this illness is usually in childhood, and there are associated features, the most prominent of which is enuresis. In fact, it often has been said that firesetting, enuresis, and cruelty to animals form a triad of behaviors in childhood which predict violent and dangerous behavior in adulthood. The predictive ability of this triad has not been established, however. It is clear, though, that enuresis is very frequently associated with Pyromania.

Psychoanalytic theory, as you may have already realized, is highly dependent on symbolism. In Pyromania the symbols are sexual, and according to Fenichel (1945) the illness represents a regression to a developmental stage of urethral eroticism. Indeed Lewis and Yarnell (1951) report in some instances masturbation and orgasm occur at the time of setting the fire.

Pyromania is a disorder of impulse control, but this does not mean that persons with this disorder act on the "spur of the moment" without prior planning. In fact, much planning may go into the setting of the fire. In Kleptomania, on the other hand, the stealing is done without much, if any, prior planning.

Differentially one must consider a variety of other possibilities before making the diagnosis of Pyromania. In childhood it is not uncommon for children to be fascinated by fire and very curious about it. A single incident of setting a fire obviously would not warrant the diagnosis of Pyromania. At the same time the setting of several fires might well be a part of a Conduct Disorder (DSM-III 312.0) and the antisocial behavior associated with this entity. Similarly, in adults one must rule out Antisocial Personality (see Chapter 13, Personality Disorders) before making a diagnosis of Pyromania.

Some schizophrenics also engage in firesetting. Usually this is associated with delusions or hallucinations, and generally it is relatively easy to differentiate between Schizophrenia and Pyromania.

Finally, one must differentiate between Pyromania and brain disease. In children, for example, a rather rare illness, the Kleine-Levin syndrome, often has firesetting as a feature (Powers & Gunderman, 1978). In this instance, periodic hypersomnia or some often bizarre psychotic-like symptoms are present. This seems to be clearly a neuropsychiatric disorder since a brief course of amphetamines seems to control the episodes.

There are, of course, other brain syndromes which may, in some instances, produce firesetting behavior. Once again, however, it is relatively easy to differentiate between Pyromania and such disorders as temporal lobe epilepsy. More will be said about the sometimes confusing or confounding aspects of organicity in the next section of this chapter which deals with the explosive disorders.

One last comment should be made here regarding firesetting behavior. The role of fire in the history of man has been a very important one. Poets and writers have given fire considerable prominence in their work, Dante and Milton, for example. Fire has also played a major part in many of the religions of the world. In these areas the symbolism of fire has been more or less clear. In our day-to-day lives fire figures prominently and directly, in terms of its survival value through its use as an energy source to keep us warm, cook our food, and provide us with a wide variety of luxuries. Most of us are to some extent fascinated by fire. Macht and Mack (1968) quote a few lines from Walt Whitman's Poems of Joy:

> I hear the alarm at dead of night,
> I hear the bells -- shouts!
> I pass the crowd -- I run!
> The sight of flames maddens me with
> pleasure.

[If you are interested in reading more about the role of fire in literature, see Axberger (1973) whose paper deals with fire in an international cross-section of literature, plays, and poetry. Also Arlow (1978) describes the role of fire specifically in the writings of the Japanese writer, Yukio Mishima.]

DSM-III gives the following criteria for making the diagnosis of Pyromania:

   A.   Recurrent failure to resist impulses to set fires.

   B.   Increasing sense of tension before setting the fire.

   C.   An experience of either intense pleasure, gratification, or release at the time of committing the act.

   D.   Lack of motivation, such as monetary gain or sociopolitical ideology, for setting fires.

   E.   Not due to an Organic Mental Disorder, Schizophrenia, Anti-social Personality Disorder, or Conduct Disorder.

Now a warning. The person who suffers from Pyromania is extremely difficult to treat. If you suspect the presence of Pyromania in a patient, he should be seen by a competent psychiatrist without delay.

QUIZ, Section IV.

1.   The triad of behaviors in childhood which some say predict violent and dangerous behavior in adulthood are:

   _____
   _____
   _____

2.   Name three psychiatric diseases which must be ruled out before one can make the diagnosis of Pyromania.

   _____
   _____
   _____

3.   You are called upon to see a 29-year-old male who has been arrested for setting a series of four fires in lumber yards and furniture stores over the last six months. He describes to you a feeling of tension which builds in him prior to setting a fire, as well as a feeling of pleasurable release at the time he sets the fire. You are informed by the police that there is evidence that he is a paid "torch" or firesetter who works for people who want to collect insurance on their property. Would the diagnosis be that of Pyromania? _____

ANSWERS, Section III._____

1. F
2. T
3. a,b,c,d
4. Schizophrenia
    Antisocial Personality Disorder
    Conduct Disorder
    Malingering

V. INTERMITTENT EXPLOSIVE DISORDER (DSM-III 312.34)
AND
ISOLATED EXPLOSIVE DISORDER (DSM-III 312.35)

This section combines two categories in the DSM-III because the diagnostic criteria differ mainly in regard to the number of episodes of violent, explosive behavior exhibited by the patient, although by implication the Isolated Explosive Disorder is much more catastrophic. More will be said about differentiation below.

A. DESCRIPTION AND DIAGNOSTIC CRITERIA

Before discussing the features of the Explosive Disorders it is important to clarify the nomenclature used in the literature. What is now called "Explosive Disorder" in the DSM-III has been variously called "Instinct Neurosis" or "Instinct Dyscontrol" in the psychoanalytic writings on acting out behavior. Deficit of the control aspect of the ego and/or the developmental failure of the superego is, in theory, the basis for the inability of the individual to delay gratification (gratification through motor activity). The symbolism of the acting out rests in the notion that the current acting out is in defense against some repressed, ego-dystonic impulse which is beginning to emerge into consciousness. Thus the acting out is in service of keeping the impulse repressed. The conflict, then, is between the ego and the external world. Accordingly the acting out behavior on the one hand may be adaptive for the individual, but on the other hand may be socially unacceptable. That is, when the acting out takes the form of assaultive behavior it is maladaptive, particularly if the assault is unprovoked or significantly out of proportion to the stimulus.

In DSM-II Explosive Personality was classified as one of the Personality Disorders. The term "aggressive personality" has often been used synonymously with Explosive Personality, as has been "Epileptoid Personality Disorder."

In a general sense anyone who displayed outbursts of hostile and aggressive behavior, either verbal or physical, which were significantly different from his or her normal behavior was likely to be diagnosed as "Explosive Personality." In DSM-III the Intermittent Explosive Disorder refers to persons who have displayed at least three "episodes of significant loss of control of aggressive impulses, that result in serious assault or destruction of property." These episodes are out of proportion to any environmental stimuli which may have elicited the aggressive behavior. The Isolated Explosive Disorder, on the other hand, refers to a single event in which the impulse to act out aggressively is expressed in a "violent, externally-directed act, that had a catastrophic impact on others." For instance, in the 1960's a young man climbed to the top of a tower in Texas and began shooting people on the ground below. Up until this event the young man gave no indication that he was a violently aggressive individual. Post-mortem examination of this young man disclosed a nut-sized tumor in the posterior thalamus.

The first of the diagnostic criteria, then, for the Intermittent Explosive Disorder is:

A.   Several discrete episodes of loss of control of aggressive impulses resulting in serious assault or destruction of property.

The first diagnostic criterion for the Isolated Explosive Disorder, on the other hand, is:

A.   A single, discrete episode in which failure to resist an impulse led to a single, violent externally directed act that had a catastrophic impact on others.

The other three criteria for these two categories are essentially the same:

B.   The magnitude of the behavior during the episode is grossly out of proportion to any psychosocial stressors which may have played a role in eliciting the episode(s) of lack of control.

C.   Between the episodes (or prior to the episode in the case of the Isolated Explosive Disorder) there are no signs of generalized impulsivity or aggressiveness.

D.   Not due to Schizophrenia, Antisocial Personality Disorder, or Conduct Disorder.

The diagnostic criteria are certainly specific for both of these categories, but the problem of diagnosis is confounded by the frequency with which a diagnosis in this category also carries a diagnosis on Axis III (Physical Disorders). Before considering this area, however, differentiation on Axis I (Psychiatric Disorders) should be considered.

Violent, explosive, impulsively driven behavior sometimes occurs among schizophrenics, particularly paranoid and catatonic schizophrenics. Ruling out Schizophrenia should be relatively easy since these individuals present symptoms which are specific to Schizophrenia, like delusions or hallucinations. (See Chapter 7, Schizophrenia.) Antisocial Personality Disorder, or Conduct Disorder (in children) usually can readily be ruled out by definition of the Explosive Disorder. In short the aggressivity and impulsivity of the Antisocial Personality or the Conduct Disorders are seen

ANSWERS, Section IV._____

1. firesetting
   enuresis
   cruelty to animals

2. Schizophrenia
   Antisocial Personality Disorder
   Conduct Disorder
   Klein-Levin syndrome
   other organic syndromes

3. No. The motivation of money rules out this diagnosis. Note, however, that many "torches" or firebugs do demonstrate the same dynamics of the pyromaniac. The "no" here is really an equivocal one.

---

between any violent episodes which may occur. In the Explosive Disorders this is not the case.

Some Dissociative Disorder episodes (see Chapter 10) may have the violent, impulsive characteristics seen in the Explosive Disorders. But usually with the Dissociative Disorder a specific stress-producing precipitating event of major consequence can be identified. In the case of the Explosive Disorders such an event is usually either absent or of a relatively minor nature.

****

GO TO VIDEOTAPE

****

B. AXIS III

The kind of behavior described by these diagnostic categories of Explosive Disorder has also been referred to as "Epileptoid Personality Disorder" in the DSM-II as a parenthetical term for Explosive Personality. Most commonly, however, in recent psychiatric literature the term, Episodic Dyscontrol Syndrome has been used (Bach-y-Rita, et al., 1971; Maletzky & Klotter, 1974; Mark & Ervin, 1970; Monroe, 1970).

Monroe (1970) defines Episodic Dyscontrol in the following manner:

> An abrupt single act or short series of acts with a common intention carried through to completion with at least a partial relief of tension or gratification of a specific need. As a subclass of the Episodic Behavioral Disorder it also has the characteristic of a maladaptive, precipitous interruption in the lifestyle or life flow of the individual (p. 26).

From examining the histories of 532 individuals who exhibited poor impulse control and periods of destructive behavior, Mark and Ervin (1970) concluded that these persons shared four characteristics: 1) physical assault, especially wife and/or child beating; 2) pathological intoxication, i.e., even a small amount of alcohol ingestion producing markedly brutal behavior; 3) impulsive sexual behavior, including in some cases sexual assault; and 4) numerous traffic violations and auto accidents.

Maletzky and Klotter (1974) described the individuals who fit this category of episodic dyscontrol in terms of the features most commonly seen. They are usually males in their 20's and 30's who have a history of hyperactivity and febrile seizures as children, delinquency as adolescents, and legal difficulties as adults. They also frequently report aurae and post-ictal phenomena as well as exhibit "soft" neurological signs and nonspecific temporal lobe EEG changes. Morrison and Minkoff (1975) conclude that what is called the Episodic Dyscontrol Syndrome in some instances, may well be etiologically related to whatever organic defect it is which affects the hyperactive child syndrome.

In their very impressive study of 130 patients who were assaultive and/or destructive Bach-y-Rita and his colleagues (1971) concluded that in many instances organic factors played an important role. They add, however, that "interacting with this impaired cerebral integrative system were obvious dynamically significant psychopathological experiences" (p. 1474).

In examining a patient who has exhibited violent, explosive, and destructive behavior, it is important to include a neurological examination. If it is possible to get a reliable history, "soft" neurological signs may emerge. For example, one might elicit a history of childhood hyperkinesis, impulse disorder, late speech, marked clumsiness, inability to develop simple athletic skills, speech peculiarities, learning problems, intellectual defect, temper tantrums (Quitkin & Klein, 1969).

EEG might reveal a lesion, particularly a temporal or frontal lobe lesion, but at least as often the EEG will be negative. This will not rule out the possibility of organicity. Mark and Ervin (1970) cite examples of normal brain activity findings until electrodes were stereotaxically implanted and recordings made. Obviously implanting electrodes is not a standard or routine procedure and is noted here only to illustrate the point that negative findings do not necessarily rule out the role of organicity in the Explosive Disorders.

The use of anticonvulsants, especially diphenylhydantoin (Dilantin), in the treatment of some Explosive Disorders has been cited in recent psychiatric literature. Specifically, Bach-y-Rita and his associates (1971) tried Dilantin, not only with any patients with abnormal EEG's, but also with patients whose histories revealed any "seizure-like outbursts," (p. 1478) with good success. Maletzky and Klotter (1974) report that of their 22 patients who were treated with Dilantin, 19 had a reduction of at least 75% in both frequency and severity of their outbursts.

In the diagnosis and in the treatment of Explosive Disorders, it is important to remember that neurological, psychological, and sociocultural factors may all play a role in the etiology and course of the illness, and all three must be given appropriate attention.

QUIZ, Section V.

Circle the correct answer(s). <u>One</u> or <u>more</u> <u>than</u> <u>one</u> answer may be correct.

1. In psychoanalytic theory, the term "acting out" when used in relation to violent, aggressive behavior refers to

    a. ego deficiency regarding control of impulses.
    b. superego deficit regarding impulsive behavior.
    c. a defense against another impulse.
    d. adaptive for the individual but maladaptive as far as society is concerned.

2. You would rule out both types of Explosive Disorder if the

    a. patient showed no remorse about his behavior.
    b. behavior was in response to a verbal direction by God.
    c. patient has no history of aggressive behavior.
    d. violent behavior was the fifth episode for this patient, but in each case has been directed at his wife only.

T   F   3. The major differences between <u>Intermittent</u> and <u>Isolated</u> Explosive Disorders are quantitative and qualitative ones.

T   F   4. Negative EEG finding will serve to rule out organicity as a factor in Explosive Disorders.

Complete the following.

5. Neurologically related considerations in the examination of persons who exhibit violent, explosive, and destructive behavior include history of:

    a. childhood _____
    b. late development of _____
    c. marked _____
    d. _____ peculiarities
    e. trouble developing simple _____ _____

6. Four characteristics identified by Mark and Ervin as being associated with persons who exhibited poor impulse control and periods of destructive behavior are:

    _____
    _____
    _____
    _____

Match the following numbered statements with the lettered disorders with regard to differentiating from the Explosive Disorders.

___7. behavior during the violent episode is only quantitatively different from usual behaviors

___8. behavior during the violent episode is clearly in response to a delusion or hallucination

___9. behavior during the violent episode is precipitated by a specific stressful event of major consequence

___10. behavior during the violent episode is in response to a relatively minor stressful event

a. Schizophrenia
b. Antisocial Personality Disorder
c. Dissociative Disorder
d. Explosive Disorder

VI.   OTHER IMPULSE CONTROL DISORDERS (DSM-III 312.39)

This category has been designated for disorders of impulse control which cannot be classified elsewhere. In short, the behavior of the individual does not meet the criteria for diagnoses such as Antisocial Personality Disorder, Conduct Disorder, or Schizophrenia, nor for any of the specific categories listed in this chapter.

ANSWERS, Section V.

1. a,b,c,d
2. a,b
3. T
4. F
5. a. hyperkinesis
   b. speech
   c. clumsiness
   d. speech
   e. athletic skills
6. a. physical assault
   b. pathological intoxication
   c. impulsive sexual behavior
   d. numerous traffic violations
7. b
8. a
9. c
10. d

POST-TEST

TRUE or FALSE: Circle the correct letter.

T   F   1.   A 25-year-old male has been diagnosed as having Intermittent
                 Explosive Disorder. EEG reveals the likelihood of a temporal
                 lobe lesion. You begin treating him with Dilantin and find that
                 both the frequency and severity of the violent episodes decrease.
                 You should include psychotherapy in his treatment regimen.

T   F   2.   Impulses to do things which are socially unacceptable (such
                 as, stealing, sexual promiscuity, fighting) are pathological.

Define the following.

3.   Define the concept of "chasing" as it is applied to pathological gamblers.

_____

_____

Circle the correct answer(s).   One or more than one answer may be correct.

4.   Impulses are sometimes

     a.   ego-syntonic.
     b.   controlled by defense mechanisms.
     c.   ego-dystonic.
     d.   converted to words (rather than action).

5.   There are two types of Explosive Personality Disorders described in
     DSM-III, Intermittent and Isolated. These are distinguished from each
     other in terms of the

     a.   quantity of the violent episodes.
     b.   presence or absence of remorse about the violent episodes.
     c.   quality of the violent episodes.
     d.   object (person or thing) of the violent episode.

6.   In the framework of learning theory, control of impulsive behavior is

     a.   referred to as passive-avoidance behavior or nonbehavior.
     b.   related to the conditioning of an aversive state of arousal.
     c.   attained through developing ego function.
     d.   usually dependent on aversive conditioning.

7.   Mark and Ervin have listed certain characteristics of individuals who
     exhibit poor impulse control along with periods of destructive behavior.
     These characteristics include which of the following?

     a.   physical assault
     b.   pathological intoxication
     c.   impulsive sexual behavior
     d.   numerous traffic violations

8. Pathological Gambling as a disorder is determined by the amount of money

    a. risked.
    b. lost.
    c. won.
    d. none of the above.

9. Control of impulses is thought to be a function of the

    a. id.
    b. ego.
    c. superego.

10. Which of the following pieces of information would be important for you to have in order to diagnose Kleptomania?

    a. whether or not the individual suffers from delusions or hallucinations
    b. the person experienced orgasm at the time of the theft
    c. whether the person was alone or with someone else at the time of the theft
    d. the usefulness of the object stolen

11. It is thought that, neuroanatomically, aggressive, attack behaviors may be interactive with

    a. autonomic nervous system.
    b. limbic system.
    c. neocortex.
    d. pineal gland.

12. Differential diagnosis of Explosive Disorders should include

    a. Schizophrenia.
    b. Antisocial Personality Disorder.
    c. Conduct Disorder.
    d. Dissociative Disorder.

13. Which of the following disorders must be ruled out before making a diagnosis of Pyromania?

    a. Schizophrenia
    b. Antisocial Personality Disorder
    c. Conduct Disorder
    d. Klein-Levin syndrome

14. Which of the following is <u>not</u> in the triad of behaviors which, when seen in children, is said to predict violent and dangerous behavior in adulthood?

    a. firesetting
    b. enuresis
    c. autism
    d. cruelty to animals

15. Psychodynamically, which of the following is (are) considered to be features of kleptomaniacs?

    a. tension
    b. anxiety
    c. conflict
    d. guilt

16. Reading the psychiatric literature on Intermittent Explosive Disorders, you will find which of the following used as synonymous for this entity?

    a. Epileptoid Personality Disorder
    b. Episodic Dyscontrol Syndrome
    c. Explosive Personality Disorder
    d. instinct dyscontrol

17. Which of the following would rule out a diagnosis of Kleptomania?

    a. an increased sense of tension prior to the act of stealing
    b. a history of six acts of stealing
    c. a concurrent diagnosis of Antisocial Personality Disorder
    d. the use of two confederates to carry out the theft

PRE-TEST ANSWERS

1. a,b,c,d
2. a,b,c
3. a,b,c,d
4. a,b,c,d
5. a,b,c,d
6. a,c
7. a,b,c,d
8. a,b,c,d
9. a,b,c,d
10. a,b

11. c,d
12. b
13. d
14. c
15. F
16. T
17. should include the idea of gambling to get even with gambling losses

POST-TEST ANSWERS

1. T
2. F
3. should include the idea of gambling to get even with gambling losses
4. a,b,c,d
5. a,c
6. a,b
7. a,b,c,d
8. d
9. b

10. a,b,c,d
11. a,b,c
12. a,b,c,d
13. a,b,c,d
14. c
15. a,b,c,d
16. a,b,c,d
17. c,d

REFERENCES

Arlow, J. Pyromania and the primal scene: A psychoanalytic comment on the work of Yukio Mishima. Psychoanalytic Quarterly, 1978, 47, 24-51.

Axberger, G. Arson and fiction: A cross-disciplinary study. Psychiatry, 1973, 36, 244-265.

Bach-y-Rita, G., Lion, J., Climent, C. & Ervin, I. Episodic dyscontrol: A study of 130 violent patients. American Journal of Psychiatry, 1971, 127, 1473-1478.

Eidelberg, L. (Ed.), Encyclopedia of psychoanalysis. New York: The Free Press, 1968.

Fenichel, O. The psychoanalytic theory of neurosis. New York: W. W. Norton & Co., 1945.

Grossbard, H. Ego deficiency in delinquents. Social Casework, 1962, 43, 171-178.

Leaff, L. Psychodynamic aspects of personality disturbances. In J. Lion (Ed.), Personality disorders: Diagnosis and Management. Baltimore: The Williams and Wilkins Company, 1974.

Lesieur, H. The compulsive gambler's spiral of options and involvement. Psychiatry, 1979, 42, 79-87.

Lewis, N., & Yarnell, H. Pathological firesetting. New York: Nervous and Mental Disease Monographs, 1951.

Lewis, D., & Balla, D. Delinquency and psychopathology. New York: Grune and Stratton, 1976.

Macht, L., & Mack, J. The firesetter syndrome. Psychiatry, 1968, 31, 277-288.

Maletzky, B., & Klotter, J. Episodic dyscontrol: A controlled replication. Diseases of the Nervous System, 1974, 35, 175-179.

Mark, V., & Ervin, F. Violence and the brain. New York: Harper and Row, 1970.

Monroe, R. Episodic behavioral disorders: A psychodynamic and neurophysiologic analysis. Cambridge, Mass.: Harvard University Press, 1970.

Morrison, J., & Minkoff, K. Explosive personality as a sequel to the hyperactive child syndrome. Comprehensive Psychiatry, 1975, 16, 343-348.

Pincus, J., & Tucker, G. Behavioral neurology. New York: Oxford University Press, 1974.

Powers, P., & Gunderman, R.   Kleine-Levin syndrome associated with fire-setting.   American Journal of Diseases of Children, 1978, 132, 786-789.

Quitkin, F., & Klein, D.   Two behavioral syndromes in young adults related to possible minimal brain dysfunction.   Journal of Psychiatric Research, 1969, 7, 131-142.

Redl, F., & Wineman, D.   The aggressive child.   Glencoe, Ill.:   The Free Press, 1957.

Redlich, F., & Freedman, D.   The theory and practice of psychiatry.   New York: Basic Books, Inc., 1966.

Satterfield, J.   The hyperactive child syndrome: A precursor of adult psychopathy?   In R. Hare, & D. Schalling (Eds.), Psychopathic behavior: Approaches to research.   New York: John Wiley and Sons, 1978.

Trasler, G.   Relations between psychopathy and persistent criminality -- Methodological and theoretical issues.   In R. Hare, & D. Schalling (Eds.), Psychopathic behavior: Approaches to research.   New York: John Wiley and Sons, 1978.

Zuckerman, M., Kolin, E., Price, L., & Doob, I.   Development of a sensation seeking scale.   Journal of Consulting Psychology, 1964, 28, 477-482.

CHAPTER 13

Personality Disorders
Donald E. Manning, M.D.

CHAPTER OUTLINE

LEARNING OBJECTIVES

After completing this chapter you will be able to:

1. Define and/or classify the following terms:

    Personality Disorder
    Ego-syntonic
    Ego-dystonic
    Entitlement
    "Fearful" cluster
    "Eccentric" cluster
    "Erratic" cluster

2. Define, characterize or classify the following Personality Disorders:

    Paranoid
    Schizoid
    Schizotypal
    Histrionic
    Narcissistic
    Antisocial
    Borderline
    Avoidant
    Dependent
    Compulsive
    Passive-Aggressive

3. Recognize the treatment approaches to Personality Disorders.

4. Identify the theories of the etiology of Personality Disorders.

PRE-TEST

For each of the following questions, one or more than one answer may be correct. Circle the correct answer(s).

1. Personality Disorders are

    a. maladaptive behavior patterns.
    b. chronic.
    c. dysfunctional.
    d. associated with distress.

2. Personality Disorders

    a. are on a continuum from normal to severe disorder.
    b. fit the concept of a medical illness.
    c. are accepted by the legal system as diseases.
    d. are frequently seen in patients with other psychiatric syndromes.

3. The number of Personality Disorders is

    a. 10 in four clusters.
    b. 12 in three clusters.
    c. 11 in three clusters.
    d. 12 in four clusters.

4. The "odd" or eccentric cluster includes

    a. Schizoid Personality Disorder.
    b. Paranoid Personality Disorder.
    c. Borderline Personality Disorder.
    d. Schizotypal Personality Disorder.

5. If a person is not distressed by his psychiatric disorder it is said to be

    a. a Personality Disorder.
    b. ego-syntonic.
    c. ego-dystonic.
    d. characterologically compatible.

6. The "fearful" cluster of Personality Disorders includes

    a. Passive-Aggressive.
    b. Compulsive.
    c. Dependent.
    d. Discordant.
    e. Obsessive.
    f. Avoidant.

7. The etiology of Personality Disorders has been attributed to

   a. psychological trauma during infancy or early childhood.
   b. social deprivation.
   c. pathological style of family interaction.
   d. biological abnormalities.
   e. genetic inheritance.

8. Appropriate treatment modalities for Personality Disorders include

   a. brief psychotherapy.
   b. intensive psychotherapy.
   c. group therapy.
   d. marital, family therapy.
   e. milieu therapy.
   f. psychopharmacotherapy.

9. Regarding persons with Paranoid Personality Disorder, which of the following statements is (are) true?

   a. Individuals belong to the "erratic" cluster of Personality Disorders.
   b. Individuals are hyperactive.
   c. Individuals are hyperalert.
   d. Individuals are mistrustful.
   e. Individuals are hypersensitive.
   f. Individuals have restricted affect.

10. Which of the following are characteristic of the Schizoid Personality Disorder?

    a. bland affect
    b. no social relationships
    c. detached from the environment
    d. intense expression of anger

11. The "erratic" cluster of Personality Disorders consists of

    a. Narcissistic Personality Disorder.
    b. Borderline Personality Disorder.
    c. Antisocial Personality Disorder.
    d. Schizoid Personality Disorder.

12. The Histrionic Personality Disorder is characterized by

    a. dramatic behavior.
    b. superficial charm.
    c. frequent physical complaints.
    d. sexually naive or inadequate behavior.

13. Which of the following are associated with the Narcissistic Personality Disorder?

    a. grandiosity
    b. exhibitionism
    c. acceptance of criticism
    d. exploitation
    e. expecting favors without reciprocation
    f. distorted empathy

14. Individuals with an Antisocial Personality Disorder

    a. violate the rights of others.
    b. see no need for rules.
    c. anticipate consequences only because they are obstacles.
    d. feel no responsibility for their actions.

15. Individuals with an Antisocial Personality Disorder

    a. frequently have symptoms before age 12.
    b. as adults may be sexually frigid.
    c. are often hobos.
    d. make up a large proportion of the prison population.

16. The Borderline Personality Disorder is characterized by

    a. intense and unstable interpersonal relationships.
    b. frequent feelings of sadness and depression.
    c. transient psychoses.
    d. chronic identity problems.

17. The individual with an Avoidant Personality

    a. is hypersensitive to rejection.
    b. is socially isolated.
    c. has low self-esteem.
    d. has symptoms which are ego-syntonic.
    e. desires to be accepted.

18. Persons with Dependent Personality Disorder are characterized by

    a. allowing others to assume responsibility for major areas of their lives.
    b. preference for being alone.
    c. no confidence.
    d. frequent anxiety.
    e. frequent depression.
    f. being emotionally "cold."

19. Compulsive Personality Disorders are characterized by

    a. decisiveness.
    b. preoccupation with rules, lists, or details.
    c. being controlled by others.
    d. incessant pursuit of pleasure to the exclusion of productivity.

20. The Passive-Aggressive Personality Disorder is characterized by

    a. indecisiveness.
    b. procrastination.
    c. obstinacy.
    d. dedication to pleasure to the exclusion of productive work.
    e. underlying hostility.

I. INTRODUCTION

Personality Disorders may be defined as deeply ingrained, inflexible, maladaptive patterns of relating to, perceiving, or thinking about the environment and oneself. In order to be considered a Personality Disorder, these pervasive patterns must be of such severity that they lead to maladaptive functioning or subjective distress.

Frequently the description of a Personality Disorder includes statements such as "he's been this way for as long as anyone can remember," "nothing seems to produce any change in his behavior," or "she only seems to get upset when things don't go her way."

Before considering the characteristics of distinct Personality Disorders, it is important to distinguish the category of Personality Disorders from other categories of psychiatric illness and from personality types or traits.

Personality Disorder is one of the few conditions coded on Axis II of the DSM-III diagnostic classification. Axis I, on the other hand, is used to encode those major, acute, or severe psychiatric conditions other than the chronic, inflexible Personality Disorders and certain other disorders seen in children. The Axis I conditions are considered the Clinical Psychiatric Syndromes and include Organic Mental Disorders, Substance Use Disorders, Schizophrenic Disorders, Paranoid Disorders, Affective Disorders, Anxiety Disorders, Somatoform and Dissociative Disorders, Psychosexual Disorders, Disorders of Childhood or Adolescence, and Disorders of Impulse Control. All of these clinical conditions have definite symptoms, a clinical course, and in many cases a definite time of onset.

This Axis II separation of Personality Disorders from the majority of psychiatric syndromes underscores the difficulties with this diagnostic category. There are several reasons for these difficulties. First, Personality Disorders do not fit the concept of "illness" which is used by most physicians, i.e., there is no beginning, clinical course, and termination to the illness. In addition, the patient may frequently have another psychiatric syndrome which can be readily diagnosed and treated. Also, the legal structure and society in general tend to regard Personality Disorders as different from other syndromes. For example, if an individual with a Personality Disorder commits a crime, he is "bad"; if a schizophrenic individual commits a crime, he is "sick" (Pierce, 1979).

There is one other difficulty in utilizing this diagnostic category. Personality traits occur on a continuum from normal personality through mild and moderate personality disorders to severe personality disorders. At the extremes of this continuum, little difficulty is encountered in making a diagnosis. Mild or moderate personality traits may be considered to be "Personality Disorders," "eccentric" or even "normal variants." Whether these individuals are diagnosed as having Personality Disorders depends on other factors: treatment setting, physician attitudes, or degree of dysfunction in the environment (Salzman, 1974).

Another important distinction must be made between Personality Disorders and personality types or personality traits. Personality Disorders are associated with dysfunction or distress. On the other hand, personality types or traits are usually connected with little or no dysfunction or distress. All humans have a personality--their technique or style for getting along with others and coping with their environment. This style will have components of one or more Personality Disorders which are discussed below. These personality types or traits can only be diagnosed as a disorder, however, when the pattern becomes dysfunctional or causes distress.

QUIZ, Section I.

Circle the correct answer(s). <u>One</u> or <u>more</u> <u>than</u> <u>one</u> answer may be correct.

1. Personality Disorders

    a. are maladaptive behavior patterns.
    b. are chronic.
    c. are dysfunctional.
    d. produce distress.

2. Axis I disorders

    a. have a definite clinical course.
    b. include Affective Disorders.
    c. include Personality Disorders.
    d. may have a definite time of onset.
    e. include most clinical psychiatric conditions.

3. Axis II disorders generally

    a. are chronic.
    b. are fixed and inflexible.
    c. are long-term.
    d. include Personality Disorders.
    e. usually have no specific time of onset.

4. Personality Disorders

    a. are on a continuum from mild to severe disorder.
    b. fit the concept of a medical illness.
    c. are accepted by the legal system as diseases.
    d. are frequently seen in patients with other psychiatric syndromes.

Match the following phrases with their appropriate descriptions.

_____ 5. associated with dysfunction or distress   a. Personality Disorder

_____ 6. present in all humans   b. personality type or traits

_____ 7. not generally accepted as legal defense   c. both of the above

_____ 8. resembles a medical illness   d. neither of the above

II. NOSOLOGY

There are 11 types of Personality Disorders which are discussed in this chapter. They may be divided into three clusters.

The first cluster may be considered the "eccentric" personality cluster. There are three disorders:

1) Paranoid Personality Disorder
2) Schizoid Personality Disorder
3) Schizotypal Personality Disorder

There are also three characteristics common to these three disorders.

1) The individuals appear "odd" or "eccentric."
2) They seem to be avoiding intimacy, are "cold."
3) The disorders are believed to be related to more severe conditions; the Schizoid and Schizotypal to chronic Schizophrenia and the Paranoid to Paranoid Schizophrenia, paranoia, or paranoid state.

Individuals with Personality Disorders in this "eccentric" cluster rarely present for treatment for their Personality Disorder. These individuals are more likely to have dysfunctional behavior than to be distressed by their disorder. In other words, the Personality Disorder may be said to be ego-syntonic; the patient is not subjectively distressed by his Personality Disorder. (If the patient was distressed by his disorder it would be referred to as ego-dystonic.) When these individuals do present for treatment it is usually because a more serious complication has developed.

The second cluster of Personality Disorders may be considered the "erratic" cluster. There are four:

1) Histrionic Personality Disorder
2) Narcissistic Personality Disorder
3) Antisocial Personality Disorder
4) Borderline Personality Disorder

There are also four characteristics common to these:

1) Appear dramatic
2) Often erratic in behavior

3) Emotionally labile
4) Interpersonal relationships that are intense, superficial, manipulative, or unstable

The third cluster, the "fearful" cluster includes four disorders:

1) Avoidant Personality Disorder
2) Dependent Personality Disorder
3) Compulsive Personality Disorder
4) Passive-Aggressive Personality Disorder

The fear or anxiety present in these individuals is usually related to their inability to cope with their dysfunctional behavior and they are therefore distressed. In other words, their symptoms are ego-dystonic.

Before discussing these specific disorders, there are several general facts that relate to all Personality Disorders.

By definition, Personality Disorders begin in childhood or adolescence and with five exceptions carry the same diagnosis at that age as they do as adults. These exceptions and the corresponding adult diagnoses are:

Disorders of Children or Adolescents	Personality Disorders
1) Conduct Disorder	1) Antisocial Personality Disorder
2) Avoidant Disorder	2) Avoidant Personality Disorder
3) Schizoid Disorder of Childhood	3) Schizoid Personality Disorder
4) Identity Disorder	4) Borderline Personality Disorder
5) Oppositional Disorder	5) Passive-Aggressive Personality Disorder

Most Personality Disorders are characteristically and classically seen in early adult life. The severity of the symptoms generally becomes less obvious in late middle age. However, it should be noted that a Personality Disorder can be exacerbated by acute physical illness or life-threatening chronic illness, and the disorder may become more obvious during old age.

As each Personality Disorder is studied, remember that the pure disorder is not common, but rather what one sees frequently in a clinical setting is a mixture of two or more Personality Disorders. Usually one disorder is more prominent with associated features of one or more disorders.

QUIZ, Section II.

Circle the correct answer(s). One or more than one answer may be correct.

1.   The "odd" or eccentric cluster includes

a.   Schizoid Personality Disorder.
b.   Paranoid Personality Disorder.
c.   Introverted Personality Disorder.
d.   Schizotypal Personality Disorder.

ANSWERS, Section I._____

1. a,b,c,d
2. a,b,d,e
3. a,b,c,d,e
4. a,d
5. a
6. b
7. c
8. d

_____

2. The eccentric group of Personality Disorders

    a. seems odd.
    b. is related to Schizophrenia and paranoia.
    c. is related to Affective Disorder.
    d. avoids intimacy.

3. If a person is not distressed by his psychiatric disorder, it is said to be

    a. a Personality Disorder.
    b. ego-syntonic.
    c. ego-dystonic.
    d. characterologically compatible.

4. The erratic cluster of Personality Disorders shares

    a. avoidance of intimacy.
    b. intense, unstable relationships.
    c. eccentric behavior.
    d. dramatic appearance.

5. The "fearful" cluster of Personality Disorders includes

    a. Passive-Aggressive.
    b. Compulsive.
    c. Dependent.
    d. Discordant.
    e. Avoidant.

6. Personality Disorders

    a. are rigid, deeply engrained behavior patterns or ways of thinking about the world.
    b. are maladaptive or dysfunctional.
    c. begin in childhood or, at the very latest, adolescence.
    d. exacerbate during illness.
    e. are commonly mixed in type of disorder.
    f. are classically seen during young adulthood.

7.   The number of Personality Disorders is

    a. 10 in four clusters.
    b. 12 in three clusters.
    c. 11 in three clusters.
    d. 12 in four clusters.

Match the following lettered items with the numbered terms.

___ 8.   schizoid   a. eccentric cluster
___ 9.   antisocial   b. erratic cluster
___10.   histrionic
___11.   schizotypal
___12.   borderline
___13.   paranoid
___14.   narcissistic

Match the following disorders of childhood with the corresponding Personality Disorders.

___15.   Schizoid Disorder of Childhood   a. Antisocial Personality Disorder
___16.   Identity Disorder   b. Avoidant Personality Disorder
___17.   Avoidant Disorder   c. Schizoid Personality Disorder
___18.   Conduct Disorder   d. Borderline Personality Disorder
___19.   Oppositional Disorder   e. Passive-Aggressive Personality
                                                Disorder

===

III. ETIOLOGY AND TREATMENT

The causes of Personality Disorders are not known. There is some tentative evidence for biological or genetic factors in the etiology of Personality Disorders. For example, certain Personality Disorders tend to have a familial pattern of occurrence, particularly the Antisocial Personality Disorder. Secondly, infants seem to have congenitally different "constitutions" or "temperaments." Rather than biological or genetic, these have been explained as a behavioral response to the parent's style of interacting with the infant. A third area of biological investigation deals with the relationship between abnormal electroencephalograms and behavioral or Personality Disorders. The research in these areas lacks the intensity and definitive data obtained from similar research with other psychiatric syndromes.

On the other hand, many writers support psychodynamic theories of the etiology of Personality Disorders. The disorder is seen as the result of a severe psychological trauma to the infant or young child. This trauma arrested or altered his normal psychological development. According to this schema, a severe disruption in psychological development at a time when the infant is attempting to separate himself from the mothering figure could lead to a Borderline Personality Disorder. If the infant fails to develop the capacity for trust, this can lead in the adult to any of the eccentric cluster of Personality Disorders. If the psychological trauma occurs during the time when the child is dealing with autonomy and control, the trauma can produce a Dependent or Compulsive Personality Disorder in the adult. Furthermore, the Antisocial Personality Disorder is considered the result of trauma during the stage when the superego (conscience) was developing.

Other writers believe social or familial factors are predominant in the development of Personality Disorders. There is a growing body of literature supporting the relationship between Personality Disorders and family pathology or social deprivation.

Treatment of individuals with Personality Disorders is difficult, and some appear impossible to help. The most commonly employed treatments are brief psychotherapy and in some patients intensive psychotherapy. Group, marital, and family therapy have been reported to be helpful. Long-term hospitalization may be helpful for severe disorders when it is combined with an interpretive milieu and intensive individual and group psychotherapy. Medications are rarely helpful and may be contraindicated in many Personality Disorders because of addictive and abuse potential.

QUIZ, Section III.

Circle the correct answer(s). One or more than one answer may be correct.

1. The etiology of Personality Disorders has been attributed to

   a. psychological trauma during infancy or early childhood.
   b. social deprivation.
   c. pathological style of family interaction.
   d. biological abnormalities.
   e. genetic inheritance.

2. Appropriate treatment modalities for Personality Disorders include

   a. brief psychotherapy.
   b. intensive psychotherapy.
   c. group therapy.
   d. marital, family therapy.
   e. milieu therapy.
   f. psychopharmacotherapy.

IV. SPECIFIC DISORDERS

A. PARANOID PERSONALITY DISORDER (DSM-III 301.00)

According to the DSM-III, individuals with a Paranoid Personality Disorder have a long-standing and pervasive suspiciousness and mistrust of
people. They are hypersensitive, easily slighted, and hypervigilant. They
are strikingly unwilling to relinquish suspicious ideas, even in the face of
irrefutable data. They rarely seek psychiatric help unless forced into it
by superiors in the military, prison, or other institution. The prevalence
is not known, but this disorder may be overrepresented among leaders of
mystical or esoteric religions, pseudoscientific and quasi-political groups.
It is probably more common among men.

Case Study: P.P., a 57-year-old male, is referred for psychiatric evaluation by his attorney, who wonders if there is a psychiatric disorder in
his client and if it is treatable. The attorney gives the history that his
client has entered into six lawsuits in the past three years, all of some
questionable validity. The attorney describes Mr. P. as a strikingly controlled, unemotional man who now wishes to sue a local department store
for "conspiracy to deprive him of his rights as a consumer." On interview,
Mr. P. confirms this history. He believes that the department store is
biased against him for reasons that are not clear to him and that the management has consistently issued bad credit reports on him. This is in spite
of his only infrequent delinquencies in paying his debts. On further questioning, there are two other areas in Mr. P.'s life that are conflicted. He
has long distrusted his next door neighbors and keeps binoculars by his
window to carefully monitor their activities. Mr. P. has had three jobs in
the last 14 years, but is currently unemployed. He left each position because of a series of events: his supervisors became disloyal and complained
about his actions to his superiors. Mr. P. contends that he was faultless
in all cases. In fact, he has always prided himself on being objective and
rational. On examination, Mr. P.'s mental status is unremarkable except for
a certain hesitation or guardedness in his response to questions and some
constriction of affect.

From the following list of diagnostic criteria, choose the positive findings
from the case study above.

Diagnostic Criteria for Paranoid Personality Disorder

The following are characteristic of the individual's current and
long-term functioning, are not limited to episodes of illness, and
cause either significant impairment in social or occupational functioning or subjective distress.

A. Pervasive, unwarranted suspiciousness and mistrust of
people as indicated by at least three of the following:

(1) expectation of trickery or harm

ANSWERS, Section II.

1.	a,b,d	11.	a
2.	a,b,d	12.	b
3.	b	13.	a
4.	b,d	14.	b
5.	a,b,c,e	15.	c
6.	a,b,c,d,e,f	16.	d
7.	c	17.	b
8.	a	18.	a
9.	b	19.	e
10.	b		

    (2) hypervigilance, manifested by continual scanning of the environment for signs of threat, or taking unneeded precautions

    (3) guardedness or secretiveness

    (4) avoidance of accepting blame even when warranted

    (5) questioning the loyalty of others

    (6) intense, narrowly focused searching for confirmation of bias, with loss of appreciation of total context

    (7) overconcern with hidden motives and special meanings

    (8) pathological jealousy

B.   Hypersensitivity as indicated by at least two of the following:

    (1) tendency to be easily slighted and quick to take offense

    (2) exaggeration of difficulties, e.g., "making mountains out of molehills"

    (3) readiness to counterattack when any threat is perceived

    (4) inability to relax

C.   Restricted affectivity as indicated by at least two of the following:

    (1) appearance of being "cold" and unemotional

    (2) pride taken in always being objective, rational, and unemotional

    (3) lack of a true sense of humor

    (4) absence of passive, soft, tender, and sentimental feelings

D.   Not due to another mental disorder such as Schizophrenia or a Paranoid Disorder.

ANSWERS to Case Study:

A   (1), (2), (3), (4), (5), (7);

B   (1), (3);

C   (1), (2);

D

B. SCHIZOID PERSONALITY DISORDER (DSM-III 301.20)

According to the DSM-III, individuals with a Schizoid Personality Disorder lack the capacity to form social relationships and have a bland or constricted affect. These are the true loners, the hermits, the hobos, the skid row bums. They seem vague and detached from their environment. They seem "in a fog," are humorless, and unable to express hostility. These individuals are usually severely impaired socially and occupationally, although females may passively marry and males may perform satisfactorily in certain occupations such as night watchmen or clerks.

****

GO TO VIDEOTAPE

****

C. SCHIZOTYPAL PERSONALITY DISORDER (DSM-III 301.22)

According to the DSM-III, individuals with this disorder show various oddities of thinking, perception, communication, and behavior. The disturbance in thinking may be magical thinking, ideas of reference, or paranoid ideation. These symptoms were discussed in the chapter on Schizophrenia, as were the perceptual disturbances: frequently illusions, depersonalization or derealization. Communication is disrupted because words are used in an odd, deviant way (neologism). As was the case with the Schizoid Personality Disorder, the individual is socially isolated and his affect is flat or inappropriate.

The differential diagnosis of Schizotypal Personality Disorder from Schizophrenia rests primarily on the short-lived nature of the schizotypal psychotic episodes (periods of bizarre behavior and oddities of thinking that approach delusions). These oddities of thinking are not present in Schizoid Personality Disorder.

Case Study: A.B., a 36-year-old single female presented for evaluation for outpatient treatment. She was referred by her mother who complained that the patient had no interests, friends, or outside activities. The patient readily admitted that these things were true, but she denied that they were a problem for her. The patient believed that her mother was concerned about her because of what might happen to the patient after the mother's death. The patient was not able to identify any recent changes in her life or emotional state that would account for her mother's insistence on treatment for her.

The patient was an only child whose father died in an auto accident prior to her birth. When she was a child, she and her mother moved to a small resort community and continue to share the home they bought there. The patient was educated in the local public schools and graduated from high school with average grades. She was not involved in extracurricular activities in school. Following graduation, the patient was tutored in art by a local retired commercial artist. She had begun sketching when she was an adolescent and continues painting and sketching erratically. She has never sold nor exhibited her works. The patient has never dated and in the past 20 years has, for the most part, stayed at home, reading and watching television.

On examination the patient was an alert, somewhat uncooperative female who appeared older than her stated age with moderately disheveled hair and clothing. Rapport during the interview was low. The patient's speech was monotonous and deliberate. She was vague and tangential in her thinking and expressed a belief that her fate lay in "the stars." She denied specific delusions. Her affect was constricted except for one episode of anger when she felt the examiner was being critical of her for not working. She denied perceptual abnormalities.

From the diagnostic criteria listed below, choose the positive findings from the case study above.

Diagnostic Criteria for Schizoid Personality Disorder

The following are characteristic of the individual's current and long-term functioning, are not limited to episodes of illness, and cause either significant impairment in social or occupational functioning or subjective distress.

A.   Emotional coldness and aloofness, and absence of warm, tender feelings for others.

B.   Indifference to praise or criticism or to the feelings of others.

C.   Close friendships with no more than one or two persons, including family members.

D.   No eccentricities of speech, behavior, or thought characteristic of Schizotypal Personality Disorder.

E.   Not due to a psychotic disorder such as Schizophrenia or Paranoid Disorder.

F.   If under 18, does not meet the criteria for Schizoid Disorder of Childhood or Adolescence.

Diagnostic Criteria for Schizotypal Personality Disorder

The following are characteristic of the individual's current and long-term functioning, are not limited to episodes of illness, and cause either significant impairment in social or occupational functioning or subjective distress.

A.   At least four of the following:

(1) magical thinking, e.g., superstitiousness, clairvoyance, telepathy, "6th sense," "others can feel my feelings" (in children and adolescents, bizarre fantasies or preoccupations)
(2) ideas of reference
(3) social isolation, e.g., no close friends or confidants, social contacts limited to essential everyday tasks
(4) recurrent illusions, sensing the presence of a force or person not actually present (e.g., "I felt as if my dead mother were in the room with me"), depersonalization, or derealization not associated with panic attacks
(5) odd speech (without loosening of association or incoherence), e.g., speech that is digressive, vague, overelaborate, circumstantial, metaphorical
(6) inadequate rapport in face-to-face interaction due to constricted or inappropriate affect, e.g., aloof, cold
(7) suspiciousness or paranoid ideation
(8) undue social anxiety or hypersensitivity to real or imagined criticism

B.   Does not meet the criteria for Schizophrenia.

ANSWERS to Case Study:
Schizoid: A; C; E
Schizotypal: A (1),(3),(5),(6),(8); B

QUIZ, Section IV. A - C.

Circle the correct answer(s). One or more than one answer may be correct.

1.   The Paranoid Personality Disorder

a.   belongs to the "erratic" cluster of Personality Disorders.
b.   individuals are hyperactive.
c.   individuals are hyperalert.
d.   individuals are mistrustful.
e.   individuals are hypersensitive.
f.   individuals have restricted affect.

2.   Characteristics of the Schizoid Personality Disorder are

a.   bland affect.
b.   no social relationships.
c.   detached from the environment.
d.   intense expression of anger.

3. The Schizotypal Personality Disorder is

    a. similar to the Schizoid Personality Disorder in affect, social isolation.
    b. dissimilar from the Schizoid Personality Disorder in bizarre thinking.
    c. related to Schizophrenia.
    d. commonly associated with perceptual disturbances.

4. Symptoms of the Schizoid Personality Disorder include

    a. brief psychoses.
    b. bland affect.
    c. social isolation.
    d. perceptual disturbance.

5. Symptoms of the Schizotypal Personality Disorder include

    a. brief psychoses.
    b. bland affect.
    c. social isolation.
    d. perceptual disturbances.

6. Symptoms of Schizophrenia include

    a. brief psychoses.
    b. bland affect.
    c. social isolation.
    d. perceptual disturbances.

7. The "eccentric" cluster of Personality Disorders consists of

    a. Paranoid Personality Disorder.
    b. Introverted Personality Disorder.
    c. Schizoid Personality Disorder.
    d. Schizotypal Personality Disorder.

8. Supporting the diagnosis of an "eccentric" Personality Disorder are all the following except

    a. few close friends.
    b. severe social and occupational impairment.
    c. bizarre thoughts.
    d. symptoms that are ego-dystonic.

Match the lettered eccentric Personality Disorder(s) associated with each of the following numbered symptoms. Lettered items may be used once or more than once.

___ 9.	difficulty getting angry
___10.	social isolation, avoid intimacy
___11.	usually forced when they come to treatment
___12.	hypervigilant
___13.	"skid row bums," hobos
___14.	flat, inappropriate, or constricted affect
___15.	bizarre thinking
___16.	symptoms are ego-dystonic

a. schizoid
b. schizotypal
c. paranoid
d. none

D.   HISTRIONIC PERSONALITY DISORDER (DSM-III 301.50)

This disorder was previously contained in a broader category of disorders known as the hysterical character or Hysterical Personality Disorder. According to the DSM-III, individuals with this disorder behave in a dramatic, overly reactive and intense way. As with other "erratic" Personality Disorders, there is an inconsistency of behavior. Superficially, these individuals may appear charming, appealing, and gregarious, but on close scrutiny they become demanding, vain, and egocentric. Sexual adjustment is poor; females are usually flirtatious, coquettish, and sexually naive. Although more common in females, males with this condition are usually promiscuous, sexually inadequate, or feminine in behavior. Individuals with this disorder often complain of physical symptoms (Somatization Disorder), are prone to depressions, substance abuse, and suicide attempts.

Case Study: J.T. was a 26-year-old female seen in the emergency room for consultation following ingestion of an overdose of minor tranquilizers. The patient stated she took the overdose in an attempt to kill herself, that she found life not worth living since her boyfriend had moved out the afternoon before. The patient was observed to be an attractive, well-dressed woman wearing makeup and nail polish. During the interview she was warm and charming, maintained good eye contact with some flirtatiousness (winking, seductive smiles), and was emotionally labile, shifting from smiling elation to tearful sadness. The patient's boyfriend was with her in the emergency room. In fact, it was he who called the ambulance after the patient had called him and told him about her overdose. He states that the reason he left the patient was because she made demands of him that he could not meet, that he never seemed able to satisfy her emotionally or sexually. In addition, he had been unable to afford the clothes she had expected him to buy for her and complained that she wanted to "go out every night and party." The day before she had lost her temper because he had wanted to play golf with a friend and he had decided to leave.

From the following diagnostic criteria, choose the positive findings for the case study above.

Diagnostic Criteria for Histrionic Personality Disorder

The following are characteristic of the individual's current and long-term functioning, are not limited to episodes of illness, and cause either significant impairment in social or occupational functioning or subjective distress.

A. Behavior that is overly dramatic, reactive, and intensely expressed, as indicated by at least three of the following:

    (1) self-dramatization, e.g., exaggerated expression of emotions
    (2) incessant drawing of attention to oneself
    (3) craving for activity and excitement
    (4) overreaction to minor events
    (5) irrational, angry outbursts or tantrums

B. Characteristic disturbances in interpersonal relationships as indicated by at least two of the following:

    (1) perceived by others as shallow and lacking genuineness, even if superficially warm and charming
    (2) egocentric, self-indulgent, and inconsiderate of others
    (3) vain and demanding
    (4) dependent, helpless, constantly seeking reassurance
    (5) prone to manipulative suicidal threats, gestures, or attempts

ANSWERS To Case Study:
A (1),(3),(5)
B (1),(3),(5)

****

GO TO VIDEOTAPE

****

E. NARCISSISTIC PERSONALITY DISORDER (DSM-III 301.81)

This condition has been described for many years as a component of other Personality Disorders, but only recently has it won general acceptance as a separate and specific Personality Disorder. The incidence and sexual prevalence are unknown. This disorder may be defined as a fixed, chronic disturbance in the individual's self-regard and in how he relates to others. According to the DSM-III, there are five essential features:

    1) A grandiose sense of self-importance or uniqueness
    2) Preoccupation with fantasies of unlimited success
    3) Exhibitionistic need for constant attention and admiration

4) When criticized, the narcissistic personality may develop a cool indifference, or may become enraged with feelings of shame, inferiority or emptiness.

5) Interpersonal relationships are characterized by several disturbances. The narcissistic personality may use others as if he were "squeezing a lemon and then dropping the remains" (Kernberg, 1975, p. 233). Entitlement is usually present; this is the expectation of special favors without assuming reciprocal responsibility. There may also be a lack of empathy or the appreciation of how others feel--the individual may also vacillate between over-idealization and devaluation.

Case Study: C.D., a 63-year-old male, presented for treatment for feelings of shame and inferiority following a forced early retirement from his job as a used car salesman. His employer stated the patient was ineffective and erratic, frequently scaring customers away with exaggerated claims and pressured selling techniques. The patient denied that this was true. He stated that to the contrary, he was the number one salesman in the state for six consecutive years, that he "made" his former company the best in the region and that the company is "headed down the tube" without him. The patient further contributed that he was too important to be summarily dismissed. To support this, he volunteered that in his capacity as a regional officer of a veteran's group, he was a security advisor to the federal government, and produced a picture of himself shaking hands with then Vice-President Nixon.

His personal life has been complicated, including several marriages and divorces. One of his greatest disappointments is that his children by his first marriage have had nothing to do with him ever since they have moved out of their mother's home. He stated that their mother prevented contact between them before but that they were obligated to "honor" him, and he was angry that they had avoided contact.

From the diagnostic criteria listed below, choose the positive findings from the case study above.

Diagnostic Criteria for Narcissistic Personality Disorder

The following are characteristic of the individual's current and long-term functioning, are not limited to episodes of illness, and cause either significant impairment in social or occupational functioning or subjective distress:

A. Grandiose sense of self-importance or uniqueness, e.g., exaggeration of achievements and talents, focus on the special nature of one's problems.

B. Preoccupation with fantasies of unlimited success, power, brilliance, beauty, or ideal love.

C. Exhibitionism: the person requires constant attention and admiration.

1.	c,d,e,f	9.	a
2.	a,b,c	10.	a,b,c
3.	a,b,c,d	11.	c
4.	b,c	12.	c
5.	a,b,c,d	13.	a
6.	b,c,d	14.	a,b
7.	a,c,d	15.	b
8.	d	16.	d

D. Cool indifference or marked feelings of rage, inferiority, shame, humiliation, or emptiness in response to criticism, indifference of others, or defeat.

E. At least two of the following are characteristic of disturbances in interpersonal relationships:

   (1) entitlement: expectation of special favors without assuming reciprocal responsibilities, e.g., surprise and anger that people will not do what is wanted
   (2) interpersonal exploitativeness: taking advantage of others to indulge own desires or for self-aggrandizement; disregard for the personal integrity and rights of others
   (3) relationships that characteristically alternate between the extremes of overidealization and devaluation
   (4) lack of empathy: inability to recognize how others feel, e.g., unable to appreciate the distress of someone who is seriously ill

ANSWERS to Case Study:
A; B; C; D; E (1), (2), (4)

F. ANTISOCIAL PERSONALITY DISORDER (DSM-III 301.70)

According to the DSM-III, this disorder may be defined as a disorder where individuals chronically violate the rights of others. These people in the past have also been diagnosed as psychopaths, psychopathic deviates, and sociopaths. There is much debate over whether this is a legitimate psychiatric illness, with some writers suggesting that the "treatment of choice" should be incarceration with other criminals. On the other hand, those who support the concept of this being a psychiatric illness believe that the condition is an outgrowth of a basic flaw in the development of the individual. This flaw in the superego (or conscience) prevents the adequate control of impulses and prevents the individual from feeling guilt or remorse. Furthermore, this defect prevents the individual from perceiving the need for rules in society nor can he anticipate the consequences of breaking rules (Winokur & Crowe, 1975).

The Antisocial Personality Disorder frequently appears before the age of 12 and invariably appears before 15. Usual presenting symptoms are lying, stealing, fighting, truancy, or other trouble at school, home, or in the community. The disorder progresses to early or aggressive sexual behavior and alcohol and drug abuse. In adulthood the prevalent behaviors are sexual promiscuity, fighting, criminality, and vagrancy. There are strong familial patterns to this disorder, and it is more common in males and in lower socioeconomic groups.

Case Study: J.C., a 20-year-old male, was referred for evaluation by his family physician. He had a history of increasing difficulty at home with frequent fights with his widowed mother and 17-year-old sister. The week before the referral he had been involved in his third fight with his sister in two months, and she had required sutures at the doctor's office. He has not worked in seven months and has been frequently unemployed since he quit high school at 16. Most of his money comes from selling drugs, although his personal use of drugs does not seem an issue.

The patient's mother stated that he was always a difficult child, running away from home, fighting at school, being expelled from school and always lying. The earliest problem she remembered was his "playing hookey" in the third grade.

She had always thought the patient was "brain damaged," but multiple evaluations had been negative.

From the diagnostic criteria listed below, choose the positive findings from the case study above.

Diagnostic Criteria for Antisocial Personality Disorder

A.   Current age at least 18.

B.   Onset before age 15 as indicated by a history of three or more of the following before that age:

(1) truancy (positive if it amounted to at least five days per year for at least two years, not including the last year of school)
(2) expulsion or suspension from school for misbehavior
(3) delinquency (arrested or referred to juvenile court because of behavior)
(4) running away from home overnight at least twice while living in parental or parental surrogate home
(5) persistent lying
(6) repeated sexual intercourse in a casual relationship
(7) repeated drunkenness or substance abuse
(8) thefts
(9) vandalism
(10) school grades markedly below expectations in relation to estimated or known IQ (may have resulted in repeating a year)
(11) chronic violations of rules at home and/or at school (other than truancy)
(12) initiation of fights

C. At least 4 of the following manifestations of the disorder since age 18:

(1) inability to sustain consistent work behavior, as indicated by any of the following: (a) too frequent job changes (e.g., three or more jobs in five years not accounted for by nature of job or economic or seasonal fluctuation), (b) significant unemployment (e.g., six months or more in five years when expected to work), (c) serious absenteeism from work (e.g., average three days or more of lateness or absence per month) (d) walking off several jobs without other jobs in sight (Note: Similar behavior in an academic setting during the last few years of school may substitute for this criterion in individuals who by reason of their age or circumstances have not had an opportunity to demonstrate occupational adjustment.)

(2) lack of ability to function as a responsible parent as evidenced by one or more of the following: (a) child's malnutrition, (b) child's illness resulting from lack of minimal hygiene standards, (c) failure to obtain medical care for a seriously ill child, (d) child's dependence on neighbors or nonresident relatives for food or shelter, (e) failure to arrange for a caretaker for a child under six when parent is away from home, (f) repeated squandering, on personal items, of money required for household necessities

(3) failure to accept social norms with respect to lawful behavior, as indicated by any of the following: repeated thefts, illegal occupation (pimping, prostitution, fencing, selling drugs), multiple arrests, a felony conviction

(4) inability to maintain enduring attachment to a sexual partner as indicated by two or more divorces and/or separations (whether legally married or not), desertion of spouse, promiscuity (ten or more sexual partners within one year)

(5) irritability and aggressiveness as indicated by repeated physical fights or assault (not required by one's job or to defend someone or oneself), including spouse or child beating

(6) failure to honor financial obligations, as indicated by repeated defaulting on debts, failure to provide child support, failure to support other dependents on a regular basis

(7) failure to plan ahead, or impulsivity, as indicated by traveling from place to place without a prearranged job or clear goal for the period of travel or clear idea about when the travel would terminate, or lack of a fixed address for a month or more

(8) disregard for the truth as indicated by repeated lying, use of aliases, "conning" others for personal profit

(9) recklessness, as indicated by driving while intoxicated or recurrent speeding

    D.   A pattern of continuous antisocial behavior in which the rights of others are violated, with no intervening period of at least five years without antisocial behavior between age 15 and the present time (except when the individual was bedridden or confined in a hospital or penal institution).

    E.   Antisocial behavior is not due to either Severe Mental Retardation, Schizophrenia, or Manic Episodes.

ANSWERS to Case Study:
A
B (1),(2),(4),(5),(11), (12)
C (1),(3),(5),(8)
D
E

****

GO TO VIDEOTAPE

****

G.   BORDERLINE PERSONALITY DISORDER (DSM-III 301.83)

The hallmark of the Borderline Personality Disorder is instability. According to the DSM-III, interpersonal relationships are intense and unstable. Behavior can be impulsive and unpredictable. Mood is unstable with a strong tendency to feelings of loneliness, anger, emptiness, or boredom. There may be a profound identity problem, either in self-image or gender identity. There may be transient episodes that resemble acute psychoses, particularly during and following periods of extreme stress.

Case Study: C.B., a 25-year-old female, was seen in the emergency room after a drug overdose and wrist cutting episode. She stated that she was furious with her husband because he was having an affair with a man who was living with them. The patient stated that her current husband was her fourth. Past history was significant in that she had run away from home when she was 16 with a rodeo clown, but left him two years later to move into an artists' commune in the Southwest. She lived there for six months with a man who taught Eastern meditation and then returned to a city near her home where she remarried. During this last marriage she was using drugs heavily and was hospitalized once for detoxification. Following this, she lived with two men who were lovers, eventually marrying one. The patient complains of long-standing feelings of depression, loneliness, emptiness, and boredom that are intermittently more severe. Her mental status examination is essentially normal except for intense anger when discussing important people in her life, and some lability of affect.

From the following diagnostic criteria, choose the ones which were observed in this case.

Diagnostic Criteria for Borderline Personality Disorder

The following are characteristic of the individual's current and long-term functioning, are not limited to episodes of illness, and cause either significant impairment in social or occupational functioning or subjective distress.

A. At least five of the following are required:

   (1) impulsivity or unpredictability in at least two areas that are potentially self-damaging, e.g., spending, sex, gambling, substance use, shoplifting, overeating, physically self-damaging acts

   (2) a pattern of unstable and intense interpersonal relationships, e.g., marked shifts of attitude, idealization, devaluation, manipulation (consistently using others for one's own ends)

   (3) inappropriate, intense anger or lack of control of anger, e.g., frequent displays of temper, constant anger

   (4) identity disturbance manifested by uncertainty about several issues relating to identity, such as self-image, gender identity, long-term goals or career choice, friendship patterns, values, and loyalties, e.g., "Who am I," "I feel like I am my sister when I am good"

   (5) affective instability: marked shifts from normal mood to depression, irritability, or anxiety, usually lasting a few hours and only rarely more than a few days, with a return to normal mood

   (6) intolerance of being alone, e.g., frantic efforts to avoid being alone, depressed when alone

   (7) physically self-damaging acts, e.g., suicidal gestures, self-mutilation, recurrent accidents or physical fights

   (8) chronic feelings of emptiness or boredom

B. If under 18, does not meet the criteria for Identity Disorder.

ANSWERS to Case Study:
A. (1),(2),(3),(5),(6),(7),(8)

****

GO TO VIDEOTAPE

****

QUIZ, Section IV. D-G.

Circle the correct answer(s). One or more than one answer may be correct.

1. The disorders that are included in the second or "erratic" cluster of Personality Disorders are

    a. Histrionic Personality Disorder.
    b. Hysterical Personality Disorder.
    c. Borderline Personality Disorder.
    d. Antisocial Personality Disorder.
    e. Narcissistic Personality Disorder.

2. The Histrionic Personality Disorder is characterized by

    a. dramatic behavior.
    b. superficial charm.
    c. frequent physical complaints.
    d. sexually naive or inadequate behavior.

3. Which of the following is/are associated with the Narcissistic Personality Disorder?

    a. grandiosity
    b. exhibitionism
    c. acceptance of criticism
    d. exploitation
    e. expecting favors without reciprocation
    f. distorted empathy

4. Individuals with an Antisocial Personality Disorder

    a. violate the rights of others.
    b. see no need for rules.
    c. anticipate consequences only because they are obstacles.
    d. feel no responsibility for their actions.

5. Individuals with an Antisocial Personality Disorder

    a. frequently have symptoms before 12.
    b. as adults may be sexually frigid.
    c. are often hobos.
    d. make up a large proportion of the prison population.

6. The Borderline Personality Disorder is characterized by

    a. intense and unstable interpersonal relationships.
    b. frequent feelings of sadness and depression.
    c. transient psychoses.
    d. chronic identity problems.

H. AVOIDANT PERSONALITY DISORDER (DSM-III 301.82)

As described by the DSM-III, the individual with an Avoidant Personality Disorder is hypersensitive to rejection, is socially withdrawn, yet desires affection and acceptance, and has low self-esteem. Another Personality Disorder, the Introverted also is socially isolated but does not desire social contact. This is the essential difference between the Avoidant and the Introverted Personality Disorders: one is ego-syntonic and the other ego-dystonic.

I. DEPENDENT PERSONALITY DISORDER (DSM-III 301.60)

An individual with this disorder has other people assume responsibility for major areas of his life, lacks self-confidence and is intensely uncomfortable when alone. Anxiety and depression are common.

Case Study: H.D., a 48-year-old single female, admitted herself for inpatient psychiatric treatment because of intense suicidal ideations. The patient related the onset of these feelings to two unrelated, simultaneous events. First, her homosexual lover of 25 years left for one month to place her elderly parents in a nursing home. Secondly, the patient's sister visited and made some comments about the patient's cooking ability which the patient interpreted as ridiculing and rejecting. Following these two events, the patient began obsessing about suicide. She thought, however, that she did not want to kill herself. She only wanted her lover to come back and her family to leave her alone.

The patient described lifelong feelings of inadequacy, inferiority, low self-esteem, and lack of self-confidence. She saw her lover as more responsible, capable and confident. In fact, she stated this was the only person she had ever allowed herself to depend on. In the relationship, the partner had the larger income, shopped, paid the bills, cooked, and kept the house. The patient, who had a masters degree in religion, did not work nor drive a car. She did, however, substitute teach a Sunday school class at a neighborhood church.

On examination, the patient was a slight, tremulous female who appeared depressed and obsessed about her need for her partner and her need to be rid of her family. Her mental status examination was otherwise unremarkable.

This case represents a Mixed Personality Disorder. Review the criteria for Avoidant and Dependent Personality Disorders, as listed below, checking those that are present in this case study.

Diagnostic Criteria for Avoidant Personality Disorder

The following are characteristic of the individual's current and long-term functioning, are not limited to episodes of illness, and cause either significant impairment in social or occupational functioning or subjective distress.

A.   Hypersensitivity to rejection, e.g., apprehensively alert to signs of social derogation, interprets innocuous events as ridicule.

B.   Unwillingness to enter into relationships unless given unusually strong guarantees of uncritical acceptance.

C.   Social withdrawal, e.g., distances self from close personal attachments, engages in peripheral social and vocational roles.

D.   Desire for affection and acceptance.

E.   Low self-esteem, e.g., devalues self-achievements and is overly dismayed by personal shortcomings.

F.   If under 18, does not meet the criteria for Avoidant Disorder of Childhood or Adolescence.

Diagnostic Criteria for Dependent Personality Disorder

The following are characteristic of the individual's current and long-term functioning, are not limited to episodes of illness, and cause either significant impairment in social or occupational functioning or subjective distress.

A.   Passively allows others to assume responsibility for major areas of life because of inability to function independently (e.g., lets spouse decide what kind of job he or she should have).

B.   Subordinates own needs to those of persons on whom he or she depends in order to avoid any possibility of having to rely on self, e.g., tolerates abusive spouse.

C.   Lack of self-confidence, e.g., sees self as helpless, stupid.

ANSWERS to Case Study:
Avoidant: A; B; C; D; E
Dependent: A; B; C

J.   COMPULSIVE PERSONALITY DISORDER (DSM-III 301.40)

As described in the DSM-III, individuals with a Compulsive Personality Disorder cannot express warm and tender emotions; they are "cold."

They are preoccupied with rules and details. They need others to submit to their way of doing things, i.e., they are controlling. They devote themselves to work and exclude pleasure. Because of an overriding need to avoid mistakes, they postpone or avoid decisions.

Case Study: W. G. was a 38-year-old male who presented for evaluation for psychotherapy with a chief complaint of a pervasive feeling of dread. He

ANSWERS, Section IV. D-G. _____

1. a,c,d,e
2. a,b,c,d
3. a,b,d,e,f
4. a,b,d
5. a,d
6. a,b,c,d

_____

gave a history of long-standing feelings of dissatisfaction in his marriage which had become worse over the last 3-4 years. He described his marriage as one where his wife was constantly making more demands for affection than he was capable of delivering. He saw this need for affection as a weakness that his wife had. On the other hand, his professional life had not been conflicted until recently. A highly successful businessman, he had worked 12-18 hours per day to build his business, but had now come to the point of having to decide whether to break up a long-standing partnership. He felt he had to make decisions about what to do with his marriage and with his partnership and found himself unable to do so. He felt that he "couldn't see the forest for the trees" and wished therapy to help him make decisions.

On examination, the patient was neatly dressed in a three-piece suit with club tie and matching handkerchief. His posture was rigid and his speech was controlled and somewhat formal. Affect was constricted and isolated. His thinking was characterized by preoccupation with accounting procedures at his work, and he was markedly circumstantial.

Review the diagnostic criteria for the Compulsive Personality Disorder below. Choose those criteria which are demonstrated in this case study.

Diagnostic Criteria for Compulsive Personality Disorder

At least four of the following are characteristic of the individual's current and long-term functioning, are not limited to episodes of illness, and cause either significant impairment in social or occupational functioning or subjective distress:

(1) restricted ability to express warm and tender emotions, e.g., the individual is unduly conventional, serious and formal, and stingy

(2) perfectionism that interferes with the ability to grasp "the big picture," e.g., preoccupation with trivial details, rules, order, organization, schedules, and lists

(3) insistence that others submit to his or her way of doing things and lack of awareness of the feelings elicited by this behavior, e.g., a husband stubbornly insists his wife complete errands for him regardless of her plans

(4) excessive devotion to work and productivity to the exclusion of pleasure and the value of interpersonal relationships

(5) indecisiveness: decision-making is either avoided, post-poned, or protracted, perhaps because of an inordinate fear of making a mistake, e.g., the individual cannot get assignments done on time because of ruminating about priorities

ANSWERS to Case Study:
(1),(2),(4),(5)

****

GO TO VIDEOTAPE

****

K.   PASSIVE-AGGRESSIVE PERSONALITY DISORDER (DSM-III 301.84)

Individuals with a Passive-Aggressive Personality Disorder are resistant to demands for acceptable behavior at work or socially. Hostility is expressed covertly, usually through procrastination, stubbornness, or inefficiency.

The diagnosis is rarely made on examination but rather from history or lengthy observation.

Diagnostic Criteria for Passive-Aggressive Personality Disorder

The following are characteristic of the individual's current and long-term functioning, and are not limited to episodes of illness.

A.   Resistance to demands for adequate performance in both occu-pational and social functioning.

B.   Resistance expressed indirectly through at least two of the following:

(1) procrastination
(2) dawdling
(3) stubbornness
(4) intentional inefficiency
(5) "forgetfulness"

C.   As a consequence of A and B, pervasive and long-standing social and occupational ineffectiveness (including in roles of housewife or student), e.g., intentional inefficiency has prevented job promotion.

D.   Persistence of the behavior pattern even under circumstances in which more self-assertive and effective behavior is pos-sible.

E. Does not meet the criteria for any other Personality Disorder, and if under age 18, does not meet the criteria for Oppositional Disorder.

****

GO TO VIDEOTAPE

****

QUIZ, Section IV. H-K.

Circle the correct answer(s). One or more than one answer may be correct.

1. The third cluster, the fearful group, of Personality Disorders consists of

    a. Avoidant Personality Disorder.
    b. Obsessive Personality Disorder.
    c. Compulsive Personality Disorder.
    d. Passive-Dependent Personality Disorder.
    e. Passive-Aggressive Personality Disorder.
    f. Dependent Personality Disorder.

2. The Avoidant Personality

    a. is hypersensitive to rejection.
    b. is socially isolated.
    c. has low self-esteem.
    d. has symptoms which are ego-syntonic.
    e. desires to be accepted.

3. Persons with Dependent Personality Disorder are characterized by

    a. allowing others to assume responsibility for major areas of their lives.
    b. preference for being alone.
    c. no confidence.
    d. frequent anxiety.
    e. frequent depression.
    f. being emotionally "cold."

4. Compulsive Personality Disorders are characterized by

    a. decisiveness.
    b. preoccupation with rules, lists, or details.
    c. being controlled by others.
    d. incessant pursuit of pleasure to the exclusion of productivity.

ANSWERS, Section IV. H-K._____

1.   a,c,e,f
2.   a,b,c,e
3.   a,c,d,e
4.   b

_____

POST-TEST

For each of the following questions, <u>one</u> or <u>more than one</u> answer may be correct. Circle the correct answer(s).

1. The Borderline Personality Disorder is characterized by

   a. intense and unstable interpersonal relationships.
   b. frequent feelings of sadness and depression.
   c. transient psychoses.
   d. chronic identity problems.

2. Regarding persons with Paranoid Personality Disorder, which of the following statements is (are) true?

   a. Individuals belong to the "erratic" cluster of Personality Disorders.
   b. Individuals are hyperactive.
   c. Individuals are hyperalert.
   d. Individuals are mistrustful.
   e. Individuals are hypersensitive.
   f. Individuals have restricted affect.

3. Compulsive Personality Disorders are characterized by

   a. decisiveness.
   b. preoccupation with rules, lists, or details.
   c. being controlled by others.
   d. incessant pursuit of pleasure to the exclusion of productivity.

4. If a person is not distressed by his psychiatric disorder it is said to be

   a. a personality disorder.
   b. ego-syntonic.
   c. ego-dystonic.
   d. characterologically compatible.

5. The etiology of Personality Disorders has been attributed to

   a. psychological trauma during infancy or early childhood.
   b. social deprivation.
   c. pathological style of family interaction.
   d. biological abnormalities.
   e. genetic inheritance.

6. The "erratic" cluster of Personality Disorders consists of

   a. Narcissistic Personality Disorder.
   b. Borderline Personality Disorder.
   c. Antisocial Personality Disorder.
   d. Schizoid Personality Disorder.

7. Individuals with an Antisocial Personality Disorder

    a. violate the rights of others.
    b. see no need for rules.
    c. anticipate consequences only because they are obstacles.
    d. feel no responsibility for their actions.

8. Personality Disorders are

    a. maladaptive behavior patterns.
    b. chronic.
    c. dysfunctional.
    d. associated with distress.

9. Persons with Dependent Personality Disorder are characterized by

    a. allowing others to assume responsibility for major areas of their lives.
    b. preference for being alone.
    c. no confidence.
    d. frequent anxiety.
    e. frequent depression.
    f. being emotionally "cold."

10. The "odd" or eccentric cluster includes

    a. Schizoid Personality Disorder.
    b. Paranoid Personality Disorder.
    c. Borderline Personality Disorder.
    d. Schizotypal Personality Disorder.

11. The individual with an Avoidant Personality

    a. is hypersensitive to rejection.
    b. is socially isolated.
    c. has low self-esteem.
    d. has symptoms which are ego-syntonic.
    e. desires to be accepted.

12. The "fearful" cluster of Personality Disorders includes

    a. Passive-Aggressive.
    b. Compulsive.
    c. Dependent.
    d. Discordant.
    e. Obsessive.
    f. Avoidant.

13. Individuals with an Antisocial Personality Disorder

    a. frequently have symptoms before age 12.
    b. as adults may be sexually frigid.
    c. are often hobos.
    d. make up a large proportion of the prison population.

14. The Passive-Aggressive Personality Disorder is characterized by

    a. indecisiveness.
    b. procrastination.
    c. obstinacy.
    d. dedication to pleasure to the exclusion of productive work.
    e. underlying hostility.

15. Which of the following are associated with the Narcissistic Personality Disorder?

    a. grandiosity
    b. exhibitionism
    c. acceptance of criticism
    d. exploitation
    e. expecting favors without reciprocation
    f. distorted empathy

16. Which of the following are characteristic of the Schizoid Personality Disorder?

    a. bland affect
    b. no social relationships
    c. detached from the environment
    d. intense expression of anger

17. The Histrionic Personality Disorder is characterized by

    a. dramatic behavior.
    b. superficial charm.
    c. frequent physical complaints.
    d. sexually naive or inadequate behavior.

18. The number of Personality Disorders is

    a. 10 in four clusters.
    b. 12 in three clusters.
    c. 11 in three clusters.
    d. 12 in four clusters.

19. Appropriate treatment modalities for Personality Disorders include

    a. brief psychotherapy.
    b. intensive psychotherapy.
    c. group therapy.
    d. marital, family therapy.
    e. milieu therapy.
    f. psychopharmacotherapy.

20. Personality Disorders

    a. are on a continuum from normal to severe disorder.
    b. fit the concept of a medical illness.
    c. are accepted by the legal system as diseases.
    d. are frequently seen in patients with other psychiatric syndromes.

PRE-TEST ANSWERS

1. a,b,c,d
2. a,d
3. c
4. a,b,d
5. b
6. a,b,c,f
7. a,b,c,d,e
8. a,b,c,d,e
9. c,d,e,f
10. a,b,c

11. a,b,c
12. a,b,c,d
13. a,b,d,e,f
14. a,b,d
15. a,d
16. a,b,c,d
17. a,b,c,e
18. a,c,d,e
19. b
20. b,c,e

POST-TEST ANSWERS

1. a,b,c,d
2. c,d,e,f
3. b
4. b
5. a,b,c,d,e
6. a,b,c
7. a,b,d
8. a,b,c,d
9. a,c,d,e
10. a,b,d

11. a,b,c,e
12. a,b,c,f
13. a,d
14. b,c,e
15. a,b,d,e,f
16. a,b,c
17. a,b,c,d
18. c
19. a,b,c,d,e
20. a,d

REFERENCES

Diagnostic and statistical manual of mental disorders (3rd Ed.). Washington: American Psychiatric Association, 1979.

Kernberg, O.F. Borderline conditions and pathological narcissism. New York: Jason Aronson, 1975.

Pierce, C. Personality disorders. In G. Usdin & J. Lewis, (Eds.), Psychiatry in general medical practice. New York: McGraw-Hill, 1979.

Salzman, L. Other character-personality syndromes: Schizoid, inadequate, passive-aggressive, paranoid, and dependent. In S. Arieti & E. Brody, (Eds.), American handbook of psychiatry, (Vol. III). New York: Basic Books, 1974.

Winokur, G. & Crowe, R. Personality disorders. In A. Freedman, H. Kaplan, & B. Sadock, (Eds.), Comprehensive textbook of psychiatry II, (Vol. II). Baltimore: Williams & Wilkins, 1975.

CHAPTER 14

Sleep Disorders

Luis A. Marco, M.D.
Patricia M. Randels, M.D.
C. Inga Taylor, M.D.

CHAPTER OUTLINE

Learning Objectives

Pre-Test

V. Dysfunctions Associated with Sleep, Sleep Stages, or Partial Arousals (Parasomnias)

   A. Sleepwalking or Somnambulism
   B. Sleep Terror (Pavor Nocturnus, Night Terrors, Incubus)
   C. Sleep-related Enuresis
   D. Other Dysfunctions
       1. Dream Anxiety Attacks (DAA)
       2 Sleep-related Epileptic Seizures
       3. Sleep-related Bruxism
       4. Sleep-related Headbanging (Jactatio Capitis Nocturnus)
       5. Familial Sleep Paralysis
       6. Impaired Penile Tumescence during Sleep
       7. Sleep-related Painful Erections
       8. Sleep-related Cluster Headaches and Chronic Paroxysmal Hemicrania
       9. Sleep-related Abnormal Swallowing Syndrome
    10. Sleep-related Asthma
    11. Sleep-related Cardiovascular Symptoms
    12. Sleep-related Gastro-esophageal reflux
    13. Sleep-related Hemolysis (Paroxysmal Nocturnal Hemoglobinuria)
    14. Asymptomatic Polysomnographic Finding

Post-Test

Pre-Test Answers

Post-Test Answers

References

LEARNING OBJECTIVES

After completing this chapter you will be able to:

1. Recognize the stages of sleep, 1, 2, 3, 4 and REM.

2. Define the following terms: hypersomnia, hyposomnia, dyssomnia, REM sleep, hypnagogic, hypnopompic, sleep drunkenness, SWS.

3. Diagnose the following syndromes: Sleep apnea, alveolar hypoventilation, nocturnal myoclonus, restless legs, narcolepsy, sudden infant death, Ondine's curse, Pickwickian and Kleine-Levin syndromes.

4. Recognize the effects on sleep of: psychophysiological states, psychiatric disorders, endocrinological dysfunction, neurologic lesions, aging and dietary factors, drugs and alcohol, and disturbance in the sleep-wake schedule.

5. Recognize the following dysfunctions associated with sleep or partial arousals: somnambulism, sleep terror, sleep-related enuresis, dream anxiety attacks, sleep-related epileptic seizures, sleep-related bruxism, sleep-related head banging, familial sleep paralysis, impaired penile tumescence, sleep-related painful erections, sleep-related cluster headaches, sleep-related abnormal swallowing, sleep-related asthma, sleep-related cardiovascular symptoms, sleep-related gastroesophageal reflux and sleep-related hemolysis.

PRE-TEST

For the following questions, <u>one</u> or <u>more</u> <u>than</u> <u>one</u> answer may be correct.
Circle the correct answer(s).

1.   Sleep disturbance occurs in

      a. less than 5% of the population.
      b. old age often.
      c. about 35% of the population.
      d. 70-80% of psychiatric patients.
      e. association with respiratory impairment in some cases.
      f. the form of excessive or insufficient sleep.
      g. patients with DIMS and DOES syndromes.
      h. patients with nocturnal pain or discomfort.
      i. Alcoholic Intoxication or Withdrawal.
      j. infants with SIDS.
      k. some cerebral infections and neurological diseases.
      l. the narcoleptic syndrome.
      m. nocturnal alveolar hypoventilation.
      n. Ondine's syndrome but not the Pickwickian syndrome.
      o. association with disorders of the motor system.
      p. hyper- and hypothyroidism.
      q. some nutritional deficiencies, but not that due to lack or deficit
          of L-tryptophan.

2.   The sleep apnea syndrome is usually diagnosed if

      a. 30 or more apneic episodes of more than 10 seconds duration occur
          during the night.
      b. a night-time sleep tape recording demonstrates alternation
          between loud snoring of abrupt onset and periods of silence.
      c. daytime hypersomnolence reinforces the above.
      d. there is EDS without night-time apnea.

3.   In the alveolar hypoventilation DIMS syndrome

      a. significant apneic pauses do not occur.
      b. there is inadequate tidal volume.
      c. hypoxia worsens as sleep progresses.
      d. there is no insomnia or repetitive arousal.
      e. the prognosis is worse than in sleep apnea.
      f. upper airway obstruction is a constant concomitant.

4.   Sleep drunkenness is often responsible for

      a. poor school performance.
      b. post-dormital headaches.
      c. learning difficulties.
      d. ethanolic breath.
      e. automatic behavior with memory blackouts.

5. If the anticholinergic potential of tricyclics is therapeutic against cataplectic attacks, one would also expect therapeutic effects from the action of

    a. thioridazine.
    b. reserpine.
    c. atropine.
    d. physostigmine.
    e. diazepam.

6. Which of the following characteristics are common to the Kleine-Levin syndrome and menstrual hypersomnolence?

    a. episodes of hypersomnia
    b. both usually in the female sex
    c. hyperphagia
    d. none of the above

7. There is an association between sleepwalking and

    a. nocturnal enuresis.
    b. sleeptalking.
    c. low intelligence.
    d. homosexuality.
    e. night terrors.

8. Often during a depressive episode there is

    a. insomnia.
    b. increased awakenings.
    c. early premature final awakening.
    d. increase in REM sleep.
    e. decrease in stage 4 of sleep.
    f. none of the above

9. Normal sleep is often disrupted by

    a. alcohol.
    b. caffeine.
    c. usual hypnotics.
    d. amphetamines.

For the following questions, circle the <u>one</u> correct response.

10.   Sleep of less than five hours per night

      a.   is characteristic of drug-induced insomnia.
      b.   is characteristic of all depressions.
      c.   can be normal for some individuals.
      d.   often occurs following Amphetamine Withdrawal.
      e.   precipitates uncontrollable sleep attack in most people.

11.   A complaint of insomnia

      a.   automatically calls for prescription of a hypnotic.
      b.   always reflects a primary sleep disorder.
      c.   should be treated first with psychotherapy.
      d.   may have multiple causes.
      e.   should be considered symptomatic of depression and treated auto-
           matically with tricyclic antidepressants.

12.   Upper airway resistance increases during obstructive sleep apnea be-
      cause of

      a.   increased tonus of intercostal muscles.
      b.   increased tonic activity of pharyngeal muscles.
      c.   decreased tonic activity of throat muscles.
      d.   constant hyperextension of neck due to upward oriented gaze of
           rapid-eye-movements tracking falling objects in the dream content.

13.   The single most frequent effect of psychoactive drugs on sleep patterns
      is

      a.   sleep regularization.
      b.   reduction of stages 1 and 2.
      c.   reduction of REM sleep.
      d.   abolition of K-complexes.

14.   Sleep drunkenness refers to

      a.   sleep of the drunkard following excessive alcohol ingestion.
      b.   usual state of "dope eaters."
      c.   state following arousal from REM sleep.
      d.   disorientation, incoordination, and grogginess observed in patients
           with sleep-induced respiratory depression upon awakening from a
           day-time sleep episode.

15.   The Pickwickian syndrome usually describes

      a.   a young chlorotic female.
      b.   an obese hypersomnolent lad.
      c.   insomnia due to Caffeine Intoxication.
      d.   a grandiose impersonation of Dickens.

16. Sleeping pills

    a. are indicated to counteract the insomnia of patients with central sleep apnea.
    b. help individuals with obstructive sleep apnea.
    c. should be given to the two categories of patients mentioned in a and b, but only for the first 2-3 days.
    d. are usually ineffective in treating most types of insomnia after the first 2-3 weeks of administration.

17. Strong emotions often serve as triggers of

    a. sleep apnea daytime hypersomnolent attacks.
    b. narcoleptic-cataplectic attacks.
    c. slow wave sleep attacks.

18. The cataplectic attacks of REM narcoleptics are due to

    a. paralysis of the respiratory center.
    b. an episode of Catatonic Schizophrenia.
    c. the normal paralysis of sleep, always with cessation of consciousness.
    d. decreased tonic activity of groups of skeletal musculature.

19. The cataplectic attacks of narcoleptics respond best to

    a. amphetamines.
    b. neuroleptics.
    c. barbiturates.
    d. tricyclic antidepressants.
    e. L-tryptophan.

20. Classical narcolepsy is a condition with strong

    a. environmental etiology.
    b. infectious contributory factors.
    c. hereditary background.
    d. intrapsychic etiology.
    e. easily demonstrable gross neurological damage.

21. The treatment of choice for sleepwalking is

    a. barbiturates.
    b. neuroleptics.
    c. environmental protection.
    d. psychotherapy.
    e. electroconvulsive therapy.
    f. none of the above.

22.   Nocturnal penile tumescence correlates best with sleep stage

    a.   REM.
    b.   stages 1 and 2.
    c.   stages 3 and 4.
    d.   never occurs during sleep but only while very awake.

Match each one of the following characteristics with the appropriate diagnosis.

    ___23.   never continent before   a.   primary enuresis
    ___24.   continent before   b.   secondary enuresis
    ___25.   male predominance
    ___26.   non-REM related
    ___27.   psychopathology is present
    ___28.   arousal or REM-related
    ___29.   usually unassociated with dreams
    ___30.   begins with burst of K-complexes
    ___31.   predominantly during the first third of night
    ___32.   responds to psychotherapy
    ___33.   managed through reassurance, bladder training, imipramine

Match the following characteristics with the appropriate diagnosis.   Lettered items may be used more than once for each question.

    ___34.   2nd half of night   a.   night terrors
    ___35.   1st third of night   b.   dream anxiety attacks
    ___36.   treated with benzodiazepines
    ___37.   more autonomic upheaval
    ___38.   deep sleep
    ___39.   good recollection
    ___40.   REM sleep-related
    ___41.   male predominance
    ___42.   female predominance

Match the following characteristics with the appropriate diagnosis.

    ___43.   swallowing   a.   nocturnal psychomotor
    ___44.   EEG seizure discharge   epilepsy
    ___45.   uncinate aura   b.   sleepwalking
    ___46.   wakeful attacks
    ___47.   handrubbing
    ___48.   usual temporal lobe focus
    ___49.   association with enuresis and night terrors

Match the following characteristics with the appropriate diagnosis.

___50. disturbance at muscle
___51. responds to tricyclics
___52. develops while patient is asleep
___53. develops at sleep-onset or on emerging from sleep
___54. often associated with hallucinations and cataplexy
___55. touching patient terminates attack
___56. central disturbance

a. narcoleptic sleep paralysis
b. familial sleep paralysis

I. INTRODUCTION

Sleep ties up about 1/3 of an average person's life (8 hours per day), that is, over 23 cumulative years will have been spent in slumber by the end of an average life span (70 years). Yet, sleep is one of man's least understood processes.

Sleep and arousal depend on very intricate and delicate neurobiological and biochemical mechanisms. Although normal and necessary, sleep is an extremely complicated mechanism which can be readily disturbed by a variety of causes. Explosive growth in understanding sleep mechanisms and their disturbances began with the discovery in 1953 by Aserinsky - a student of Kleitman - of a fundamental fact of far-reaching theoretical and clinical significance: the association of dreams with a stage of sleep in which rapid eye movements (REM) occur. Other areas of research over the last decade have focused on the phylogenetic (evolutionary) and ontogenetic (developmental) aspects of sleep. However much of the physiology and neurochemistry of sleep remains to be elucidated.

A concept of the different sleep stages is needed in order to understand the multiple sleep and arousal disorders described in subsequent pages. There are five distinct stages in normal sleep which can be differentiated in terms of the EEG and eye-movement patterns. During wakefulness, the EEG is low in amplitude and is characterized by alpha activity in the 8 to 10 Hz range. As the person goes to sleep, there are many changes in the EEG as the sleeper passes through different sleep stages.

1) <u>Stage 1</u> is the lightest stage of sleep and is a transition from waking to sleep. It is the first pattern in a normal sleep cycle.

2) <u>Stage 2</u> makes up about half the total normal sleep time. It is characterized by the periodic appearance of 12-14 Hz or EEG spindle waves and high-amplitude sharp negative waves called "K-complexes."

3) <u>Stage 3</u> is characterized by a mixture of spindle and high-amplitude slow waves ($\frac{1}{2}$-3 Hz activity) in the EEG. The most widely used criterion for stage 3 sleep is when 20% of the EEG record shows slow waves.

4) <u>Stage 4</u> -- deep sleep -- is characterized by slow waves during at least 50 percent of the EEG record. Both stages 3 and 4 usually occur during the first half of one's sleep period. During stage 4 peak secretion of growth hormone takes place.

5) <u>Stage REM</u> -- REM sleep, (desynchronized sleep, dream sleep, or D-sleep) refers to rapid eye movement sleep. In humans its depth is similar to stage 2 sleep. After about 90 minutes of the first four stages of sleep (collectively called non-REM or NREM sleep), the first period of REM sleep occurs. During REM sleep there is an almost total absence of tone in the skeletal musculature. The

waves of the EEG are of low amplitude and fast frequency, and the EEG resembles that of wakefulness. Most dreaming occurs during this stage. In males, nocturnal erections occur almost exclusively during REM sleep, and in females there is increased vaginal blood flow. A large percentage of normal sleep is REM during the later part of a period of sleep, i.e., early morning in a person with a nocturnal sleep pattern.

Sleep disturbances occur commonly. About 35% of the population suffer from insomnia. This incidence is even greater with increasing age and during anxiety and depressive syndromes. Among psychiatric patients, the incidence may be as high as 70-80%. Sleep disorders are among the most common and difficult problems to manage for the physician. Some sleep disorders are primary, while others may be secondary to other disturbances. The result of these aberrations may be either too little sleep (hyposomnia, insomnia), too much (hypersomnia), or an altered quality of sleep (dyssomnia). Numerous chemical factors (particularly drugs), environmental settings (jet lag), and medical disorders (especially psychiatric and neurological), may lead to acute or chronic sleep disturbances.

Hyper-, hypo- and dys-somnia are only symptoms, not disease conditions. The physician must scrutinize the causes and diseases to which such symptoms are related. This is the only way to provide rational therapy for sleep disorders. Prescribing hypnotics, stimulants, or other drugs before a diagnosis is firmly established may be harmful.

Complete agreement on an over-all classification of sleep disorders is not yet available since the physiological and biochemical processes involved in the sleep-wake cycle are not sufficiently elucidated. We will follow the classification proposed by the Diagnostic and Statistical Manual of Mental Disorders (DSM-III). In this manual, sleep and arousal disorders are classified into four major categories: 1) Disorders of initiating and maintaining sleep (DIMS); 2) Disorders of excessive somnolence (DOES); 3) Disorders of the sleep-wake schedule; and 4) Dysfunctions associated with sleep, sleep stages, or partial arousals. The Association for the Psychophysiological Study of Sleep has also recently published a comprehensive nosology of the sleep disorders (Roffwarg, 1979).

II.   DISORDERS OF INITIATING AND MAINTAINING SLEEP (DIMS)

One may also think of these disorders as "difficulty in initiating and maintaining sleep." Either way, it can be expressed - short-hand - by the acronym DIMS. Other frequent and partly equivalent expressions are "difficulty in falling asleep or sleep-onset insomnia." Insomnia as a complaint is by far the most common symptom of the sleep disorders and also the most frequently encountered sleep complaint by psychiatrists and family practitioners. In about 10% of insomnias, specific causes may be determined upon close scrutiny. Some of the more frequent ones are listed below. Some patients have trouble falling asleep but can maintain their sleep, others have no difficulty falling asleep but readily wake up much too often. Some people may have both problems. Young people have greater proclivity for difficulty in falling asleep, while older persons are prone to complain of difficulty in remaining asleep. The physician must take a detailed history and address the individual needs. Some people get along with about 4 hours of sleep at night, but others may need 10 to feel fully well during the day. Some patients may think that they do not get enough sleep, yet all night sleep monitoring (by EEG) may indicate that they sleep 7-8 hours. Short sleepers do not necessarily require medical attention if they offer no complaints.

The causes of insomnia are multiple. The most relevant to the clinician are reviewed below.

A. PSYCHOPHYSIOLOGICAL

Psychophysiological arousability exists when the patient is subject to such overactivity of the mechanisms of arousal (reticular activating system or RAS) that the mechanisms of initiating or maintaining sleep are overpowered and thus covertly causes DIMS.

Pain or discomfort will usually cause DIMS, but repeated awakenings may also occur, depending on the nature and exacerbation patterns of the pain. Whether insomnia is transient (less than 3 weeks) or persistent will depend on the remission or chronicity of the painful condition (i.e., toothache vs. inoperable cancer). Sometimes the pain may not interfere with performance during the day, but it might alter sleep at night.

If one is not sufficiently tired, sleeplessness may result. Simple colds, mental overwork, mental stimulation from the radio, moving pictures or television, environmental disturbances (traffic sounds, hot or cold room, a spouse with kicking spasms or snoring, lack of adequate humidity in the bedroom causing dryness and obstruction of nasal mucosae), emotional excitement of any sort, the expectation of Santa Claus before bed-time, insistence upon sleep when there is no desire for it, or heavy evening meals or hunger, may all be contributory factors to insomnia.

Other events loosely related to sleep - full urine bladder - may produce the symptom of insomnia. These will be described later.

B. PSYCHIATRIC DISORDERS

A frequent presenting symptom of anxiety or depression is insomnia. With anxiety there is usually difficulty in falling asleep, while the depression of middle-aged and older people presents more often with trouble remaining asleep, especially during the latter half of the night which may lead to early final awakening. In depression there is also a reduction of stages 3 and 4 of sleep and many sleep stage shifts and body movements. Some 97% of depressed patients suffer from sleep disturbance. The most typical disorders are middle-of-the-night awakening and early morning awakening. The sleep of the depressed patient may not reach stage 4, while REM sleep is significantly increased during the most serious phase of the illness. REM latency (the time from sleep onset to first REM period) is decreased in severe primary depression. For a more detailed description, see the chapter on Affective Disorders. Mania and hypomania are associated with sleeplessness. The manic patient, however, is not likely to complain of insomnia. He will rather boast that he needs no sleep or that he never gets tired enough to go to bed. Indeed, sleep during mania is quite short, and total REM sleep time is disproportionately even shorter. The same bipolar (manic-depressive) patients in their depressed phase may have an increased REM sleep and decreased REM latency. In the depression following Amphetamine Withdrawal there is also greatly increased total sleep time and REM sleep time.

C.   DRUG EFFECTS

Moderate use or abuse of stimulants of various kinds may cause insomnia of sleep-onset or sleep-maintenance type. Caffeine disturbs the normal sleep pattern and in high doses produces insomnia. Excessive caffeine ingestion before bed-time shifts the bulk of REM sleep toward the early part of the night, thus delaying the normal concentrations of early delta or deep sleep.

Withdrawal from hypnotic drugs, particularly the barbiturates and alcohol, typically causes dramatic insomnia, often with vivid dreams and nightmares. The duration of withdrawal insomnia correlates positively with the duration of ingestion of the hypnotic drug withdrawn. Understanding the occurrence of these withdrawal phenomena might prevent the patient from using the drug again. Withdrawal from neuroleptics, tricyclic antidepressants and benzodiazepines is less often associated with insomnia than withdrawal from barbiturates. Nighttime Nicotine Withdrawal associated with heavy smoking has been observed occasionally in the form of repeated awakenings 1-4 hours after sleep-onset. Reducing the number of cigarettes smoked daily should help improve the insomnia.

Sleeping pills (sedative hypnotics), often prescribed for insomniacs without the benefit of etiological scrutiny, are bound to lose their effectiveness and to exacerbate the insomnia for which they were originally intended if they are continued for a period longer than few days or weeks. Sometimes the first good night of sleep will follow withdrawal of the sleeping pill. For patients with either porphyria or sleep apnea (see below) the administration of sleeping pills of both barbiturate and benzodiazepine type can be extremely dangerous and life threatening, even if prescribed for a few days. Patients with either of these two conditions occasionally come to the attention of the psychiatrist and may present with other neuro-psychiatric problems which may have insomnia as a symptom. Therefore, a thorough history and differential diagnosis are necessary.

D.   SLEEP-INDUCED RESPIRATORY IMPAIRMENT

   1.   Sleep Apnea Syndrome.
        This refers to a pathophysiological mechanism consisting of interference with breathing. Patients with this condition have short sleep latencies, usually falling asleep within minutes. However, they wake up many times during the night either gasping for air or with a sense of choking. The polysomnogram shows a pathological number

of apneic episodes. There are three types of sleep apnea. The more frequent is central apnea in which there is a cessation of breathing attempts during REM and NREM sleep. The second is obstructive (upper airway) apnea in which attempts to breathe fail, despite desperate efforts. The third type is mixed, central and obstructive. In obstructive sleep apnea, blockage is overcome intermittently by a gradually increasing intrathoracic pressure. At these times there is loud snorting and snoring coinciding with respiratory excursion and then awakening. This cycle is repeated many times throughout most of the night. With sleep apnea there is: a) a decreased tonus of intercostal, laryngeal, pharyngeal, and tongue muscles which may cause obstruction of upper airways, b) diaphragmatic paralysis which recovers before the relief of the obstruction and which then causes a terrific increase in intrathoracic pressure, sometimes as much as 300%(!). The arousal coincides with a loud snore through a partially obstructed larynx. These powerful impediments may eventually lead to right and left cardiac failure and arrhythmia. It predominates in males (male/female ratio 20:1). During the day, hypersomnolence (see below) is its most common manifestation, presumably due to the extensive disruption of nocturnal sleep. But daytime examination of respiratory function of these patients generally yields negative results. A sleep apnea syndrome is usually diagnosed if, during seven hours of sleep, at least 30 apneic episodes of more than 10 seconds duration are recorded. In the absence of polysomnographic instrumentation to monitor various physiological processes simultaneously, a close-to-the-mouth tape recording of the entire night or part of it may be crucial for the diagnosis. A patient with daytime hypersomnia who is not apneic at night, may be suffering from analeptic drug dependence, brain tumor, other CNS abnormalities, or from a psychiatric disorder. Sleep apnea is not a common cause of insomnia (at night). In the USA the prevalence is estimated to be about 50,000. Considering that affected patients rarely, if ever, complain of respiratory distress, but rather of excessive daytime sleepiness and snoring, higher prevalence figures are likely. Since sleep apnea can be life-threatening and may require tracheostomy, it is crucial that the physician be aware of this syndrome. Chronic tracheostomy in obstructive cases is very effective for daytime somnolence, insures comfortable nocturnal sleep, and is effective for normalization of arterial and pulmonary artery pressures. Apneic episodes are also greatly relieved. On the other hand, tracheostomy may be difficult to accept and may be considered a drastic procedure if the affliction is not life-threatening.

Studies of normal individuals are enlightening in understanding the relationship between sleep and respiratory physiology. In a study of 70 normal subjects, 2/3 showed periodic breathing during sleep onset that fluctuated in respiratory rate and tidal volume. Some individuals exhibited total apnea from 20 to 60 sec. During REM sleep, some normal individuals also exhibit apnea and a Cheyne-Stokes pattern of breathing (crescendo-descrescendo fluctuations).

The ventilatory response to CO_2 is also invariably decreased. Thus, highly irregular breathing patterns are often observed during sleep onset (Mills & Dement, 1980).

An adult disorder of the sleep apnea type used to be seen in early, mild, chronic, or residual bulbar poliomyelitis. The apneic episodes would last 4-12 seconds. During the day these patients exhibited an irregular breathing pattern which was of prognostic value. After acute polio, patients often required artificial respiration and showed markedly decreased responsiveness to 5% CO_2 inhalation. Post-mortem evaluation often showed inflammatory changes and areas of necrosis in the ventrolateral regions of the medullary reticular formation.

The "crib death," now called sudden infant death syndrome or SIDS, is another condition in which death occurs during sleep, silently, without a gasp, cough, or stridor. Full term babies show an incidence for SIDS of 3% (about 10,000 per year in the USA), while premature babies have an incidence of 20%, that is 6-7 times higher. These figures suggest that prematurity is an important factor in SIDS. The incidence of SIDS in siblings of affected infants is 5 times greater than in the normal population. SIDS represents the greatest single cause of death during the first year of life. SIDS, however, has no code in the International Classification of Diseases (ICD) or in DSM-III, and thus the true incidence may be even higher (18,000 ?). Polygraphic recordings in "near miss" infants show prolonged apnea during upper respiratory infections or nasopharyngitis, often for 2 sec. or more and sometimes for 15 sec. or more. SIDS occurs more frequently during REM sleep when the automatic inspiratory-expiratory cycle becomes disrupted by recurrent apnea. Apnea is normal in full-term babies and adults (as described above), but in susceptible infants it is more frequent and prolonged, to the point of compromising O_2 uptake and possibly causing death. There is presumably a maturational lag factor of the CNS which causes a functional abnormality of the respiratory center and which is difficult to treat. Recent evidence suggests that a lack of development of laryngeal structures might be linked to the syndrome. Arousal or direct resuscitation may be the only recourse. Otherwise progressive anoxia, cyanosis, elevation of CO_2, and cardiac arrest will supervene. Children who have survived the threat of a SIDS may have respiratory tract obstruction such as hypertrophied adenoids, enlarged tonsils, and thyroid enlargement (intrathoracic goiter). Surgical removal often helps. Correction of cranio-vertebral anomalies involving C_1 and C_2 or of platibasia with basilar invagination and micrognathia may be indicated.

A relationship has been established recently between the SIDS and intoxication by Clostridium botulinum (CB). It appears that many strains of CB produce significant thiaminase-I. Thus, this anaerobe could produce or precipitate a thiamine deficiency by decomposition in the gut of low concentrations of ingested thiamine. The neurological effects of thiamine deficiency are, although milder, very similar to those of botulinum toxin. Both neurological syndromes resembled the signs of the SIDS, especially the characteristic apnea. This discovery is all the more meaningful considering that thiamine intake may be marginal in breast-fed infants or those fed pasteurized milk, which contains about half the thiamine present in fresh cow's milk. Thiamine triphosphate appears to have an important role in the function of excitable membranes such as respiratory neurons. In summary then, the possibility of a SIDS on a toxicologic-nutritional basis must be kept in mind (Rogers, 1979).

2. Alveolar Hypoventilation DIMS Syndrome.
    Unlike the preceding syndrome, significant apneic pauses do not occur, but there is inadequate tidal volume or respiratory rate during sleep, particularly during REM sleep. Hypoventilation tends to worsen as sleep progresses, and, concomitantly with this deterioration, sleep stages 3 and 4 tend to disappear. The presenting symptoms may include complaints of insomnia and repetitive arousal which coincide with the onset of normal respiration. Polysomnographic recordings, that is all-night-sleep monitoring of various physiological processes, are necessary for a definite diagnosis which is based on low arterial oxygen levels and exclusion of sleep apnea or partial obstruction of the upper airway. The pathogenesis may involve a variety of contributing factors, including muscle and neurological disease. This condition appears to be related to sleep apnea although it is considered to have a better prognosis.

Another disorder consisting of primary alveolar hypoventilation, presumably due to an abnormality in the respiratory center, is the so-called Ondine's curse syndrome. It receives this romantic name from the German legend of a water nymph, Ondine, who having been jilted by her mortal lover, puts a curse on him that "he must always voluntarily remember to breathe." He finally succumbs by falling asleep and since breathing under Ondine's spell is no longer automatic, he dies. The syndrome of Ondine's curse was first described to occur after high bilateral cervical cordotomy or following low brainstem surgery for relief of chronic pain. It is a very rare condition, with only 40 cases so far described. Although primarily an alveolar hypoventilation during the day, it may become sleep apnea at night and cause death. The ventilatory response to inhaled CO_2 during the daytime is always decreased, but more so at night, such that failure of the automatic ventilatory control is always a nocturnal risk. Fifty per cent of those affected also have diurnal hypersomnolence with periodic apnea during sleep. Sleep-respiratory disorders are now viewed as a derangement of CNS control mechanisms. Whether or not these patients might represent "near miss" survivors of SIDS is still under investigation.

E.   SLEEP-RELATED SYNDROMES

1.   Nocturnal Myoclonus.
This term refers to sudden muscle contractions (myoclonus) at night (nocturnal). One or more muscle groups, usually of the leg(s), may repeatedly contract during sleep. Each isolated jerk, at 20-40 sec. intervals, lasts 0.5-10 sec. and typically includes extension of the big toe and partial flexion of the ankle, knee, and, less frequently, the hip (triple withdrawal) often followed by partial arousal or full awakening. These episodes may repeat themselves for up to one hour or more before there is a full arousal. The patient is usually unaware and unlikely to complain of myoclonus. He usually complains of frequent nocturnal awakenings, unrefreshing sleep, or excessive daytime sleepiness. Sometimes the patient may present no complaints of his own but the bedpartner may complain of violent kicking. It predominates among middle-aged and older people. Sleep electromyography of the anterior tibialis muscles will usually establish the diagnosis. This condition typically occurs during sleep. More generalized body jerks during drowsiness, sleep-onset, or after arousal from sleep (so called hypnic jerks), should not be included under the diagnosis of nocturnal myoclonus. Nocturnal myoclonus must also be differentiated from other waking or nocturnal myoclonic conditions of neurological origin or neuropathies, and differential diagnosis from a neurologist and a sleep specialist is desirable. The psychiatrist must differentiate between primary nocturnal myoclonus and nocturnal myoclonus secondary to administration of tricyclic antidepressants, or to withdrawal from sedatives and anticonvulsants of various types. Frequency of body movements during sleep increases as a result of amphetamine ingestion. Limited success in the treatment of nocturnal myoclonus is afforded by diazepam (Valium), clonazepam (Clonopin), or diphenhydramine. This condition is often observed in association with other sleep disorders such as narcolepsy, sleep apnea, drug abuse, and restless legs (see below).

2.   Restless Legs Syndrome (RLS).
This problem occurs during waking (sitting or lying down) as opposed to myoclonus, but RLS is almost always found in patients who also exhibit nocturnal myoclonus. The syndrome consists of usually painless but disagreeable, creeping, deep dysesthesias of the calf muscles, sometimes also involving the foot, thigh, or arm muscles. These sensations cause an irresistible urge to move or exercise the muscles in order to relieve the discomfort. Although these dysesthesias are associated with the waking state, they will prevent sleep even when drowsiness tends to overcome the patient. The RLS is exacerbated by sleep deprivation and thus may start a vicious circle which may, in addition, lead to serious depression. Vigorous exercise relieves the discomfort only temporarily and the dysesthesias recur with termination of exercise. The cause is unknown, but in one-third of those affected, a familial pattern can be disclosed by history (autosomal dominant trait with low penetration). The RLS

is not to be confused with neuroleptic-induced akathisia (see chapter on psychopharmacology), painful leg cramps related to iron or calcium deficiencies or other causes, the restless legs phenomenon of chronic uremia, the growing pains in children, and the agitation or restlessness of anxious patients.

F. MEDICAL, TOXIC, AND ENVIRONMENTAL CONDITIONS

1. Endocrinological Dysfunction.
Hyperthyroidism and thyrotoxicosis cause fragmented, short sleep which is often complained of as insomnia. This pattern manifests itself in all-night-sleep EEG recordings with a high percentage of stages 3 and 4 sleep. Recovery may be very gradual after successful treatment of the endocrinological condition. Hypothyroidism (myxedema) on the other hand causes excessive sleepiness and lack or decrease of stages 3 and 4 sleep.

2. Neurologic Lesions.
Gross or subtle brain stem (reticular activating system), third ventricle, or hypothalamic damage usually causes insomnia (by irritative lesion) and sometimes sleepiness (by interference due to neuronal loss). Etiological factors include: neoplasms, vascular pathology, infection, degenerative conditions, trauma, toxic encephalopathies, and peripheral pathology in muscles and nerves.

3. Aging.
Normally, aging is associated with a decrease in sleep time, an increase in number of night awakenings, and not feeling rested in the morning. This biological fact, however, does not justify the assumption that older people need less sleep than younger individuals. Although elderly individuals commonly report as little as five hours of sleep, the most healthy elderly persons continue to secure almost as much sleep as in their younger years. Considerable variation is the rule among the older population as well as for younger persons and, indeed, a sizable minority of older people sleep longer with increasing age. Another biological fact is that in older people, deep sleep (stages 3 and 4) occupies a smaller percentage of the total sleep time and that REM sleep is also decreased. It is tempting to point out that sleep stage 4 has been associated with increase in growth hormone (GH) secretion. Thus, there is a correlation between old age, decrease in stage 4, and decrease in GH secretion. There is also another intriguing correlation between decrease in slow wave and REM sleep and decrease in cognitive performance in the elderly. Perhaps changes in neuro-transmitter levels (acetylcholine, serotonin), enzyme activity (monoamine oxidase), and hormonal output (growth hormone), might be associated with the sleep changes which occur with advancing age.

4. Dietary Factors.
Many claims have been made involving the role of malnutrition and some mineral and metal deficiencies in insomnia, but more research

is required. One nutritionally-determined deficiency which appears to play a role in insomnia is that of insufficient tryptophan intake among rural Mexicans and Latin Americans who may consume only corn (very low in tryptophan) as their total source of protein. This amino acid is the precursor of serotonin (see chapter on psychopharmacology) and thus insufficient concentrations of this brain monoamine will be synthesized. This clinical insight - the resulting insomnia - is compatible with current thinking postulating an important role for serotonin and serotonergic neurons of the brain stem raphe nucleus in slow-wave sleep mechanisms. It would also be in agreement with the claimed hypnotic effect of pharmacologic doses of L-tryptophan which have been shown to significantly decrease sleep latency by some investigators (Hartmann, 1977). Others, however, have been unable to demonstrate a sleep-promoting effect of L-tryptophan. Salicylate (aspirin), which increases the levels of plasma tryptophan, is also known to be a short-term hypnotic. At the experimental level, cats with lesions of the raphe nuclei (which harbors the serotonin-containing neurons) or when given parachlorophenylalanine (which blocks serotonin formation) exhibit insomnia. Most hypnotics have diminished efficacy when given continuously for a few weeks and REM sleep is reduced by almost all hypnotics. L-tryptophan, on the contrary, in doses of 1-5 Gm produces short-term hypnotic effects: reduction of sleep onset latency without reduction in REM sleep.

QUIZ, Section II.

Circle the correct answer(s). <u>One</u> or <u>more</u> <u>than</u> <u>one</u> answer may be correct.

1. Sleep disturbance occurs in

    a. less than 5% of the population.
    b. 70-80% of psychiatric patients.
    c. association with respiratory impairment in some cases.
    d. the form of excessive or insufficient sleep.
    e. patients with DIMS and DOES syndromes.
    f. patients with nocturnal pain or discomfort.
    g. Alcoholic Intoxication or Withdrawal.
    h. infants with SIDS.
    i. some patients with cerebral infections and neurological diseases.
    j. the narcoleptic syndrome.
    k. nocturnal alveolar hypoventilation.
    l. Ondine's syndrome but not the Pickwickian syndrome.
    m. association with disorders of the motor system.
    n. hyper- and hypothyroidism.
    o. some nutritional deficiencies, but not that due to lack or deficit of L-tryptophan.

2. The sleep-induced respiratory syndrome(s) is/are

    a. central sleep apnea.
    b. impaired penile tumescence.
    c. obstructive sleep apnea.
    d. jet lag.

3. The sleep apnea syndrome is usually diagnosed if

    a. thirty or more apneic episodes of more than 10 seconds duration occur.
    b. a nighttime sleep tape recording demonstrates alternation between loud snoring of abrupt onset and periods of silence.
    c. daytime hypersomnolence reinforces the above (a,b).
    d. there is excessive daytime sleepiness without nighttime apnea.

4. In the alveolar hypoventilation DIMS syndrome,

    a. significant apneic pauses do not occur.
    b. there is inadequate tidal volume.
    c. hypoxia worsens as sleep progresses.
    d. there is no insomnia or repetitive arousal.
    e. the prognosis is worse than in sleep apnea.
    f. upper airway obstruction is a constant concomitant.

5. Often during a depressive episode there is

    a. insomnia.
    b. increased awakenings.
    c. early premature final awakening.
    d. increase in REM sleep.
    e. decrease in stage 4 of sleep.

6. Normal sleep is often disrupted by

    a. alcohol.
    b. caffeine.
    c. usual hypnotics.
    d. amphetamines.

7. Sleep in depressed patients is characterized by

    a. intermittent wakefulness and early-morning awakening.
    b. REM latency is decreased in severe primary depression.
    c. consistent shortening of REM sleep periods.

8. In obstructive sleep-induced apnea,

    a. daytime physical examination usually yields negative respiratory findings.
    b. tracheostomy may be indicated.
    c. excessive daytime sleepiness is the rule.
    d. the male/female ratio is 20:1.

9. The indications for tracheoplasty in obstructive sleep apnea are

    a. always clear.
    b. the presence of obvious cardiovascular complications.
    c. the sleep apnea seriously interferes with adjustment.
    d. only when the patient is obese and has a short neck.

10. Other helpful approaches to obstructive sleep-induced apnea may be

    a. weight reduction.
    b. adenoidectomy and tonsillectomy.
    c. hypnotics to alleviate the insomnia.
    d. diaphragmatic pacemaker.

11. Sleep in mania is characterized by

    a. increase in REM.
    b. low threshold for arousal from sleep.
    c. reduction of stage 4 sleep.
    d. reduced total sleep time.

12. A previously dependable nurse has started making serious errors with administration of medications to patients following a new work schedule requiring a change in shift each week. You suspect

    a. incipient psychosis.
    b. homicidal tendencies.
    c. circadian mismatch with sleep-wake cycle.
    d. interference of daytime traffic noise and activity with her sleep.

Circle the letter corresponding to the <u>one</u> correct response.

13. Sleep of less than five hours per night

    a. is characteristic of drug-induced insomnia.
    b. is characteristic of all depressions.
    c. can be normal for some individuals.
    d. often occurs following Amphetamine Withdrawal.
    e. precipitates uncontrollable sleep attack in most people.

14. Elderly individuals

    a. have deeper sleep than more youthful people.
    b. commonly report five hours of nighttime sleep.
    c. have higher threshold for arousal from sleep.
    d. have higher correlation of penile tumescence with REM sleep periods.
    e. have lower heart rate during REM sleep.

15. A complaint of insomnia

    a. automatically calls for prescription of hypnotics.
    b. always reflects a primary sleep disorder.
    c. should be treated first with psychotherapy.
    d. may have multiple causes.
    e. should be considered symptomatic of depression and treated automatically with tricyclic antidepressants.

16. Normal sleep stage sequence requires that

    a. REM be first, following sleep onset.
    b. about 90 minutes of other sleep stages precede the first REM period.
    c. 75% of total sleep time be spent in stage 4.
    d. stage 3 appears in the EEG at sleep onset.

17. Obstructive (upper airway) sleep apnea is more prevalent in

    a. cigar smokers.
    b. young females with history of lung disease.
    c. middle-aged obese men with history of loud snoring and excessive daytime sleepiness.
    d. hysterical women with bolus hystericus.

18. Upper airway resistance increases during obstructive sleep apnea because of

    a. increased tonus of intercostal muscles.
    b. increased tonic activity of pharyngeal muscles.
    c. decreased tonic activity of throat muscles.
    d. constant hyperextension of neck due to upward oriented gaze of rapid eye movements tracking falling objects in the dream content.

19 The single most frequent effect of psychoactive drugs on sleep patterns is

    a. sleep regularization.
    b. reduction of stages 1 and 2.
    c. reduction of REM sleep.
    d. abolition of K-complexes.

III. DISORDERS OF EXCESSIVE SOMNOLENCE (DOES)

Much attention has been paid in the past few years to hypersomnolence or hypersomnia. This interest has been partly generated by the conviction that DIMS (insomnias) and DOES (hypersomnias) are more interrelated pathophysiologically than they might have appeared on first consideration, despite their apparent opposition. DOES may refer to excessive amount of night sleep or excessive daytime sleepiness. These two symptoms are sometimes separable, but often appear in the same patient. DOES is much less

frequent than DIMS but by no means rare. Narcolepsy combined with drug-
and alcohol-related conditions makes hypersomnolence a very common symptom.
The number of narcoleptics in the USA only is estimated at over 100,000.
As with insomnia, the physician must assume that hypersomnolence is a
symptom rather than a disease condition. As such, it has many causes which
must be ruled out before treatment for the symptom is prescribed. The
most common conditions responsible for hypersomnolence are narcolepsy,
alcohol, drugs, depression, and sleep apnea.

A. PSYCHOPHYSIOLOGICAL DISORDERS

Transient or situational psychophysiological disorders usually last 1 day to
3 weeks at most and are of little clinical significance since most of the times
the individual is aware of the contributing factors and eager to correct the
deficiency (lack of rest, physical exertion, all-night duty, etc.).

More persistent hypersomnolence on psychophysiological bases may come to
the attention of the physician (i.e., boredom in class or at the job may lead
to hypersomnolence and repercussions with teacher or supervisor).

B. PSYCHIATRIC DISORDERS

1. Affective Disorders.
    Serious depression, whether psychotic or neurotic, is usually as-
    sociated with sleep disturbance. While insomnia is more frequent
    in Affective Disorders than hypersomnia, there are subgroups of
    depressed patients (bipolar, unipolar, neurotic, and simple mourn-
    ing) who show hypersomnia and increased REM time.

2. Schizophrenic and Schizoaffective Disorders.
    Young people in these categories may exhibit periods of excessive
    sleep. But the symptoms may be secondary to neuroleptic treat-
    ment.

C. DRUG- AND ALCOHOL-RELATED DISORDERS

Excessive sleep time and daytime sleepiness often follow use or abuse of
alcohol, other central nervous system (CNS) depressants, or even CNS
stimulants such as amphetamines. The so-called Amphetamine Withdrawal
Organic Mental Disorder (see chapter on Organic Mental Disorders) courses
with depression and excessive daytime sleepiness. Withdrawal from caffeine
or other stimulant drugs may cause similar effects. When drugs or alcohol
are suspected in the face of denial, blood levels of the presumed agents may
be required for a definitive diagnosis.

Alcohol-related sleep disorders are extremely common and complex among
chronic alcoholics in particular, but also, although to a lesser extent, among
nonalcoholics acutely abusing alcohol. The disturbances are due either to
intoxication or withdrawal effects on the CNS and range from brief and mild
to protracted and severe. Blood alcohol concentration, whether it is rising

or falling, and duration of exposure are factors which shape the likelihood of onset of disturbance and its nature: insomnia, hypersomnia, poor sleep, increased daytime napping, fragmentation or increased nightly awakenings, nightmares, and delirium. The entire kaleidoscope of EEG disruptions may be observed: instability or fragmentation of the circadian and ultradian sleep rhythms reflected in frequent EEG stage changes, shifts in REM and SWS percentage, reduction or absence of characteristic sleep stage landmarks such as K-complexes and sleep spindles. Alcohol withdrawal leaves its prolonged mark in EEG tracings with SWS reductions of sometimes months and even years. Thus the folk wisdom belief that alcohol improves sleep is a gross oversimplification. The treatment however should address the alcohol intoxication or withdrawal primarily rather than the secondary sleep disturbance. Hypno-sedatives in particular should be discouraged (see the chapter on Organic Mental Disorders).

Somnolence often follows excessive doses of antipsychotics or tricyclic antidepressants, particularly of the sedating types. Early after initiation of pharmacotherapy, somnolence may follow even moderate daily doses.

Table 14-1 summarizes the main effects of a list of pertinent drugs in psychiatry on important sleep parameters. Arrows pointing upward indicate an increase, down-oriented arrows a decrease, and blank spaces indicate that no definitive statement can be made.

TABLE 14-1

KNOWN DRUG EFFECTS ON NOCTURNAL SLEEP AND ITS EEG PARAMETERS

Substance	Spindling	Spindle %	K-complexes	Delta	Delta %	Theta	Alpha	Beta	REM %	REM Latency	Total Sleep Time	Awakenings	Sleep Latency
Benzodiazepines	↑	↑	↓	↓	↓			↑	↓	↑	↑	↓	↓
Barbiturates		↑						↑	↓	↓	↑	↓	↓
Chloral Hydrate											↑		↓
Neuroleptics Normal Subjects	↓	↓			↑			↑	↓	↑			↓
Neuroleptics Schizophrenics		↑	↓ CPZ↑	↓	↑			↑	↓	↑			↓
Tricyclics	↑	↑		↓	↑	↓		↑	↓			↓	
MAOI				↑					↓				
Lithium		↑			↑				↓	↑	↑		
Ethanol			↓	↓	↑				↓		↓	↓	↓
Marijuana		↑			↓								↑
Methaqualone	↓			↓	↓			↑	↓				↓
Opioids					↓				↓				↑
Amphetamines		↑			↓				↓	↑			
Caffeine	↓							↓			↓	↑	↑

1. b,c,d,e,f,g,h,i,j,k,m,n   11. b,c,d
2. a,c   12. c,d
3. a,b,c   13. c
4. a,b,c   14. b
5. a,b,c,d,e   15. d
6. a,b,c,d   16. b
7. a,b   17. c
8. a,b,c,d   18. c
9. b,c   19. c
10. a,b

D. SLEEP-INDUCED RESPIRATORY IMPAIRMENT

Daytime sleepiness is the usual counterpart of the sleep apnea struggles and insomnia during the night (as described previously), sometimes to the point of abrupt and unexpected sleep attacks which are reminiscent of narcolepsy (see below). Contrary to the short refreshing effect of the typical narcoleptic naps, the daytime sleep attacks of the sleep apnea DOES syndrome are prolonged (>1 hour) and unrefreshing. During the sleep episode these patients are difficult to arouse from slumber and, upon awakening, they are often disoriented, uncoordinated, and feel foggy (sleep drunkenness, see below). In children, this may be responsible for enuresis, learning difficulties, poor school performance, and motor hyperactivity. Older persons may complain of persistent postdormital headaches, malaise, night sweats, and heat intolerance. Obesity is a classical, although inconsistent, accompaniment.

The Pickwickian syndrome was first described in 1956 after Charles Dickens' famous fictitious characterization in the "Posthumous Papers of the Pickwick Club" of a hypersomnolent, rotund, and red-faced bar lad called Joe, who could not manage to stay awake and was thought to be a "dope eater." It is characterized by diurnal hypersomnolence, hypoventilation which often leads to cyanosis and polycythemia, and cardio-respiratory disorder with sleep apneic episodes of up to 3 minutes. These individuals may spend up to 75% of their total sleep time in apnea. Sometimes the syndrome starts with sleep apneic episodes for about 10 years prior to the other clinical manifestations of a typical Pickwickian syndrome. These individuals are partly insensitive to inspired 5% CO_2. Other signs include hypoxia, hypercapnia, and twitching. Uncorrected, the lethargy may deepen into stupor due to CO_2 narcosis, and papilledema (choked disks) may be seen in some with impairment of consciousness and confusion. The diagnosis can be made from blood gas measurements (hypoxemia, hypercapnia), lung volume measurements (decreased vital capacity, reduced respiratory reserve volume), and measurements of thoracic compliance which is reduced to below normal levels. The differential diagnosis of the Pickwickian syndrome usually is with hepatic coma (asterixis), brain tumor (longstanding increase in intracranial pressure), polycythemia, heart disease and sickle cell anemia when O_2 tension is lowered. Chlorimipramine, a tricyclic which is not available for prescription in the USA, has been recommended for this condition but pro-triptyline (Vivactil), another tricyclic which is available, may be equally effective. Amphetamines also improve the daytime sleepiness but not the syndrome per se, except perhaps by their effect on appetite and eating. Improvement often goes parallel with loss of weight. However, the Pickwick-ian syndrome is no longer viewed as a unique, discrete entity. Indeed, most, if not all, disorders of the daytime hypersomnolence - sleep apnea spectrum have these in common:

1) diurnal hypersomnolence
2) respiratory abnormalities during sleep
3) hypotonia of nasopharyngeal and laryngeal muscles during sleep

Thus, they can all be considered together as hypersomnolence with periodic sleep apnea. The differences appear to rest on the degree of severity of each one of the abnormalities listed above. Apneic episodes during sleep may be of:

1) central or diaphragmatic origin if there is cessation of air inflow for more than 10 seconds and no respiratory effort;
2) obstructive nature: no air flow through upper airway despite persistent diaphragmatic contractions leading to incredible rise in intrathoracic pressure, until suddenly the obstruction is lifted, and there is cacophonous snorting and snoring with which the apnea is momentarily resolved;
3) mixed type or complex: central followed by obstructive but never in the reversed order.

Patients with central sleep apnea usually complain of daytime tiredness and occasionally of excessive daytime sleepiness. As described earlier in the DIMS section, the majority of patients also complain of chronic insomnia and frequent awakenings but rarely of difficulty in falling asleep. Prescription of sleeping pills will only aggravate the condition by depressing the respir-atory center. Obstructive and central sleep apnea are sometimes associated with narcolepsy (3% of narcoleptics). There is no satisfactory treatment. Diaphragmatic pacing, based on instrumentation similar to cardiac pacemak-ers, as a therapeutic approach, is a promising possibility, but is still at the experimental level.

Patients with obstructive (upper airway) sleep apnea usually complain of sleep attacks, excessive daytime somnolence, and daytime tiredness. Their spouses report loud snoring (air-starved snorers) and motorically violent sleep (the bed often looks like a battlefield in the morning). This is caused by the respiratory and concomitant motor struggle to overcome the obstruc-tion. The apnea episodes may arouse the patient more than a hundred times in the course of the night. A constellation of other manifestations can be found among patients with obstructive sleep apnea. These are sleep walking, hypnagogic hallucinations, personality changes, decreased intellectual activ-ity, difficulty in concentration, decreased libido, frontal headaches, and automatic behavior syndrome (ABS). ABS manifestations may last for hours with retrograde amnesia for the episode. Patients with obstructive sleep apnea often exhibit a hypertrophic or double chin composed of excessive muscle tissue rather than fat as opposed to obese people. The fact that these patients are frequently overweight may render difficult the identification of the "double chin." Micrognathia, hypertrophic tonsils or adenoids, and soft-palate abnormalities may be aggravating factors which can be eliminated by surgical correction. Other physiological concomitants of the sleep apnea syndrome are cardiac arrhythmias, bradycardia during the apnea episode and tachycardia at the onset of renewed breathing. The cycle repeats every 60 to 120 seconds. Prolonged asystoles of up to 6 seconds and antrioventricular block have also been reported. The treatment of obstructive sleep apnea is based on diet geared toward weight loss and corrective surgery or permanent tracheostomy if the patient exhibits obvious cardiovascular and psychological problems.

Although the association of hypersomnolence with sleep apnea has been known for many years, it has been extensively studied only for the last decade. Respiration during sleep has long been taken completely for granted. We breathe ever so blissfully, yet recent neurophysiological research indicates that alpha motoneurons of lower pons and medulla oblangata which control automatic respiration are subject to delicate interactions dependent on respiratory periodicity and fluctuations of the sleep-waking cycle with marked firing rate changes during the transitions from waking to sleep. These should make us wonder how we manage to continue breathing when we fall asleep and realize how vulnerable the respiratory adjustment is in this intriguing transition from wakefulness to sleep. It appears that the body's automatic control of breathing breaks down in the shift from wakefulness to sleep, particularly deep sleep. This transition seems to reduce respiratory drive. This lack of control can immobilize the diaphragm, rib cage, and throat muscles to the point of stoppage of air flow. The apnea quickly cuts off oxygen supply to the blood and brain and alters acid-base balance. This luckily wakes up the brain sufficiently to facilitate respiratory physiology again. Since the throat has collapsed, the lungs may not fill with air immediately. The victim's struggle causes further arousal with which more tone returns to the throat muscles. This, plus the incredible intrathoracic pressure developed, finally resumes air exchange with a loud snore and the cycle repeats as deep sleep sets in again. Daytime sleepiness is often a source of problems in school, at work, and within the family. Secondary anxiety, irritability, depression, and even despair to the point of suicide may result.

Daytime sleepiness is often the presenting symptom in alveolar hypoventilation, nocturnal myoclonus, and the restless legs syndrome and should be listed as a DOES with these syndromes (for more details see the DIMS section).

E. NARCOLEPSY

Daytime sleepiness and sleep attacks are prominent manifestations of narcolepsy. In normal individuals the first REM sleep episode as measured by the EEG at night usually occurs 90 minutes after sleep onset. In the narcoleptic, a REM sleep episode may initiate a sleep period either at night or during the day. Accidents may ensue from such episodes and may involve dropping a hand into a pan of burning oil or automobile accidents. Some patients develop stratagems to stay awake in dangerous situations or in hostile environments. The usual daytime sleepiness of the narcoleptic may be relieved episodically by a sudden fit of sleep from which the patient awakens feeling refreshed and refractory to sleepiness for several hours. Signals of a sleep attack are: physical exhaustion, blurred vision, burning eyes, and sudden headaches. The normal REM stage of sleep occurs with a decrease or collapse of muscle tone. In narcolepsy, this striking physiology explains cataplexy, which is the second and most frequent accompanying sign (66-95%) of the tetrad constituting classical narcolepsy. Cataplexy refers to a collapse of voluntary and postural musculature. As a result, the individual may dangerously plummet to the floor if he is standing or may slump in his chair or driver's seat. This loss of tone of the musculature during REM sleep normally occurs well into the night when the individual is secure in bed. Without this safety device, animal research suggests that during REM sleep brain activity would move the body and propel the sleeper leaping, thrashing, and acting out his dreams. Muscle paralysis in the narcoleptic may be rather circumscribed (head tilts, knees buckle, jaw drops), or may be limited to a fleeting sensation of weakness of some muscles, or may be quite generalized. Some muscle groups are not affected: extraocular muscles (palpebral muscles also affected), middle ear muscles, sphincters, and diaphragm. The REM sleep attack may coincide with the cataplectic component, leaving no memory of the occurrence, or short cataplectic attacks may occur without sleep and with full consciousness. In this case, speech becomes impaired and vision is blurred. Emotions such as laughter and anger, love-making, playing sports, stress, fatigue, and heavy meals may trigger the cataplectic attack.

The frequency of cataplectic attacks varies greatly, from 1/week to 4 or more/day. During a cataplectic attack there may be not only abolition of muscle strength and tone, but also of EMG potentials and tendon reflexes. Motor inhibition is presumably due to tonic postsynaptic inhibition of spinal motoneurons concomitant with REM sleep. This effect may be mediated by a cholinergic corticobulbospinal pathway originating in the frontal cortex. Conceivably a complementary limbico-orbital pathway may be responsible for triggering cataplectic attacks during episodes of emotion such as laughter or anger. The cholinergic nature of this pathway may explain the favorable response of the cataplectic component of narcolepsy to tricyclic antidepressants, some of which have a substantial built-in anticholinergic action, and all of which greatly decrease measures of REM sleep. The cholinergic involvement in REM sleep is fairly well-documented and supported by the REM-blocking effects of atropine.

Two more signs complete the narcoleptic tetrad: hypnagogic hallucinations (20-50%) and sleep paralysis (17-57%). Hypnagogic hallucinations are vivid dream-like experiences at sleep onset. If the hallucinations occur on awakening, they are called hypnopompic. These dream perceptions are frightening and anxiety-laden, particularly the first few times after the onset of the condition. The hallucinations can be visual, auditory, or tactile - in fact they are often mixed. If the patient has an escape or avoidance response, he may, in his terrified condition, move into danger. If unable to move, the experience can be even more unpleasant and terrifying. These features can serve as cues for a differential diagnosis with hysterical attacks in which the proclivity to get hurt is rare. Luckily, individuals suffering from these misperceptions usually realize quickly the hallucinatory quality of their experience. But younger patients may refuse to sleep to avoid what they may call "daytime nightmares."

Sleep paralysis, as is the case with the hallucinations, is experienced at sleep onset or on emerging from sleep. In the latter case, there is a conscious inability to move the entire body or talk for a period ranging from seconds up to 20 minutes. Touching the patient or calling his name will often terminate the attack.

The "narcoleptic tetrad," that is all four manifestations together, is found in about 11% of all narcoleptics. The prevalence of narcolepsy is estimated at 4-9 per 10,000, and the total number of affected individuals in the USA at over 100,000. There are no sex differences in the incidence of this condition, but a hereditary factor is suggested by a 60 to 200-fold greater risk of narcolepsy among relatives of diagnosed narcoleptics than in the general population. Narcolepsy-cataplexy has been described in female toy poodles. These animals go limp and collapse when excited. Breeding attempts are being made with affected pets referred by their masters to develop an animal model for the study of this condition.

Rigorous diagnosis of narcolepsy requires all-night polysomnography to demonstrate the sleep onset REM pattern and to rule out other confounding diagnoses (i.e., sleep apnea, epilepsy, hysterical trance, etc.). Although this sleep onset REM pattern is the most widely accepted diagnostic criterion, other conditions associated with sleep onset REM must be ruled out (i.e., drug withdrawal, previous REM sleep deprivation, rapid travel across time zones). Short REM sleep latency in dubious cases is suggestive of the diagnosis of classical narcolepsy. The Hoffmann or H reflex is very valuable as an ancillary diagnostic procedure. It tests the monosynaptic contraction of calf muscles elicited by percutaneous electrical stimulation in the popliteal fossa. This reflex is absent during REM sleep in normal individuals and during narcoleptic and cataplectic attacks.

The pathology and pathophysiology of narcolepsy are not yet clear. Narcolepsy characteristically begins at a point of maturational crisis such as puberty (about age 15) or pregnancy (about age 25) in 77% of those affected. In only 18% it begins after the age of 30 and in scarcely 5% before 10 years of age. Narcolepsy often begins with daytime drowsiness and sleep spells. The triad of cataplexy, sleep paralysis, and hypnagogic hallucinations may precede daytime sleepiness for 10 years or more. A deficit or inability of the α-noradrenergic system to inhibit REM sleep is conceivably involved in narcolepsy. This speculation is in keeping with the observation that substances with noradrenergic potential are therapeutic.

Amphetamines and methylphenidate (up to 40-60 mg/day) usually curb sleep attacks and daytime sleepiness, but do not influence the other manifestations of the tetrad. Amphetamines cause a reduction in REM sleep time, but this is probably not their mechanism of action in their curtailment of sleep episodes. As will be seen below, tricyclic antidepressants, which also reduce REM time in long- as well as short-term studies, are effective against the accessory manifestations of the narcoleptic tetrad but have little effectiveness against the sleep attacks themselves. Amphetamines must be avoided in the evening. Scheduling short naps at times when the patient feels the most compelling need for sleep may reduce the use or abuse of amphetamines and their side effects (i.e., increased blood pressure, addiction, depression, psychosis, paradoxical increase in daytime sleepiness with increased dose). Methylphenidate has less drastic effects on REM sleep than amphetamines and also fewer side effects, particularly on blood pressure. Provisos to avoid large meals, with their usual sequela of postprandial drowsiness, are also helpful.

Cataplectic attacks and the other auxiliary symptoms of narcolepsy are best treated with tricyclic antidepressants, especially imipramine, protriptyline, and chlorimipramine. But tricyclics have little effect on daytime sleepiness or sleep attacks. For the auxiliary symptoms, tricyclics are also more effective the first year after inception of treatment than later when the effect is not as convincing. This therapeutic effect may be related to their REM suppressant efficacy because other antidepressants without influence on REM (i.e., trimipramine, iprindole) lack efficacy. Narcoleptics who do not respond to the approaches outlined above may be given a trial of monoamine oxidase inhibitors (MAOI) such as phenelzine, which in doses of 15 mg tid, causes striking reductions in cataplectic attacks, in sleep paralysis episodes, hypnagogic hallucinations, and even in sleepiness and sleep attacks. Phenelzine has been reported to suppress REM for over one year. Caution must be exercised however in the use of MAOI. Abrupt MAOI withdrawal is bound to be followed by complete nocturnal insomnia and persistent frightening visual hallucination in the midst of darkness. Caution must also be exerted if tricyclics are used in combination with amphetamines (see chapter on Psychopharmacology).

F. IDIOPATHIC CNS HYPERSOMNOLENCE

This condition resembles narcolepsy in the seriousness of hypersomnolence and the sleep attacks, but it lacks the sleep onset REM stage in the EEG which is typical of classical narcolepsy. It is also referred to by a variety of other names such as independent, idiopathic, functional, mixed, or harmonious hypersomnia. Some 12-15% of the patients with excessive daytime sleepiness are thought to have idiopathic CNS hypersomnolence.

Patients with excessive daytime sleepiness are often misperceived as being "lazy" and as not presenting a legitimate medical diagnosis. This stigma may haunt them for 10-15 years from the earliest manifestations to the time of definitive diagnosis. Excessive sleep is complained of in about 45% of the referrals and chronic insomnia in about about 48%. It is obviously a significant public health problem.

G. HYPERSOMNOLENCE ASSOCIATED WITH OTHER MEDICAL, TOXIC, AND ENVIRONMENTAL CONDITIONS

Head trauma may cause excessive daytime sleepiness and excessive nighttime sleep some 6 to 18 months after the accident.

Infections and inflammatory conditions, such as trypanosomiasis and viral encephalitis of von Economo, can cause hypersomnolence, but are rare nowadays in the USA.

Other more transient febrile illnesses may cause excessive sleepiness. Metabolic and toxic conditions such as elevated urea nitrogen and other poisons may cause encephalopathies with hypersomnolence.

Hydrocephalus and hypothyroidism in children and adults can increase night sleep and daytime sleepiness. In feeble newborn infants there may be a disposition to constant sleep even without brain disease.

The normal aged individual has a greater prevalence for daytime somnolence, as well as for reduced nocturnal sleep than other age groups. This may be a sign of cerebral deterioration or may represent an expression of an associated abnormal sleep-wake schedule (see p. 655).

H. OTHER DOES CONDITIONS

1. Intermittent DOES (Periodic) Syndrome.
    The Kleine-Levin syndrome is characterized by recurrent periods of hypersomnia, usually associated with morbid hunger (hyperphagia). This disorder affects mainly young men. The sleep is prolonged and deep, such that arousal is difficult, but this sleep does not guarantee a refreshed and productive day. On the contrary, during wakefulness the patient is apathetic, irritable, confused, withdrawn, and eager to return to bed. Besides the classical association of hypersomnia and hyperphagia, there are other associated features. Anorexia may rarely replace the more usual voracious consumption of large quantities of food. Behavioral abnormalities are common. The social withdrawal may also be replaced by a bizarre loss of sexual inhibitions with inappropriate sexual advances or public exhibitionism. Delusions and hallucinations, excitation or depression, frank impairment of cognitive function (i.e., disorientation, amnesia, incoherent speech), metabolic and EEG abnormalities, and unexplained febrile illness prior to the period of hypersomnia have often led most authors to attribute this condition to an intermittent, organic dysfunction of limbic or hypothalamic structures which disappears spontaneously. But the etiology is unknown, the nature is obscure and puzzling, and there is controversy as to whether it is a definite classical entity. There are no specific treatment measures available for this relatively uncommon disturbance.

Although this condition was originally described in adolescent boys of schizoid personality among whom it predominates, a similar syndrome has subsequently been reported in few young and middle-aged normal women at the premenstrual phase. The similarities in cardinal findings as well as associated features are so striking that DSM-III has chosen to list them together. The menstruation-associated DOES syndrome is reserved for women in whom the hypersomnolence occurs intermittently but invariably at the time of menses (menstrual) or shortly before the onset of irregular menses (premenstrual). The hypersomnolence and hyperphagia are often associated with depression in the milder form (premenstrual tension) and with diminished amounts of REM sleep and nonspecific EEG abnormalities similar to those found in the Kleine-Levin syndrome in the more severe form during menstruum. Suggestions of an etiological role played by increased brain serotonin turnover and cyclic increases in progesterone secretions require further research. Regularization of menses, either spontaneously or through the use of hormonal supplements such as estrogen-progesterone compounds, has been reported to clear the daytime hypersomnolence. Periodic drowsiness secondary to the use of sedating analgesics during painful menses may mask the more pure forms of the menstrual-related hypersomnolence. Thorough neurological examination and EEG should be taken to rule out hypersomnolence caused by abnormal discharges from lesions in the temporal lobe or limbic structures at the time of menses.

2. Insufficient Sleep.
Insufficient sleep at night is bound to produce excessive daytime sleepiness. The individual is voluntarily, but often unwittingly, chronically sleep deprived. Examination reveals no inability to fall asleep or remain asleep suitably. Polysomnography shows a normal sleep structure except for an increase in deep NREM (stages 3 and 4) sleep and a high ratio and intensity of REM sleep. This diagnosis is often made among factory workers holding two jobs or hospital guards who stay up late nightly with friends but have to be at work at 7 a.m. Secondary symptoms are irritability, difficulty in concentration, reduced vigilance, distractibility, reduced motivation, depression, fatigue, restlessness, incoordination, malaise, loss of appetite, weight loss, gastrointestinal disturbance, dry mouth, painful muscles, and diplopia. These secondary symptoms become the focus of concern and the patient is quite unaware that more sleep will be recuperative in and of itself.

3. Disorder of Initiating Wakefulness (Sleep Drunkenness).
Sleep drunkenness is an abnormal form of awakening in which the lack of a clear sensorium in the transition from sleep to full wakefulness is prolonged and exaggerated. Essential to this diagnosis is the absence of sleep deprivation. Thus, a differential diagnosis is often presented with some patients with sleep apnea who experience post-sleep disorientation, fogginess, dulling of the sensorium, incoordination, and periods of automatic behavior for which no

recollection can be demonstrated (blackouts), probably due to their sleepiness. These are typical manifestations of sleep drunkenness. The patient is usually hard to arouse from sleep. Regressive behavior is likely to re-emerge in children during such episodes (i.e., enuresis, learning difficulties, decreased school performance, hyperactivity). Headaches, general malaise, obesity, drenching night sweats, and heat intolerance are frequent concomitants of sleep drunkenness in adults. There is a preponderance for males in the reports and the syndrome has an affinity for certain families. Sleep deprivation, physical exertion leading to extreme tiredness, and hypnotic medication enhance the potential of an episode.

I. NO DOES ABNORMALITY

There are individuals who normally sleep more hours than most ("long sleepers") but present no complaints and exhibit no daytime sleepiness. Some individuals may have cycles of unusual lengths of several days which replace the normal circadian cycle. In such condition, insomnia and somnolence may appear in sequence and last several days. There are still others who subjectively complain of DOES but exhibit no objective findings to support such diagnosis.

QUIZ, Section III.

TRUE or FALSE: Indicate which of the following statements are true (T) and which are false (F) by circling the appropriate letter.

T   F   1.   DOES is much less frequent than DIMS but by no means rare.

T   F   2.   Narcolepsy is a DOES syndrome.

T   F   3.   Hypersomnolence is a disease condition.

T   F   4.   Narcolepsy, alcohol abuse, drugs, depression, and sleep apnea are among the most common conditions causing DOES.

T   F   5.   In depression one never sees hypersomnia.

T   F   6.   There are no animal models of narcolepsy.

T   F   7.   Amphetamine use or withdrawal never causes hypersomnolence.

T   F   8.   The treatment of choice of alcohol-induced sleep disturbances is administration of hypnotics.

T   F   9.   Both the daytime naps of the typical narcoleptic and the daytime sleep episodes of the sleep-induced apnea patient have equally refreshing effects.

Circle the letter corresponding to the <u>one</u> correct response.

10. Sleep drunkenness resembles most

   a. the sleep of the drunkard following excessive alcohol ingestion.
   b. the usual state of "dope eaters."
   c. the state following arousal from REM sleep.
   d. the disorientation, incoordination, and grogginess observed in patients with sleep-induced respiratory depression upon awakening from a daytime sleep episode.

11. The Pickwickian syndrome usually describes

   a. a young chlorotic female.
   b. an obese hypersomnolent lad.
   c. insomnia due to Caffeine Intoxication.
   d. a grandiose impersonation of Dickens.

12. In the mixed or complex type of sleep apnea, the correct sequence is

   a. obstructive followed by central.
   b. central followed by obstructive.
   c. obstructive and central types of apnea occurring simultaneously.
   d. cataplexy precedes and ushers the apneic episode.

13. Respiratory drive is higher during

   a. SWS.
   b. alertness.
   c. state of narcosis.
   d. severe acute Alcoholic Intoxication.

14. Sleeping pills

   a. are indicated to counteract the insomnia of patients with central sleep apnea.
   b. help individuals with obstructive sleep apnea.
   c. should be given to the two categories of patients mentioned in a and b but only for the first 2-3 days.
   d. are usually ineffective in treating most types of insomnia after the first 2-3 weeks of administration.

15. The cataplectic attacks of REM narcoleptics are due to

   a. paralysis of the respiratory center.
   b. an episode of Catatonic Schizophrenia.
   c. the normal paralysis of sleep, always with cessation of consciousness.
   d. decreased tonic activity of groups of skeletal musculature.

16. The cataplectic attacks of narcoleptics respond best to

    a. amphetamines.
    b. neuroleptics.
    c. barbiturates.
    d. tricyclic antidepressants.
    e. L-tryptophan.

17. Classical narcolepsy is a condition with strong

    a. environmental etiology.
    b. infectious contributory factors.
    c. hereditary background
    d. intrapsychic etiology.
    e. easily demonstrable gross neurological damage.

Circle the correct answer(s). One or more than one answer may be correct.

18. Sleep drunkenness is often responsible for

    a. poor school performance.
    b. post-dormital headaches.
    c. learning difficulties.
    d. ethanolic breath.
    e. automatic behavior with memory blackouts.

19. Who is more likely to be in possession of information that will lead to an accurate diagnosis of obstructive sleep apnea?

    a. patient
    b. spouse
    c. sleeping companion
    d. roommate
    e. marital counselor
    f. social worker

20. Muscles not affected in the collapse of tonic activity during a cataplectic attack are

    a. palpebral muscles.
    b. extraocular muscles.
    c. sphincters (anus and bladder).
    d. diaphragm.
    e. myocardium.
    f. jaw muscles.

21. The therapeutic action of tricyclics against the cataplexy of narcoleptics is best explained on the basis of their

    a. antidepressant properties.
    b. blockage of serotonin and norepinephrine nerve terminal uptake.
    c. built-in anticholinergic potential.

22. If the anticholinergic potential of tricyclics is therapeutic against cataplectic attacks, one would also expect therapeutic effects from the action of

    a. thioridazine.
    b. reserpine.
    c. atropine.
    d. physostigmine.
    e. diazepam.

23. Condition(s) capable of causing daytime hypersomnolence is/are

    a. trypanosomiasis.
    b. Von Economo viral encephalitis.
    c. hydrocephalus.
    d. hypothyroidism.
    e. hyperthyroidism.

24. Common to the Kleine-Levin syndrome and menstrual hypersomnolence is/are

    a. episodes of hypersomnia.
    b. both usually in the female sex.
    c. hyperphagia.

25. Associate sign(s) of the Pickwickian syndrome is/are

    a. relative insensitivity to inspired 5% CO_2.
    b. hypoxia, hypercapnia, twitching.
    c. a decrease in vital capacity.
    d. cyanosis, polycythemia.

26. Some 3% of narcoleptics

    a. are so-called REM narcoleptics.
    b. also have central sleep apnea.
    c. have cataplectic attacks.
    d. exhibit the entire narcoleptic tetrad.

27. Diaphragmatic pacing, although still at an experimental stage, appears promising for

    a. obstructive sleep apnea.
    b. central sleep apnea.
    c. cataplexy.
    d. the restless legs syndrome.

28. Strong emotions often serve as triggers of

    a. sleep-apnea daytime hypersomnolent attacks.
    b. cataplectic attacks.
    c. slow-wave sleep attacks.

29. Diagnostic criteria of classical REM narcolepsy is/are

    a. sleep-onset REM pattern.
    b. short REM sleep latency.
    c. associated cataplexy, and perhaps sleep paralysis and hypnagogic hallucinations.
    d. absence of the H-reflex during an attack.
    e. onset at puberty or pregnancy.

IV. DISORDERS OF THE SLEEP-WAKE SCHEDULE

The characteristic disturbance here is not DIMS or DOES but rather one of the sleep-wake cycle. This may be transient or persistent.

Rapid time zone change ("jet lag") syndrome: Rapid east-west travel can produce temporary hypersomnia during the wake period or insomnia during the sleep period which usually resolves within several days after adjustment to a new time zone. Body temperature normally reflects a low point in the early morning and a peak in the afternoon. This circadian rhythm may be altered following rapid travel across the time zones and detection of this disruption may be helpful in the diagnosis of such phase-shifts. Patients who suffer from jet lag usually need approximately one day to readjust for every hour of time zone shift. Irregular bed and arising times can lead to a chronic phase shift in the absence of rapid travel across time zones. Regularization of those times will normalize sleep after a couple of weeks.

Circadian rhythmicity entails greatest somnolence, poorest performance, and lowest body temperature in the pre-dawn hours; greatest alertness, best performance, and highest body temperature during the daytime. Neuro-endocrinological function also waxes and wanes in a predictable circadian fashion. Thus, growth hormone peak release occurs within the first two hours of sleep onset when maximal concentration of stages 3/4 sleep occurs; highest plasma and urine cortisol occur during the last third of nocturnal sleep time; prolactin release rises during non-REM sleep and falls off just before each REM period; luteinizing hormone also follows ontogenetic and circadian evolution with first increases concomitant with sleep during early puberty. All these physiological and neuroendocrine rhythmicities are probably related to the sleep disturbances following rapid travel across time zones, with a misalignment of bedtime to a local clock time.

Less transient and more repeated or almost continuous may be the form of sleep disorder in shift workers who must adapt to variable sleep and work schedules ("work shift" changes in conventional sleep-wake schedule) or to periodically "rotating shift work."

In the delayed sleep phase syndrome there is a perpetuated involuntary asynchrony between the person's interval sleep-wake phase schedule and clock time (phase lag), without alteration in work shifts or travel across time zones.

In the advanced sleep phase syndrome there is an evening inability to stay awake and early morning wakefulness. Typically, the patient may go to bed and sleep from 8 p.m. to 3 a.m. This is sometimes seen in elderly patients and is frequently associated with, or confounded by, symptoms of depression.

The non-24-hour sleep-wake syndrome is a free running sleep pattern which may be intermittent or continuous in the progression. Impaired performance may be marked in attempts to participate in scheduled social activities because the individual may reach peak alertness and efficiency only late in the waking day.

An irregular sleep-wake pattern exists when there is a loss of zeitgebers (time or scheduling indicators) and the patient exhibits frequent daytime naps at irregular times, excessive bedrest, sleep at night is of inadequate length, and subjective DIMS. But total 24-hour sleep is normal for age.

V. DYSFUNCTIONS ASSOCIATED WITH SLEEP, SLEEP STAGES, OR PARTIAL AROUSALS (PARASOMNIAS)

These dysfunctions encompass a heterogeneous group of episodic nocturnal events which may be disturbing to the sleeper himself or to others. The first three of the following categories of dysfunctions are stage 4 parasomnias.

A. SLEEPWALKING OR SOMNAMBULISM

This condition is characterized by onset of a paroxysmal burst of high voltage SWS and rising out of bed, ambulation, and other complex patterns of purposive motor behavior during sleep with eyes open, usually in the first third of the night and lasting 1/2 to several minutes, but possibly up to 30-40 minutes. Confusion, temporal disorientation, and amnesia follow awakening. Gaining the patient's attention and awakening him are extremely difficult. This is because sleepwalking occurs in the midst of stage 4 or deep sleep during which the arousal threshold is very high. For this reason too, while seemingly capable of climbing through windows or driving a car, these patients are very vulnerable and prone to have serious accidents.

1. T	12. b	23. a,b,c,d
2. T	13. b	24. a,c
3. F	14. d	25. a,b,c,d
4. T	15. d	26. b
5. F	16. d	27. b
6. F	17. c	28. b
7. F	18. a,b,c,e	29. a,b,c,d,e
8. F	19. b,c,d	
9. F	20. b,c,d,e	
10. d	21. c	
11. b	22. a,c	

Old wives' tales and even pseudoscientific notions have often purported the sleepwalker as acting out dreams. But psychological conflicts do not cause this condition, which in most cases disappears spontaneously by the third decade. Popular notion also holds that these individuals enjoy a high level of awareness during the sleepwalking episode and that they never harm themselves. But reality is quite contrary to this notion and these patients need protection during the episode. There is no impairment, however, of waking mentation or behavior.

Adult sleepwalking is much less prevalent than in childhood, usually occurs in persons with a history of sleepwalking in childhood or adolescence, and is more chronic and associated with psychiatric disturbance than childhood sleepwalking. The condition is fairly common, 1-6% in the general population, and 15% of all children, particularly frequent between the ages of 6 and 12. Boys are more frequently affected than girls, and there seems to be a strong genetic influence which may be elicited from the family history. Some 56% of sleepwalkers have relatives who also walk in their sleep. Nocturnal or daytime psychomotor epileptic seizures and fugue states, although capable of exhibiting similar automatic motor behaviors, can easily be ruled out by means of EEG.

There are pharmacological means (diazepam, flurazepam) of reducing the deep stages of sleep, which would be expected to decrease the incidence of sleepwalking episodes. But these drugs do not appear to be effective and prevention of accidents is usually the only measure required (safe bedroom, windows, etc.). As seen from the demographics above, many children outgrow the disorder, which seems to suggest a delay in CNS maturation. Perhaps because of this maturational lag, there is a relationship between sleepwalking and enuresis. Some 62% of adult somnambulists have current or past history of nocturnal enuresis, as opposed to only 23% of the controls. Thirty-eight percent of somnambulists have a family history of enuresis versus 17% of controls. Sleeptalking sometimes accompanies somnambulism and night-terrors (described below). CNS depressants are to be avoided since deep stage of sleep, confusional sleepwalking, and risk of accidents may be enhanced by these agents.

B. SLEEP TERROR (PAVOR NOCTURNUS, NIGHT TERRORS, INCUBUS)

This disturbance also occurs early in the night, some 15-30 minutes after sleep onset, during arousal from stages 3 or 4. An attack usually occurs during the first or second non-REM sleep period of the night. A K-complex (brief high voltage slow wave discharge) or a burst of delta waves presages the attack onset. The patient usually sits up or gets out of bed. This is quickly followed by alpha activity, investigative (undirectional) eye movements repeated at 15-second intervals, and a sharp increase in heart and respiratory rates. Sleep continuity and the attack itself are usually broken by a blood-curdling scream prompted by a feeling of terror, often described as agonizing dread or chest pressure which is probably due to a period of apnea. There are hardly any memories of a frightening dream, but there are agitated thrashings, intense global muscle contractions with feelings of paralysis, hypermotility, confused talking, intense anxiety, choking noises and sensations, profuse perspiration and sympathetic activation (tachycardia, tachypnea, pupillary dilatation). An expression of intense fear and emotion or confusion is typical in combination with unresponsiveness and feelings of impending doom. Amnesia is the rule on awakening in the morning or, if the patient has recall, memory traces exist only for an isolated hallucination, rather than an elaborate story. The dream content is usually fearful (being chased or attacked, fear of falling). The whole episode lasts usually 1-2 minutes, but possibly up to 20 minutes or more. It is a common condition at ages 3 to 5 (then called pavor nocturnus) and decreases in frequency beyond this age range, but some adults (in whom it is called incubus attacks) continue to experience the terrors throughout their lives and exhibit an association between incubus and psychopathology. Sleep terror suggests an impaired mechanism of arousal out of stages 3 or 4 of sleep. Sleep terror and ordinary dream anxiety attacks are subjectively and objectively distinguishable (see Table 14-2). Specific treatment is usually not required. Diazepam 5-20 mg at bedtime will greatly reduce the chance of a night terror attack, perhaps by decreasing stage 4 sleep in some of the afflicted individuals. But in some, such clear correlation between decrease in the attacks and use of the benzodiazepine has not been observed.

C. SLEEP-RELATED ENURESIS

Primary enuresis usually refers to bed wetting in a child who has never been totally dry for several consecutive months since infancy. It is often familial and much more common in boys than in girls. It is found in 10-15% of children 4-5 years old. Dryness is achieved in about 90% and 97% of 7 and 12 year olds, respectively. But 1-3% of 17 to 28 year olds are still prone to wetness. A misconception that it is a REM-bound defect often appears in some textbooks. Primary enuresis is not related to REM sleep, but if the child is left wet after the episode, subsequent REM dream contents are bound to incorporate the perception of wetness. This is to be distinguished from secondary enuresis in which bed wetting has reappeared after a dry period, often involves psychological problems, and the episode does not necessarily occur during stages 3 and 4 but will occur during arousal or REM. Primary enuresis is usually unassociated with dreams or dream recall. On a polysomnographic recording, the primary enuretic episode begins by a burst of rhythmic waves (K-complex) preponderantly during the first third of the night, with a series of bladder contractions and general body movement, suddenly increased muscle tone, tachycardia, and tachypnea or apnea during stage 3 or 4 of sleep. This then changes to stage 2 or 1 when micturition occurs, and the patient may wake up, but usually returns to sleep and remains amnesic for the episode.

The first task in evaluation and therapy is to determine whether it is primary or secondary enuresis. If it is primary, the approach should be lenient and should avoid the generation of guilt and anxiety in either child or parents. If secondary, psychological evaluation is required. No urological procedures should be entertained unless there is a strong specific indication for them. Physiological treatments usually involve drinking lots of fluids during the day, holding micturition, partial urination followed by holding in midstream, and resumption of urination. Children enjoy these exercises which are engineered to increase the urine retaining capacity of the bladder. Treatment may range from psychotherapy for secondary enuresis, through reassurance in milder cases of primary enuresis, to behavioral approaches or pharmacological treatment with imipramine, which also increases the urine-retaining capacity of the bladder, in the more severe cases of primary enuresis.

There is a linkage between somnambulism, night terrors, and enuresis. Some authors have lumped these three syndromes together under the concept of disorders of arousal from deep sleep. Both the pavor nocturnus of children and the incubus attacks of adults develop out of the same deep stage of sleep. About 1/3 of somnambulists suffer from night terrors and about 1/6 from enuresis.

D. OTHER DYSFUNCTIONS

    1. Dream Anxiety Attacks (DAA).
        These can be distinguished from night terrors (see above). In this case the sleeper, usually a woman, awakens from a dream (REM sleep) and is fully aware of its frightening impact and content. Autonomic activation may be minimal or nonexistent. Mean age at onset is in the late teens but the range is quite wide (4-52 years old), which suggests no relationship between DAA and development. Incidence in children is about 3% but in adults is over 20 times higher. The frequency of DAA is usually 3 attacks per week, and the second half of the night offers a greater likelihood of occurrence. Insomnia (REM-interruption insomnia) is observed as an associated complaint in about 1/3 of cases. There is a familial trend and an association with psychopathology and somnambulism in DAA. The typical DAA has the same duration as the typical dream but is loaded with more apprehension, fear, misfortune, death, attack, and physical activity, and with less happiness than normal dreaming. It is also often of a recurrent nature. DAA are responsive to benzodiazepines but the mechanism of action is not clear. Table 14-2 makes the differential diagnosis between night terrors and DAA.

TABLE 14-2

DIFFERENTIAL DIAGNOSIS BETWEEN NIGHT TERRORS
AND DREAM ANXIETY ATTACKS

	Night Terrors	Dream Anxiety Attacks
Night Time	1st 1/3	2nd 1/2
Incidence	Less	More
Sex predominance	Males	Females
Emotion	More terrifying	Less
Mental state on awakening	Confused	Clear
Intensity	More	Less
Heart & respiratory rate	More increase	Less
Memory	None or little	Long, vivid dream
Are dreams?	"Of course not"	"Of course they are"
Other verbal reports	Less complete dream report	More complete dream report
EEG	Stages 3 and 4	REM stage
Treatment	Benzodiazepines	Benzodiazepines

2. Sleep-related Epileptic Seizures.
   Epileptic seizures and psychomotor epileptic seizures, usually of the temporal lobe within the amygdala, or of frontal lobe origin occasionally occur at night (nocturnal seizures) and cause confused automatic behavior similar to that of sleepwalking. The differential diagnosis between nocturnal epilepsy and sleepwalking can be made on the basis of Table 14-3.

TABLE 14-3

DIFFERENTIAL DIAGNOSIS BETWEEN NOCTURNAL
EPILEPSY AND SLEEPWALKING

	Nocturnal Epilepsy	Sleepwalking
Temporal, amygdala, frontal lobe pathology	Usually present	Absent
EEG	Seizure discharge	No seizure discharge
Confused automatic behavior	Present	Present
Swallowing	Present	Absent
Handrubbing	Present	Absent
Return to bed	Uncommom	Usual
Wakeful attacks	Common	Absent

3. Sleep-related Bruxism.
   Symptoms of this disorder include a grinding, gnashing, and clenching of the teeth during sleep due to unusually powerful contractions of masseter and pterygoid muscles. A mild degree of bruxism is normal and relatively common (13-15% of people). But it may become more severe and pathological to the point of causing teeth

damage. The noise produced by teeth grinding can be disturbing, even to those outside the room of the sleeper. Bruxism can occur during any stage of sleep but it predominates during stage 2, in contrast to the predominantly stage 4-related disturbances called somnambulism, pavor nocturnus, and enuresis and to the dream anxiety attacks which occur during REM sleep. The cause is unknown, but physical defects of the teeth (malocclusion), psychological factors (tension, anxiety, suppressed anger), and habits (alcohol intake) may be contributing factors which, following elucidation, would suggest the most appropriate treatment.

4. Sleep-related Headbanging (Jactatio Capitis Nocturnus).
Rhythmic head banging against the bed or mattress is often seen in healthy infants and children in their second and third year, particularly when they are bored, tired, or irritated. Within certain limits it is thus a normal phenomenon. When excessive in intensity or duration, it may be a sign of mental retardation or emotional problems and may require further investigation. The habit is usually practiced shortly after the child is put to bed while he is still partially awake and in some cases even during sleep. This habit is rarely injurious to the child. It usually clears away by the fourth year of life. No treatment is indicated other than ascertaining that there are no sharp objects or toys on the bed. Pillows between the bedside and walls may be helpful. Related rhythmic motor habits (i.e., head rocking or rolling, bed rocking) are often seen together with head banging during sleep. The baby often gets up on his hands and knees and rocks back and forth or bangs his head. Undernourishment, chronic illness, minimal brain dysfunction, head nodding (Spasmus Nutans) with possibly rickets and nystagmus, eye or ear abnormalities with head tilting and possibly absence of the corpus callosum, and choreoathetosis must all be ruled out. Salaam spasm, characterized by a rhythmic series of head nods, is associated with brain damage, sometimes with epilepsy. The abnormal eye movements of Spasmus Nutans disappear on covering the eyes, during sleep, or in the supine position. A special form of movement habit to be differentiated is that in which the child, usually 1 to 3 years of age, climbs out of bed and deliberately bangs his head on the hard floor with a resounding noise, inflicting injury to the head. In these cases emotional disturbance is likely and must be ruled out.

5. Familial Sleep Paralysis.
Familial sleep paralysis is listed as a dysfunction associated with sleep because, as a rule, the paralysis develops at night when the patient is in bed asleep. The post-dormital period is the most favored point of occurrence of the attacks. Respiration is usually uncompromised. Episodes last several minutes but may be terminated by external stimulation (i.e. touch, voice) or, in some patients, by vigorous movement of the eyes which often are the only spared voluntary movements.

It is a rare condition, found in probably less than 3% of the population. The incidence is heredofamilial as a dominant trait bound to the X chromosome transmitted by the mother.

Another form of sleep paralysis is that associated with narcolepsy and the accessory signs of this tetrad (see earlier). One last but important differentiation is with familial periodic (hypokalemic) paralysis which also occurs in genetically disposed individuals. In this condition prodromal findings may be recorded the preceding evening in the form of drowsiness, numbness, tingling in the legs, excessive appetite or thirst, and a sense of heaviness or fatigue. When the patient awakens in the morning he discovers his paralysis. The weakness begins usually in the legs and extends to the arms and finally to the trunk and neck. Although intercostal and accessory respiratory muscles are always paralyzed in a severe attack, the diaphragm is rarely affected. Prevention of hypokalemic paralysis can be accomplished by means of low-carbohydrate, high-potassium diet and thiamine. Insulin and glucose should be avoided.

6. Impaired Penile Tumescence during Sleep.
Males, whether they are 3 or 80 years old, have four or five penile erections nightly, lasting 20 to 25 minutes each. The erections occur during 80-90% of the episodes of REM sleep in young adults. Thus, organic disorders associated with erectile failure can now be objectively diagnosed by means of polysomnography rather than depending almost exclusively on the patient's own report which is of questionable accuracy. Male erectile impotence is defined as inability to obtain and/or maintain erection for vaginal penetration and successful ejaculation inside the vagina. Potency assumes an erection of sufficient rigidity to effect penetration and completion of coitus. This rigidity can be evaluated by devices that measure changes in the diameter of the penis and the pressure required to buckle the erect organ.

Impaired waking penile tumescence can thus be inferred from all-night polygraphic recordings if insufficient or no tumescence is observed during REM sleep. Factors responsible for this impairment are multiple. Age is crucial since levels of impotence gradually increase from age 40. Impotence reaches epidemic proportions by the age of 80, at which age most males are either partially or totally impotent. With adult-onset diabetes mellitus of six years duration or more there is a 50% prevalence of impotence. Diabetic impotence is said to respond little or none to treatment of diabetes. End-stage renal disease under dialysis has a prevalence between 33 and 100% of impotence. Other causes of impotence are neuromuscular, endocrine, respiratory, hematological abnormalities, neurological disease (multiple sclerosis, peripheral neuropathy, pernicious anemia, syphilis, paraplegia), vascular, cardiovascular, metabolic disease, surgical complications (prostatectomy, vascular, and back surgery), trauma (disk and spinal cord), urologic problems (phimosis, Peyronie's disease or induration of the corpora cavernosa of the penis), congenital abnormalities (Klinefelters syndrome, hypospadias), and some psychiatric disorders. Psychiatric disease, according to some authors, accounts for about 90% of all cases of impotence, but other sources claim organic factors to be involved 60% of the time. Anxiety and Schizophrenia are presumed to cause psychogenic or functional impotence until proven otherwise. But it now appears that many endogenously depressed patients have impaired nocturnal penile tumescence. Ingestion of certain drugs is also often responsible for impotence. Prominent among them are antihypertensives, antipsychotics, tricyclic antidepressants, alcohol, barbiturates, antimuscarinics, narcotics, sympathomimetics, and monoamine oxidase inhibitors. Of course psychogenic and organogenic factors can, and do indeed, interact. Patients who complain of impotence but have normal nocturnal penile tumescence are likely to suffer psychogenic impotence, and in these cases a complete psychological evaluation should be made.

7. Sleep-related Painful Erections.
Priapism is a disorder characterized by permanent or inordinately sustained erection of the penis not accompanied by sexual desire. It is most frequent in the 3rd-4th decades but infantile and senile priapism have been described. Little boys or even nursing babies may exhibit priapism due to local excitations (i.e., phimosis, balanitis, oxyuriosis, bladder calculi) or neurological disease (i.e., severe epilepsy, encephalitis, mental subnormality). In the elderly or senile, neurological disease (i.e., cerebellar, median lobe) or even more, prostatism are the main causes of priapism, particularly in the early morning. Two types of priapism are recognized. One is the sustained and the other is the recurrent nocturnal type - REM sleep dependent - which is the one we are considering here. Recurrent, nonsustained, painful sleep-related priapism is of unknown etiology; although, as in the elderly, it is often associated with prostatitis. It frequently subsides spontaneously or as the triggering pathology improves. Its associated pain tends to awaken the individual. This disorder is very uncommon but striking when it occurs. It does not interfere with sexual function and erections in the awake state. The awakenings typically occur during REM sleep and may eventually progress to a DIMS complaint.

Early morning erection, due to a full bladder, is normal although it may be uncomfortable and may prevent sleep for several hours, usually in the latter part, but sometimes earlier during the night. Again, it can become more severe due to prostatic, urethral, visceral, or anal lesions.

The REM sleep-related painful erections must be distinguished from a variety of other forms of priapism which are more sustained and usually due to diagnosable organic factors. For example, involvement of the posterior roots of the uppermost segments of the spinal cord usually gives rise to pain in the back of the head and neck. Hyperreflexia, priapism and vasomotor disturbances commonly occur.

Tumors of the conus medullaris commonly result in a flaccid paralysis which affects principally the gluteal muscles and the anteroexternal muscles which lift the foot. Pain is located in the back, the sciatic region or perineum. There is incontinence or retention with overflow of urine. Priapism, involuntary ejaculation, or insensibility with impossibility of ejaculation are observed, depending upon the exact location of the lesion.

8. Sleep-related Cluster Headaches and Chronic Paroxysmal Hemicrania. Attacks occur most frequently during REM sleep and are characterized by sudden onset of orbital pain of short duration, abrupt resolution, and multiple daily recurrences. Prodromal (preheadache) symptoms are: scotomata, drowsiness, mood changes, and gastrointestinal disturbances. Concomitant signs include: eye redness, lacrimation, stuffiness of the nostrils or rhinorrhea, swelling of the temporal vessels on the only affected side (hemicrania), and vascular dilation of the painful area. The pain frequently radiates from the original orbital area to the temple, nose, upper jaw, and neck. Because typical attacks can be triggered by injection of a small dose of histamine monophosphate, this condition has also received the name histaminic (Horton's) cephalalgia. Prophylaxis is provided by methysergide maleate (Sansert), 4-8 mg daily in divided doses with meals. Frequent spontaneous long remissions call for equally frequent evaluations of the need for continued preventive therapy. Methysergide is contraindicated in pregnancy, peripheral vascular disease, and arteriosclerosis. REM sleep-suppressing agents are also indicated and taken prior to sleep.

9. Sleep-related Abnormal Swallowing Syndrome.
There is hyperactivity of the gag reflex and of swallowing during sleep. Although sedative agents for its treatment or to improve insomnia may temporarily suppress its hyperactivity, when the gag reflex breaks out from this type of suppression the new eruption is usually even more severe. It is conceivable that this hyperactivity of the gag reflex during sleep is interrelated in a complex manner with both the recumbent position and the sleep-related gastroesophageal reflux (see below) because the lower esophageal sphincter is the barrier to reflux of gastric juice into the esophagus. This sphincter relaxes during swallowing, regurgitation, belching, and vomiting.

In this condition there is inadequate swallowing which results in aspiration of saliva, coughing, and choking. It is intermittently associated with brief arousal or awakenings. Polysomnographic recordings elicit no pathological sleep apnea but the short-lived episodes of coughing and gagging follow periods of "gurgling" sounds suggestive of pooling of saliva in the hypopharynx.

10. Sleep-related Asthma.
Nocturnal respiratory distress may take the form of unpleasant disruption of sleep or, worse, sleep-depriving asthma attacks.

These may occur at any hour of sleep in adults except during stages 3/4, but only during the last two-thirds of the night in children. It can be provoked by bronchial asthma appearing in adult life for the first time and by airway obstruction due to para-tracheal tumors. In patients with emphysema, breathing difficulty may be aggravated upon awakening, perhaps because of abnormally increased alveolar CO_2 tension and reduced arterial oxygen saturation.

11. Sleep-related Cardiovascular Symptoms.
These derive from disorders of cardiac rhythm, myocardial incompetence, coronary artery insufficiency, and blood pressure variability which may be exacerbated by sleep-altered cardiovascular physiology. The extent however to which clinically significant increases in blood pressure occur during REM or other sleep stages is under current intensive revision. Preliminary observations suggest that:

1) the peak time of cardiac deaths attributable in part to myocardial infarction and of nocturnal angina may be at the REM sleep-rich interval of 5-6 a.m.,
2) a small proportion of episodes of angina may occur during deep NREM (stages 3/4) sleep, probably due to the low systemic blood pressure prevailing during that sleep stage,
3) there is an unmistakable association between reduced blood oxygenation, serious cardiac dysthymias, and sleep, and
4) a considerable number of patients at certain times appear to have exacerbations of cardiovascular symptoms during sleep, including cerebrovascular accidents.

12. Sleep-related Gastro-Esophageal Reflux (Reflux Esophagitis, Peptic Esophagitis).
During REM sleep, patients with duodenal ulcer may secrete 3 to 20 times as much gastric acid as normal individuals, which explains how nocturnal attacks of ulcer can unpleasantly disrupt sleep. Heavy, fatty, or spicy meals are bound to cause discomfort with heartburn or pyrosis (substernal burning, cramping, severe pain or pressure). Heartburn is due to gastro-esophageal reflux of gastric juice into the esophagus which causes an intermittent sensation beneath the lower sternum which spreads upwards in a wave-like fashion to the throat or even the mouth. This causes an abnormal esophageal motor response, effortless appearance of esophageal or gastric contents in the mouth (regurgitation), sour taste, and increased salivation. All together it probably triggers excessive swallowing and/or gagging, most often during the first part of the night, but if unrelieved, even toward the early morning hours. This nocturnal discomfort may cause restless sleep or insomnia. The symptoms are aggravated by recumbency and increase of abdominal pressure and relieved by the upright position because the pathophysiology includes a permanently or intermittently incompetent

lower esophageal sphincter. This symptom may be diagnosed by means of a positive Bernstein (acid infusion) test, an overnight pH study, a standard acid clearance test to appraise acid clearance during sleep, a standard acid reflux test, or endoscopic or histological evidence of esophagitis when symptoms become more severe with progression of the reflux toward physical sequelae.

Hiatal hernia may be present since it is extremely common (15-35% of persons over 50) and may aggravate the condition. It is often asymptomatic unless reflux of gastric contents can be demonstrated to occur repeatedly. Both gastro-esophageal reflux and symptoms of diaphragmatic hernia are aggravated by eating and by lying down.

13. Sleep-related Hemolysis (Paroxysmal Nocturnal Hemoglobinuria). This is a rare and chronic anemic disorder of variable severity. It courses with perpetual hemosiderinuria and paroxysmal intravascular hemolysis and hemoglobinuremia which increase during sleep. Hemoglobinuria (brownish-red urine) will usually be detected on awakening in the morning. An attack of hemoglobinuria is sometimes ushered by abdominal, lumbar, or substernal pain. It may first appear at any age but usually between ages 20-40. The factors that activate hemolysis during sleep are unknown, but the fundamental abnormality is in the membrane of the erythrocyte which renders the cell sensitive to the normal lytic action of serum complement. A traditional diagnostic test for this condition is the Ham test which introduces hemolysis of the patient's erythrocytes by slight acidification of the serum. In typical cases, weakness, pallor, and anemia coupled with dark urine in the morning will suggest the diagnosis. Hemoglobinuria may be the first sign of the disease. The disorder may terminate fatally several years from diagnosis, it may be compatible with life for many years, or may even disappear spontaneously. Transfusions may be required. Exacerbations are associated with infection, menstruation, surgery, transfusions, vaccination, oral iron, and liver extract injections.

14. Asymptomatic Polysomnographic Finding.
These are to be listed when they appear on a routine examination, even if the subject presents no specific complaints (Roffwarg, 1979).

QUIZ, Sections IV and V.

TRUE or FALSE: Circle the correct letter.

T   F   1. Normally peak body temperature is recorded in the early morning.

T   F   2. Neuroendocrinological function is at steady-state level around the clock.

T   F   3. In jet lag the amount of time required to readjust is inversely related to the number of hours of time zone shift.

T   F   4. Growth hormone levels directly correlate best with deep sleep.

T   F   5. Somnambulists can tell precisely what they are doing and why during their sleepwalking episodes.

T   F   6. Peak performance is normally exhibited in the predawn hours.

T   F   7. Sleepwalkers are difficult to arouse from their somnambulistic episodes.

T   F   8. High arousal threshold in sleepwalking is due to deep (stage 4) sleep.

T   F   9. Sleepwalking is a pattern that never clears away with maturation.

T   F   10. An Organic Mental Disorder is always present during the waking hours of sleepwalkers.

T   F   11. Childhood and adolescence are the favored ages for sleepwalking.

T   F   12. Boys and girls are equally affected by somnambulism and there is no indication of genetic influence.

T   F   13. Clear-headedness is always observed following both a night terror or a dream anxiety attack.

T   F   14. Sleep terrors are often called incubus attacks in children and pavor nocturnus in adults.

T   F   15. Persistence of incubus attacks throughout life is frequently associated with psychopathology.

T   F   16. For enuresis, the most important prognostic and therapeutic distinction is to determine whether it is primary or secondary.

T   F   17. A diagnosis of impotence can be made if there is complete absence of penile tumescence during REM sleep.

T   F   18. Presence of penile tumescence during REM sleep rules out a psychogenic cause of impotence.

T   F   19. The buckling pressure is a measure of ego strength.

T   F   20. Buckling pressure increases with age beyond 40 because tissues become more rigid with age.

T   F   21. Polysomnography has increased the percentage of organic factors contributing to impotence and decreased that of psychogenic etiology.

T   F   22. In priapism, sexual desire is greater than during a normal erection because of the inordinate duration of erection.

T   F   23. The greater incidence of priapism during the 3rd-4th decades suggests this age range as the peak of sexual power.

T   F   24. Recurrent, nonsustained, painful sleep-related priapism is often associated with prostatitis.

T   F   25. Sleep-related cluster headaches appear most frequently during sleep due to eye-redness which becomes a trigger.

T   F   26. Sedative agents are curative for sleep-related abnormal swallowing.

T   F   27. The lower esophageal sphincter relaxes during swallowing, which may explain the increased gag reflex and gastroesophageal reflux during sleep.

T   F   28. A diagnosis of paroxysmal nocturnal hemoglobinuria can be reinforced by demonstration of perpetual hemosiderinuria.

T   F   29. Although sometimes fatal, sleep-related hemolysis has been observed to disappear spontaneously.

Circle the correct answer(s). One or more than one answer may be correct.

30. The differential diagnosis of sleepwalking is usually with

     a. psychomotor epilepsy.
     b. fugue states.
     c. catatonia.
     d. severe depression.
     e. none of the above.

31. There is an association between sleepwalking and

     a. nocturnal enuresis.
     b. sleeptalking.
     c. low intelligence.
     d. homosexuality.
     e. night terrors.
     f. none of the above.

32. So-called disorders of arousal from deep sleep include

    a. dream anxiety attacks.
    b. jet lag.
    c. night terrors.
    d. bruxism.
    e. primary enuresis.
    f. somnambulism.

33. Sleep-related head banging

    a. is also called jactatio capitus nocturnus.
    b. is never seen in healthy infants.
    c. may be a sign of mental retardation or emotional problems.
    d. often occurs early after bedtime while the child is still awake.
    e. usually clears away by age 4.
    f. must be differentiated from deliberate headbanging.

Circle the letter corresponding to the <u>one</u> correct response.

34. The treatment of choice for sleepwalking is

    a. barbiturates.
    b. neuroleptics.
    c. environmental protection.
    d. psychotherapy.
    e. electroconvulsive therapy.
    f. none of the above.

35. Sleep terrors correlate highly with

    a. early part of the night.
    b. arousal from deep sleep.
    c. non-REM sleep.
    d. K-complexes ushering attack onset.
    e. high autonomic activation.
    f. concomitant strong negative emotions.
    g. poor recollection of the event.
    h. all of the above.

36. Sleep-related bruxism is a disorder involving

    a. muscle jerks.
    b. apneic episodes.
    c. insomnia.
    d. teeth-grinding.
    e. none of the above.

37.   Nocturnal penile tumescence correlates best with sleep stage

    a.   REM.
    b.   stages 1 and 2.
    c.   stages 3 and 4.
    d.   never occurs during sleep but only while very awake whether there is a female companion or not.

Match the following items with the appropriate diagnosis.

    ____38.   never continent before   a.   primary enuresis
    ____39.   continent before   b.   secondary enuresis
    ____40.   male predominance
    ____41.   non-REM related
    ____42.   psychopathology
    ____43.   arousal or REM-related
    ____44.   usually unassociated with dreams
    ____45.   begins with burst of K-complexes
    ____46.   predominantly during first third of night
    ____47.   responds to psychotherapy
    ____48.   managed by reassurance, bladder training, imipramine

Match the following items with the appropriate diagnosis, one or both diagnoses may be matched.

    ____49.   2nd half of night   a.   night terrors
    ____50.   1st third of night   b.   dream anxiety attacks
    ____51.   treated with benzodiazepines
    ____52.   more autonomic upheaval
    ____53.   deep sleep
    ____54.   good recollection
    ____55.   REM sleep
    ____56.   male predominance
    ____57.   female predominance

ANSWERS, Sections IV and V.

1.	F	20.	F	39.	b
2.	F	21.	T	40.	a
3.	F	22.	F	41.	a
4.	T	23.	F	42.	b
5.	F	24.	T	43.	b
6.	F	25.	F	44.	a
7.	T	26.	F	45.	a
8.	T	27.	T	46.	a
9.	F	28.	T	47.	b
10.	F	29.	T	48.	a
11.	T	30.	a,b	49.	b
12.	F	31.	a,b,e	50.	a
13.	F	32.	c,e,f	51.	a,b
14.	F	33.	a,c,d,e,f	52.	a
15.	T	34.	c	53.	a
16.	T	35.	h	54.	b
17.	T	36.	d	55.	b
18.	F	37.	a	56.	a
19.	F	38.	a	57.	b

POST-TEST

For the following questions, circle the <u>one</u> correct response.

1. The treatment of choice for sleepwalking is

    a. barbiturates.
    b. neuroleptics.
    c. environmental protection.
    d. psychotherapy.
    e. electroconvulsive therapy.
    f. none of the above.

2. Sleep drunkenness refers to

    a. sleep of the drunkard following excessive alcohol ingestion.
    b. usual state of "dope eaters."
    c. state following arousal from REM sleep.
    d. disorientation, incoordination, and grogginess observed in patients with sleep-induced respiratory depression upon awakening from a daytime sleep episode.

3. Sleep of less than five hours per night

    a. is characteristic of drug-induced insomnia.
    b. is characteristic of all depressions.
    c. can be normal for some individuals.
    d. often occurs following Amphetamine Withdrawal.
    e. precipitates uncontrollable sleep attack in most people.

4. Strong emotions often serve as triggers of

    a. sleep apnea daytime hypersomnolent attacks.
    b. narcoleptic-cataplectic attacks.
    c. slow wave sleep attacks.

5. A complaint of insomnia

    a. automatically calls for prescription of a hypnotic.
    b. always reflects a primary sleep disorder.
    c. should be treated first with psychotherapy.
    d. may have multiple causes.
    e. should be considered symptomatic of depression and treated automatically with tricyclic antidepressants.

6. The cataplectic attacks of REM narcoleptics are due to

    a. paralysis of the respiratory center.
    b. an episode of Catatonic Schizophrenia.
    c. the normal paralysis of sleep, always with cessation of consciousness.
    d. decreased tonic activity of groups of skeletal musculature.

7. Upper airway resistance increases during obstructive sleep apnea because of

    a. increased tonus of intercostal muscles.
    b. increased tonic activity of pharyngeal muscles.
    c. decreased tonic activity of throat muscles.
    d. constant hyperextension of neck due to upward oriented gaze of rapid eye movements tracking falling objects in the dream content.

8. Nocturnal penile tumescence correlates best with sleep stage

    a. REM.
    b. stages 1 and 2.
    c. stages 3 and 4.
    d. never occurs during sleep but only while very awake.

9. The Pickwickian syndrome usually describes

    a. a young chlorotic female.
    b. an obese hypersomnolent lad.
    c. insomnia due to Caffeine Intoxication.
    d. a grandiose impersonation of Dickens.

10. Classical narcolepsy is a condition with strong

    a. environmental etiology.
    b. infections contributory factors.
    c. hereditary background.
    d. intrapsychic etiology.
    e. easily demonstrable gross neurological damage.

11. The cataplectic attacks of narcoleptics respond best to

    a. amphetamines.
    b. neuroleptics.
    c. barbiturates.
    d. tricyclic antidepressants.
    e. L-tryptophan.

12. Sleeping pills

   a. are indicated to counteract the insomnia of patients with central sleep apnea.
   b. help individuals with obstructive sleep apnea.
   c. should be given to the two categories of patients mentioned in a and b but only for the first 2-3 days.
   d. are usually ineffective in treating most types of insomnia after the first 2-3 weeks of administration.

13. The single most frequent effect of psychoactive drugs on sleep patterns is

   a. sleep regularization.
   b. reduction of stages 1 and 2.
   c. reduction of REM sleep.
   d. abolition of K-complexes.

For the following questions, one or more than one answer may be correct. Circle the correct answer(s).

14. Sleep drunkenness is often responsible for

   a. poor school performance.
   b. post-dormital headaches.
   c. learning difficulties.
   d. ethanolic breath.
   e. automatic behavior with memory blackouts.

15. The sleep apnea syndrome is usually diagnosed if

   a. thirty or more apneic episodes of more than 10 seconds duration occur during the night.
   b. a nighttime sleep tape recording demonstrates alternation between loud snoring of abrupt onset and periods of silence.
   c. daytime hypersomnolence reinforces the above.
   d. there is excessive daytime sleepiness without nighttime apnea.

16. Normal sleep is often disrupted by

   a. alcohol.
   b. caffeine.
   c. usual hypnotics.
   d. amphetamines.

17. Which of the following characteristics are common to the Kleine-Levin syndrome and menstrual hypersomnolence?

   a. episodes of hypersomnia
   b. both usually in the female sex
   c. hyperphagia
   d. none of the above

18. In the alveolar hypoventilation DIMS syndrome,

    a. significant apneic pauses do not occur.
    b. there is inadequate tidal volume.
    c. hypnoxia worsens as sleep progresses.
    d. there is no insomnia or repetitive arousal.
    e. the prognosis is worse than in sleep apnea.
    f. upper airway obstruction is a constant concomitant.

19. There is an association between sleepwalking and

    a. nocturnal enuresis.
    b. sleeptalking.
    c. low intelligence.
    d. homosexuality.
    e. night terrors.

20. If the anticholinergic potential of tricyclics is therapeutic against cata-plectic attacks, one would also expect therapeutic effects from the action of

    a. thioridazine.
    b. reserpine.
    c. atropine.
    d. physostigmine.
    e. diazepam.

21. Often during a depressive episode there is

    a. insomnia.
    b. increased awakenings.
    c. early premature final awakening.
    d. increase in REM sleep.
    e. decrease in stage 4 of sleep.
    f. none of the above.

22. Sleep disturbance occurs in

    a. less than 5% of the population.
    b. old age often.
    c. about 35% of the population.
    d. 70-80% of psychiatric patients.
    e. association with respiratory impairment in some cases.
    f. the form of excessive or insufficient sleep.
    g. patients with DIMS and DOES syndromes.
    h. patients with nocturnal pain or discomfort.
    i. Alcoholic Intoxication or Withdrawal.
    j. infants with SIDS.
    CONTINUED ON NEXT PAGE

k. some cerebral infections and neurological diseases.
l. the narcoleptic syndrome.
m. nocturnal alveolar hypoventilation.
n. Ondine's syndrome but not the Pickwickian syndrome.
o. association with disorders of the motor system.
p. hyper- and hypothyroidism.
q. some nutritional deficiencies but not that due to lack or deficit of L-tryptophan.

Match each one of the following characteristics with the appropriate diagnosis:

___23. responds to psychotherapy
___24. begins with burst of K-complexes
___25. non-REM related
___26. continent before
___27. psychopathology is present
___28. managed by reassurance, bladder training, imipramine
___29. predominates during the first third of night
___30. usually unassociated with dreams
___31. never continent before
___32. male predominance
___33. arousal or REM-related

a. primary enuresis
b. secondary enuresis

Match the following characteristics with the appropriate diagnosis. Lettered items may be used more than once for each question.

___34. REM sleep-related
___35. male predominance
___36. 2nd half of night
___37. more autonomic upheaval
___38. female predominance
___39. deep sleep
___40. good recollection
___41. 1st third of night
___42. treated with benzodiazepines

a. dream anxiety attacks
b. night terrors

Match the following characteristics with the appropriate diagnosis

___43. usual temporal lobe focus
___44. handrubbing
___45. wakeful attacks
___46. association with enuresis and night terrors
___47. swallowing
___48. EEG seizure discharge
___49. uncinate aura

a. nocturnal psychomotor epilepsy
b. sleepwalking

Match the following characteristics with the appropriate diagnosis.

___50. responds to tricyclics
___51. often associated with hallucinations and cataplexy
___52. touching patient terminates attack

a. familial sleep paralysis
b. narcoleptic sleep paralysis

PRE-TEST ANSWERS

1.	b,c,d,e,f,g,h,i,j,k,l,m,o,p	20.	c	39.	b
2.	a,b,c	21.	c	40.	b
3.	a,b,c	22.	a	41.	a
4.	a,b,c,e	23.	a	42.	b
5.	a,c	24.	b	43.	a
6.	a,c	25.	a	44.	a
7.	a,b,e	26.	a	45.	a
8.	a,b,c,d,e	27.	b	46.	a
9.	a,b,c,d	28.	b	47.	a
10.	c	29.	a	48.	a
11.	d	30.	a	49.	b
12.	c	31.	a	50.	b
13.	c	32.	b	51.	a
14.	d	33.	a	52.	b
15.	b	34.	b	53.	a
16.	d	35.	a	54.	a
17.	b	36.	a,b	55.	a
18.	d	37.	a	56.	a
19.	d	38.	a		

POST-TEST ANSWERS

1.	c	20.	a,c	39.	b
2.	d	21.	a,b,c,d,e	40.	a
3.	c	22.	b,c,d,e,f, g,h,i,j,k, l,m,o,p	41.	b
4.	b			42.	a,b
5.	d	23.	b	43.	a
6.	d	24.	a	44.	a
7.	c	25.	a	45.	a
8.	a	26.	b	46.	b
9.	b	27.	b	47.	a
10.	c	28.	a	48.	a
11.	d	29.	a	49.	a
12.	d	30.	a	50.	b
13.	c	31.	a	51.	b
14.	a,b,c,e	32.	a	52.	b
15.	a,b,c	33.	b		
16.	a,b,c,d	34.	a		
17.	a,c	35.	b		
18.	a,b,c	36.	a		
19.	a,b,e	37.	b		
		38.	a		

REFERENCES

Hartmann, E. L-tryptophane as an hypnotic agent: A review. <u>Waking and Sleeping</u>, 1977, <u>1</u>, 155-161.

Mills, L. E., & Dement, W. C. Sleep and Aging. <u>Sleep</u>, 1980, <u>3</u>, 119-220.

Roffwarg, H. P. Diagnostic classification of sleep and arousal disorders. <u>Sleep</u>, 1979, <u>2</u>, 1-137.

Rogers, E. F. Sudden infant death. <u>Science</u>, 1979, <u>203</u>, 1197.

CHAPTER 15

Disorders of Infancy, Childhood, and Adolescence

Lorenz Villeponteaux, Ph.D.
Jonathan M. Stein, M.D.

CHAPTER OUTLINE

Learning Objectives

Pre-Test

I. Introduction

II. Intellectual

    A. Cognitive
    B. Mental Retardation

III. Behavioral

    A. Attention Deficit Disorders
    B. Conduct Disorders

IV. Emotional

    A. Anxiety Disorders of Infancy, Childhood, or Adolescence
       1. Separation Anxiety Disorder
       2. Avoidant Disorder of Childhood or Adolescence
       3. Overanxious Disorder

    B. Other Disorders of Infancy, Childhood, or Adolescence
       1. Reactive Attachment Disorder of Infancy
       2. Schizoid Disorder of Childhood or Adolescence
       3. Elective Mutism
       4. Oppositional Disorder
       5. Identity Disorder

V. Physical

    A. Eating Disorders
       1. Anorexia Nervosa
       2. Bulimia
       3. Pica
       4. Rumination

    B. Stereotyped Movement Disorders
       1. Transient Tic Disorder
       2. Chronic Motor Tic Disorder
       3. Tourette's Disorder
       4. Atypical Stereotyped Movement Disorder

LEARNING OBJECTIVES

After completing this chapter you will be able to:

1. Name the Diagnostic Criteria for the disorders found in this Chapter.

2. Define the term Mental Retardation.

3. Name the four major stages of cognitive development according to Jean Piaget.

4. List 10 known causes of Mental Retardation.

5. List three limitations of intelligence tests.

6. Name at least two factors which may cause pseudoretardation.

7. Name four terms used synonymously with Attention Deficit Disorder.

8. Differentiate between <u>state</u> and <u>trait</u> hyperactivity in terms of the effect of environmental changes.

9. Name four disorders which should be differentiated from Attention Deficit Disorder.

10. Define, as used in relation to Conduct Disorders, the terms:
    a. aggressive and nonaggressive
    b. socialized and undersocialized

11. Describe the relationships between separation anxiety and:
    a. object permanence
    b. anaclitic depression
    c. attachment figure
    d. school phobia

12. Differentiate between Separation Anxiety Disorder and Avoidant Disorder.

13. Name the two general ways this disorder manifests itself.

14. Name two key psychosocial factors which often play a role in the development of this disorder.

15. Name three other mental disorders from which Schizoid Disorder must be differentiated.

16. Name two mental disorders which may include oppositional type behavior.

17. Name three somatic symptoms often found in Anorexia Nervosa.

18. Name the predominant area of psychological distortion of the patient with Anorexia Nervosa.

19. Name four physical disorders which may produce findings similar to Anorexia Nervosa.

20. Name the common fear formed in patients with Bulimia.

21. Cite two theories of causation of Pica.

22. Name three eating disorders which may result in death.

23. Name six motor disturbances from which tics must be differentiated.

24. Differentiate between Transient Tic Disorder and Chronic Motor Tic Disorder in terms of duration of symptoms.

25. Name two personality characteristics which seem to be present in Tourette's Disorder.

26. Name three behaviors which are called Atypical Stereotyped Movement Disorder.

27. Differentiate between primary and secondary Enuresis.

28. Name three physical disorders which may have incontinence as a symptom.

29. Name two patterns of Functional Encopresis in terms of the child's awareness of the need to defecate.

30. Identify the stage of sleep when sleepwalking and sleep terrors most often occur.

31. Differentiate between sleep terrors and nightmares.

32. Name the two most common symptoms seen in Infantile Autism.

33. Differentiate between Infantile Autism and Childhood Onset Pervasive Developmental Disorder.

34. Name three other frequently found symptoms in Infantile Autism.

35. Name three characteristics shared by children with Infantile Autism and children with Childhood Onset Pervasive Developmental Disorder.

36. Name four possible etiological explanations for Developmental Reading Disorder and for Developmental Arithmetic Disorder.

37. Name two types of Developmental Language Disorder.

PRE-TEST

Use the following key to answer questions 1-4:

    a. Concrete operations
    b. Sensorimotor period
    c. Formal operations
    d. Pre-operational period

1. Piaget's stages of cognitive development in chronological order are:

    ___ First stage
    ___ Second stage
    ___ Third stage
    ___ Fourth stage

2. The attainment of the ability to solve conservation problems comes during the ___ period.

3. The ability to perform propositional operations and think abstractly is characteristic of the ___ period.

4. The ability to form mental representations of objects, that is, to use symbols is a milestone of the ___ period.

For each of the following questions, one or more than one answer may be correct. Circle the correct answer(s).

5. Which of the following statements about Mental Retardation is(are) true?

    a. Approximately 200 causes of Mental Retardation have been identified.
    b. Prevalence rates are set at about 1%.
    c. Significantly more boys than girls are retarded.
    d. Over half of the mentally retarded fall in the severe and profound categories.
    e. Approximately 10% of the mentally retarded are institutionalized.

6. Which of the following biological factors is(are) thought to be causal in Mental Retardation?

    a. phenylketonuria
    b. cri du chat
    c. fetal alcohol syndrome
    d. anoxia
    e. lead poisoning
    f. congenital blindness
    g. placenta previa
    h. cleft palate

7. Which of the following statements about intelligence tests is(are) true?

    a. They are limited in predicting occupational success.
    b. They provide a measure of innate capacity.
    c. They predict nonacademic skills.
    d. They are unreliable for long-range prediction.

8. "Significantly subaverage intellectual functioning" refers to a score of below ___ on an individually administered I.Q. test.

    a. 100
    b.   90
    c.   70
    d.   50

9. Match the following.

    ___ resistant to environmental change   a. trait hyperactivity
    ___ susceptible to environmental change   b. state hyperactivity

10. Incidence rates of Attention Deficit Disorder are estimated at various rates. Probably the most realistic rate is

    a. 20%.
    b. 10%.
    c.   5%.
    d.   3%.
    e. 0.1%.

11. Which of the following statements is (are) true regarding children with Attention Deficit Disorders?

    a. Abnormal EEG's are found in 20% to 50% of hyperkinetic children.
    b. Lead poisoning may be causal in some children.
    c. Stimuli normally found in the environment tend to increase activity and distractibility.
    d. It is commonly thought that environmental factors, such as psycho-pathology in family members, play an important primary role in the origin of the disorder.

12. In Attention Deficit Disorders the most common symptom expressions which seem to be heightened by environmental stimuli are all of the following except

    a. motor activity.
    b. autonomic nervous system arousal.
    c. inattention.
    d. impulsivity.

13. Differential diagnosis of Conduct Disorders will often include

    a. Attention Deficit Disorder.
    b. Childhood Onset Pervasive Developmental Disorder.
    c. Isolated Antisocial Act.
    d. Organic Mental Disorder.

14. Match the following symptom dimensions with the descriptions of behavior.

    ___ violation of rights of others   a. socialized
    on a face-to-face basis with
    the victim
    ___ violation of rights of others   b. aggressive
    without face-to-face confron-
    tation with the victim
    ___ no bond of affection or empathy   c. undersocialized
    with others has been established
    ___ some sense of loyalty to others   d. nonaggressive
    exists, especially to a specific
    group such as a gang

15. A young child who shows signs of withdrawal, psychomotor retardation, sleep and eating problems, and social detachment probably is suffering from what Spitz called

    a. anaclitic depression.
    b. school phobia.
    c. Agoraphobia.
    d. Separation Anxiety.

16. Separation Anxiety is

    a. not unlike Agoraphobia in adults.
    b. a normal response to early forced separation (like hospitalization).
    c. a disorder often involving school refusal.
    d. best treated by forcing separation through hospitalization of the child.

17. Passive, withdrawn, limited eye contact, and overinhibited are all terms which are applied to children with

    a. Separation Anxiety Disorder.
    b. Avoidant Disorder.
    c. Overanxious Disorder.
    d. Schizoid Disorder.

18. Although apparently unable to do so a child with _____ Disorder wishes he could extend himself to others and be accepted and appreciated by them.

    a. Avoidant
    b. Overanxious
    c. Separation Anxiety
    d. Schizoid

19. Match the following disorders with the source of anxiety.

    ___ anxiety about performance and achievement   a. Separation Anxiety Disorder

    ___ anxiety about facing new situations or people   b. Avoidant Disorder

    ___ anxiety about being away from parents   c. Overanxious Disorder

20. Children with Overanxious Disorders

    a. usually are intellectually bright.
    b. often are middle children.
    c. frequently have somatic complaints.
    d. usually behave quite independently.
    e. worry a great deal about future events.

21. Which of the following is(are) applicable to Reactive Attachment Disorder of Infancy?

    a. failure to thrive
    b. body weight below the 3rd percentile
    c. delayed or absent development such as smiling, sucking, rooting, eye tracking, etc.
    d. maternal deprivation or neglect
    e. may be seen in adolescents or occasionally in adults

22. Which of the following disorders is(are) differential diagnoses for Reactive Attachment Disorder of Infancy?

    a. certain physical disorders (GI, cardiac, etc.)
    b. severe Mental Retardation
    c. Schizoid Disorder
    d. Infantile Autism
    e. Tourette's Disorder

23. A 12-year-old child who appears withdrawn and socially isolated could be suffering from

    a. Avoidant Disorder.
    b. Depression.
    c. Schizoid Disorder.
    d. Oppositional Disorder.
    e. Adjustment Disorder (with withdrawal).

24. Which of the following statements is (are) true regarding children with Elective Mutism?

    a. They will speak to a few selected people.
    b. They often do not have the ability to speak.
    c. They appear shy, withdrawn, and retiring.
    d. They often have difficulty understanding the speech of others.
    e. They are often mentally retarded.

25. In the child with Oppositional Disorder the behavior may be characterized as

    a. argumentative.
    b. quarrelsome.
    c. passive-aggressive.
    d. negativistic.

26. Which of the following statements is(are) true regarding Adolescence and Identity Disorder?

    a. Onset of Identity Disorder is typically in adolescence.
    b. Our modern, technological, industrialized society tends to shorten the adolescent period.
    c. Identity Disorder is defined by subjectively determined stress over issues regarding identity.
    d. A teenager may feel distress over identity issues but not have Identity Disorder.

27. Probably the <u>most</u> outstanding physical sign in Anorexia Nervosa is

    a. bradycardia.
    b. bulimic episodes.
    c. cachexia.
    d. amenorrhea.

28. Anorexia may be secondary to

    a. hypothyroidism.
    b. hyperthyroidism.
    c. panhypopituitarism.
    d. cerebral tumor.

29. A diagnostic criterion of Anorexia Nervosa is a weight loss of at least ___% of body weight (considering projected growth if the patient is under 18 years of age).

    a. 5%
    b. 10%
    c. 15%
    d. 20%
    e. 25%

30. Frequently found in the patient with Bulimia is (are)

    a. rigid diets.
    b. vomiting.
    c. use of laxatives and diuretics.
    d. fear of being underweight.
    e. lack of awareness that eating habits are abnormal.

31. The eating "binge" is most characteristic of

    a. Anorexia Nervosa.
    b. Bulimia.
    c. Pica.
    d. Rumination.

32. Pica behavior may be

    a. normal in an 18-month-old child.
    b. related to nutritional deficit.
    c. an attempt to satisfy oral needs (in psychoanalytic terms).
    d. a feature of Infantile Autism.

33. Rumination

    a. sometimes spontaneously remits.
    b. has a mortality rate of as much as 25% if it is persistent.
    c. may be caused by GI anomalies.
    d. usually has its onset in the first year of life.

34. Transient Tic Disorder

    a. is a rare disorder.
    b. may last for as long as one year.
    c. usually is seen in preschool children.
    d. may be voluntarily controlled for a limited period of time.

35. Tourette's Disorder

    a. begins as a single tic in about half the cases.
    b. includes coprolalia in 90% of the patients.
    c. typically begins with eye, face, or neck area tics.
    d. often is a part of a schizophrenic process.
    e. includes vocal tics.

36. Atypical Stereotyped Movement Disorder(s)

   a. are basically tics.
   b. are intentional or voluntary.
   c. are sometimes symptoms of Mental Retardation.
   d. appear to be pleasurable for the child.

37. Stuttering is

   a. a "speech flow" defect.
   b. an articulation disorder.
   c. transient with spontaneous recovery in a large number of cases.
   d. typically increased by stress.

38. Enuresis is more likely (but certainly not always) to have an organic basis if it

   a. is nocturnal only.
   b. is diurnal only.
   c. is both nocturnal and diurnal.
   d. varies between nocturnal and diurnal.

39. Enuresis

   a. is seen in a particular kind of personality pattern.
   b. usually disappears by adolescence if not sooner.
   c. is most frequently associated with an underlying mental disorder.
   d. occasionally may be seen in adults.

40. Usually, but not always, Encopresis

   a. is seen in males.
   b. occurs in late afternoon or evening.
   c. has its onset with school entry (6-7 years of age).
   d. is associated with night terrors.

41. Regarding Sleepwalking Disorder, which of the following statements is(are) correct?

   a. It is seen in as many as 1-6% of children.
   b. Episodes typically occur during REM sleep.
   c. When seen in adults, it is more often associated with other mental disorders.
   d. The memory of the episode of sleepwalking, upon awakening, is absent in about 1/3 of the patients.

42. Sleep Terror Disorder

   a. occurs typically during stage 3 or 4 of NREM sleep.
   b. is accompanied by intense autonomic nervous system arousal.
   c. is associated with mildly abnormal EEG findings.
   d. ends abruptly when the child screams and wakes up.

43. The three symptoms present in virtually all children with Infantile Autism are

     a. repetitive, stereotyped movements.
     b. profound failure to develop social relationships.
     c. toilet training problems.
     d. language retardation (including muteness).
     e. ritualistic or compulsive behavior.

44. Diagnostic criteria for Infantile Autism include

     a. onset before 2½ years of age.
     b. lack of responsiveness to other people.
     c. attachment to one parent (usually).
     d. delusions or hallucinations.

45. Diagnostic criteria for Childhood Onset Pervasive Developmental Disorder include

     a. extensive impairment in social relations.
     b. mutism in 1/3 to 1/2 of the children with this disorder.
     c. absence of delusions and hallucinations.
     d. onset before 12 years of age and after 2½ years.

46. The more disabling type of Language Disorder is

     a. expressive.
     b. receptive.

I. INTRODUCTION

The disorders discussed in this chapter may be divided into two groups. The first group is made up of disorders which are peculiar to non-adults. Reactive Attachment Disorder of Infancy, for example, is diagnosed in infants up to eight months of age. The second group is made up of disorders which usually have their onsets in pre-adult years but are frequently seen in adults. For example, Anorexia Nervosa most often has its onset during adolescence but commonly is seen in young and middle-aged adults.

Before looking at the specific disorders in this chapter (of which there are more than three dozen) some general historical comments may be helpful.

Until well into the 19th century, "possession by the devil" was often the explanation of choice for many forms of deviant behavior. Mental patients were chained, incarcerated, and frequently physically punished. Looking back further in time, infants were believed to be born evil, stained by original sin, and particularly vulnerable to possession by the devil. Because of his great propensity for evil the young child was bound, swaddled, tied into virtual immobility lest he "tear its ear off, scratch its eyes out, break its legs, or touch its genitals" (deMause, 1974, p. 11). Until the Reformation period the ceremony of baptism incorporated the ritual of exorcism of the devil (Thomas, 1971).

A number of what are now considered treatable disorders were for centuries considered manifestations of possession. For example, one way in which changelings (young children possessed by the devil) were identified as such in the 15th century was through the fact that they were "always ailing and crying yet the milk of five women is not enough to satisfy them" (Malleus Maleficarum, 1487). Today a competent physician would consider such things as esophageal hernia, failure to thrive syndrome, allergic reactions, and intestinal parasites.

As the child grew older, physical bonds were replaced with threats that ghosts, ghouls, witches, devils, or assorted monsters were waiting to do their worst to the child who misbehaved. After the Reformation, God Himself became the threat used by parents, teachers, and clergy to terrify the child (Holliday, 1968). Even today threats commonly are used to control the behavior of children. Santa Claus does not bring presents to bad little boys and girls. DeMause (1974) documents well the use of ghost-like figures to frighten children throughout recorded history and in various cultures.

The point of all of this is that children were seen as being extremely vulnerable to deviance in some very mysterious ways. There has always been acknowledgement that, contrary to what some writers suggest, children are different from adults (Knoblock & Pasamanik, 1974). On the other hand, it is clear that for centuries high value was placed on "correcting" their childishness by shaping children as quickly as possible into little adults.

A great many other factors, of course, have played major roles in determining how children were reared, treated, depicted and, generally, how they were esteemed. The industrial revolution, for example, had a profound effect on the course of history, and certainly on the role of children in society. The industrial revolution provided the groundwork for children to become providers of cheap labor for industry (factories, coal mines, etc.) accelerating them into miniature adults.

The practice of psychiatry is less than a century old and is the first area of the practice of modern medicine to be concerned with matters which could not easily be measured, felt, probed, or touched. Simultaneously with the emergence of psychiatry in the 19th century, psychology as a discipline was developing out of elements of philosophy, physiology, physics, and Darwinian theory. The initial concerns of psychiatry were clinical mysteries, such as paralyses which did not follow neural pathways, phobias, and compulsive repetition of strange acts. Psychology grew out of efforts to answer questions about how and why normal behaviors developed.

In spite of a considerable amount of resistance within the medical profession, specialization in medicine began to emerge in the United States toward the end of the 19th century. It was only in the 1930's, however, that specialization began to be formalized. The first psychiatry board was established in 1934. What is now the subspecialty of child psychiatry developed in a somewhat paradoxical way. It grew out of the specialty of psychiatry, but for a period of time followed a very different path. Most child psychiatrists practiced in multidisciplinary mental health and child guidance clinics rather than in hospitals. Their concerns were as much with community and social problems as with "medical" problems. It was not until 1959 that the first subspecialty examination was given in child psychiatry, at which time child psychiatry moved toward a course more parallel with its parent specialty.

It is interesting to note within this historical context that the search for answers about human behavior, in both psychiatry and psychology, turned toward the study of children. Freud's psychoanalytic theories, for example, are based almost entirely on the events of childhood. In fact his basic theory makes no mention of adults insofar as the origins of behavior are concerned.

Before the midpoint of this century it was clear that it was important for psychiatry to define more precisely its area of competence. A major first step in this direction was the development of a system of classifying the disorders which come under the purview of psychiatry.

READING NOTE: For a most interesting and well-documented account of varying views of childhood throughout history, see The History of Childhood, Lloyd deMause, Editor, 1974.

The classification or systematic arrangement of mental disorders evolved from essentially one-dimensional concepts, such as lunacy or neurosis or psychosis, to the multidimensional, phenomenological approach used in the DSM-III (1980).

This evolution of a system of nosology for mental disorders reflects at least three major interrelated processes: (1) the state of knowledge about human behavior, including the identification of biological, as well as psychosocial, factors which impinge on both normal and abnormal human behavior; (2) clinical experience with individuals who exhibit aberrant behavior; and (3) theoretical propositions offered to explain observed behavioral phenomena, again, both normal and abnormal.

The major goals of classifying mental disorders are: (1) the efficient diagnosis of mental disorders, presumably leading to the implementation of effective treatment procedures; (2) the facilitation of communication among mental health personnel and non-psychiatrist physicians about the diagnosis and treatment of mental disorders; and (3) the provision of a structure against which theoretical constructs may be tested.

The first edition of the Diagnostic and Statistical Manual of Mental Disorders appeared in 1952. In this manual there was no differentiation between disorders of children and disorders of adults. The DSM-II was published in 1968, nine years after the first child psychiatry board examinations. This edition did provide special categories of disorders seen in children, but was not greeted with overwhelming enthusiasm from all quarters. While the inclusion of separate categories of disorders of children and adolescents was an important step forward, some thought that the categories were woefully inadequate, and more importantly that diagnosis still depended for the most part on the "adult" categories (Silver, 1969).

Since 1952 there have been a number of efforts to establish valid, reliable, and useful diagnostic categories. One ongoing effort is worth noting here. The World Health Organization has published the ninth revision of its International Statistical Classification of Diseases, Injuries and Causes of Death (1977), referred to as ICD-9. Although the first edition of the ICD was published at the beginning of the 20th century, it was not until the middle of this century (6th revision) that a separate section on mental disorders was included. The ICD-8 (1965) included one category of mental disorders specific to children - behavior disorders.

The ICD-9, published in 1977, includes a number of categories of disorders specific to children. The important concept of diagnosis on several axes is also introduced in this ninth revision, growing out of the work of the World Health Oganization in the 1960's (Rutter et al., 1969).

In summary, then, the notion that there is a greater propensity for deviance among children has historical roots in superstition, and although the beginnings of a modern scientific approach to the study of mental disorders appropriately has focused on early development, attempts at classifying mental disorders have been disproportionately inadequate regarding children.

At the heart of the difficulty has been an issue which seems to perpetuate, at least in modified form, society's view of children; that is, the wish to make children subject to the same societal expectations as adults. The implication is that there is an inability or unwillingness to recognize fully that children, by the nature of their status as children, are rapidly changing -- they are developing. Put another way, what may be appropriate behavior for a 5-year-old child may be outside of that expected of a 12-year-old.

An important point in this regard -- an obvious one to be sure -- is that children are different from adults in terms of behavioral expectations. Moreover, the differences are often accounted for by the fact that during nearly the first two decades of life, human beings are changing at such a rapid rate. It is only after adolescence that development slows at times to an almost imperceptible pace compared with pre-adolescent development.*

It would seem to follow logically that, with regard to children, diagnostic criteria for mental disorders and, indeed, the kinds of mental disorders themselves should be different from those applied to adults. This is true only in part. There are certainly mental disorders which seem to be age-related; in fact, there are disorders which are seen only in non-adults, and these disorders are specifically related to incongruities of development in the pre-adult.

At the same time, some disorders seem to run through childhood, adolescence, and adulthood. Weiner and Del Gaudio (1976), in a study of 1,334 adolescent patients, including a 10-year follow-up study, wrote that, "aspects of the data demonstrate continuity in adolescent and adult psychopathology..." (p. 187). Rutter and associates (1969), in a report on a World Health Organization seminar on classification of mental disorders in childhood, clearly indicate that in some instances there is comparability between childhood and adult disorders.

This brings us to the DSM-III and the classification of mental disorders in the 1980's.

II. INTELLECTUAL

The first group of disorders in this chapter are deficits in intellectual development and functioning - mental retardation. In one sense, the various disorders are merely variations in degree of a single disorder; however, in another sense the single disorder of mental retardation is a very complex one, particularly when viewed along such dimensions as etiology or treatment.

Knobloch and Pasamanick (1974) use the term "mental subnormality" to

---

*Note that development is used here in the broadest sense to include both psychosocial and physical development, and incorporates the concept of the entire life span of human beings.

include both mental <u>deficiency</u> and mental <u>retardation</u>. They use "retardation" in reference to those individuals who are functioning below their intellectual potential. "Deficiency," on the other hand, is used to refer to "some pathologic condition of the brain which precludes normal development" (p. 149). Common usage today employs the term "mental retardation" as an all-encompassing one for persons whose intellectual functioning, for whatever reason, is below normal. The distinction, however, between deficiency and retardation is a conceptually useful one.

Mental retardation is defined by the American Association on Mental Deficiency in the following way:

> Mental retardation refers to significantly sub-average general intellectual functioning existing concurrently with deficits in adaptive behavior and manifested during the developmental period (Richmond, Tarjan, & Mendelsohn, 1974, p. 1).

The major point here is that mental retardation is a multifactorial phenomenon and not a matter of lower than average IQ; and furthermore, the aspect of time is an important factor. Note, too, that the question of etiology is not directly addressed in this definition.

A. COGNITIVE

The most comprehensive and most systematically elaborated theory of cognitive development is that of Jean Piaget. While it is not the purpose of this chapter to provide a detailed review of the work of Piaget and his colleagues, it may be useful in understanding mental retardation to have as background a relatively brief summary of Piaget's work.

First, Piaget clearly recognizes the role of organic factors in determining intellectual or cognitive development. According to Piaget and Inhelder (1969), "Mental growth is inseparable from physical growth: The maturation of the nervous and endocrine systems, in particular, continues until the age of sixteen" (p. vii). They go on to point out that environmental factors must be given equal weight in considering cognitive development, including "exercise or acquired experience as well as social life in general" (p. viii). This position epitomizes, in a sense, the etiological dilemma regarding mental retardation, the age-old issue of nature versus nurture. We shall return later to this question, but first consider the developmental stages of cognitive development as described by Piaget.

Piaget considers intelligence a reflection of adaptive behavior (and thought) by the individual. Beginning in infancy with reflexive behavior, the individual goes through stages or periods of cognitive development until, if all goes well, he attains in adolescence or young adulthood the ability to think logically, conceptually, and abstractly.

The first stage of intellectual development is called the sensorimotor period-- from birth to about two years of age. Piaget sub-divides the period into six substages, but in essence the child moves from reflexive behavior to acquire the ability to organize stimuli from the environment and to interact with these stimuli. By the end of the period the child normally has learned to do some rudimentary thinking and has incorporated a large number of adaptive behaviors. The most important step he has taken, perhaps, has been the beginning of the incorporation of the concept of the permanent object.

At some point during the second half of the first year of life for example, a child will look for an object which is placed out of his perceptual field. If you cover with a blanket an object in which he is interested, he will attempt to look under the blanket. Prior to this time an object which was placed out of his perceptual field ceased to exist. Now, however, the object has permanence.*

The second period of cognitive development, called the pre-operational period, lasts from about two years to approximately seven years. During this period a fundamental milestone in cognitive development is reached in the acquisition of the ability to form mental representations of objects, i.e., the ability to use symbols.

What Piaget calls "deferred imitation" is one of the first signs that the child is developing this ability to symbolize. The two-year-old may imitate the behavior of another some time after the fact. Then comes symbolic play on a very elementary level as the child, for example, pretends to sleep or eat. The clearest evidence of the ability to form mental pictures comes with language, as the child represents a cow, for example, by saying "Moo."

Another important feature of this period is what Piaget once called "egocentrism" and later referred to as "centering on the self," or the inability to put oneself in the place of another. The process of "decentering" comes later with the gradual incorporation of concepts of time and space.

The third period is called the period of concrete operations, a period lasting from about seven until about eleven years of age. The period is characterized by the attainment of the ability to use logical thought. The child learns to arrange things in classes. He learns to separate, for example, the red objects from the green objects, the round from the square, the big from the small (seriation).

Related to the ability to classify and number is the ability to solve problems of "conservation." Prior to this time the child could not perceptually deal with weight, size, shape, quantity, etc. Six ounces of liquid in a tall, thin beaker, for example, looks like more than six ounces of liquid in a short, fat beaker. Even though the child sees the liquid poured from one beaker to another, he is unable to make the logical transformation. Now, during the period of concrete operations, he becomes able to mentally deal with such problems, but only in fairly concrete ways.

The last stage of cognitive development begins at about eleven or twelve years of age and is called the period of formal or propositional operations. Reasoning ability, as in the case of conservation problems, no longer will

---

*Note that the related concept of object constancy, and the formation of "object relations," is a central one in psychoanalytic theory of development.

require objects in order to arrive at solutions. The adolescent (usually) can formulate hypotheses and can reason without the necessity of the concrete objects. The basic principles of causal thinking are acquired. If $\underline{A}$ is bigger than $\underline{B}$ and $\underline{B}$ is smaller than $\underline{C}$ is a proposition that can be solved inside one's mind without any need for the letters to represent anything concrete.*

The stages of cognitive development must be gone through successively, each stage or period deriving from the previous one and simultaneously providing preparation for the next one. When failures occur in the process of intellectual development, the question of etiology comes immediately to the forefront. These failures may be identified in any of the periods of intellectual development, as defined by Piaget. In the infant who is profoundly retarded, lags may be apparent immediately in reflexive behavior. The young child may be unable to use symbolism at the appropriate time; the deficit may show up in the form of delayed speech development or in the inability to play the games expected of the child. The deficits may not become apparent until the school years when the child seems to have significant trouble in areas of classification and seriation.

****

GO TO VIDEOTAPE

****

B.   MENTAL RETARDATION

According to the American Medical Association's handbook Mental retardation (Richmond, Tarjan, & Mendelsohn, 1974), there have been approximately 200 causes of Mental Retardation identified. In most instances, however, the etiology of specific cases is not identifiable.

The general rule is that the more severe forms of mental retardation are identified early in the life of the child; the less severe forms are diagnosed later in life, most often in the school years. Prevalence rate for mental retardation is thought to be about 1% of the general population, with three-fourths or more falling in the mild and borderline categories.

As noted earlier, the multifactorial nature of mental retardation makes this disorder a very complex one. The condition may be directly related to biological factors, to environmental factors, or to a combination of the two.

Biological factors are many. The following list is by no means an exhaustive one, but provides some of the better known causal factors in mental retardation (for more details see Cytryn & Lourie, 1980).

---

*This entire section is, of course, a very oversimplified summary of the stages of intellectual development as defined by Piaget. For more detailed discussions, see Piaget and Inhelder (1969) and Baldwin (1967).

A. Metabolism
    1. Amino Acid Metabolism - Phenylketonuria
    2. Fat Metabolism - Cerebromacular degeneration
    3. Carbohydrate Metabolism - Galactosemia

B. Chromosomal Aberrations
    1. Down's syndrome
    2. Cri du chat syndrome
    3. Klinefelter's syndrome

C. Pregnancy Related
    1. Infections
        a. syphilis
        b. rubella
    2. Toxemias (fetal alcohol syndrome)
    3. Anoxia of fetus
        a. placenta previa
        b. premature separation of placenta

D. Perinatal Factors
    1. Prematurity (central nervous system disorders related)
    2. Trauma at birth
    3. Anoxia (around delivery)

E. Postnatal Factors
    1. Meningitis
    2. Lead poisoning
    3. Malnutrition

Environmental factors may play an important role - positive or negative - in Mental Retardation. A child who is handicapped intellectually by genetic endowment, for instance, may be further debased by environmental influences (lack of stimulation or deprivation). On the other hand, a nurturing, stimulating environment may mitigate to some extent the effects of biological deficits. It is clear that lower socioeconomic classes of people tend to provide the least enriching environments for stimulation of cognitive development; and, indeed, estimates are that as many as 75% of all mentally retarded individuals are to be found in the families of the lower socioeconomic levels. It is important to remember that these are the milder degrees of retardation; the clear-cut biological causes, like Down's syndrome, are not discriminated by socioeconomic class.

Put another way, it appears likely, although it is certainly not established, that the vast majority of the mildly retarded are more influenced by environment than by biological factors. The notion that cognitive growth could be stimulated among the environmentally deprived was the basis for such projects as Head Start.

To reiterate an earlier statement, the diagnosis of the more severe degrees of Mental Retardation is often relatively straightforward. On the other hand, determining causation for the milder forms is much more difficult. In either case, however, the primary physician can contribute much to the optimal care of the retarded individual. Not only can he provide medical management, but he can also serve as a kind of liaison between social agencies, schools, special programs, etc. and the family.

The use of the individually administered I.Q. test may be very helpful in the establishment of a diagnosis of Mental Retardation. Even though one of the three major diagnostic criteria given in DSM-III is related to a score on an I.Q. test, it must be emphasized that a great many factors may influence the test results. The motivation of the patient, the cultural background of the patient (there are no truly culture-fair I.Q. tests), the emotional state of the patient at the time of testing, and other factors may well play a role in the way a particular person performs. The Wechsler Intelligence Scale for Children (W.I.S.C.) and the Stanford-Binet are the most commonly used instruments for measuring I.Q. today. For the younger child, or the child who lacks verbal ability, it is often necessary to use developmental scales, like the Bayley Scales, to estimate intellectual functioning.

The standardized, individually administered I.Q. test may provide important diagnostic information regarding the diagnosis of mental retardation; however, most professionals agree today that it is crucial for the psychologist to consider "potential" with the score obtained on a test. Clinical observation is one important factor in estimating potential. This includes assessment of the child's (or adult's, for that matter) motivation, concentration, and sensorium at the time of test administration. It also includes the assessment of the presence or absence of emotional problems, since other mental disorders often will tend to lower the individual's performance on an I.Q. test. In addition, the competent psychologist will carefully examine the various subtests of the I.Q. test, since the interrelation of sub-test scores may provide important clues to potential levels of intellectual functioning.

The use of intelligence tests with infants and young children demands an even more guarded posture. The developmental scales, of course, rely heavily on motor behavior as opposed to verbal behavior. Thus a child with motor deficits may in later life score considerably higher on I.Q. tests which have large verbal components.

Sattler (1974) provides information about some of the limitations of intelligence tests, pointing out that they:

1. are limited in predicting occupational success,
2. are limited in predicting nonacademic skills,
3. do not provide a measure of innate capacity,
4. provide limited information about the domain of cognitive functions,
5. do not measure the process underlying test responses,
6. may penalize unconventional responses and do not measure creativity, and
7. may be unreliable for long-range predictions.

A number of states or conditions or disorders may have the effect of making the individual appear retarded. As noted earlier, many children who come from deprived backgrounds may appear retarded - and indeed may be functioning at a level far below their potential. Provided with the proper stimulation, these individuals may acquire the skills and knowledge to function at the normal or above normal range of intelligence.

Emotional problems, as already noted, may have the effect of lowering intellectual functioning. For example, the depressed child may be unable to perform at an appropriate intellectual level. Children with specific developmental disorders in speech or language or reading or math may appear to be retarded.

One of the most confounding areas of differential diagnostic problems has been with the autistic child and the child with Childhood Onset Pervasive Developmental Disorder. The diagnostic question often is related to how much of the child's behavior is due to organic problems, how much to mental retardation, and how much to the psychiatric disorder. Early in the treatment this distinction is less important since such severe disorders usually require care aimed at achieving a manageable level of socialization. This is not to say, of course, that the best possible diagnostic assessment should not be made.

Chronic illnesses which limit interactions with the environment, and especially those which require frequent or prolonged parent-child separations, may lower the intellectual functioning of the child.

Handicaps in vision, hearing, or speech also may have the effect of producing lowered I.Q. scores. It is not uncommon for children to be thought of as "slow" if such handicaps are present but undetected, when in fact they may have normal intellectual ability. The same is true for children with certain organic brain syndromes which produce the inability to write or to read.

The definition of mental retardation given earlier in this chapter refers to "deficits in adaptive behavior." This term is usually taken to mean social adaptation. The adaptive behavior of the individual, of course, is age-related. Deficits may be seen in such things as eating, talking, walking, learning, as examples. There are no truly valid, reliable, objective means of measuring social adaptation, and clinical judgment is the basic tool for assessment, although there are some instruments which are helpful in making the judgment. It is important for the physician to assess the adaptive behavior of the individual over time, rather than rely on a single period of observation.

The diagnostic criteria for Mental Retardation given in the DSM-III are:

A. Significantly subaverage intellectual functioning (70 or below on an individually administered I.Q. test) or clinical judgment of such a deficit in younger children.

B. Concurrent deficits or impairments in adaptive behavior, taking the person's age into consideration.

C. Onset before 18 years of age.

There are five (5) subtypes of this disorder based on the degree of retardation. The DSM-III uses the I.Q. criteria of the American Association on Mental Deficiency:

Mild -   I.Q. of 50 to 70 (probably as much as 80% of the mentally retarded fall in this category).

Moderate -   I.Q. of 35 to 49 (making up 10 to 12% of the mentally retarded).

Severe -   I.Q. of 20 to 34 (approximately 7 to 9% of the mentally retarded).

Profound -   I.Q. of below 20 (less than 1% of the mentally retarded population).

Unspecified -   A category used when "there is a strong presumption of mental retardation" but the individual cannot be tested at the time (DSM-III, p. 40).

The mildly retarded may function reasonably well through half or more of the 12 grades of the public school system before their deficits become serious problems. Many develop adequate social and employment skills to function reasonably well in the community.

The moderately retarded are more limited in social and occupational skills, but later may be able to function in a relatively protected environment such as a sheltered workshop in which close supervision is provided. Developmental delays are present, with such milestones as speech and locomotion acquisition coming significantly later than expected.

The severely retarded are even more delayed developmentally and may never truly acquire more than minimal ability to communicate and care for themselves. They require very close supervision and often are placed in institutions. The profoundly retarded are almost always institutionalized since they require virtually constant supervision.

Today only about 10% of the mentally retarded are placed in institutions (Richmond, Tarjan, & Mendelsohn, 1974), most of these coming, of course, from the lower levels of intellectual functioning. Many factors play a part in the decision to institutionalize the individual: the ability of the family to adapt to the retarded member; the presence or absence (and degree) of other problems, like hyperactivity, aggressiveness, organic impairments; and the availability of supportive services in the community, like special classes, sheltered workshops, speech and hearing clinics, psychological and social services, and nursing care.

Quiz, Section II.

Fill in the blanks for Questions 1-12.

1. According to Piaget the first stage of intellectual development is the _____ period.

2. This period lasts from birth to about ____ years of age.

3. The beginning of the incorporation of the concept of the permanent object takes place during the _____ period of development.

4. The child begins to use logical thought during the period of _____ operations.

5. It is during the period of _____ operations that the child learns concepts like serialization and conservation.

6. The ability to think abstractly and propositionally comes during the period of _____ operations.

7. Approximately _____ causes of Mental Retardation have been identified.

8. Estimates are that as many as ____% of all mentally retarded individuals come from families of the lower socioeconomic levels.

9. It is (more, less) _____ likely that in cases of severe or profound retardation an identifiable cause can be identified.

10. Mildly retarded persons have I.Q. scores between _____ and _____.

11. Moderately retarded persons have I.Q. scores between ____ and ____.

12. Less than ____% of the mentally retarded population fall into the profoundly retarded category.

13. Intellectual functioning as measured by I.Q. may be lowered by

   a. environmental deprivation.
   b. emotional problems.
   c. chronic illness.
   d. sensory handicaps.

III. BEHAVIORAL

The disorders in this section are divided into two main categories, Attention Deficit Disorders and Conduct Disorders. Both categories have as major features overt behavioral manifestations of the disorders.

A. ATTENTION DEFICIT DISORDERS

There are three disorders in this category: (1) Attention Deficit Disorder with Hyperactivity, (2) Attention Deficit Disorder without Hyperactivity, and (3) Attention Deficit Disorder, Residual Type. According to DSM-III the residual classification is used for an individual who at one time met the criterion of hyperactivity but no longer does so even though the other criteria for Attention Deficit Disorder are met.

A wide variety of terms has been applied to the Attention Deficit Disorders, most focusing on the hyperactive behavior so often associated with the disorders: hyperkinesis, hyperkinetic syndrome, hyperkinetic impulse disorder, Attention Deficit Disorder, minimal cerebral dysfunction, minimal brain dysfunction, learning disability, hyperactive child syndrome, neurologically handicapped child. In looking at the literature one finds a great many terms used to describe the child with an Attention Deficit Disorder: impulsive, irritable, distractible, short attention span, low frustration tolerance, visual-motor difficulties, poor academic achiever, motor restlessness, emotional lability (Laufer & Denhoff, 1957; O'Malley & Eisenberg, 1973).

The Attention Deficit Disorders are a group of disorders far from homogeneous in terms of etiology, clinical manifestations, or effective treatment. There is even a significant amount of disagreement regarding prevalence and incidence, which is certainly understandable in view of the diagnostic difficulty.

Incidence rates are estimated as high as 20% of school aged children and as low as 0.1% (Laufer & Shetty, 1980), but probably are realistically around 3% as suggested by the DSM-III. This disparity is directly related to the multivariate aspects of the disorders, some of which will be briefly noted.

There is often disagreement about the differentiation between normal childhood activity, distractibility, restlessness, etc. and pathological levels of such behaviors. Certainly the children who fall at either end of the spectrum are easily distinguished from each other, but those in the large grey area in the middle may or may not be diagnosed as having a psychiatric disorder.

The problems of maintaining attention may vary with the setting in which the child finds himself. It is not uncommon, for example, for a child to have difficulty in school but not at home, or at home but not in school. Loney (1980) refers to trait hyperactivity versus state hyperactivity, with the former being resistant to environmental changes and the latter susceptible to such changes.

One of the most important areas of disagreement has to do with the etiology of the disorders, leading, of course, to a variety of treatment approaches. There seems to be a considerable amount of evidence that, particularly with the hyperactive group, there is an organic basis for the behavior. In a review article on organic factors in hyperkinesis, Dubey (1976) reports that EEG abnormalities of one kind or another appear in 20% to 50% of hyperkinetic children. Obviously, however, 50% to 80% of the children do not have abnormal EEGs.

With the administration of dextroamphetamine or methylphenidate, hyperactivity diminishes dramatically in the majority of these children, approximately 70% (Satterfield, Cantwell, & Satterfield, 1975). In fact, Jenkins (1969) says that, "some clinicians consider a favorable response to cerebral stimulants and an unfavorable response to phenobarbital as clinical evidence of organic brain dysfunction" (p. 1033). On the other hand, Werry (1982) reports that recent studies show that children with no demonstrable psychopathology and children with Attention Deficit Disorder respond equally well to stimulant drugs. That is, cognitive and intellectual functioning seems to be enhanced in both groups.

Until recently this positive response to stimulants was referred to as a "paradoxical" effect. Now, however, many believe that the effect is not paradoxical, but rather that the medication has an aborting effect and "enables the child to focus his attention on his work and hence be less distractible and hyperactive" (Snyder, 1980, p. 157).

More specifically, the theory is that the children who respond positively to stimulants have dysfunctional reticular activating systems. "The...neurophysiological theory is one of low arousal and insufficient inhibitory controls over motor outflow and sensory input" (Satterfield, Cantwell, & Satterfield, 1975).

Coleman (1974) reports that in her studies more than 80% of the children diagnosed as hyperactive have been found to have lowered levels of 5-hydroxytryptamine (5-HT) in whole blood and that with increased serotonin levels, the hyperactive and distractible behaviors disappear. Even though the studies of Coleman and her colleagues have not been replicated there is certainly logic to her work. Animal experiments have demonstrated that destruction of raphe nuclei, where serotonin is so highly concentrated, leads to insomnia and that replacement through the use of tryptophan induces the animals to sleep (Snyder, 1980).

Environmental factors have been investigated as possible determinants of Attention Deficit Disorders. Cantwell (1972), for example, found that families of hyperkinetic children tend to have higher rates of such things as alcoholism, hysteria, and sociopathy than do families of controls. Few people today think that environmental factors play a primary role in the origins of Attention Deficit Disorders; there is considerable evidence, however, that the environment plays a very important role in terms of the exacerbation of symptoms.

Put another way, the preponderance of evidence is that this group of disorders has an organic basis; stimuli from the environment seem to heighten the symptom expressions of motor activity, inattention and impulsivity. The environmental factors may be in the form of numerous stimuli normally found in the school or home setting which the child is unable to screen out; or may be in the form of instability of the home environment which increases the undesirable responses of the disorder. Furthermore, the effect of the disorders seems to have a profound effect on the development of the child. Social immaturity, poor peer relations, poor parent-child relations, and academic underachievement are commonly seen in children with these disorders.

ANSWERS, Section II. _____

1.	sensorimotor	8.	75
2.	two	9.	more
3.	sensorimotor	10.	50,70
4.	concrete	11.	35,49
5.	concrete	12.	1
6.	formal or propositional	13.	a,b,c,d
7.	200		

Two other areas of causality should be mentioned. The first is the possibility of lead poisoning in some children. The ingestion of lead in mice has led to significant increases in motor activity levels (as well as to significant deficits in development). At any rate, as Eisenberg (1979) suggests, the diagnostic assessment of children who exhibit symptoms of hyperactivity should include a careful history of the child's exposure to lead in the environment.

The second area has to do with allergies as causative in hyperkinesis in children. Feingold (1975) has hypothesized that children with this disorder often respond to diet strategies aimed specifically at eliminating artificial food coloring and flavoring. Studies do not appear to support the theory that food additives cause hyperactivity in the majority of children, but they may well play a role in a small group of these children.

As noted at the beginning of this chapter, children with Attention Deficit Disorders do not make up a homogeneous group. They are indeed a heterogeneous group in terms of symptom constellations, most likely in terms of etiology, and certainly in terms of the course of the disorder (Loney, 1980).

Another confounding dimension is best cast in terms of differential diagnosis. First, if organic problems can be clearly identified as causative the diagnosis should be made on Axis III. According to the DSM-III this will occur in approximately 5% of the cases of Attention Deficit Disorder. In certain other neurological disorders symptoms of Attention Deficit Disorder may be present, e.g., cerebral palsy, hypoglycemia, and epilepsy. Again the diagnosis should be made on Axis III.

Children who are mentally retarded may exhibit symptoms of Attention Deficit Disorder. DSM-III criteria rule out the diagnosis of Attention Deficit Disorder if the retardation is severe or profound, but not if it is mild or moderate.

Anxiety Disorders, especially the overanxious type, may be misdiagnosed as an Attention Deficit Disorder since excessive motor activity is frequently a symptom of anxiety. If a child meets the criteria of both disorders, both diagnoses should be made even though one of the disorders may be secondary to the other.

Depression (Affective Disorder) may also bring with it symptoms of an Attention Deficit Disorder in the form of agitated behavior (motor and verbal behavior), difficulty concentrating, and apparent inattention. Ossofsky

(1974) reports a study of 220 children between one and 12 years of age who were treated with imipramine for a variety of disorders, all of whom were also depressed. She notes that all of the one to five year age group and those in the six to seven year age group were referred initially because of hyperactivity. She goes on to report that hyperactivity was controlled in all of the children by using imipramine and that hyperactivity (as well as inattention and sleep problems) re-emerged with the withdrawal of the drug.

If the diagnosis of Affective Disorder can be established and the symptoms of Attention Deficit Disorder are secondary to the depression, the diagnosis of Affective Disorder is made.

Finally, it is not uncommon to find Attention Deficit Disorders in children who also have Conduct Disorders, especially the Aggressive type disorder (Laufer & Shetty, 1980). In fact, Loney (1980) comments that some clinicians think that "there are no valid distinctions between hyperkinetic children and other children referred to clinics, especially those with Aggressive Conduct Disorders" (p. 29). These children often display signs of impulsivity and a poor tolerance for frustration. In any event both Conduct Disorder and Attention Deficit Disorder should be diagnosed if warranted.

The following are the diagnostic criteria for Attention Deficit
Disorder with hyperactivity according to the DSM-III:

Diagnostic Criteria for Attention Deficit Disorder with Hyperactivity

A.   Inattention.   At least three of the following:

(1) often fails to finish things he or she starts
(2) often doesn't seem to listen
(3) easily distracted
(4) has difficulty concentrating on schoolwork or other tasks requiring sustained attention
(5) has difficulty sticking to a play activity

B.   Impulsivity.   At least three of the following:

(1) often acts before thinking
(2) shifts excessively from one activity to another
(3) has difficulty organizing work (this not being due to cognitive impairment)
(4) needs a lot of supervision
(5) frequently calls out in class
(6) has difficulty awaiting turn in games or group situations

C.   Hyperactivity.   At least two of the following:

(1) excessively runs about or climbs on things
(2) has difficulty sitting still or fidgets excessively
(3) has difficulty staying seated

(4) moves about excessively during sleep
(5) is always "on the go"or acts as if "driven by a motor"

D.   Onset before the age of seven.

E.   Duration of at least six months.

F.   Not due to Schizophrenia, Affective Disorder, or Severe or Profound Mental Retardation.

The diagnostic criteria are exactly the same for Attention Deficit Disorder without Hyperactivity with the exception of Criterion C.

The residual type of Attention Deficit Disorder is applied to an individual who once met the criteria for Attention Deficit Disorder, but no longer meets the hyperactivity criterion (Criterion C). The specific criteria for this disorder are:

Diagnostic Criteria for Attention Deficit Disorder, Residual Type

A.   The individual once met the criteria for Attention Deficit Disorder with Hyperactivity. This information may come from the individual or from others, such as family members.

B.   Signs of hyperactivity are no longer present, but other signs of the illness have persisted to the present without periods of remission, as evidenced by signs of both attentional deficits and impulsivity (e.g., difficulty organizing work and completing tasks, difficulty concentrating, being easily distracted, making sudden decisions without thought of the consequences.)

C.   The symptoms of inattention and impulsivity result in some impairment in social or occupational functioning.

D.   Not due to Schizophrenia, Affective Disorder, or Severe or Profound Mental Retardation.

The multivariate nature of the Attention Deficit Disorders dictates that treatment approaches be multidimensional. Satterfield, Cantwell, and Satterfield (1975) say that "For management purposes, the hyperactive child is best considered a multihandicapped child requiring a multiple modality treatment approach" (p. 321).

There is clear and compelling evidence regarding the efficacy of the use of stimulant drugs, particularly dextroamphetamine (Dexedrine) and methylphenidate (Ritalin). As usual one begins with a low dose and increases until optimal effects are obtained, i.e., a dosage level which reduces the symptoms but does not produce lethargy, drowsiness, or, on the other hand, an increase in motor activity. In addition, Werry (1982) suggests that there may be a role for antipsychotic drugs in these disorders (in low doses), especially when stimulant drugs have been ineffective.

Because these children seem to increase activity and distractibility with an increase in external stimuli, some degree of environmental manipulation is often a helpful part of a treatment regimen. Parents and teachers may need some direct advice regarding ways of minimizing stimulation from the environment.

Finally, other therapy often may be indicated. Behavioral treatment has proven to be effective in helping the child control his disruptive behavior, both in the classroom and at home (see Chapter 18, Behavioral Treatment).

Psychotherapy is often used to help deal with the child's lowered self-esteem, whether the lowered self-esteem is a result of the disorder or plays a role in the exacerbation of the disorder. In either case, whether cause or effect, individual and/or family therapy may be indicated to help alter former patterns of interaction. It is also of paramount importance to allow the child and his family to explore the meaning of taking medication on a long-term basis. The fact that the child may be taking a pill in school every day adds even further meaning to the medication.

This section on Attention Deficit Disorders is necessarily somewhat vague at times since so little presently is known about these disorders. Fortunately, from a clinical standpoint, however, "it is generally accepted that organic etiology does not preclude response to psychological treatment, nor do disorders of psychogenic etiology fail to respond to pharmacological treatment" (Loney, 1980, p. 32).

****

GO TO VIDEOTAPE

****

B.   CONDUCT DISORDERS

Because of the close relationship between Conduct Disorders and juvenile delinquency some data on delinquency will be used to help define these disorders.

The term juvenile delinquency is a sociolegal term and not a medical or psychiatric term. A delinquent is a person below a legally specified age (17 years in most states) who commits an act which, if he were an adult, would be considered criminal; or a person who violates a law which applies only to juveniles (truancy, running away from home, etc.). The latter group of offenses are usually referred to as "status" offenses, i.e., offenses which are offenses only because of the individual's status as a minor.

The DSM-III gives four diagnostic categories (plus one "atypical" category) of Conduct Disorders into which most juvenile delinquents fall. On the other hand, it is important to understand that not every person who is diagnosed as having a Conduct Disorder is necessarily an adjudged delinquent.

Conduct Disorders are found in males far more often than in females. Most agree that the ratio is 4 or 5:1, males to females, although the DSM-III indicates that the ratio may be as high as 12:1. Prevalence and incidence rates are not precisely known, although Conduct Disorders are thought to be relatively common. To give you some better idea of rates, it is conservatively estimated in the United States that about 3% of children between 10 and 17 years of age will enter the Juvenile Justice System in any given year (Winslow, 1976).

Rates will vary by geographic location, with the highest rates found in larger cities and lowest rates in rural areas. Rates also tend to be influenced by socioeconomic class, with highest rates found in the lower classes; and by instability of the family, with highest rates found in homes which are broken by separation or divorce or by serious or violent marital disharmony.

There are a great many theories about the causation of Conduct Disorders. Genetic theories suggest that in some instances chromosomal aberrations, such as the XYY constellation found in some highly aggressive males, may account for some Conduct Disorders. Jacobs et al. (1965) for example, reported that 3.5% of a population of 197 violent criminal patients displayed some chromosomal aberration, usually the XYY configuration. Learning theorists, on the other hand, suggest that Conduct Disorders are the result of faulty learning, i.e., these children have "learned" (through operant conditioning) antisocial and aggressive responses. There is mounting evidence that organic factors play a role in aggression, especially among the more violent delinquents. Lewis and her colleagues (1981), for example, found that the most violent children in their study of 97 violent delinquent boys had grossly abnormal EEG tracings and/or a history of grand mal seizures. Furthermore, these children also revealed histories which included witnessing extremely violent behavior among their parents.

Sociocultural theories of causation emphasize the role of the subculture in the development of some Conduct Disorders. Sutherland's (1955) theory of "differential association" refers to an individual's isolation from pro-social patterns of behavior and association with persons in a subculture whose patterns of behavior are antisocial.

Psychodynamic theories of causation focus attention on defects in personality structure. Earlier hypotheses suggested that many of conduct-disordered children suffer from superego defects (Johnson, 1949), but the emphasis today seems to be on ego deficiency (Grossbard, 1962; Redl & Wineman, 1957). In a very succinct paper, Grossbard (1962) makes the point that delinquents so often have not developed the internal controls, a function of the ego, necessary to convert impulses into socially acceptable behaviors like fantasy or language. Instead many children with Conduct Disorders act on their impulses.

The truth of the matter is that Conduct Disorders, not unlike Attention Deficit Disorders, are multidimensional. There is no single cause of Conduct Disorders and many of the theories of causation probably have limited validity. Genetic endowment, cultural heritage, socioeconomic class, organic factors, parental attitudes and child-rearing practices, as well as others may well, in various combinations, play roles in the development of Conduct Disorders.

Attention Deficit Disorders often are associated with Conduct Disorders. This certainly does not mean that all children with behavior disorders have Attention Deficit Disorders; nor does this mean that all children with Attention Deficit Disorders will develop behavior disorders. From a practical standpoint this means: (1) that the differential diagnosis may be difficult at times, and (2) that it may be appropriate to make both diagnoses in some instances. The same thing is true of some of the specific developmental disorders, particularly the Developmental Reading Disorder. A significant number of children with Conduct Disorders are unable to read at a level appropriate to their age and I.Q.

The most difficult differential diagnosis to make is often between a single, isolated act of antisocial behavior and a Conduct Disorder. It is not unusual for a child to commit a single antisocial act, usually, but not necessarily, against property. Some of these children get caught and end up in the juvenile justice system or in a psychiatrist's office. The differentiation is relatively easy in most instances, but children with Conduct Disorders will often deny the repetitive aspects of their behavior and may be supported in the denial by their parents.

Conduct Disorders are categorized along two dimensions, aggression and socialization, yielding the four types of Conduct Disorders seen in Figure 1 below. There is, in addition, an atypical Conduct Disorder for persons who do not fit one of the four categories but now meet the major criteria of aggression or undersocialization.

The aggressive dimension refers to the violation of the rights of other persons in a face-to-face manner, i.e., actual physical aggression or stealing directly from a victim. Nonaggression refers to the violation of the rights in a nonconfrontive manner, e.g., stealing, vandalism, etc. in which the victim is not directly encountered.

The socialization dimension refers to the relationships the individual has established with others. Undersocialized refers to a, "failure to establish a normal degree of affection, empathy or bond with others" (DSM-III, p. 45).

This usually means that the individual does not seem to feel guilt or remorse about his behavior, does not seem to be anxious, and is not restrained from acting impulsively. Socialized means that the individual demonstrates that he has loyalties to some persons, such as a gang or specific group of persons, but may lack the ability to be empathic with persons outside this group.

Obviously the undersocialized, aggressive type is the most severe disorder in this group. It is not uncommon to see a history of this disorder in adults with Antisocial Personality Disorders. The socialized, nonaggressive type clearly is the least severe, and many of these children make relatively good adjustments in adult life. The other two categories, socialized aggressive and undersocialized nonaggressive fall in between the other two and many children in these categories make only marginal adjustments in adult life.

FIGURE 15-1
TYPES OF CONDUCT DISORDERS

	Aggressive	Nonaggressive
Undersocialized	Most Severe	Moderately Severe
Socialized	Moderately Severe	Least Severe

Marguerite Q. Warren and her associates developed a system of nosology for delinquents based on "Interpersonal Maturity Levels" or "I-Levels" (Palmer, 1971). Translating the categories of the I-levels into the four DSM-III categories indicates that over half of the Conduct Disorders probably fall in the less severe categories, while only a small percentage (estimated 1% to 5%) fall in the undersocialized, aggressive category.

It is important to note that "pure" types of conduct disordered children are seldom seen and that the types probably are best viewed on a continuum. Treatment implications generally conform to a kind of continuum in which the more severe disorders usually need a greater amount of external controls imposed by society (institutions or well-run day treatment programs) and the least severe disorders require fewer external controls.

The Diagnostic Criteria (from DSM-III) for the Conduct Disorders are as follows:

Conduct Disorder, Undersocialized, Aggressive (312.00)

A. A repetitive and persistent pattern of aggressive conduct in which the basic rights of others are violated, as manifested by either of the following:

(1) physical violence against persons or property (not to defend someone else or oneself), e.g., vandalism, rape, breaking and entering, fire-setting, mugging, assault
(2) thefts outside the home involving confrontation with the victim (e.g., extortion, purse-snatching, gas station robbery)

B. Failure to establish a normal degree of affection, empathy, or bond with others as evidenced by no more than one of the following indications of social attachment:

  (1) has one or more peer-group friendships that have lasted over six months

  (2) extends himself or herself for others even when no immediate advantage is likely

  (3) apparently feels guilt or remorse when such a reaction is appropriate (not just when caught or in difficulty)

  (4) avoids blaming or informing on companions

  (5) shares concern for the welfare of friends or companions

C. Duration of pattern of aggressive conduct of at least six months.

D. If 18 or older, does not meet the criteria for Antisocial Personality Disorder.

Conduct Disorder, Undersocialized, Nonaggressive (312.10)

A. A repetitive and persistent pattern of nonaggressive conduct in which either the basic rights of others or major age-appropriate societal norms or rules are violated, as manifested by any of the following:

  (1) chronic violations of a variety of important rules (that are reasonable and age-appropriate for the child) at home or at school (e.g., persistent truancy, substance abuse)

  (2) repeated running away from home overnight

  (3) persistent serious lying in and out of the home

  (4) stealing not involving confrontation with a victim

B. Failure to establish a normal degree of affection, empathy, or bond with others as evidenced by no more than one of the following indications of social attachment:

  (1) has one or more peer-group friendships that have lasted over six months

  (2) extends himself or herself for others even when no immediate advantage is likely

  (3) apparently feels guilt or remorse when such a reaction is appropriate (not just when caught or in difficulty)

  (4) avoids blaming or informing on companions

  (5) shows concern for the welfare of friends or companions

C. Duration of pattern of nonaggressive conduct of at least six months.

D.   If 18 or older, does not meet the criteria for Anti-social Personality Disorder.

Conduct Disorder, Socialized, Aggressive (312.23)

A.   A repetitive and persistent pattern of aggressive conduct in which the basic rights of others are violated, as manifested by either of the following:

(1) physical violence against persons or property (not to defend someone else or oneself), e.g., vandalism, rape, breaking and entering, fire-setting, mugging, assault
(2) thefts outside the home involving confrontation with a victim (e.g., extortion, purse-snatching, gas station robbery)

B.   Evidence of social attachment to others as indicated by at least two of the following behavior patterns:

(1) has one or more peer-group friendships that have lasted over six months
(2) extends himself or herself for others even when no immediate advantage is likely
(3) apparently feels guilt or remorse when such a reaction is appropriate (not just when caught or in difficulty)
(4) avoids blaming or informing on companions
(5) shows concern for the welfare of friends or companions

C.   Duration of pattern of aggressive conduct of at least six months.

D.   If 18 or older, does not meet the criteria for Anti-social Personality Disorder.

Conduct Disorder, Socialized, Nonaggressive (312.21)

A.   A repetitive and persistent pattern of nonaggressive conduct in which either the basic rights of others or major age-appropriate societal norms or rules are violated, as manifested by any of the following:

(1) chronic violations of a variety of important rules (that are reasonable and age-appropriate for the child) at home or at school (e.g.,

persistent truancy, substance abuse)
(2) repeated running away from home overnight
(3) persistent serious lying in and out of the home
(4) stealing not involving confrontation with a victim

B. Evidence of social attachment to others as indicated by at least two of the following behavior patterns:

(1) has one or more peer-group friendships that have lasted over six months
(2) extends himself or herself for others even when no immediate advantage is likely
(3) apparently feels guilt or remorse when such a reaction is appropriate (not just when caught or in difficulty)
(4) avoids blaming or informing on companions
(5) shows concern for the welfare of friends or companions

C. Duration of pattern of nonaggressive conduct of at least six months.

D. If 18 or older, does not meet the criteria for Anti-social Personality Disorder.

****

GO TO VIDEOTAPE

****

QUIZ, Section III.

Fill in the blanks for Questions 1-3.

1. The three most prominent symptoms expressed in Attention Deficit Disorders are motor activity, inattention, and _____.

2. While it is most likely that Attention Deficit Disorder has an organic basis, environmental factors also play a role in the _____ of symptoms.

3. Organic causes are clearly identified in approximately _____% of the cases of Attention Deficit Disorder.

    a. 1%
    b. 5%
    c. 10%
    d. 25%
    e. 50%

Match the following numbered items with the lettered responses.

___ 4. Cerebral palsy and ADD	a. Axis I only (ADD not diagnosed)
___ 5. Epilepsy and ADD	b. Axis III only
___ 6. Mild Mental Retardation and ADD	c. Axis I and III
___ 7. Profound Mental Retardation and ADD	d. Both on Axis I
___ 8. Affective Disorder and ADD	
___ 9. Schizophrenia	

Circle the correct answer(s).

10. In instances where chromosomal aberrations are associated with Conduct Disorders the most common constellation is

     a. xyy.
     b. xxyy.
     c. xxy.
     d. xo.

Fill in the blanks below.

11. The most severe form of Conduct Disorder is the Undersocialized, _____ type.

12. The least severe is usually the _____ Nonaggressive type.

IV. EMOTIONAL

There are two groups of disorders in this section. The first is a group of three disorders in which anxiety is the most prominent feature: (1) Separation Anxiety, (2) Avoidant Disorder, and (3) Overanxious Disorder. The second group is a kind of "catch-all" group containing five disorders: (1) Reactive Attachment Disorder, (2) Schizoid Disorder, (3) Elective Mutism, (4) Oppositional Disorder, and (5) Identity Disorder.

A. ANXIETY DISORDERS OF INFANCY, CHILDHOOD, OR ADOLESCENCE

Recall that anxiety is an emotion shared by all human beings and that anxiety is closely related to fear. Remember, too, that anxiety is a multifactorial phenomenon with components which may derive from genes, instincts, cognition, central and peripheral nervous system factors, environmental factors, and unconscious processes (including, of course, defense mechanisms). You should review Chapter 9, Anxiety Disorders, if you do not recall the concepts of anxiety which you learned in relation to the other disorders of anxiety.

    1. Separation Anxiety Disorder.

        The concept of separation anxiety as a naturally occurring phenomen has been elaborately expounded in the literature, especially by Bowlby (1969, 1973) and by Mahler, Pine, and Bergman (1975). The concept is based in the natural dependency of the child on caregivers and the anxiety produced by loss or threat of loss of the caregiver. It is perhaps obvious that one cannot suffer the pains of separation without first having formed an attachment. Separation, then, refers to perceived loss of what Bowlby (1973) calls the "attachment figure," usually the mother. The child, beginning in infancy, experiences brief separations from the attachment figure with the accompanying anxiety which is behaviorally expressed in crying, reaching, searching for the lost figure.

The anxiety is lessened, but not totally abated, when the young child incorporates a sense of object permanence, i.e., the concept that an object (including persons) still exists although the object is outside of the field of vision. Part of the normal developmental process is the growing ability to tolerate longer and longer periods of separation from attachment figures. The process of separation is detailed in the work of Mahler (1968; 1975) who divided the process into stages or sub-phases. When the child's response to separation from the attachment figure is outside of what is expected or is more than a passing phenomenon, intervention is often necessary. A forced separation, as in the case of hospitalization or institutionalization of the child, may precipitate a Separation Anxiety Disorder in infancy or early childhood. In this instance, if the separation is prolonged, the disorder may take the form of anaclitic depression as defined by Rene Spitz (1946) in which the child exhibits signs of withdrawal, psychomotor retardation, sleep and eating problems, and eventually becomes detached and may literally waste away and die. Most often the brief separations from the attachment figure include loud protest, despair, and withdrawal which diminish shortly after the child is reunited with the attachment figure.

The most frequently occurring form of separation anxiety is seen in the child of school or pre-school age who becomes anxious and agitated at being separated from the attachment figure (again, usually mother) in order to enter nursery school, kindergarten, or the first grade. The term school phobia has been used to describe this disorder, but most often separation anxiety is the more appropriate term. (If there is something specific about the school which the child actually fears, rather than separation from mother, then the term phobia is appropriate).

In general, the symptoms of the disorder are not unlike those of Agoraphobia. That is, the anticipation of anxiety about being separated from the security of home (mother) leads to feelings of dread, fears that danger is waiting, increase in autonomic nervous system activity, and limitations of social activity.

ANSWERS,   Section   III.   _____

1.	impulsivity	7.	a
2.	exacerbation	8.	a
3.	b	9.	a
4.	b	10.	a
5.	b	11.	aggressive
6.	d	12.	socialized

_____

For the child this means such things as somatic complaints, (stomach pain, headaches, dizziness, etc.), limited peer group interactions, fear and panic reactions to new situations, a feeling of dread that something bad is going to happen to those close to him, and sleep difficulties (including nightmares).

The specific diagnostic criteria for Separation Anxiety Disorder are:

A. Excessive anxiety concerning separation from those to whom the child is attached, as manifested by at least three of the following:

(1) unrealistic worry about possible harm befalling major attachment figures or fear that they will leave and will not return

(2) unrealistic worry that an untoward calamitous event will separate the child from a major attachment figure, e.g., the child will be lost, kidnapped, killed, or be the victim of an accident

(3) persistent reluctance or refusal to go to school in order to stay with major attachment figures or at home

(4) persistent reluctance or refusal to go to sleep without being next to a major attachment figure or to go to sleep away from home

(5) persistent avoidance of being alone in the home and emotional upset if unable to follow the major attachment figure around the home

(6) repeated nightmares involving theme of separation

(7) complaints of physical symptoms on school days, e.g., stomachaches, headaches, nausea, vomiting

(8) signs of excessive distress upon separation, or when anticipating separation, from major attachment figures, e.g., temper tantrums or crying, pleading with parents not to leave (for children below the age of six, the distress must be of panic proportions)

(9) social withdrawal, apathy, sadness or difficulty concentrating on work or play when not
with a major attachment figure

B. Duration of disturbance of at least two weeks.

C. Not due to a Pervasive Developmental Disorder,
Schizophrenia, or any other psychotic disorder.

D. If 18 or older, does not meet the criteria for Agoraphobia.

Treatment of separation anxiety is usually focused on parental
involvement in terms of reassurance to the child about the parents'
love and affection and a clear message of support for the child's
developing a more independent pattern of behavior. When school
refusal is a feature of the disorder, it is necessary to elicit the
cooperation and the support of the school, specifically a person
(teacher, principal) who will reassure the child while he is in
school. It is crucial that the child be returned to school as soon
as possible.

Drugs are sometimes used initially to help with sleep problems and
anxiety, but these should be used only in the context of an overall
therapeutic program. Behavior modification techniques have been
found useful as a part of such a program. In cases when the child
does not respond relatively quickly, referral to a specialist is
indicated. In those very resistant cases, imipramine has been
shown to be effective (Gittleman-Klein, 1975-76).

2. Avoidant Disorder of Childhood or Adolescence.

A key word in this disorder is "shyness" since this is the impression the children or adolescents give to the observer. They
tend to be quite passive and withdrawn, speak very softly (when
they do speak), often avoid eye contact, and tend to avoid interaction with others (adults or peers). In short, they tend to be
overinhibited. The increase in anxiety comes in virtually any social
situation or any activity which necessitates interaction with others,
particularly, but not limited to, situations where strangers are
involved.

Remember that in the normal course of development the child at
6-12 months of age, shows for the first time anxiety in the presence
of strangers (stranger anxiety) and certainly expresses anxiety
at the prospect of separation from attachment figures. The child
usually manages in time to overcome the anxiety associated with new
situations and with strangers. This achievement is a kind of hallmark in the development of social interactions.

For the child who suffers from an Avoidant Disorder, the overinhibited response to strangers persists. Obviously peer relations are dramatically reduced, if indeed they develop at all. At the same time these children are able to maintain relatively close relationships with persons who are familiar to them - family members and perhaps a few people outside the family. Another distinguishing characteristic of the child with Avoidant Disorder is his wish to be able to extend himself to others in order to be accepted and appreciated. This is in marked contrast to the child with a Schizoid Disorder, for example, who apparently has no wish to form relationships outside of a very limited number of persons (one or two).

As in the case of the child with Separation Anxiety Disorder, the predominant affect is anxiety when confronted with what is perceived as the threat of facing social interactions with strangers or relative strangers such as peers.

The diagnostic criteria for the Avoidant Disorder of Childhood or Adolescence are:

A. Persistent and excessive shrinking from contact with strangers.
B. Desire for affection and acceptance, and generally warm and satisfying relations with family members and other familiar figures.
C. Avoidant behavior sufficiently severe to interfere with social functioning in peer relationships.
D. Age at least 2½. If 18 or older, does not meet the criteria for Avoidant Personality Disorder.
E. Duration of the disturbance of at least six months.

Many times the mild form of this disorder is untreated since some children can form relationships with a few peers. In more severe forms, however, psychotherapy is the treatment of choice (Werkman, 1980). In younger children particularly, involvement of parents is essential since they will have to play a role in supporting the child's move toward independence and away from dependence on them.

Generally treatment is more successful in cases where the precipitant of the disorder is based on something like an early chronic illness of the child which led to parental overprotection and social isolation of the child. This is in marked contrast to the parents whose character structures have led to overprotective behaviors.

Psychotropic drugs are of little value in the treatment of Avoidant Disorders, and, in fact, may be contraindicated since they may serve only to mask the anxiety and reinforce the withdrawn behavior of the child (Werkman, 1980).

3. Overanxious Disorder.

The third of the Anxiety Disorders is the Overanxious Disorder. While the child with Separation Anxiety Disorder responds to separation from attachment figures, and the child with Avoidance Disorder responds to facing new situations or people, the child with Overanxious Disorder responds with anxiety in a generalized way. He worries about the future and about whether or not he will be able to perform adequately - on a test, in a ball game, at a dance, etc. He has many of the characteristics of the obsessive person who makes great demands upon himself in a perfectionistic, ruminative way. There is some evidence that children with this disorder are children whose parents are demanding in terms of achievement and performance. The child translates the parental attitude to mean that his (the child's) worth is contingent upon performance rather than upon his value as a person (Jenkins, 1973). The upshot is that the child, in order to maintain his acceptance in the family, must excel, perhaps even become perfect, and anxiety about failing leads to a diffuse anxiety.

The child becomes hypersensitive to criticism by others, exhibits an approval-seeking kind of dependence, and displays autonomic nervous system hyperactivity in the form of stomach pain, headaches, dizziness, etc. Perhaps most noteworthy is a virtually constant seeking of acceptance by others - peers, teachers, coaches, etc.

Most of these children are bright, tend to come from families in the upper socioeconomic levels, frequently are firstborn, and actually do achieve well in school. Many never require therapeutic intervention. Stressful life events, however, may escalate their symptoms to the point where they are unable to function adequately (in school, for example).

It is not unusual for these children to bite their nails, pull their hair, suck their thumbs, etc.; nor is it unusual for them to have frequent somatic complaints. It is important to examine them carefully since the disorder does not rule out the possibility of physical illness.

If a clear relationship between anxiety and a recent psychosocial stressor (Axis IV) is present, the diagnosis will most often be Adjustment Disorder with Anxious Mood. The differential diagnosis must consider a variety of disorders, like Major Depression and Schizophrenia, but most often diagnostic questions will center around Obsessive Compulsive Disorder.

The diagnostic criteria for the Overanxious Disorder are:

A. The predominant disturbance is generalized and persistent anxiety or worry (not related to concerns about separation), as manifested by at least four of the following:

(1) unrealistic worry about future events
(2) preoccupation with the appropriateness of the individual's behavior in the past

        (3) overconcern about competence in a variety of areas, e.g., academic, athletic, social

        (4) excessive need for reassurance about a variety of worries

        (5) somatic complaints, such as headaches or stomachaches, for which no physical basis can be established

        (6) marked self-consciousness or susceptibility to embarrassment or humiliation

        (7) marked feeling of tension or inability to relax

B.   The symptoms in A have persisted for at least six months.

C.   If 18 or older, does not meet the criteria for Generalized Anxiety Disorder.

D.   The disturbance is not due to another mental disorder, such as Separation Anxiety Disorder, Avoidant Disorder of Childhood or Adolescence, Phobic Disorder, Obsessive Compulsive Disorder, Depressive Disorder, Schizophrenia, or a Pervasive Developmental Disorder.

Treatment of choice is psychotherapy and, especially in preadolescents, family involvement in therapy. Werkman (1980) notes that these children often do well in psychotherapy because of their intelligence and thus ability to deal with unconscious material. Pharmacotherapy may be useful at times of particular stress, but should not substitute for an overall treatment program for the child.

B. OTHER DISORDERS OF INFANCY, CHILDHOOD, OR ADOLESCENCE

There are five disorders in this group. There is no really unifying theme like "anxiety" in the group of disorders immediately preceding this one. They are all classified, rather loosely, in the DSM-III under the general category of disorders in which the "predominant area of disturbance" (p. 35) is emotional.

1.   Reactive Attachment Disorder of Infancy.

In the section on Separation Anxiety, it was noted that in order to have problems separating from a mother figure it was necessary first for the child to form an attachment. When there is failure in the bonding of the child and the attachment figure, a Reactive Attachment Disorder of Infancy may ensue.

This disorder is manifested in two ways: (1) developmental failures in emotional and psychosocial areas, and (2) developmental failures in physical growth. For nearly half a century the term "Failure to Thrive syndrome" has been used to describe this disorder, the emphasis having been on retarded physical development. The obvious presenting symptom is frequently the failure of the infant to gain weight, although often the parent brings the child to the physician complaining of an infection or some other symptom. It is indeed a disorder more frequently diagnosed by pediatricians than by psychiatrists (Reinhart, 1979), and there is abundant literature in both pediatrics and psychiatry under such titles as "hospitalism" (Spitz, 1946), "maternal deprivation" (Ainsworth, 1962), and "failure to thrive" (Reinhart, 1972; 1979; Smith & Berenberg, 1970).

Physical findings may be due to organic factors alone (GI, cardiac, renal, etc.), but it is estimated that in at least one half of the infants who are significantly underweight (below the third percentile) physical findings are secondary to psychosocial factors (Hannaway, 1970).

Psychosocial factors, then, play a major role in the development of this disorder. Specifically, maternal deprivation and neglect, for whatever reason, are key factors; and diagnostic assessment should include an evaluation of parent-infant interactions. The deprivation may stem from ignorance of child care methods; psychopathology in the maternal figure; fear and anxiety in parents; family stress and crises; circumstances such as early hospitalization of the infant for a prolonged period. The general rule is that the earlier the deprivation, the more severe the disorder.

A great deal has been written about the attachment process and what the necessary ingredients are for the successful accomplishment of this crucial relationship. Schulhofer speaks of the necessity of "the breast and the breath" in the adequate development of the parent-infant relationship, i.e., the provision of necessary nutrients along wth closeness and warmth.* Each is probably useless without the other.

To make an adequate assessment of the infant's functioning, a thorough understanding of the process of normal growth and development is essential. Even though there are degrees of severity of the disorder, the infant with Reactive Attachment Disorder shows marked delays or even absences of those behaviors which usually provide evidence of mother-infant attachment (eye tracking, crying, sucking, rooting, smiling, body orientation, etc.)

The diagnostic criteria for Reactive Attachment Disorder are:

A.   Age at onset before eight months.

---

*Dr. Edith Schulhofer, personal communication.

B.   Lack of the type of care that ordinarily leads to the development of affectional bonds to others, e.g., gross emotional neglect, imposed social isolation in an institution.

C.   Lack of developmentally appropriate signs of social responsivity, as indicated by at least several of the following (the total number of behaviors looked for will depend on the chronological age of the child, corrected for prematurity):

(1) lack of visual tracking of eyes and faces by an infant more than two months of age
(2) lack of smiling in response to faces by an infant more than two months of age
(3) lack of visual reciprocity in an infant of more than two months; lack of vocal reciprocity with caretaker in an infant of more than five months
(4) lack of alerting and turning toward caretaker's voice by an infant of more than four months
(5) lack of spontaneous reaching for the mother by an infant of more than four months
(6) lack of anticipatory reaching when approached to be picked up by an infant more than five months of age
(7) lack of participation in playful games with caretaker by an infant of more than five months

D.   At least three of the following:

(1) weak cry
(2) excessive sleep
(3) lack of interest in the environment
(4) hypomotility
(5) poor muscle tone
(6) weak rooting and grasping in response to feeding attempts

E.   Weight loss or failure to gain appropriate amount of weight for age unexplainable by any physical disorder. In these cases usually the failure to gain weight (falling weight percentile) is disproportionately greater than failure to gain length; head circumference is normal.

F.   Not due to a physical disorder, Mental Retardation, or Infantile Autism.

G. The diagnosis is confirmed if the clinical picture is reversed shortly after institution of adequate caretaking, which frequently includes short-term hospitalization.

Treatment of the child with Reactive Attachment Disorder must focus first on his physical well-being, and hospitalization may be necessary to treat effectively the nutritional deficits (protein deficits, vitamin deficiency, electrolyte imbalances, and so forth), as well as to assess thoroughly attendant physical disorders. Concomitantly the family, in particular the "mothering" figure, must receive attention in the treatment of this disorder. If neglect and/or abuse are factors, a not unusual finding, then these issues must be addressed. Simply removing the child from the custody of his parents is a less than ideal solution if there is any hope that they are amenable to the necessary changes in behavior toward the child.

Early in the course of the disorder a change to a warm and loving approach to the child will bring dramatic results, and the child will respond affectively as well as physically. If treatment is delayed, the results can be devastating. It is often wise for the physician to call upon resources in the community for assistance in the management of the disorder (public health nurses, child welfare workers, Family Service Agency, Family Court, etc.). A firm yet nonpunitive approach to the parents is important if the child is to be protected and treatment of the family is to be effective.

2. Schizoid Disorder of Childhood or Adolescence.

This disorder is characterized by withdrawn and isolated demeanor. In fact, the GAP report (1966) refers to this disorder as "isolated personality" because of the tendency to be distant and detached and to form no truly close relationships with either family or friends. The word "loner" is frequently used to describe the children or adolescents with this disorder.

These youngsters tend to avoid peer relationships, both in organized activities and in informal interactions. This, in turn, tends to reinforce the isolation and offers little opportunity for the acquisition and development of social skills.

The diagnosis of the disorder is a very difficult one to make since the key feature of withdrawn behavior is present in a number of disorders. In Avoidant Disorders the individual, because of anxiety, may appear withdrawn and socially isolated. In this instance, however, the child or adolescent wishes to participate in peer group activity but, again, because of the anxiety, he is unable to reach out to peers. Also in the case of Avoidant Disorders, warm, close relationships within the family are usually present.

Depression also may present with withdrawal and social isolation. In younger children the differential diagnosis may be quite difficult to make if the depression is characterized by withdrawn, isolated behavior. In adolescence the diagnosis may also be difficult, but often the premorbid state will include normal, healthy peer relationships. The final diagnostic test, in some instances, may be the depressed patient's response to antidepressant medication. In any case, remember that Schizoid Disorder and Depression may co-exist (La Vietes, 1980).

In younger children, the diagnosis of psychosis (Pervasive Developmental Disorder, Schizophrenia, and, less often, Autism) may carry similar features of isolation and withdrawal. In the case of Schizoid Disorder, however, the youngster is not functioning outside of reality (even though there may be instances when he behaves in erratic and impulsive ways). There is no hard evidence that schizoid children are pre-psychotic, although "some...under the stress of puberty and adolescence, become overtly psychotic" (Finch & Green, 1979).

Children with Conduct Disorder, particularly undersocialized non-aggressive type, may be isolated and may appear withdrawn. In these children, however, the predominant feature is repetitive anti-social behavior; in Schizoid Disorders, episodes of antisocial behavior do not have the persistence seen in Conduct Disorders.

Finally, some children may suffer from Adjustment Disorder (with withdrawal) and may present a clinical picture similar to the child with Schizoid Disorder. The identification of a psychosocial stressor as a precipitant is present in the Adjustment Disorder. Once again the premorbid state of the youngster is an important factor in diagnosis.

Although there is no clear evidence that the Schizoid Disorder "becomes" a Schizoid Personality in adulthood, there is some indication that with continued isolation and withdrawal this may be the case.

The diagnostic criteria for Schizoid Disorder are:

A. No close friend of similar age other than a relative or a similarly socially isolated child.

B. No apparent interest in making friends.

C. No pleasure from usual peer interactions.

D. General avoidance of nonfamilial social contacts, especially with peers.

E. No interest in activities that involve other children (such as team sports, clubs).

F.   Duration of the disturbance of at least three months.

G.   Not due to Pervasive Developmental Disorder; Conduct Disorder, Undersocialized, Nonaggressive, or any psychotic disorder, such as Schizophrenia.

H.   If 18 or older, does not meet the criteria for Schizoid Personality Disorder.

In general, treatment of the child or adolescent with Schizoid Disorder should be multifaceted. The treatment of choice is psychotherapy, the form depending on the age of the child and the degree of impairment. Behavior modification techniques may be helpful in terms of reinforcing social interactions. As is true with virtually all childhood disorders, the treatment program should involve the family of the child. Medication has not been found to be of value in the treatment of Schizoid Disorder.

3.   Elective Mutism.

Just as with Reactive Attachment Disorder and Schizoid Disorder, the child with this disorder appears withdrawn, shy, and retiring. The major feature of the disorder is a refusal to speak to all but a selected few people (usually to family members, outside the presence of others, and to a few peers). Although the disorder typically begins earlier, referral usually does not come until the time of school entry (Silver, 1980).

It is not uncommon for these children to function well on a nonverbal basis, and clearly they have the ability to speak. They may learn well in school, particularly if they have a teacher and peers who will tolerate their muteness. There may be, however, an attendant academic problem.

Theories of etiology of the disorder include: (1) a traumatic event, either physical or emotional; (2) regression or fixation at the anal retentive level of development (and indeed many of these children suffer from enuresis, encopresis, fecal retention, etc.); (3) reinforcement of the "cute" shy behavior by parents (Laybourne, 1979; Silver, 1980). It also has been noted that some of these children will speak to one parent, usually mother, and not the other. This is thought to be a reflection of family pathology in which the child is allied with one parent against the other, and the mutism is interpreted to be punitive toward the ignored parent.

The diagnosis is relatively easy to make from the history and clinical signs and symptoms. It is important to rule out such disorders as Mental Retardation, congenital deafness, Pervasive Developmental Disorder, Childhood Psychosis, Schizoid Disorder, and Avoidant Disorder. The diagnosis of Avoidant Disorder may be the most difficult to differentiate, but the distinguishing feature is that in Elective Mutism the mutism is the primary symptom.

The diagnostic criteria for Elective Mutism are:

A. Continuous refusal to talk in almost all social situations, including at school.

B. Ability to comprehend spoken language and to speak.

C. Not due to another mental or physical disorder.

Treatment may, depending on the individual assessment, involve psychotherapy and or family therapy. Techniques of behavior modification have been found to be very useful in many instances.

4. Oppositional Disorder.

In the course of normal development of children, a certain amount of aggressive behavior is necessary, not hostile aggression, but certainly assertive aggression. Without assertive aggression, the desired move on the part of the child toward separation and independence can only be chaotic.

Thus far in this section you have learned about several disorders in which the behavior of the child may be characterized, in some form, as withdrawn and in some sense passive. In the child with Oppositional Disorder the behavior is characterized as more openly aggressive - in the form of provocative, argumentative, negativistic attitudes.

The behavior is reminiscent of the normal negative period of the 1½ to 2½ year old, the "terrible two's," which developmentally represents one of the first strivings for independence. In the case of the Oppositional Disorder, however, the negative, provocative behavior has persisted and increased in intensity to the extent that the "more overt manifestations are quarrelsomeness, rebelliousness, teasing, temper tantrums, fighting, and delinquent acts" (LaVietes, 1980, p. 2618).

There are features of passive-aggressiveness commonly found in these children, and frequently they are described as children who "forget" to perform tasks, are often late, procrastinate, and fail to fully complete assignments. The opposition may be active and/or passive, and the objects of the expression of aggression are usually authority figures such as parents and teachers. Sometimes the behavior is extended to peers as well. The disorder is much more common in boys than in girls.

The theory of etiology is related to family interactions which early in the life of the child center around issues of power, authority, and control. These are initially parental issues which directly conflict with the developmental process of attaining autonomy. It is easy to see that direct, open opposition may not be successful in the face of parental power, and that passive-aggressive opposition may eventually become the primary technique in the struggle with authority. It is also easy to see that such a manner of behaving can become a fixed characterological trait leading in adult life to Passive-Aggressive Personality Disorder.

Other Mental Disorders may include oppositional behavior as a feature - childhood psychosis, Mental Retardation, some forms of Organic Mental Disorders, for examples. The most difficult differential diagnosis is often Conduct Disorder (in which the rights of others or major norms of society are violated).

The diagnostic criteria for Oppositional Disorder are:

A. Onset after 3 years of age and before age 18.

B. A pattern, for at least six months, of disobedient, negativistic, and provocative opposition to authority figures, as manifested by at least two of the following symptoms:

    (1) violations of minor rules
    (2) temper tantrums
    (3) argumentativeness
    (4) provocative behavior
    (5) stubbornness

C. No violation of the basic rights of others or of major age-appropriate societal norms or rules (as in Conduct Disorder), and the disturbance is not due to another mental disorder, such as Schizophrenia or a Pervasive Developmental Disorder.

D. If 18 or older, does not meet the criteria for Passive-Aggressive Personality Disorder.

Treatment of choice generally is individual psychotherapy for the child and collateral work with the parents. The very nature of the disorder, however, makes treatment difficult since missed appointments and uncooperative behavior tend to make these children somewhat less than ideal candidates for therapy.

5. Identity Disorder.

From your knowledge of normal development you will recall that the major tasks of the adolescent period are: (1) to achieve a reasonable measure of independence and autonomy from parental authority and control; and (2) to attain a sense of identity. The two are inextricably bound to each other and have developmental roots which reach back to virtually all previous stages. During the period of adolescence there is a consolidation of previous childhood "identities," but more importantly there also should emerge in the individual a sense of ego identity which is the true springboard into mature adulthood.

Erik Erikson has made the major contribution to the understanding of adolescence and specifically to the concept of identity. He saw the achievement of ego identity as the major task of adolescence, and failure in this developmental task as resulting in "role diffusion" (Erikson, 1950). In defining ego identity, Erikson (1964) writes that it is "more than the sum of childhood identifications (but rather) the accrued confidence that the inner sameness and continuity prepared in the past are matched by the sameness and continuity of one's meaning for others, as evidenced in the tangible promise of a career" (p. 250).

Identity Disorder typically has its onset during adolescence, and therefore is found in the group of disorders related to adolescence. Just as typically the disorder extends into young adulthood and not uncommonly into the middle years.

Etiologically, Identity Disorders develop during adolescence on the basis of failures in earlier developmental periods which then undermine the final striving for identity during adolescence. Put another way, deficiencies in the relatively orderly process of ego development during infancy and childhood may lead to failure to establish a sense of ego identity during adolescence.

Confounding the problem today is our society itself. Lidz (1976) points out that in our industrialized, technologically oriented society the movement from childhood to adulthood often requires much more time and experience than this transition did in previous, less complex societies. In other words it is not unusual for the adolescent period to be extended in some measure by prolonged educational and training efforts.

According to DSM-III, Identity Disorder is defined by subjective distress on the part of the adolescent over the inability to synthesize an acceptable identity in terms of such things as value systems, career choice, sexual orientation, and so forth. The distress is severe and is more than the normal transient crises of adolescence. Note that the diagnosis may be made beyond adolescent age range and may be - usually in milder forms - the basis of what has been called the middle age crisis.

The stress of the disorder is frequently accompanied by anxiety and/or depression. The diagnosis is not made if the patient is suffering from an Affective Disorder or an Anxiety Disorder. The distress of the Identity Disorder also frequently interferes with social functioning and may be confused with Borderline Personality Disorder. If the individual meets the criteria of this disorder then Identity Disorder is not diagnosed.

The diagnostic criteria for Identity Disorder are:

A. Severe subjective distress regarding uncertainty about a variety of issues relating to identity, including three or more of the following:

(1) long-term goals
(2) career choice
(3) friendship patterns
(4) sexual orientation and behavior
(5) religious identification
(6) moral value systems
(7) group loyalties

B. Impairment in social or occupational (including academic) functioning as a result of the symptoms in A.

C. Duration of the disturbance of at least three months.

D. Not due to another mental disorder, such as Affective Disorder, Schizophrenia, or Schizophreniform Disorder.

E. If 18 or older, does not meet the criteria for Borderline Personality Disorder.

The treatment of choice for Identity Disorder is individual and/or group psychotherapy aimed at overcoming developmental failures. Feinstein (1980) points out that this is not unlike the most effective therapy used in the treatment of Borderline Personality Disorders in which a kind of corrective developmental experience is used within the context of a transference relationship with the therapist.

QUIZ, Section IV.

Circle the correct answer(s). <u>One</u> or <u>more</u> <u>than</u> <u>one</u> answer may be correct.

1.   Signs of anaclitic depression include

     a. psychomotor retardation.
     b. sleep disturbance.
     c. withdrawal.
     d. eating problems.

Fill in the blanks with the correct answers.

2.   "School phobia" usually is, in reality, a form of _____ anxiety.

3.   Avoidant Disorder cannot be diagnosed before the age of _____ .

TRUE or FALSE: Circle the correct letter.

T   F   4.   The child with Avoidant Disorder has no real desire to extend
                himself to others and to develop peer relationships.

Fill in the blanks with the correct answers.

5.   In Avoidant Disorder when the child is faced with social interactions the
     predominant affect is _____ .

6.   For whatever reason the parent or parents of the child with Avoidant
     Disorder tend to be _____ .

Circle the correct answer(s). <u>One</u> or <u>more</u> <u>than</u> <u>one</u> answer may be correct.

7.   Which of the following usually may be applied to the child with Over-
     anxious Disorder?

     a. perfectionistic
     b. generalized anxiety response
     c. hypersensitive to criticism
     d. somatic complaints
     e. intellectually bright

Fill in the blanks for Questions 8-10.

8.   Most often differential diagnosis of Overanxious Disorder will be _____
     _____ disorder.

9.   The age of onset for Reactive Attachment Disorder of Infancy must be
     before _____ _____ .

10. Reactive Attachment Disorder of Infancy has often been referred to as the _____ to _____ syndrome.

Circle the correct answer(s). One or more than one may be correct.

11. Anxiety is the key feature in which of the following disorders?

    a. Avoidant Disorder
    b. Reactive Attachment Disorder
    c. Separation Anxiety Disorder
    d. Schizoid Disorder

12. Etiologically, Reactive Attachment Disorder of Infancy may be related to which of the following?

    a. maternal deprivation
    b. neglect
    c. early hospitalization
    d. paternal abandonment

Fill in the blanks for Questions 13-14.

13. Schizoid Disorder of Childhood or Adolescence is characterized by withdrawn and _____ demeanor.

14. The child or adolescent with Schizoid Disorder is frequently labeled as a _____.

Circle the correct answer(s). One or more than one answer may be correct.

15. Disorders from which Schizoid Disorder of Childhood or Adolescence must be differentiated (in terms of withdrawn behavior) may include

    a. Depression.
    b. Avoidant Disorder.
    c. Adjustment Disorder.
    d. Childhood Onset Pervasive Developmental Disorder.
    e. Overanxious Disorder.

TRUE or FALSE: Circle the correct letter.

T   F   16. Most children with Elective Mutism have at least a mild speech impediment.

T   F   17. Elective Mutism in some cases may be reinforced by parents who think the shy behavior is "cute".

T   F   18. Onset of Elective Mutism may be physical or emotional trauma.

T   F   19. In Oppositional Disorder the "opposition" may take the form of passive behavior.

T   F   20. It is not uncommon for the child with Oppositional Disorder to become an adult who has Passive-Aggressive Personality Disorder.

Circle the correct answer(s). One or more than one answer may be correct.

21. Identity Disorder typically has an onset in

     a. pre-school years.
     b. latency age.
     c. adolescence.
     d. young adulthood.

22. Identity Disorder involves the inability to resolve issues in such areas as

     a. values.
     b. career choice.
     c. sexual orientation.

V. PHYSICAL

The disorders in this group all have physical manifestations and are divided into three categories: (A) disorders of eating; (B) disorders of movement, specifically tics; and (C) a miscellaneous group of disorders having to do with speech, elimination, and sleep.

A. EATING DISORDERS

There are four Eating Disorders in this section: Anorexia Nervosa, Bulimia, Pica, and Rumination. In addition, there is an atypical category reserved for disturbances of eating behavior which do not fit into the other categories. The Eating Disorders may be life-threatening, particularly Anorexia Nervosa and Rumination; and Pica may have very serious life-long effects if lead-containing substances like paints and plaster are ingested.

     1. Anorexia Nervosa.

Sir William Gull named the syndrome of Anorexia Nervosa in 1874. For centuries before that psychological aspects of the disorder were virtually unrecognized and treatment was focused on the assumption of organic etiology. It is probably fair to speculate that patients with severe weight loss from Anorexia Nervosa were treated for consumption.

The disorder is found predominantly in females, although a small percentage of males is found in the Anorexia Nervosa population (probably in the vicinity of 5%). Bruch (1970) noted that cachexia is the most outstanding physical symptom, and indeed the weak and emaciated appearance of the patient with Anorexia Nervosa is quite startling. Other frequent somatic symptoms include constipation, amenorrhea, bradycardia, and dry, cool skin. Episodes of bulimia are not uncommon in these patients.

The psychological symptoms are often just as startling, particularly the patient's denial of her illness. This includes a contention on the part of the patient that she is overweight in the face of being 25% or more below the weight appropriate for her age and height. These patients do seem to suffer from what Bruch (1970) refers to as "body-image disturbances of delusional proportions" (p. 23). Patients also tend to resist all treatment efforts, often to the point of very direct action to circumvent the therapeutic regimen, especially regarding calorie intake.

Paradoxically, patients with Anorexia Nervosa often extend their preoccupation with food to preparing elaborate meals for others, collecting recipes, and taking over the feeding responsibilities for their families.

Bruch (1970) describes this disorder as "a state of self-inflicted starvation and relentless pursuit of thinness" (p. 3). This pursuit in the patient with Anorexia Nervosa extends from literally starving herself to induced vomiting, to the use of laxatives and diuretics, and to exhaustive exercises.

The distinction is made by Bruch (1970) between primary anorexia and secondary anorexia. In a study of 51 anorexic patients, she found that in 14 the refusal to eat was secondary to neurotic or schizophrenic conflicts. Anorexia, of course, may be secondary to a variety of physical disorders. Sours (1979) provides the following examples:

1. Cerebral tumors of the frontal lobe, fourth ventricle or diencephalon
2. Hypothyroidism
3. Hyperthyroidism
4. Panhypopituitarism
5. Granulomatous disease of the small bowel

There are, of course, other diseases which are accompanied by anorexia, the most notable examples, perhaps, being many of the forms of cancer.

The etiology of Anorexia Nervosa is not clearly established. Sours (1979) reports that there are some who feel that the basis of the disorder is pituitary and/or hypothalamus dysfunction. If clear evidence were to emerge to support this hypothesis, however, one would still have to consider the distinct possibility that psychogenic factors lead to the dysfunction. Though there is some evidence of familial relationship with Anorexia Nervosa, no genetic-chromosomal link has been found. Mortality rates for Anorexia Nervosa are reported at 15% to 21% (Miller et al., in press).

ANSWERS, Section IV.

1. a,b,c,d
2. separation
3. 2½ years
4. F
5. anxiety
6. overprotective
7. a,b,c,d,e
8. obsessive-compulsive
9. eight months
10. failure, thrive
11. a,c

12. a,b,c
13. isolated
14. loner
15. a,b,c,d
16. F
17. T
18. T
19. T
20. T
21. c
22. a,b,c

Most authorities today hold the view that the disorder is developmentally determined. Parental attitudes, early in the life of the child, seem to emphasize delay of gratification (except, perhaps oral gratification) and stringent self-control. As Sours (1979) writes, "The conceptual and perceptual attainment of absolute power and control of body, self, parents, and other significant object relations is central to the syndrome" (p. 577). The result for the child is not entirely unlike some of the characteristics of the obsessive-compulsive in terms of control of impulses. In fact, Bruch (1970) notes that the Anorexia Nervosa patient seeks to achieve "autonomy through this bizarre control over the body and its functions" (p. 21).

The diagnostic criteria of Anorexia Nervosa are

A. Intense fear of becoming obese, which does not diminish as weight loss progresses.

B. Disturbance of body image, e.g., claiming to "feel fat" even when emaciated.

C. Weight loss of at least 25% of original body weight or, if under 18 years of age, weight loss from original body weight plus projected weight gain expected from growth charts may be combined to make the 25%.

D. Refusal to maintain body weight over a minimal normal weight for age and height.

E. No known physical illness that would account for the weight loss.

It must be recognized that there are some adolescents who experience brief, transient episodes of food refusal. It also must be recognized that some individuals do diet and exercise in order to maintain a very slim physique, but the maintenance is not out of control and these individuals do not meet the three basic criteria which Bruch (1970) says are the sine qua non of Anorexia Nervosa:

1. Disturbance of body-image and body concept;
2. Disturbance in the recognition of stimuli, especially the recognition of hunger and appetite and fatigue;
3. Sense of ineffectiveness beneath a sense of helplessness at being externally controlled and unable to internalize controls over such things as eating.

Treatment of the patient with Anorexia Nervosa must include a careful monitoring of physiological functioning. Because of the potentially grave outcome of the disorder, hospitalization and I.V. feeding may be necessary. Most of the physical concomitants of the disorder are correctable -- hypothermia, dehydration, hypotension, bradycardia, amenorrhea, anemia, electrolyte imbalance, etc.

Individual psychotherapy alone has not proven to be the most efficacious treatment choice. A behavioral approach has proven to be a very helpful adjunct to treatment in terms of modifying the eating behavior itself. Family therapy is often another important part of the treatment program. Psychoactive drugs also may be helpful. Positive responses to chlorpromazine (Thorazine) have been reported (Halmi, 1980).

****

GO TO VIDEOTAPE

****

2. Bulimia.

Halmi (1980) defines Bulimia as "an episodic, uncontrolled, rapid ingestion of large quantities of food over a short period of time (binge eating)" (p. 2600). The episodes are followed immediately by feelings of guilt, self-deprecation, and depression. The eating binge is "terminated by abdominal pain, interruption by others, sleep, or self-induced vomiting" (Miller et al., in press). Many of these patients then enter a period of weight loss efforts including rigid diets, vomiting, and the use of laxatives and diuretics. The common fear expressed by bulimic patients is that they will be unable to control their binges.

The disorder was recognized only relatively recently, probably because patients with the disorder: (1) are aware of the abnormality of the eating behavior, (2) attempt to hide their binges from others, and (3) seldom have significant fluctuations in weight and appearance. In severe cases, the frequent vomiting may lead to dehydration and problems with electrolyte imbalance. These patients seem to have an exaggerated fear of weight gain.

The onset of the disorder is usually during adolescence or young adulthood and is seen predominantly in females. Body weight is usually within normal limits although the desired weight often is below these limits and these patients often express concerns about how they appear to other people. Little is known at this time about the prevalence of the disorder, but there is reason to suspect that it is not rare. Recent popular discussion in the news media about Bulimia has led to a great many women seeking help for the disorder.

Little is known about the etiology of the disorder. Speculation has been drawn from the frequent themes of patients about loss of control and feelings of depression. Psychodynamic theory has long hypothesized that eating may be used as a counter-depression mechanism.

Patients with Anorexia Nervosa may also become bulimic at times, but Bulimia is not diagnosed if the patient meets the criteria of Anorexia Nervosa.

The diagnostic criteria for Bulimia are:

A. Recurrent episodes of binge eating (rapid consumption of a large amount of food in a discrete period of time, usually less than two hours).

B. At least three of the following:

(1) consumption of high-caloric, easily ingested food during a binge
(2) inconspicuous eating during a binge
(3) termination of such eating episodes by abdominal pain, sleep, social interruption, or self-induced vomiting
(4) repeated attempts to lose weight by severely restricted diets, self-induced vomiting, or use of cathartics and/or diuretics
(5) frequent weight fluctuations greater than ten pounds due to alternating binges and fasts

C. Awareness that the eating pattern is abnormal and fear of not being able to stop eating voluntarily.

D. Depressed mood and self-deprecating thoughts following eating binges.

E. The bulimic episodes are not due to Anorexia Nervosa or any known physical disorder.

Because of the limited clinical experience and dearth of literature about the disorder, little is known at this time regarding treatment of Bulimia. Homogeneous group therapy may become the method of

choice for the time being, i.e., until more is known about the disorder.

****

GO TO VIDEOTAPE

****

3. Pica.

    This is a rather rare disorder defined as the persistent eating of
    nonnutritive substances such as dirt, paint, wood, paper, insects,
    or feces. While rare, the eating of nonfood has been reported
    from every part of the world and has been known for many hun-
    dreds of years.

    Beginning in infancy, taste and touch occupy a prominent place in
    the exploration of the environment. Young children typically touch
    objects and spontaneously put them to their mouths. Up until ap-
    proximately 1½ to 2 years of age this behavior is considered normal,
    and parents invest considerable energy in keeping harmful material
    out of the reach of children. Some children, however, focus on
    nonfood substances and continue to put them in their mouths and
    swallow them. The Pica behavior is not a substitute for food at
    meal time; i.e., children with this disorder continue to eat normal
    nutritive meals.

    Halmi (1980) notes that there are two theories of causality regarding
    Pica: (1) the presence of a specific nutritional deficit which leads
    to the ingestion of substances to make up the deficit, and (2) a
    faulty mother-child relationship resulting in unusual oral needs and
    leading to a persistent ingestion of substances to satisfy these
    needs.

    At any rate, the continuation of the Pica behavior beyond a month
    in duration warrants the diagnosis. If the behavior is a
    feature of another disorder such as Infantile Autism or Schizophre-
    nia, Pica is not diagnosed separately.

    The diagnostic criteria for Pica are:

    A. Repeated eating of a nonnutritive substances for at
        least one month.

    B. Not due to another mental disorder, such as Infan-
        tile Autism or Schizophrenia, or a physical disor-
        der, suc as Kleine-Levin syndrome.

    The treatment of the disorder involves several factors: environmen-
    tal, in terms of protecting the child from such substances as paint

or plaster which contain lead; educational in terms of helping parents understand the long-range danger of ingestion of harmful substances; behavioral management of the child's Pica, including the involvement of the parents in the child's behavioral modification program. Treatment may also include the remediation of mineral deficiencies in the child which possibly play some role in the Pica.

This is a disorder of early childhood, but there are some intractable cases which persist into adolescence or even adulthood. It is likely that the behavior in the older patient (adolescent or young adult) has taken on a meaning different from the initial behavior.

****

GO TO VIDEOTAPE

****

4. Rumination.

This is a disorder of infancy which is rarely seen but which has the potential of being life threatening. Rumination, or as it is sometimes called, Merycism, refers to voluntary regurgitation of food from the stomach, re-chewing the food, and then either swallowing it again or spitting it out. Most often some of the food is spit out and some re-swallowed. The behavior appears to be quite purposeful and after successful regurgitation the infant appears to derive great satisfaction from "re-eating" the food.

In the process some food is lost, and malnutrition often follows. If the disorder is not treated, death may follow from malnutrition. On very rare occasions, the disorder is seen in adults, but malnutrition is usually not a factor in this instance. Although it seems that spontaneous remission occurs in some cases, persistent rumination has a death rate of as much as 25 percent (Halmi, 1980). The onset is usually in the first year of life, coming after the normal feeding process has been established.

In making the diagnosis one has to be aware that the infant, early in life, regurgitates food to some extent. Furthermore, certain anomalies of the GI tract (hiatal hernia and pyloric stenosis, for example) can produce similar symptoms.

Etiology of the disorder is unknown, but there is evidence, based on successful treatment of the disorder, that there is some disturbance in the mother-child relationship, specifically in the feeding process.

The diagnostic criteria for Rumination are:

A. Repeated regurgitation without nausea or associated gastrointestinal illness for at least one month following a period of normal functioning.

B. Weight loss or failure to make expected weight gain.

Treatment has involved provision of virtually continuous attention by a caregiver or caregivers leading to a decrease in the behavior and an increase in weight. Behavior modification techniques have proved to be much more successful in terms of the rapidity with which the child responds (O'Neil et al., 1979).

B. STEREOTYPED MOVEMENT DISORDERS

The common theme of these disorders is <u>movement</u>. This does not refer to the types of movement seen in the hyperactive child syndrome, but to more specific gross motor behavior. All of the disorders in this group involve tics with the exception of the Atypical Stereotyped Movement Disorder. The three other disorders, Transient Tic Disorder, Chronic Motor Tic Disorder, and Tourette's Disorder, DSM-III notes, may be separate disorders or may represent varying degrees of the same condition.

A tic is defined as "an involuntary, repetitive movement of a muscle or group of muscles" (Lucas, 1979). According to Kanner (1972) "tics manifest themselves in a practically unlimited number of varieties" (p. 402), but most often are seen in the head and neck region.

Shapiro et al. (1976) provide an excellent, succinct description of tics:

The essential features are involuntary movements of functionally related groups of skeletal muscles in one or more parts of the body, involuntary noises, or words. These symptoms are frequent, rapid, sudden, unexpected, repetitive, purposeless, stereotypic, of variable intensity, and occur at irregular intervals (p. 277).

1. Transient Tic Disorder.

In its transient form the disorder is not an uncommon one. It is seen most frequently in the latency age range of 6 to 12 years. Redl (1966) points out that during the preadolescent years tics from earlier years may reappear briefly in relation to normal developmental processes. This represents a re-emergence of old anxieties, fears, and conflicts as the child personality "loosens up" in preparation for adolescence.

The transient tic may last for weeks or months but usually disappears spontaneously. After a year the tic is considered to be chronic. The transient tic involves only one or two movements and begins before adolescence, or during early adolescence. Most people have experienced brief, transient tic behavior in their lives. By adolescence these tics have disappeared in most persons, although they may persist throughout the life span of the individual. In either the transient or chronic form of the disorder the symptoms vary in intensity within the individual. Although the etiology is not clearly determined, an increase in the motor behavior seems to accompany stress. The tic temporarily may be voluntarily controlled, but the discharge of energy in the form of tic behavior seems to follow an increase in tension from controlling the behavior.

Clinical experience and research regarding tics have not revealed a clearly established etiology. Lucas (1979) notes that a variety of factors have been examined: hereditary; metabolic; toxic, infectious; perinatal trauma; nutritional; and psychodynamic. Sweet et al. (1975) have suggested that an increase in catecholamine activity may be one common factor in people with tics. Male ticquers outnumber females at a ratio of 3 or 4:1. While tics do seem to appear in families there is a suggestion (Lucas, 1979) that onset of some tics may be from imitation of adults or older siblings which then becomes habitualized.

Shaw (1966) points out that tics must be differentiated from: generalized motor restlessness (which actually may be hyperactivity, or may fall in the category of Atypical Stereotyped Movement); choreiform movements (especially Sydenham's chorea), which involve a variety of muscle groups in irregular, involuntary activity, and athetoid movement, a continual, recurrent, slow changing of hands, feet, fingers, etc. DSM III lists a number of motor disturbances which must be differentiated from tics.

Transient Tic Disorder must also be differentiated from Chronic Motor Tic Disorder and from Tourette's Disorder. Chronic Motor Tic Disorder differs from Transient Tic Disorder in terms of duration, age at onset, and intensity of the symptoms.

TABLE 15-1

DIFFERENTIATION BETWEEN TRANSIENT AND
CHRONIC MOTOR TIC DISORDERS

	Transient	Chronic
Duration	1-12 months	More than 12 months
Onset	Childhood or early adolescence	Childhood or after age 40
Intensity	Variable over weeks or months	Unvarying over weeks or months

The differentiation between Transient Tic Disorder and Tourette's Disorder is relatively easy since Tourette's Disorder includes vocal tics, and the duration of the symptoms is more than a year. Note, however, that Tourette's Disorder begins with a single tic in half of these patients.

The diagnostic criteria for Transient Tic Disorder are:

A.   Onset during childhood.

B.   Presence of recurrent, involuntary, repetitive, rapid, purposeless motor movements (tics).

C.   Ability to suppress the movements voluntarily for minutes to hours.

D.   Variation in the intensity of the symptoms over weeks or months.

E.   Duration of at least one month but not more than one year.

2. Chronic Motor Tic Disorder.

   Much of what has been said here regarding Transient Tic Disorder also will apply to Chronic Motor Tic Disorder. Shapiro et al. (1976) note that chronic multiple tic disorders may be differentiated from Tourette's Disorder since symptoms persist after adolescence in the latter. This is not a DSM-III diagnostic criterion.

   Diagnostic Criteria for Chronic Motor Tic Disorder are:

   A. Presence of recurrent, involuntary, repetitive, rapid, purposeless motor movements (tics) involving no more than three muscle groups at any one time.

   B. Unvarying intensity of the tics over weeks or months.

   C. Ability to suppress the movements voluntarily for minutes to hours.

   D. Duration of at least one year.

3. Tourette's Disorder.

   This disorder was named after Georges Gilles de la Tourette who described nine of these patients in the late 19th century. Shapiro et al. (1973)* write that onset of the disorder is almost invariably before the age of 13, (half the patients before 6.5 years). The disorder begins with a single tic in half the patients. Others begin with from two to eight symptoms often including vocal tics such as grunts, yelps, snorts, etc. (Shapiro et al. 1976).

   According to Woodrow (1975) the symptoms usually begin with eye blinking, facial twitching, or neck movement and progress cephalocaudally to (1) shoulders, upper extremities, and chest, and (2) lower extremities. Months to years later, vocal tics typically appear. At one time it was thought that coprolalia was always a symptom of this disorder. Coprolalia is present in about one-half (Woodrow, 1975) to 60% (Shapiro et al., 1976) of the patients.

   Symptom shifts will occur periodically; some drop out to be replaced by others or additional symptoms are added. The intensity of the symptoms will vary across time. Woodrow (1975) points out

---

*Arthur Shapiro and his associates have written extensively about this disorder. For a very succinct and yet comprehensive description of Tourette's Disorder see: Shapiro et al. in Volume 14 of Advances in Neurology.

that an increase of activity seems to come when the patient is under stress, is tired, is angry or excited; and symptom activity will tend to decrease with sleepiness, fever, or relaxation.

The differential diagnosis must include a variety of disorders which have associated abnormal motor activity. Woodrow (1975) specifically mentions the stereotypic or perseverative motor activity seen in some schizophrenics and in patients with Amphetamine Intoxication. A great many neurological disorders have unusual motor activity associated but do not include vocal tic.

There is some controversy over whether or not certain personality factors play a role in the etiology of this disorder. Woodrow (1975) notes that two clusters of personality characteristics seem to be present: (1) Extroversion, and (2) Compulsivity. He goes on to describe them as, "obedient, well-behaved, perfectionistic, and anxious, with marked difficulty in the overt expression of anger" (p. 462).

On the other hand, Shapiro et al. (1976) say that there is no evidence that Tourette's patients have "Schizophrenia, underlying psychosis, inhibited aggression, obsessive compulsive neurosis, hysteria, common premorbid personalities, psychopathology or personality characteristics" (p. 279). Silver (1980) states that the most likely cause of Tourette's Disorder is some type of central nervous system disorder.

The diagnostic criteria of Tourette's Disorder are:

A. Age at onset between 2 and 15 years.

B. Presence of recurrent, involuntary, repetitive, rapid, purposeless motor movements affecting multiple muscle groups.

C. Multiple vocal tics.

D. Ability to suppress movements voluntarily for minutes to hours.

E. Variations in the intensity of the symptoms over weeks or months.

F. Duration of more than one year.

The treatment of choice for Tourette's Disorder is pharmacological. Specifically, haloperidol (Haldol) is used to control both the motor and vocal tics. The effective dosage will vary individually so the dosage must be titrated beginning at 0.25 mg per day. Since the half life of this butyrophenone compound, a neuroleptic, is four days, increases of 0.25 mg per day can be made at five day intervals until a therapeutic level is established. It is important also to prescribe benztropine mesylate (Cogentin) in order to prevent dystonic reactions to the haloperidol (Shapiro et al., 1978).

The consensus is that the patient with Tourette's Disorder should also be followed in psychotherapy if for no other reason than to help the individual deal with the psychosocial aspects of the disorder which can be quite serious - social isolation, academic-problems, depression, lowered self-esteem, etc.

4. Atypical Stereotyped Movement Disorder.

    This group of disorders is distinguishable from the three previous disorders by intentionality, i.e., these disorders are voluntary movements such as head banging, rocking, and repetitive hand movements. In some children the behavior is relatively benign and disappears spontaneously or with a minimum of intervention. In other instances the behavior may be symptomatic of a serious disorder such as Mental Retardation or Pervasive Developmental Disorder.

    Not only are these behaviors voluntary, but they also seem to be pleasurable for the child and to furnish him some form of relief-presumably from tension.

    Head banging may be rhythmic, hitting on the mattress or crib side or may take the form of what Silver (1980) calls tantrum banging which is a part of a temper tantrum.

    Hand movements are rhythmic fluttering or shaking movements which seem to be pleasurable for the child. A similar type of hand movement is often seen in children with Pervasive Developmental Disorder and in Autistic children. The behavior may well be relatively innocuous, however.

    Rocking has the same rhythmic, pleasurable, voluntary features as head banging and hand movements. It is most often seen in the child just before he goes to sleep.

****

GO TO VIDEOTAPE

****

C. OTHER DISORDERS WITH PHYSICAL MANIFESTATIONS

The disorders in this group are related to a variety of physical functions: speech; elimination; and sleep. DSM-III points out that these disorders are included because they traditionally have been considered symptoms of other mental disorders, although consensus is now that most of the children with these disorders do not have other mental disorders.

1. Stuttering (Stammering).

    "The literature on stutterers and stuttering (or stammering) is ancient, vast, contradictory, and inconclusive" (Eisensen, 1963, p. 216). The disorder is viewed by speech pathologists as a "defect of speech-flow" (Perkins, 1977). A large number of people experience transient episodes of stuttering. Between 50% and 80% of diagnosable stutterers recover spontaneously (DSM-III, 1980). Perkins (1977) notes that the incidence of stuttering is about 1% of the total population, most of whom are children since there is such a high recovery rate.

    Onset of the disorder is most often between 2 and 7 years of age (Perkins, 1977) with the biggest incidence at around 3 years (Rousey, 1979). The onset is usually gradual, with syllables and words being fragmented. There may be weeks or months during which the child has no difficulty; then there may be periods of severe fragmentation and repetition of syllables and words.

    There have been a great many theories of etiology offered to explain stuttering. Eisenson (1963) summarizes into three groups the theories of causation of stuttering:

    a. Unconscious need to stutter based in neurotic conflict.
    b. Emotional or constitutional vulnerability to the breakdown of neuromuscular and intellectual coordination needed in order to effectively speak.
    c. Learned act in which the anticipation of stuttering increases the likelihood of further stuttering.

    Schwartz (1976) makes a very convincing or at least thought-provoking argument for a genetic role in stuttering. He notes that the concordance rate for monozygotic twins is 90% (7% in dizygotics); that the ratio of male to female stutterers is 4:1 (sex linked?); and that about three-fourths of adult stutterers have a familial history of stuttering 7½ times greater than that of nonstutterers who have a stutterer in the family.

    Most authorities do acknowledge, regardless of theoretical orientation, that stress tends to increase stuttering. The stress may be situational, may be connected with a specific fear, may be physical, or may be internally idiosyncratically derived. The stress, whatever the source, does seem to produce laryngospasm which leads to the stuttering (Schwartz, 1976).

    The diagnostic criteria for Stuttering are:

    Frequent repetitions or prolongations of sounds, syllables, or words; or frequent, unusual hesitations and pauses that disrupt the rhythmic flow of speech.

2. Functional Enuresis.

An individual above the age of four years who repetitively and involuntarily urinates in his bed while asleep (nocturnal) or his clothes while awake (diurnal) is said to be enuretic. Some persons suffer from both nocturnal and diurnal enuresis. Enuresis occurs far more frequently in males than in females, in the range of 2:1.

Enuresis is described as either primary or secondary. Primary enuresis refers to an individual who has never developed sustained urinary continence (for at least one year). Secondary enuresis refers to the individual who has been continent for a period of at least a year and then becomes incontinent. Secondary enuresis is often associated with neurotic conflict (e.g., the birth of a sibling, separation from a parent) or with emotionally stressful life events (e.g., move to a new city, school entry). In any case secondary enuresis is viewed as a regressive phenomenon (Pierce, 1980).

This designation of primary and secondary enuresis may be somewhat confusing because some authors (Ritvo et al., 1969) refer to secondary enuresis as being secondary to demonstrable organic causes. Indeed incontinence can be traced to central nervous system disorders (spinal tumors, spina bifida, epilepsy, etc.) or genitourinary tract problems (anomalies of the urethra, kidney stones, cystitis, etc.) or a variety of other organic causes (diabetes insipidus, intestinal parasites,etc.). The number of children presenting with symptoms of enuresis for which an organic cause is later demonstrated is very small.

The diagnosis of Functional Enuresis is usually relatively easy to make on the basis of the history and physical examination. You should continue to be alert, of course, to the possibility of an organic cause later becoming evident. The combination of nocturnal and diurnal wetting increases the possibility of an underlying organic cause (Pierce, 1980).

It is not unusual for enuresis to be associated with sleepwalking and with night terrors.

> Note: See Chapter 14, Sleep Disorders, for additional information regarding Functional Enuresis.

The diagnostic criteria for Functional Enuresis are:

A.   Repeated involuntary voiding of urine by day or at night.

B.   At least two such events per month for children between the ages of five and six, and at least one event per month for older children.

C. Not due to a physical disorder, such as diabetes or a seizure disorder.

Treatment of this disorder is most frequently managed by the pediatrician or the family practitioner. As a group, children with enuresis do not fit a specific personality pattern. There are, however, a great many psychoanalytic theories of causation mostly related to the symbolism of the behavior, and treatment of persistent Functional Enuresis until recent years has centered around psychotherapy.

Pharmacological approaches to the problem have been many, including belladonna and other anticholinergic drugs, various tranquilizers, and antidepressants. Imipramine has been effective with some enuretic patients. Werry (1982), on the other hand, contends that the behavioral approach (bed-buzzer device) is superior to the use of imipramine.

Short-term and long-term psychotherapy also have had mixed results, as has psychoanalysis. It is likely that when there is an underlying mental disorder these treatment methods are more effective; in the majority of enuretic children, however, no such disorder is identifiable.

Most recently a resurgence in the use of techniques of behavior modification has been seen in the treatment of enuresis. Werry and Cohrssen (1965) report a 30% success rate among a group of severe, primary enuretic children with the use of the "bed-buzzer". This and other such devices sound an alarm when the child wets the bed. In this way the child is conditioned to wake up when he senses the need to urinate. Eventually the buzzer is not needed. Remember that in the majority of cases the enuresis remits spontaneously. Virtually all patients become continent by adolescence, although a very small percentage remain enuretic into adulthood.

3. Functional Encopresis.

Normally in our culture bowel control is established in a child by the age of two or three years. Certainly by the fifth birthday a child is expected to no longer defecate in his clothes. Primary and secondary distinguish two types of encopresis, just as with enuresis. That is, primary encopresis refers to a person above the age of four years who has never attained fecal continence, and secondary encopresis to a person who was "toilet trained" for a period of at least a year but began soiling his clothes again. Onset of secondary encopresis is usually between 4½ and 5 years of age (Hoag, et al., 1971).

In a well-designed study, Levine (1975) reported on 102 encopretic children. He found that excitement or stress seemed to be an important factor in episodes of fecal incontinence with a significant number of these children. He also reported associated Functional Enuresis in about one-third of his subjects. The children in the study were predominantly males at a ratio of nearly 6:1. Pierce (1980) and Levine (1975) both report that episodes of fecal incontinence usually occur in late afternoon and early evening. Nocturnal encopresis is unusual, just the opposite of the pattern of enuresis.

There seem to be two patterns of encopresis in terms of the child's awareness of the need to defecate. In some instances the child puts off going to the bathroom until it is too late; in others he denies anticipatory awareness of the need to have a bowel movement (Fisher, 1979).

Etiology is not established for this disorder. Ruling out organic causes (anatomical anomalies, gastroenteritis, for examples), one is left with speculation about psychological causation. Most of the speculation has centered around the mother-child relationship, often specifically around toilet training. In secondary encopresis, the behavior has been viewed as regressive, i.e., the expression of a wish to be dependent again like an infant. Other views have noted the anal retentive aspects in terms of the parent-child struggle over control.

Three theories of etiology emerge frequently in the literature: that of early and aggressive toilet training procedures by the mother; traits of compulsivity and neatness on the part of the mother (and often the child himself); and lack of warmth or at least ambivalence about the maternal role.

The diagnostic criteria for Functional Encopresis are:

A. Repeated, voluntary or involuntary passage of feces of normal or near-normal consistency into places not appropriate for that purpose in the individual's own sociocultural setting.

B. At least one such event a month after the age of four.

C. Not due to a physical disorder, such as aganglionic megacolon.

The pediatrician or family physician is the person who most often deals with this problem. Patients who do not respond or remit spontaneously are then referred to psychiatrists. This happens most frequently at school entry when social pressure comes very forcibly to bear.

Regardless of who treats the encopretic child, the physiological aspects of the disorder must be given some attention (constipation, megacolon, etc.). The treatment regimen must also include some educational aspects regarding bowel movements for the child as well as the parents. Even after a successful course of psychotherapy the behavior may remain until very practical aspects of bowel control are learned. This may be done by helping the child learn the cues necessary for bowel training (the fecal mass moving into the rectum, for example, may have to be learned by the child as a cue to the need to go to the toilet to defecate).

4. Sleepwalking Disorder (Somnambulism).

    Ablon and Mack (1979) and Broughton (1968) describe a typical sleepwalking episode:

    a. child sits up abruptly
    b. eyes are open but he appears not to see things
    c. leaves the bed (or in a brief episode may remain sitting up in bed)
    d. moves about, opening drawers, doors, etc.
    e. returns to bed
    f. difficult to awaken

    In a review article on sleep disorders in infants and children, Anders and Weinstein (1972) note that perhaps as many as 15% of all children between 5 and 12 years of age have had at least one episode of sleepwalking. Persistent sleepwalking occurs in 1-6% of the population, mostly in children and more often in males than females. Numerous authorities have noted the association among enuresis, sleepwalking, and sleep terrors (Anders & Weinstein, 1972; Broughton, 1968; Kales & Kales, 1974).

    All of these disorders seem to occur primarily during stage 4 of NREM sleep prior to cycling back to REM sleep. Thus the disorders of sleep, sleepwalking and sleep terrors, are considered to be arousal disorders.

    In children no specific psychopathology is consistently found among sleepwalkers, and developmental delays in CNS maturation are hypothesized for many of these children. Indeed the great majority of these children "outgrow" the disorder (Kales & Kales, 1974). Adults, on the other hand, frequently demonstrate specific mental disorders such as Schizophrenia, schizoid personalities, and neurotic disorders (Sours et al., 1963).

    NOTE: See Chapter 14, Sleep Disorders, for additional information regarding sleepwalking.

    The diagnostic criteria for Sleepwalking Disorder are:

    A. There are repeated episodes of arising from bed during sleep and walking about for several minutes to a half hour, usually occurring between 30 and 200 minutes after onset of sleep (the interval of sleep that typically contains EEG delta activity, sleep stages 3 and 4).

B.   While sleepwalking, the individual has a blank staring face; is relatively unresponsive to the efforts of others to influence the sleepwalking or to communicate with him or her; and can be wakened only with great difficulty.

C.   Upon awakening (either from the sleepwalking episode or the next morning), the individual has amnesia for the route traversed and for what happened during the episode.

D.   Within several minutes of awakening from the sleepwalking episode, there is no impairment of mental activity or behavior (although there may initially be a short period of confusion or disorientation).

E.   There is no evidence that the episode occurred during REM sleep or that there is abnormal electrical brain activity during sleep.

Treatment of the disorder is usually not necessary, but adults need to be instructed to provide a safe environment (locked windows, removal of potentially harmful objects, etc.). In intractible cases psychotherapy may be indicated. Diazepam (Valium) has been used on the basis of its ability to suppress stages 3 and 4 sleep. However, Kales and Kales (1974) indicate that they have found no "clear-cut decrease in the incidence of sleepwalking episodes" (p. 489).

5.   Sleep Terror Disorder (Pavor Nocturnus).

Sleep Terror is characterized by intense autonomic nervous system arousal, intense anxiety, motility, loud vocalizations, and amnesia for the episode (Ablon & Mack, 1979; Anders & Weinstein, 1972). Nightmares are far less intense than Sleep Terrors, produce less anxiety, and occur during REM stage sleep; in addition, memory for the dream is often present with nightmares. The Sleep Terror, like Sleepwalking and Enuresis, typically occurs during stages 3 and 4 of NREM sleep, and, like Sleepwalking, is considered a sleep arousal disorder.

The disorder is seen most frequently in preschool children, but may have an onset during or continue into adulthood. Generally no treatment is needed, but diazepam often is given in severe cases in an effort to suppress stage 4 NREM sleep.

The diagnostic criteria for Sleep Terror Disorder are:

A.   Repeated episodes of abrupt awakening (lasting 1-10 minutes) from sleep, usually occurring between 30 and 200 minutes after onset of sleep (the interval of sleep that typically contains EEG delta activity, sleep stages 3 and 4) and usually beginning with a panicky scream.

B. Intense anxiety during the episode and at least three of the following signs of autonomic arousal:

(1) tachycardia
(2) rapid breathing
(3) dilated pupils
(4) sweating
(5) piloerection

C. Relative unresponsiveness to efforts of others to comfort the individual during the episode and, almost invariably, confusion, disorientation, and perseverative motor movements (e.g., picking at pillow).

D. No evidence that the episode occurred during REM sleep or of abnormal electrical brain activity during sleep.

QUIZ, Section V.

Circle the correct answer.

1. One diagnostic criterion for Anorexia Nervosa is that the patient must be below ___% of the body weight appropriate for age and height.

    a. 10%
    b. 15%
    c. 25%
    d. 30%
    e. 40%

TRUE or FALSE: Circle the correct letter.

T   F   2. Patients with Anorexia Nervosa usually realize that they are seriously underweight.

T   F   3. Mortality rates for Anorexia Nervosa may be as high as 21%.

Circle the correct answer(s). One or more than one answer may be correct.

4. Some of the most common physical concomitants of Anorexia Nervosa include

      a. hyperthermia.
      b. hypertension.
      c. amenorrhea.
      d. bradycardia.
      e. dehydration.

5. Anorexia may be secondary to

      a. Schizophrenia.
      b. hypothyroidism.
      c. hyperthyroidism.
      d. certain cerebral tumors.
      e. panhypopituitarism.

Fill in the blank.

6. The common fear expressed by patients with Bulimia is that they will be unable to control their _____ .

TRUE or FALSE: Circle the correct answer.

T   F   7. Bulimic episodes are often present in patients with Anorexia Nervosa.

T   F   8. Patients with Bulimia usually are aware that their eating patterns are abnormal.

Circle the correct answer(s). One or more than one answer may be correct.

9. The greatest danger from Pica is

      a. malnutrition.
      b. poisoning.

10. Mortality rates associated with Rumination are estimated to be as high as ____%.

      a. 10%
      b. 15%
      c. 25%
      d. 35%

TRUE or FALSE: Circle the correct answer.

T   F   11. In Rumination the regurgitation of food appears to be a voluntary behavior.

Circle the correct answer(s). One or more than one answer may be correct.

12. Which of the following statements is (are) TRUE regarding tics?

   a. Transient Tic Disorder usually disappears spontaneously.
   b. A tic is said to be chronic after 6 months.
   c. A tic usually can be controlled temporarily on a voluntary basis.
   d. Tics may persist throughout the life span of the individual.

13. Coprolalia is present in about ____ of the patients with Tourette's Disorder.

   a. 1/4
   b. 1/3
   c. 1/2
   d. 3/4

14. Multiple vocal tics are present in Tourette's Disorder

   a. always.
   b. usually.
   c. about one-half of the time.
   d. seldom.

15. Spontaneous recovery from diagnosable stuttering occurs in about _____% of the cases.

   a. 10-25%
   b. 20-45%
   c. 50-80%
   d. 75-90%

16. Enuresis may be "secondary" to

   a. conflicts (e.g., birth of a sibling).
   b. stressful life events (e.g., school entry).
   c. CNS disorders (e.g., spina bifida, epilepsy).
   d. GU tract problems (e.g., kidney stones).

17. Regarding Functional Enuresis, which of the following is(are) TRUE?

   a. The ratio is 2:1; male:female.
   b. There is usually a demonstrable organic cause for the enuresis.
   c. The combination of nocturnal and diurnal enuresis increases the likelihood of an organic cause for the enuresis.
   d. Diagnosis of enuresis is most frequently made in the three to four year age range.

18. Which of the following statements is(are) <u>TRUE</u> regarding Functional Encopresis?

    a. The ratio is 3:1; boys:girls.
    b. Episodes usually occur in late afternoon or early evening.
    c. Nocturnal encopresis is very unusual.
    d. The diagnosis of Functional Encopresis rules out the diagnosis of Functional Enuresis.

19. The concept of sleepwalking (and sleep terror) as an "arousal" disorder is related to the fact that the episode usually takes place during _____ sleep.

    a. REM
    b. Stage 1 of NREM
    c. Stage 2 of NREM
    d. Stage 4 of NREM

TRUE or FALSE: Circle the correct answer.

T   F   20. Sleepwalking seen in children is associated with other mental disorders, such as Schizophrenia or schizoid disorders.

T   F   21. A sleep terror is essentially the same as a nightmare.

T   F   22. Sleep Terror Disorder usually requires treatment in the form of intensive psychotherapy.

VI. DEVELOPMENTAL

There are two subgroupings of disorders in this section, Pervasive Developmental Disorders and Specific Developmental Disorders. The common theme, of course, is that all of the disorders in this section of the chapter are highlighted by deficits or failures in the development process.

A. PERVASIVE DEVELOPMENTAL DISORDERS

The disorders in this category are Infantile Autism and Childhood Onset Pervasive Developmental Disorder, each of which has two forms (full syndrome is present or residual, i.e., the full syndrome was once present). In addition, there is a third disorder, the Atypical Pervasive Developmental Disorder.

The World Health Organization Seminar on Psychiatric Disorder in 1967 (Rutter et al., 1969) developed a system of classification of psychoses seen in children. DSM-III in essence follows this categorization system:

   a. Infantile Psychosis (Infantile Autism in DSM-III);
   b. Disintegrative Psychosis (Childhood Onset Pervasive Developmental Disorder in DSM-III);
   c. Schizophrenia (Adult criteria of DSM-III);
   d. Other Psychoses (various other psychotic disorders of DSM-III).

A crucial differentiating feature is the age of onset of the disorder. Infantile Autism has its onset before 2½ years of age; Childhood Onset Pervasive Developmental Disorder postulates a period of normal development prior to onset of symptoms (Kolvin, 1971; Rutter et al., 1969).

   1. Infantile Autism.

In 1943 Leo Kanner described and named this disorder early infantile autism. His description of the disorder nearly 40 years ago has been altered very little, "an instance almost unexampled in child psychology" (Eisenberg, 1971, p. 2).

Rutter (1975) reports that work by him and his colleagues basically confirms the description of the disorder by Kanner. There are three symptoms which are present in virtually all autistic children: "profound and general failure to develop social relationships; language retardation with impaired comprehension, echolalia, and pronominal reversal; and ritualistic or compulsive phenomena" (p. 329). In addition there are four other symptoms listed which are frequently found in autistic children: repetitive, stereotyped movements, especially of the hands; short attention span; a tendency to self-inflicted injuries (like head banging); and toilet training problems (Rutter, 1975).

The failure to develop social relationships is quite dramatic in that these children fail to respond to human beings, often from birth. They become fascinated by objects (inanimate) and ignore or "look through" people as though the people were not present.

ANSWERS, Section V. _____

1.	c	12.	a,c,d
2.	F	13.	c
3.	T	14.	a
4.	c,d,e	15.	c
5.	a,b,c,d,e	16.	a,b,c,d
6.	binges	17.	a,c
7.	T	18.	b,c
8.	T	19.	d
9.	b	20.	F
10.	c	21.	F
11.	T	22.	F

They are frequently mute; Kanner (1972) says that about one-third of them do not learn to speak. Their language impairment and failure to respond to others lead one to think initially that they are either deaf or profoundly retarded. In truth, deafness among autistic children is no more common than in the normal population. When it does develop, language of the autistic child is quite idiosyncratic. Echolalia is often present as is reversal of pronouns ("you" for "I," for example). The communication deficits extend to gestures and non-verbal communication. It is generally thought that 2/3 to 3/4 of autistic children will perform throughout life on a retarded level (Rutter, 1970).

The life of the autistic child is highly ritualized. He wants nothing moved or changed in his environment and becomes quite upset if schedules or even furniture placement is altered, particularly if changes are made in his own personal environment (his room).

The etiology of Infantile Autism is unknown. Although the disorder is rare (DSM-III says 2-4/10,000) a great deal of research has been done on this fascinating disorder. Until relatively recently (the last 10-15 years) the cause of the disorder was generally considered psychogenic and placed at the feet of cold, aloof, perfectionistic parents. There is now evidence, although far from conclusive at this point, that organic factors play a major role.

Hier et al., (1979) report that computerized brain tomography revealed that the right parieto-occipital region is wider than the left in 57% of the autistic children in their study. They speculate that the location of the asymmetry near the posterior language area may account for the language deficit.

Biochemical research is being carried on, with promising leads but no definitive results at this time (Piggott, 1979). Being studied are such things as catecholamines (lowered dopamine-B-hydroxylase (DBH) serum levels in autistic children), indoleamines (serotonin metabolism and blood serotonin levels), enzymes and immunologic system deficiencies.

The cognitive deficits certainly suggest the possibility of organic problems from genetic transmission, trauma, infection or some other cause. Rutter (1975) summarizes the possible outcomes of research into three general areas:

a. single cause condition (like PKU),
b. a behavioral syndrome with a common biological outcome but no single cause (like cerebral palsy),
c. interactive cause including both biological and psychosocial factors.

Differential diagnosis must include the various developmental deviations (hearing, language, etc.), Mental Retardation (which may co-exist), Schizophrenia, and Childhood Onset Pervasive Developmental Disorder.

The diagnostic criteria for Infantile Autism are:

A. Onset before 30 months.

B. Pervasive lack of responsiveness to other people (autism).

C. Gross deficits in language development.

D. If speech is present, peculiar speech patterns such as immediate and delayed echolalia, metaphorical language, pronominal reversal.

E. Bizarre responses to various aspects of the environment, e.g., resistance to change, peculiar interest in or attachments to animate or inanimate objects.

F. Absence of delusions, hallucinations, loosening of associations, and incoherence as in Schizophrenia.

The treatment of Infantile Autism in recent years has focused on a behavioral approach "applied more in a developmental context" (Rutter, 1975, p. 349). That is to say the goals of treatment have aimed at helping the autistic child develop social and language skills which more nearly approximate the norms of expected behavior. Parental involvement in behavioral treatment, as well as in political and community action, has increased dramatically in the last decade (Reichler & Schopler, 1976).

Largely through the efforts of parents and professionals, educational programs have sprung up around the United States, programs designed to meet the needs of autistic children. One of the earliest and most successful has been the League School in Brooklyn, New York; however, smaller communities have developed behavioral-educational schools which have become an important part of the treatment for autistic children.

As with any significantly disabling disorder for which no definitive treatment has been established, a wide variety of treatment approaches emerge. Many of these are attempts at "one-shot-cures" for the disorder. Infantile Autism is no different, in this sense, from such disorders as rheumatoid arthritis or cancer. Such things as megavitamin therapy, hemodialysis, and body patterning have been tried without success.

The children who make significant progress in treatment most often continue to have a psychiatric diagnosis, that of Infantile Autism, Residual State. The diagnostic criteria for this disorder are:

A.   The child once had an illness that met the criteria for Infantile Autism.

B.   The current clinical picture no longer meets the full criteria for Infantile Autism, but signs of the illness have persisted to the present, such as oddities of communication and social awkwardness.

2.   Childhood Onset Pervasive Developmental Disorder (COPDD).

This diagnosis is reserved for children who have developed relatively normally for at least the first 2½ years of life and then experience what seems to be a disintegration of behavior, emotion, and relationships with others. There is often a regression of certain functions such as speech and bowel control.

Mahler (1968) has differentiated between Kannerian early infantile autism and what she calls symbiotic psychosis in essentially developmental terms. In short, the child with Infantile Autism has never reached the normal symbiotic phase (beginning at 2-3 months of age) - "that state of undifferentiation, of fusion with mother" (Mahler, 1968, p. 9). In symbiotic psychosis the child either becomes fixated at the symbiotic stage or regresses to that stage.

In general this concept fits with the concept of "disintegration psychosis" in the World Health Organization classification system (Rutter et al., 1969) and with the category of Childhood Onset Pervasive Developmental Disorder (COPDD) in DSM-III.

Phenomenologically, there are similarities between Infantile Autism and Childhood Onset Pervasive Developmental Disorder, but clear differences as well. In both instances there are severely impaired social relations, but in COPDD there is also clinging behavior (usually with mother or substitute). Age of onset is different, below 2½ years for autism and above 2½ years for COPDD. Affective response is often grossly inappropriate in COPDD, as is true in autism, but often the autistic child simply does not respond at all. Both disorders share such things as a compulsive devotion to sameness in the environment, unusual motor behavior and fascination for and attachment to objects.

One very essential difference is in the area of language development. It has been noted that in the autistic child language may not develop at all, and when it does the use of it is usually idiosyncratic and the impairment extends to nonverbal communication. The child with COPDD also has peculiarities of language, but these are often peculiarities of expression such as odd inflections or lack of inflection.

The adult syndrome of Schizophrenia may also be diagnosed in children if the criteria are met. We have some doubt that this will ever be done appropriately in young children given the differences in development between adults, or even older children, and young children. Note, too, that a criterion for diagnosis of either Infantile Autism or Childhood Onset Pervasive Developmental Disorder is the absence of hallucinations and delusions. You will recall that these are prominent features of Schizophrenia.

The diagnostic criteria for Childhood Onset Pervasive Developmental Disorder are:

A.   Gross and sustained impairment in social relationships, e.g., lack of appropriate affective responsivity, inappropriate clinging, asociality, lack of empathy.

B.   At least three of the following:

(1) sudden excessive anxiety manifested by such symptoms as free-floating anxiety, catastrophic reactions to everyday occurrences, inability to be consoled when upset, unexplained panic attacks
(2) constricted or inappropriate affect, including lack of appropriate fear reactions, unexplained rage reactions, and extreme mood lability
(3) resistance to change in the environment (e.g., upset if dinner time is changed), or insistence on doing things in the same manner every time (e.g., putting on clothes always in the same order)
(4) oddities of motor movements, such as peculiar posturing, peculiar hand or finger movements, or walking on tiptoe
(5) abnormalities of speech, such as questionlike melody, monotonous voice
(6) hyper- or hypo-sensitivity to sensory stimuli, e.g., hyperacusis
(7) self-mutilation, e.g., biting or hitting self, head banging

C.   Onset of the full syndrome after 30 months of age and before 12 years of age.

      D.   Absence of delusions, hallucinations, incoherence, or marked loosening of associations.

This, like Infantile Autism, is a profound disorder with a generally poor prognosis for normal functioning. The prognosis is probably somewhat better for COPDD than for Infantile Autism.

Treatment for COPDD is not unlike that described for Infantile Autism in terms of a behavior approach, parent involvement, and special education programs.

There is also a diagnostic category of Atypical Pervasive Developmental Disorder which is used when a child has serious developmental deviations in the areas of social relationships and language, but does not meet the criteria of either Infantile Autism or Childhood Onset Developmental Disorder.

****

GO TO VIDEOTAPE

****

B.   SPECIFIC DEVELOPMENTAL DISORDERS

    Note: These are diagnosed on Axis II because they so often co-exist with other disorders even though they are not due to other disorders.

These disorders represent failures or deviations in the development of specific abilities such as reading, talking, computation, etc. We will provide here brief descriptions of these disorders and the DSM-III diagnostic criteria for them. DSM-III notes the controversy surrounding the inclusion of these categories as mental disorders since often no other psychopathology exists and treatment is usually carried out in settings such as schools and speech clinics.

    1.   Developmental Reading Disorder.

        The written word is an invention of man. The ability to read is a complex developmental task involving visual, to some extent auditory, and cognitive skills. Other factors, such as motivation, organic integrity, and intellectual level, all play important roles in the acquisition and proficiency of reading ability.

        Probably the best single predictor of reading ability is intelligence. However, a reading level below that expected on the basis of age, amount of instruction (school), and intelligence defines Reading Disorder.

A number of explanations for the disorder have been offered, but generally fall into one of the following categories:

    a. organic brain dysfunction (minimal brain dysfunction), usually undefined by neurological examination or EEG, particularly, it is speculated, in the left hemisphere

    b. sensory deficits, particularly visual and/or auditory

    c. sociocultural factors, related to identification with a subcultural value system and leading to decreased motivation

    d. emotional factors which lead to such things as decreased attention, low energy level, or increased anxiety

    e. a combination of more than one of these

Reading Disability may have a significant effect, of course, on all areas of academic achievement and frequently leads to decreased self-esteem and social isolation.

Dysfunction in reading ability is often a part of mental disorders such as Attention Deficit Disorders. If this is the case the diagnosis of Reading Disability is also made. In the case of Pervasive Developmental Disorders the reading dysfunction is considered a part of the disorder and is not diagnosed separately. The same is true for a diagnosis of Mental Retardation.

The diagnostic criteria for Reading Disorder are:

Performance on standardized, individually administered tests of reading skill is significantly below the expected level, given the individual's schooling, chronological age, and mental age (as determined by individually administered IQ test). In addition, in school, the child's performance on tasks requiring reading skills is significantly below his or her intellectual capacity.

2. Developmental Arithmetic Disorder.

In terms of theories of causation, what has been said about Reading Disorder generally will apply to Arithmetic Disorder. This disorder, however, is more unusual and does not seem to have the same social and academic consequences as Reading Disorder. It is not unusual for a child to experience both disorders.

The diagnostic criteria for Arithmetic Disorder are:

Performance on standardized, individually administered tests of arithmetic achievement is significantly below expected level, given the individual's schooling, chronological age, and mental age (as determined by an individually administered IQ test). In addition, in school, the child's performance on tasks requiring arithmetic skills is significantly below his or her intellectual capacity.

3. Developmental Language Disorder.

DSM-III notes that language problems may be: a failure to develop language (as in some cases of profound mental retardation and of Pervasive Developmental Disorders); a loss of language ability, usually as the result of an organic disorder; or "delayed language acquisition" (p. 95).

The diagnosis of Developmental Language Disorder is in the delayed language acquisition category. There are two types described, expressive and receptive. The expressive type of Developmental Language Disorder is much more common than the receptive type. Stevenson and Richman (1976) report between 5 and 6 nonretarded children per 1,000 in the expressive type and Howlin (1981) suggests that there are less than 1 per 10,000 in the receptive category. Howlin also notes that children in the receptive category often have a concomitant partial hearing loss.

The child with expressive type of language disorder will be able to understand spoken language but will be unable to verbalize. This is not unlike the normal pattern of language development in which comprehension precedes expression. Children (and adults learning a new language), to put it another way, have a larger passive vocabulary than an active one.

The more disabling of these two disorders is the receptive type, since failure to develop adequately the ability to understand language is accompanied by a failure to express language.

The diagnostic criteria for Developmental Language Disorder, Expressive Type, are:

A. Failure to develop vocal expression (encoding) of language despite relatively intact comprehension of language.

B. Presence of inner language (the presence of age-appropriate concepts, such as understanding the purpose and use of a particular household object).

C. Not due to Mental Retardation, Childhood Onset Pervasive Developmental Disorder, hearing impairment, or trauma.

The diagnostic criteria for Developmental Language, Receptive Type, are:

A. Failure to develop comprehension (decoding) and vocal expression (encoding) of language.

  B. Not due to hearing impairment, trauma, Mental Retardation, or Childhood Onset Pervasive Developmental Disorder.

4. Developmental Articulation Disorder.

This disorder, popularly known as "speech defect" has to do with the inability to pronounce certain sounds. There are varying degrees of the disorder, and many children make adequate adjustment if the disorder is mild. The inability to articulate certain sounds does not effect comprehension or abilities in grammar or writing.

Sometimes articulation problems are mechanically determined (tongue, palate, or vocal organs) and can be corrected surgically (Howlin, 1981).

The diagnostic criteria for Developmental Articulation Disorder are:

  A. Failure to develop consistent articulations of the later-acquired speech sounds, such as r, sh, th, f, z, l, or ch.

  B. Not due to Developmental Language Disorder, Mental Retardation, Childhood Onset Pervasive Developmental Disorder, or physical disorders.

There are two other categories in this group: Mixed Specific Developmental Disorder, which is used when there is more than one of the Specific Developmental Disorders present but none is dominant; and Atypical Specific Developmental Disorder, a residual category for Specific Developmental Disorders not covered in the other categories.

Treatment of the Specific Developmental Disorders generally is not medical unless the distress (anxiety, depression, etc.) over the disorder requires attention. Most of these children are seen in speech and hearing clinics and/or special remedial education programs.

QUIZ, Section VI.

Circle the correct answer.

1. Three of the following symptoms are found in virtually all children with Infantile Autism. Which one is <u>not</u> (although it may be seen frequently)?

  a. profound and general failure to develop social relationships
  b. repetitive, stereotyped movements
  c. language retardation
  d. ritualistic or compulsive phenomena

TRUE or FALSE: Circle the correct answer.

T   F   2.   Childhood Onset Pervasive Developmental Disorder is the same as Schizophrenia in adults.

Circle the correct answer(s).   <u>One</u> or <u>more</u> <u>than</u> <u>one</u> answer may be correct.

3.   Infantile Autism and Childhood Onset Pervasive Developmental Disorders share which of the following?

   a.   same age at onset
   b.   same language impairment
   c.   relate to people in the same manner
   d.   neither experiences delusions or hallucinations

Match each numbered item with the correct lettered responses.

4.   ___ Attention Deficit Disorder

5.   ___ Childhood Onset Pervasive Developmental Disorder

6.   ___ Mental Retardation

7.   ___ Infantile Autism

   a.   Reading Disorder diagnosed on Axis II
   b.   Reading Disorder diagnosed on Axis I
   c.   Reading Disorder not diagnosed

Circle the correct answer(s).   <u>One</u> or <u>more</u> <u>than</u> <u>one</u> answer may be correct.

8.   In Developmental Language Disorder which of the following statements is(are) <u>true</u>?

   a.   Receptive type is seen less often than the expressive type.
   b.   Expressive type is more disabling.
   c.   Receptive type includes expressive disability.
   d.   Expressive type includes receptive disability.

9.   Children with Developmental Articulation Disorder frequently have problems with

   a.   verbal comprehension.
   b.   writing skills.
   c.   grammar concepts.
   d.   enuresis.
   e.   none of these.

ANSWERS, Section VI. _____

1. b
2. F
3. d
4. a
5. c

6. c
7. c
8. a,c
9. e

POST TEST

For each of the following questions, <u>one</u> or <u>more than one</u> answer may be correct. Circle the correct answer(s).

1. Which of the following biological factors are thought to be causal in Mental Retardation?

   a. phenylketonuria
   b. cri du chat
   c. fetal alcohol syndrome
   d. anoxia
   e. lead poisoning
   f. congenital blindness
   g. placenta previa
   h. cleft palate

2. Which of the following statements about Mental Retardation is(are) true?

   a. Approximately 200 causes of Mental Retardation have been identified.
   b. Prevalence rates are set at about 1%.
   c. Significantly more boys than girls are retarded.
   d. Over half of the mentally retarded fall in the severe and profound categories.
   e. Approximately 10% of the mentally retarded are institutionalized.

3. Which of the following statements is(are) true regarding children with Attention Deficit Disorders?

   a. Abnormal EEG is found in 20% to 50% of hyperkinetic children.
   b. Lead poisoning may be causal in some children.
   c. Stimuli normally found in the environment tend to increase activity and distractibility.
   d. It is commonly thought that environmental factors, such as psychopathology in family members, play an important primary role in the origin of the disorder.

4. "Significantly subaverage intellectual functioning" refers to a score below _____ on an individually administered I.Q. test.

   a. 100
   b. 90
   c. 70
   d. 50

5. Differential diagnosis of Conduct Disorders will often include

   a. Attention Deficit Disorder.
   b. Childhood Onset Pervasive Developmental Disorder.
   c. Isolated Antisocial Act.
   d. Organic Mental Disorder.

6. Passive, withdrawn, limited eye contact, and overinhibited are all terms which are applied to children with

    a. Separation Anxiety Disorder.
    b. Avoidant Disorder.
    c. Overanxious Disorder.
    d. Schizoid Disorder.

7. Incidence rates of Attention Deficit Disorder are estimated at various rates. Probably the most realistic rate is

    a. 20%.
    b. 10%.
    c. 5%.
    d. 3%.
    e. 0.1%.

8. In Attention Deficit Disorders the most common symptom expressions which seem to be heightened by environmental stimuli are all of the following except

    a. motor activity.
    b. autonomic nervous system arousal.
    c. inattention.
    d. impulsivity.

9. Which of the following statements about intelligence tests is(are) true ?

    a. They are limited in predicting occupational success.
    b. They provide a measure of innate capacity.
    c. They predict nonacademic skills.
    d. They are unreliable for long-range prediction.

10. Although apparently unable to do so, a child with _____ Disorder wishes he could extend himself to others and be accepted and appreciated by them.

    a. Avoidant
    b. Overanxious
    c. Separation Anxiety
    d. Schizoid

11. Children with Overanxious Disorders

    a. usually are intellectually bright.
    b. often are middle children.
    c. frequently have somatic complaints.
    d. usually behave quite independently.
    e. worry a great deal about future events.

12. A 12-year-old child who appears withdrawn and socially isolated could be suffering from

     a. Avoidant Disorder.
     b. Depression.
     c. Schizoid Disorder.
     d. Oppositional Disorder.
     e. Adjustment Disorder (with withdrawal).

13. Which of the following is(are) applicable to Reactive Attachment Disorder of Infancy?

     a. failure to thrive
     b. body weight below the 3rd percentile
     c. delayed or absent development such as smiling, sucking, rooting, eye tracking, etc.
     d. maternal deprivation or neglect
     e. may be seen in adolescents or occasionally in adults

14. A young child who shows signs of withdrawal, psychomotor retardation, sleep and eating problems, and detachment probably is suffering from what Spitz calls

     a. anaclitic depression.
     b. school phobia.
     c. Agoraphobia.
     d. Separation Anxiety.

15. Which of the following disorders are differential diagnoses for Reactive Attachment Disorder of Infancy?

     a. certain physical disorders (GI, cardiac, etc.)
     b. severe Mental Retardation
     c. Schizoid Disorder
     d. Infantile Autism
     e. Tourette's Disorder

16. In the child with Oppositional Disorder the behavior may be characterized as

     a. argumentative.
     b. quarrelsome.
     c. passive-aggressive.
     d. negativistic.

17. Which of the following statements is(are) true regarding Adolescence and Identity Disorder?

    a. Onset of Identity Disorder is typically in adolescence.
    b. Our modern, technological, industrialized society tends to shorten the adolescent period.
    c. Identity Disorder is defined by subjectively determined stress over issues regarding identity.
    d. A teenager may feel distress over identity issues but not have Identity Disorder.

18. Separation anxiety is

    a. not unlike Agoraphobia in adults.
    b. a normal reponse to early forced separation (like hospitalization).
    c. a disorder often involving school refusal.
    d. best treated by forcing separation through hospitalization of the child.

19. Which of the following statements is (are) true regarding children with Elective Mutism?

    a. They will speak to a few selected people.
    b. They often do not have the ability to speak.
    c. They appear shy, withdrawn, and retiring.
    d. They often have difficulty understanding the speech of others.
    e. They are often mentally retarded.

20. Anorexia may be secondary to

    a. hypothyroidism.
    b. hyperthyroidism.
    c. panhypopituitarism.
    d. cerebral tumor.

21. Probably the most outstanding physical symptom in Anorexia Nervosa is

    a. bradycardia.
    b. bulimic episodes.
    c. cachexia.
    d. amenorrhea.

22. Rumination

    a. sometimes spontaneously remits.
    b. has a mortality rate of as much as 25% if it is persistent.
    c. may be caused by GI anomalies.
    d. usually has its onset in the first year of life.

23. A diagnostic criterion of Anorexia Nervosa is a weight loss of at least ____% of body weight (considering projected growth if the patient is under 18 years of age).

    a. 5%
    b. 10%
    c. 15%
    d. 20%
    e. 25%

24. Frequently found in the patient with Bulimia is (are)

    a. rigid diets.
    b. vomiting.
    c. use of laxatives and diuretics.
    d. fear of being underweight.
    e. lack of awareness that eating habits are abnormal.

25. Atypical Stereotyped Movement Disorder(s)

    a. are basically tics.
    b. are intentional or voluntary.
    c. are sometimes symptoms of Mental Retardation.
    d. appear to be pleasurable for the child.

26. Transient Tic Disorder

    a. is a rare disorder.
    b. may last for as long as one year.
    c. usually is seen in preschool children.
    d. may be voluntarily controlled for a limited period of time.

27. The eating "binge" is most characteristic of

    a. Anorexia Nervosa.
    b. Bulimia.
    c. Pica.
    d. Rumination.

28. Pica behavior may be

    a. normal in an 18-month-old child.
    b. related to nutritional deficit.
    c. an attempt to satisfy oral needs (in psychoanalytic terms).
    d. a feature of Infantile Autism.

29. Tourette's Disorder

    a. begins as a single tic in about half the cases.
    b. includes coprolalia in 90% of the patients.
    c. typically begins with eye, face, or neck area tics.
    d. often is a part of a schizophrenic process.
    e. includes vocal tics.

30. Stuttering is

    a. a "speech flow" defect.
    b. an articulation disorder.
    c. transient with spontaneous recovery in a large number of cases.
    d. typically increased by stress.

31. Enuresis

    a. is seen in a particular kind of personality pattern.
    b. usually disappears by adolescence if not sooner.
    c. is most frequently associated with an underlying mental disorder.
    d. occasionally may be seen in adults.

32. Regarding Sleepwalking Disorder, which of the following statements is(are) correct?

    a. It is seen in as many as 1-6% of children.
    b. Episodes typically occur during REM sleep.
    c. When seen in adults, it is more often associated with other mental disorders.
    d. The memory of the episode of sleepwalking, upon awakening, is absent in about 1/3 of the patients.

33. Enuresis is more likely (but certainly not always) to have an organic basis if it

    a. is nocturnal only.
    b. is diurnal only.
    c. is both nocturnal and diurnal.
    d. varies between nocturnal and diurnal.

34. Usually, but not always, Encopresis

    a. is seen in males.
    b. occurs in late afternoon or evening.
    c. has its onset with school entry (6-7 years of age).
    d. is associated with night terrors.

35. Diagnostic criteria for Infantile Autism include

    a. onset before 2½ years of age.
    b. lack of responsiveness to other people.
    c. attachment to one parent (usually).
    d. delusions or hallucinations.

36. Sleep Terror Disorder

    a. occurs typically during stage 3 or 4 of NREM sleep.
    b. is accompanied by intense autonomic nervous system arousal.
    c. is associated with mildly abnormal EEG findings.
    d. ends abruptly when the child screams and wakes up.

37. The three symptoms present in virtually all children with Infantile Autism are

    a. repetitive stereotyped movements.
    b. profound failure to develop social relationships.
    c. toilet training problems.
    d. language retardation (including muteness).
    e. ritualistic or compulsive behavior.

38. Diagnostic criteria for Childhood Onset Pervasive Developmental Disorder include

    a. extensive impairment in social relations.
    b. mutism in 1/3 to 1/2 of the children with this disorder.
    c. absence of delusions and hallucinations.
    d. onset before 12 years of age and after 2½ years.

39. The more disabling type of Language Disorder is

    a. expressive.
    b. receptive.

40. Match the following.

    ___ resistant to environmental change   a. trait hyperactivity
    ___ susceptible to environmental change   b. state hyperactivity

41. Match the following symptom dimensions with the descriptions of behavior.

    ___ violation of rights of others   a. socialized
        on a face-to-face basis with
        the victim
    ___ violation of rights of others   b. aggressive
        without face-to-face confron-
        tation with the victim
    ___ no bond of affection or empathy   c. undersocialized
        with others has been established
    ___ some sense of loyalty to others   d. nonaggressive
        exists, especially to a specific
        group such as a gang

42. Match the following disorders with the source of anxiety.

    ___ anxiety about performance   a. Separation Anxiety Disorder
        and achievement
    ___ anxiety about facing new   b. Avoidant Disorder
        situations or people
    ___ anxiety about being   c. Overanxious Disorder
        away from parents

Use the following key to answer questions 43-46:

    a. Concrete operations
    b. Sensorimotor period
    c. Formal operations
    d. Pre-operational period

43. The attainment of the ability to solve conservation problems comes during the ___ period.

44. The ability to form mental representations of objects, that is, to use symbols is a milestone of the ___ period.

45. Piaget's stages of cognitive development in chronological order are:

    ___ First stage
    ___ Second stage
    ___ Third stage
    ___ Fourth stage

46. The ability to perform propositional operations and think abstractly is characteristic of the ___ period.

PRE-TEST ANSWERS

1. b,d,a,c	16. a,b,c	31. b
2. a	17. b	32. b,c,d
3. c	18. a	33. a,b,c,d
4. d	19. c,b,a	34. b,d
5. a,b,e	20. a,c,e	35. a,c,e
6. a,b,c,d,e,g	21. a,b,c,d	36. b,c,d
7. a,d	22. a,b,d	37. a,c,d
8. c	23. a,b,c,e	38. c
9. a,b	24. a,c	39. b,d
10. d	25. a,b,c,d	40. a,b
11. a,c	26. a,c,d	41. a,c
12. b	27. c	42. a,b
13. a,c	28. a,b,c,d	43. b,d,e
14. b,d,c,a	29. e	44. a,b
15. a	30. a,b,c	45. a,c,d
		46. b

POST-TEST ANSWERS

1. a,b,c,d,e,g
2. a,b,e
3. a,c
4. c
5. a,c
6. b
7. d
8. b
9. a,d
10. a
11. a,c,e
12. a,b,c,e
13. a,b,c,d
14. a
15. a,b,d

16. a,b,c,d
17. a,c,d
18. a,b,c
19. a,c
20. a,b,c,d
21. c
22. a,b,c,d
23. e
24. a,b,c
25. b,c,d
26. b,d
27. b
28. b,c,d
29. a,c,e
30. a,c,d

31. b,d
32. a,c
33. c
34. a,b
35. a,b
36. a,b
37. b,d,e
38. a,c,d
39. b
40. a,b
41. b,d,c,a
42. c,b,a
43. a
44. d
45. b,d,a,c
46. c

REFERENCES

Ablon, S., & Mack, J. Sleep disorders. In J. Noshpitz (Ed.), _Basic handbook of child psychiatry_ (Vol. II). New York: Basic Books, Inc., 1979.

Ainsworth, M. _The effects of maternal deprivation_. Public Health Paper 14. Geneva: World Health Organization, 1962.

Anders, T., & Weinstein, P. Sleep and its disorders in infants and children. _Pediatrics_, 1972, _50_ (2), 312-322.

Baldwin, A. _Theories of child development_. New York: John Wiley & Sons, Inc., 1967.

Bowlby, J. _Attachment and Loss_ (Vol. 1) New York: Basic Books, Inc., 1969.

Bowlby, J. _Separation: Anxiety and anger_. New York: Basic Books, Inc., 1973.

Broughton, R. Sleep disorders: Disorders of arousal? _Science_, 1968, _159_, 1070-1078.

Bruch, H. Changing approaches to anorexia nervosa. _International Psychiatric Clinics_, 1970, _7_, 3-24.

Cantwell, D. P. Psychiatric illness in the families of hyperactive children. _Archives of General Psychiatry_, 1972, _27_, 414-417.

Coleman, M. Serotonin and central nervous system syndromes of childhood: A review. In S. Chess & A. Thomas (Eds.), _Annual progress in child psychiatry and child development_. New York: Brunner/Mazel, 1974.

Cytryn, L., & Lourie, R. Mental retardation. In H. Kaplan, A. Freedman, & B. Sadock (Eds.). _Comprehensive textbook of psychiatry_ (Vol. 3). Baltimore: Williams and Wilkins, 1980.

deMause, L. The evolution of childhood. In L. deMause (Ed.), _The history of childhood_. New York: The Psychohistory Press, 1974.

Dubey, D. Organic factors in hyperkinesis: A critical evaluation. _American Journal of Orthopsychiatry_, 1976, _46_ (2), 353-366.

Eisenberg, L. Introduction. In M. Rutter (Ed.), _Infantile autism: Concepts, characteristics and treatment_. Edinburgh: Churchill Livingstone, 1971.

Eisenberg, L. Hyperkinetic reactions. In J. Noshpitz (Ed.), _Basic handbook of child psychiatry_ (Vol. II). New York: Basic Books, Inc., 1979.

Eisensen, J. The nature of defective speech. In W. Cruickshank (Ed.), _Psychology of exceptional children and youth_ (2nd Edition). Englewood Cliffs, N.J.: Prentice-Hall, Inc., 1963.

Erikson, E. <u>Childhood and society</u>. New York: W.W. Norton & Co., 1950.

Erikson, E. Eight ages of man. In C. Stendler (Ed.), <u>Readings in child behavior and development</u> (2nd Edition). New York: Harcourt, Brace and World, Inc., 1964.

Feingold, B. F. <u>Why your child is hyperactive</u>. New York: Random House, 1975.

Feinstein, S. Identity and adjustment disorders of adolescence. In H. Kaplan, A. Freedman, & B. Sadock (Eds.), <u>Comprehensive textbook of psychiatry</u> (Vol. 3). Baltimore: Williams and Wilkins, 1980.

Finch, S., & Green, J. Personality disorders. In J. Noshpitz (Ed.), <u>Basic handbook of child psychiatry</u> (Vol. II). New York: Basic Books, Inc., 1979.

Fisher, S. Encopresis. In J. Noshpitz (Ed.), <u>Basic handbook of child psychiatry</u> (Vol. II). New York: Basic Books, Inc., 1979.

Gittleman-Klein, R. Pharmacotherapy and management of pathological separation anxiety. <u>International Journal of Mental Health</u>, 1975-76, <u>4</u>, 255-271.

Grossbard, H. Ego deficiency in delinquents. <u>Social casework</u>, 1962, <u>43</u>, 171-178.

Group for the Advancement of Psychiatry. <u>Psychopathological disorders in childhood: Theoretical considerations and a proposed classification</u>. New York: 1966.

Halmi, K. Eating disorders. In H. Kaplan,, A. Freedman, & B. Sadock (Eds.), <u>Comprehensive textbook of psychiatry</u> (Vol. 3). Baltimore: Williams and Wilkins, 1980.

Hannaway, P. Failure to thrive: A study of 100 infants and children. <u>Clinical Pediatrics</u>, 1970, <u>9</u>, 96-99.

Hier, D., LeMay, M., & Rosenberg, P. Autism and unfavorable left-right asymmetrics of the brain. <u>Journal of Autism and Developmental Disorders</u>, 1979, <u>9</u> (2), 153-159.

Hoag, J., Norris, N., Himeno, E., & Jacobs, J. The encopretic child and his family. <u>Journal of the American Academy of Child Psychiatry</u>, 1971, <u>10</u>, 242-256.

Holliday, C. <u>Women's life in colonial days</u>. Williamstown, Mass: Corner House, 1968.

Howlin, P. Language. In M. Rutter (Ed.), <u>Scientific foundations of developmental psychiatry</u>. Baltimore: University Park Press, 1981.

Jacobs, P., Brunton, M., Melville, M., Britton, R., & McClemont, W. Aggressive behavior, mental subnormality, and the XYY male. Nature, 1965, 208, 1351-1352.

Jenkins, R. Classification of behavior problems of children. American Journal of Psychiatry, 1969, 125, 1032-1039.

Jenkins, R. Behavior disorders of childhood and adolescence. Springfield, III: Charles C. Thomas, 1973.

Johnson, A. Sanctions for superego lacunae of adolescents. In K. Eissler (Ed.), Searchlights on delinquency. New York: International Universities Press, 1949.

Kales, A., & Kales, J. Sleep disorders: Recent findings in the diagnosis and treatment of disturbed sleep. New England Journal of Medicine, 1974, 290 (9), 487-498.

Kanner, L. Child psychiatry (Fourth edition). Springfield, III: Charles C. Thomas, 1972.

Knobloch, H., & Pasamanick, B. (Eds.). Gesell and Amatura's developmental diagnosis (third edition). Hagerstown, MD: Harper and Row, 1974.

Kolvin, I. Psychoses in childhood. In M. Rutter (Ed.), Infantile autism: Concepts, characteristics and treatment. Edinburgh: Churchill Livingstone, 1971.

Laufer, M., Denhoff, E., & Solomons, G. Hyperkinetic impulse disorders in children's behavior problems. Psychosomatic Medicine, 1957, 19, 38-49.

Laufer, M., & Shetty, T. Attention deficit disorders. In H. Kaplan, A. Freedman, & B. Sadock (Eds.), Comprehensive textbook of psychiatry (Vol. 3). Baltimore: Williams and Wilkins, 1980.

LaVietes, R. Schizoid disorder. In H. Kaplan, A. Freedman, & B. Sadock (Eds.), Comprehensive textbook of psychiatry (Vol. 3). Baltimore: Williams and Wilkins, 1980.

LaVietes, R. Oppositional disorder. In H. Kaplan, A. Freedman, & B. Sadock (Eds.), Comprehensive textbook of psychiatry (Vol. 3). Baltimore: Williams and Wilkins, 1980.

Laybourne, P. Elective mutism. In J. Noshpitz (Ed.), Basic handbook of child psychiatry (Vol. II). New York: Basic Books, Inc., 1979.

Levine, M. Children with encopresis: A descriptive analysis. Pediatrics, 1975, 56 (3), 412-416.

Lewis, D., Shanok, S., & Pincus, J. The neuropsychiatric status of violent male juvenile delinquents. In D. Lewis (Ed.), Vulnerabilities to delinquency. New York: Spectrum Publications, 1981.

Lidz, T. The person (Revised edition). New York: Basic Books, Inc., 1976.

Loney, J. Hyperkinesis comes of age: What do we know and where should we go? American Journal of Orthopsychiatry, 1980, 50 (1), 28-42.

Lucas, A. Tic: Gilles de la Tourette's Syndrome. In J. Noshpitz (Ed.), Basic handbook of child psychiatry (Vol. II). New York: Basic Books, Inc., 1979.

Mahler, M. On human symbiosis and the vicissitudes of individuation (Vol. I: Infantile psychosis). New York: International Universities Press, Inc., 1968.

Mahler, M., Pine, F., & Bergman, A. The psychological birth of the human infant. New York: Basic Books, Inc., 1975.

Malleus Maleficarum (M. Summers, translator). New York: Benjamin Blonn, Inc., 1970 (Original edition, 1487).

Miller, P., O'Neil, P., Malcolm, R., & Currey, H. Eating disorders. In H. Adams & P. Sutker (Eds.), Comprehensive handbook of psychopathology. New York: Plenum Press, in press.

O'Malley, J., & Eisenberg, L. The hyperkinetic syndrome. Seminars in Psychiatry, 1973, 5 (1), 95-103.

O'Neil, P., White, J., King, C., & Carek, D. Controlling childhood rumination through differential reinforcement of other behavior. Behavior Modification, 1979, 3 (3), 355-372.

Ossofsky, H. Endogenous depression in infancy and children. Comprehensive Psychiatry, 1974, 15 (1), 19-25.

Palmer, T. California's community treatment program for delinquent adolescents. Journal of Research in Crime and Delinquency, 1971, 8, 74-92.

Perkins, W. Speech pathology (second edition). St. Louis: C.V. Mosby Co., 1977.

Piaget, J., & Inhelder, B. The psychology of the child. New York: Basic Books, Inc., 1969.

Pierce, C. Enuresis. In H. Kaplan, A. Freedman, & B. Sadock (Eds.), Comprehensive textbook of psychiatry (Vol. 3). Baltimore: Williams and Wilkins, 1980.

Pierce, C. Encopresis. In H. Kaplan, A. Freedman, & B. Sadock (Eds.), Comprehensive textbook of psychiatry (Vol. 3). Baltimore: Williams and Wilkins, 1980.

Piggott, L. Overview of selected basic research in autism. Journal of Autism and Developmental Disorders, 1979, 9 (2), 199-217.

Redl, F. When we deal with children. New York: The Free Press, 1966.

Redl, F., & Wineman, D. The aggressive child. Glencoe, Ill: The Free Press, 1957.

Reichler, R., & Schopler, E. Developmental therapy: A program model for providing individualized services in the community. In E. Schopler & R. Reichler (Eds.), Psychopathology and child development. New York: Plenum Press, 1976.

Reinhart, J. Failure to thrive: A 50 year followup. Journal of Pediatrics, 1972, 81, 1218-1219.

Reinhart, J. Failure to thrive. In J. Noshpitz (Ed.), Basic handbook of child psychiatry (Vol. II). New York: Basic Books, Inc., 1979.

Richmond, J., Tarjan, G., & Mendelsohn, R. (Eds.). Mental retardation: A handbook for the primary physician. Chicago: American Medical Association, 1974.

Ritvo, E., Ornitz, E., Gottlieb, F., Poussaint, A., Marion, B., Ditman, K., & Blinn, K. Arousal and nonarousal enuretic events. American Journal of Psychiatry, 1969, 126 (1), 77-84.

Rousey, C. Disorders of speech. In J. Noshpitz (Eds.), Basic handbook of child psychiatry (Vol. II). New York: Basic Books, Inc., 1979.

Rutter, M. Autistic children: Infancy to adulthood. Seminars in Psychiatry, 1970, 2, 435-450.

Rutter, M., Lebovici, S., Eisenberg, L., Sneznevskiy, A., Sadoun, R., Brooke, E., & Lin, T. A tri-axial classification of mental disorders in childhood: An international study. Journal of Child Psychology and Psychiatry, 1969, 10, 41-61.

Rutter, M. The development of infantile autism. In S. Chess & A. Thomas (Eds.), Annual progress in child psychiatry and child development. New York: Brunner/Mazel, 1975.

Satterfield, J., Cantwell, D., & Satterfield, B. Pathophysiology of the hyperactive child syndrome. In S. Chess & A. Thomas (Eds.), Annual progress in child psychiatry and child development. New York: Brunner/Mazel, 1975.

Sattler, J. Assessment of children's intelligence. Philadelphia: W.B. Saunders, 1974.

Schwartz, M. Stuttering solved. Philadelphia: J.B. Lippincott Co., 1976.

Shapiro, A., Shapiro, E., & Wayne, H. The symptomatology and diagnosis of Gilles de la Tourette's syndrome. Journal of the American Academy of Child Psychiatry, 1973, 12, 702-723.

Shapiro, A., Shapiro, E., Bruun, R., & Sweet, R. Gilles de la Tourette's Syndrome. New York: Raven Press, 1978.

Shapiro, A., Shapiro, E., Bruun, R., Sweet, R., Wayne, H., & Solomon, G. Gilles de la Tourette's Syndrome: Summary of clinical experience with 250 patients and suggested nomenclature for tic syndromes. In R. Eldridge & S. Fahn (Eds.), Advances in neurology: Dystonia (Vol. 14). New York: Raven Press, 1976.

Shaw, C. The psychiatric disorders of childhood. New York: Appleton-Century-Crofts, 1966.

Silver, L. DSM-II and child and adolescent psychopathology (Letter to the editor). American Journal of Psychiatry, 1969, 125, 1267-1269.

Silver, L. Stereotyped movement and speech disorders. In H. Kaplan, A. Freedman, & B. Sadock (Eds.), Comprehensive textbook of psychiatry (Vol. 3). Baltimore: Williams and Wilkins, 1980.

Smith, C., & Berenberg, W. The concept of failure to thrive. Pediatrics, 1970, 46, 661-662.

Snyder, S. Basic science of psychopharmacology. In H. Kaplan, A. Freedman, & B. Sadock (Eds.), Comprehensive textbook of psychiatry (Vol. 1). New York: Williams and Wilkins, 1980.

Sours, J. The primary anorexia nervosa syndrome. In J. Noshpitz (Ed.), Basic handbook of child psychiatry (Vol. II). New York: Basic Books, Inc., 1979.

Sours, J., Frumkin, P., & Indermill, R. Somnambulism. Archives of General Psychiatry, 1963, 9, 112-125.

Spitz, R. Hospitalism: A follow-up report. Psychoanalytic Study of the Child (Vol. II), 1946.

Stevenson, J., & Richman, N. The prevalence of language delay in a population of three-year-old children and its association with general retardation. Developmental Medicine and Child Neurology, 1976, 18, 431-441.

Sutherland, E. Principles of criminology (4th edition). New York: J.B. Lippincott Co., 1945.

Sweet, R., Bruun, R., Shapiro, E., & Shapiro, A. Presynaptic catecholamine antagonists as treatment for Tourette's syndrome: Effects of alpha methyl paratyrosine and tetrabenazine. In S. Chess & A. Thomas (Eds.), Annual progress in child psychiatry and child development. New York: Brunner/Mazel, 1975.

Thomas, K. Religion and the decline of magic. New York: Charles Scribner's Sons, 1971.

Weiner, I., & Del Gaudio, A. Psychopathology in adolescence: An epidemiological study. Archives of General Psychiatry, 1976, 33, 187-193.

Werkman, S. Anxiety disorders. In H. Kaplan, A. Freedman & B. Sadock (Eds.), Comprehensive textbook of psychiatry (Vol. 3). Baltimore: Williams and Wilkins, 1980.

Werry, J. An overview of pediatric psychopharmacology. Journal of Child Psychiatry, 1982, 21 (1), 3-9.

Werry J., & Cohrssen, J. Enuresis - an etiologic and therapeutic study. Journal of Pediatrics, 1965, 67, 423-430.

Winslow, R. (Ed.). Juvenile delinquency in a free society (third edition). San Diego: Dickenson Publishing Co., 1976.

Woodrow, K. Gilles de la Tourette's disease - A review. In S. Chess & A. Thomas (Eds.), Annual progress in child psychiatry and child development. New York: Brunner/Mazel, 1975.

World Health Organization. International statistical classification of diseases, injuries, and causes of death (8th revision). Geneva, 1965.

World Health Organization. International statistical classification of diseases, injuries, and causes of death (9th revision). Geneva, 1977.

Section III

Treatments

Three general categories of treatment approaches are provided in the chapters of this section: (1) psychopharmacological, (2) psychosocial, and (3) behavioral. In addition, a fourth chapter deals with some of the more frequently encountered methods (hypnosis, electroconvulsive therapy, etc.) which do not fit in the categories of the first three chapters of the section.

The goal of this section is to provide you with *familiarity* with treatment methods, not to teach you in four lessons to become experts in the treatment of mental disorders. For this reason, no attempt has been made to provide a truly exhaustive description of techniques.

Chapter 16 will serve as a good guide to the uses of phychoactive drugs. We urge you to check the literature before prescribing the medications discussed in this chapter since changes do occur frequently in this area as new knowledge becomes available.

Chapter 17, Psychosocial Treatments, is based essentially on psychodynamic theory. It goes beyond the traditional individual psychotherapy, including, for example, family therapy and group therapies. A thorough understanding of the material in Chapter 2, Psychodynamic Considerations and Defense Mechanisms, will make this chapter much more understandable.

Chapter 18, Behavioral Treatment, is based primarily on the principles of operant conditioning. Basic principles of learning theory are provided, and some of the specific techniques used in behavioral treatment are outlined.

Chapter 19 has two major categories of treatments, somatic therapies (electroconvulsive therapy, psychosurgery and narcotherapy) and hypnotherapy. Rarely are these modalities used exclusively in the treatment of mental disorders. In general, they are used adjunctively with other treatment methods.

CHAPTER 16
Psychopharmacology
Luis A. Marco, M.D.

CHAPTER OUTLINE

LEARNING OBJECTIVES

After completing this chapter you will be able to:

1. Classify the drugs used in the treatment of psychiatric disorders.

2. Use these drugs:

    a. For the appropriate disorder.
    b. In proper dosage for an adequate length of time.

3. Recognize and treat the important side effects of these drugs.

4. Describe currently entertained mechanisms of action of psychotherapeutic agents.

PRE-TEST

For the following questions, <u>one</u> or <u>more</u> <u>than</u> <u>one</u> answer may be correct. Circle the correct answer(s).

1. Which of the following statements about phenothiazines is (are) correct?

    a. Phenothiazines are drugs of choice for treating anxiety.
    b. Side effects of phenothiazines such as sedative or hypnotic effects are often considered therapeutic effects in treating agitated patients.
    c. Increasing doses of phenothiazines are required with increasing age of the patient to obtain a therapeutic response.
    d. The main therapeutic effect of phenothiazines is the antipsychotic effect.

2. Which of the following statements is (are) correct?

    a. Phenothiazines used at lower doses (1-10 mg) are more likely to induce parkinsonian-like side effects than those used at higher doses (100-500 mg).
    b. Sedating, hypotensive and anticholinergic side effects of phenothiazines are usually inversely related to parkinsonian-like symptomatology.
    c. Thioridazine is the most anticholinergic of the phenothiazines.
    d. Nonphenothiazine anticholinergic agents are usually employed to treat phenothiazine-induced parkinsonian-like symptomatology.

3. Which of the following statements is (are) correct?

    a. Antipsychotics are additive with each other.
    b. Chlorpromazine in larger doses counteracts amphetamine intoxication or psychosis.
    c. MAOI-phenothiazine combinations may produce arterial hypotension and severe extrapyramidal symptoms.
    d. Phenothiazines combined with other phenothiazines cause enhanced sedation and respiratory depression.

4. Phenothiazines usually have some effects similar to

    a. nicotine.
    b. muscarine.
    c. physostigmine.
    d. atropine.

5. Pigmentary retinopathy may result from overdose of

    a. thioxanthenes.
    b. trifluoperazine (Stelazine).
    c. chlorpromazine (Thorazine).
    d. thioridazine (Mellaril).

6. Phenothiazines vary in

    a. dosage.
    b. sedative effect.
    c. anticholinergic effect.
    d. capacity for extrapyramidal reactions.

7. Amphetamines are not used for serious depressions because of

    a. significant incidence of toxic reactions.
    b. toxic reactions with other drugs.
    c. paradoxical sedation.
    d. ineffectiveness.

8. The anticholinergic effects of tricyclics suggest caution in their use with
    patients who have

    a. prostatic hypertrophy.
    b. spastic colon.
    c. certain types of glaucoma.
    d. complaints of chronic pain.

9. Tricyclic drugs used to treat depression vary most in

    a. effectiveness.
    b. dose.
    c. unwanted reactions.
    d. degree of sedative effect.

10. If most tricyclic drugs are ineffective at the upper limit of their dosage
    range,

    a. dosage should be increased.
    b. another tricyclic should be added.
    c. an MAOI inhibitor should be added.
    d. electroconvulsive therapy may be indicated.

11. Which of the following may be useful in treating mania?

    a. barbiturates
    b. phenothiazines
    c. benzodiazepines
    d. lithium carbonate

12. Phenothiazines are not a good first choice to treat anxiety because

    a. they are ineffective.
    b. withdrawal reactions are more serious than with other drugs.
    c. dependency and addiction occur more readily than with other drugs.
    d. they have more serious side effects than antianxiety drugs.

13. Drug choice primarily depends on

    a. diagnosis.
    b. dynamic formulation.
    c. specific signs or symptoms.
    d. an understanding of the doctor-patient relationship.

14. Complications of concern in lithium therapy include

    a. nephrotoxicity.
    b. neurotoxicity.
    c. interference with antidiuretic hormone function.
    d. respiratory insufficiency.

15. Which of the following produce <u>severe</u> physiological addiction?

    a. benzodiazepines
    b. phenothiazines
    c. amphetamines
    d. barbiturates

16. Haloperidol is useful in the treatment of

    a. Schizophrenia.
    b. mania.
    c. Organic Brain Syndromes with psychosis of the elderly.
    d. Gilles de la Tourette syndrome.

17. Tardive dyskinesia

    a. usually emerges late after a protracted period of antipsychotic use.
    b. is characterized by stereotyped involuntary movements, especially of the mouth, face and shoulder muscles.
    c. has no effective treatment.
    d. in some patients behaves as an irreversible process despite total withdrawal of the neuroleptic.

18. The "central anticholinergic syndrome" occurring with concomitant signs of peripheral muscarinic receptor blockade is characterized by

    a. impaired cognitive functioning.
    b. restlessness.
    c. impaired consciousness.
    d. impaired perception.

19. The "central anticholinergic syndrome" is dramatically reversed by

    a. physostigmine, 2 mg I.V.
    b. chlorpromazine, 100 mg po.
    c. Valium, 10 mg I.V.
    d. imipramine, 50 mg po.

20. Side effects of reserpine include

    a. hypotension.
    b. depression.
    c. nausea and vomiting.
    d. impotence.

For the following questions, circle the letter corresponding to the one correct answer.

21. Your patient has been started on 200 mg of chlorpromazine tid for treatment of an acute episode of agitation, delusions, and threatening gestures. These appear to be responding well to chlorpromazine, but within a few days he develops a severe skin rash thought to be an allergic reaction to the phenothiazine. Select the one best alternative from the following.

    a. Increase the dose of chlorpromazine since it is antihistiminic.
    b. Reduce chlorpromazine by half.
    c. Switch to haloperidol 4 mg tid.
    d. Leave chlorpromazine as is and add an anticholinergic agent.
    e. Leave chlorpromazine as is and recommend suntanning.

Use the following case study to answer questions 22-24.

A 60-year-old female comes to your office complaining that she has lost control of her tongue which keeps darting inside and outside of her mouth. Inspection further reveals that she also exhibits facial grimaces, winking and sudden jerks of the head and shoulder to one side. She further volunteers that she was discharged from the state hospital two months ago with a diagnosis of Schizophrenia and a prescription for Stelazine (trifluoperazine) and Haldol (haloperidol) which she has been taking for the last 20 years until about three weeks ago when she ran out of medication. She exhibits no evidence of psychosis at this time.

22. The most likely diagnosis for the above signs is

    a. Gilles de la Tourette syndrome.
    b. hysteria.
    c. levodopa-induced tardive dyskinesia.
    d. neuroleptic-induced tardive dyskinesia.
    e. Schizophrenia.

23. What is the likely trigger of this syndrome at this point?

    a. discharge from the hospital
    b. the anxieties of being on her own
    c. a return to the stresses at home
    d. abrupt cessation of antipsychotic medication
    e. none of the above

24. Which of the following options would you choose at this time?

    a. Place her back on Stelazine and Haldol.
    b. Administer anticholinergics.
    c. Explain that at this juncture it is better to wait without medication and see whether signs will worsen or improve and whether her mental condition will require medication later.
    d. Advise immediate return to the state hospital.

Use the following case study to answer questions 25-27.

A 70-year-old female comes to your office with complaints of decreased appetite and energy, loss of interest in activities, and cessation of involvement with friends and neighbors. These have gradually become worse for the last three months. Another doctor has treated her with amitriptyline 75 mg daily for the past two months without much improvement. There have been no previous similar episodes or other past psychiatric disturbances. Mental Status: Thinking logical, no delusions or hallucinations.

25. You decide to treat her with

    a. haloperidol 5 mg qid.
    b. amitriptyline 150 mg daily.
    c. thyroid 30 mg daily.
    d. multivitamins.
    e. lithium carbonate 300 mg tid.

26. A week later she reports, stating that she feels much worse. She now appears confused, disoriented, and has visual hallucinations. You decide to

    a. increase haloperidol to 10 mg qid.
    b. increase amitriptyline to 250 mg daily.
    c. switch her to imipramine.
    d. discontinue amitriptyline and observe closely every two days.
    e. increase lithium to 600 mg daily.

27. Two days later thinking is clear and there are no hallucinations or disorientation but presenting symptoms remain as on the first visit. You decide the patient has been suffering from

    a. depression with added central anticholinergic delirium during the last few days.
    b. Multi-infarct Dementia for the last three months.
    c. plain depression with exacerbation lately.
    d. hysterical neurosis.
    e. Schizophrenia.

28. From the following, select the therapeutic lithium level to treat mania.

    a. 1.0 mEq/L
    b. 2.0 mEq/L
    c. .1 mEq/L
    d. 2.5 mEq/L
    e. 3.0 mEq/L

29. In regard to drug therapy of psychoses, which of the following statements is true?

    a. Only one variety of chemical compounds is useful in improving the manifestations of psychoses.
    b. Simultaneous use of drugs belonging to two or more categories is frequently advisable because most studies show that combinations are better than a single agent.
    c. Use of multiple drugs will decrease the number and types of side effects.
    d. Oligopharmacy is generally preferable to using multiple drugs.
    e. Adverse drug interactions are rare.

30. A 19-year-old student is admitted to the hospital because he hears accusatory voices telling him he is a faggot and that he is to die soon. Speech is incoherent, rushed, and inappropriate. He appears very anxious, fearful, and suspicious. Prior to admission he had not been eating, sleeping, or going to class for several days. At this point the best approach would be:

    a. Valium, 5 mg tid.
    b. fluphenazine, 2 mg daily.
    c. electroconvulsive therapy.
    d. chlorpromazine and thioridazine combined, 100 mg of each daily.
    e. chlorpromazine, 50 mg orally, followed by 100 mg every hour until relaxation or drowsiness occurs.

31. If specific treatment of phenothiazine-induced hypotension is required, use

    a. norepinephrine.
    b. epinephrine.
    c. isoproterenol.
    d. reserpine.
    e. levodopa.

Use the following case study to answer question 32.

An elderly man with severe arterial hypertension has been maintained with fair success on the antihypertensive guanethidine for a long period. Recently he became so psychotic as to pose the need for specific medication.

32. Your choice for the treatment of this psychosis is

    a. imipramine.
    b. chlorpromazine.
    c. amitriptyline.
    d. reserpine.
    e. none of the above.

33. Imipramine, amitriptyline, and chlorpromazine have in common which of the following?

    a. release all norepinephrine, dopamine, and serotonin from neurons
    b. blockade of guanethidine uptake into noradrenergic neurons
    c. hypotensive; therefore, more effective in combination with guanethidine
    d. decrease blood volume through diuresis
    e. none of the above

Match the following disorders with the lettered items. Lettered items may be used once, more than once, or not at all.

___34. pseudoparkinsonism   a. mechanism not clear
___35. akathisia   b. norepinephrine blockade
___36. dystonia   c. dopamine blockade plus acetylcholine activation

I. INTRODUCTION

People under psychological or emotional distress are often helped by drugs called psychotherapeutic agents. The body of knowledge and understanding about these drugs is called psychopharmacology. A psychopharmacological, psychotropic, or better yet, psychotherapeutic agent is to be distinguished from psychotomimetic or psychotogenic and psychedelic agents. The distinctions are easy until one begins to define the terms; then difficulties arise. Let us therefore just illustrate. Psychotherapeutic implies an influence on the psyche which is medically beneficial. Psychotomimetic refers to an agent whose influence mimics psychotic manifestations. Psychotogenic refers to the capacity of the agent to cause psychosis. Psychedelic implies that the influence is pleasurable or welcome ("good LSD trip"). Thus, the same compound, LSD, may be seen as psychedelic (good trip) or as psychotomimetic (bad or frightening trip).

Four main psychopathological syndromes are often treated with psychotherapeutic drugs. These syndromes are schizophrenia, depression, mania, and anxiety. Other psychopathological conditions such as dependence, regression, transference, abnormal sexual impulses, and personality disorders are not usually treated with drugs. This indicates that one must make a diagnosis before instituting drug therapy. Thus, the first two steps in initiating drug therapy are: making a proper diagnosis and choosing the appropriate drug according to the diagnosis. Most drugs used to treat psychopathological syndromes are effective over time at optimal doses. Inadequate dosage or an insufficient duration of treatment may cause drug therapy to fail. Insufficient dose may fail to decrease or abolish the symptoms or signs. Excessive dose is likely to cause or exacerbate otherwise more tolerable side effects. The third consideration, then, is using the drug in its proper dose and duration, before you change it.

Drugs interact; they may potentiate one another or have opposing mechanisms of action. Therefore, one must know what drugs a patient has been receiving before starting another drug. One must always take a drug history. Another rule deriving from the fact that drugs interact is that drugs should not be used in combination if at all possible. Multiple drug administration (polypharmacy) is more dangerous and less desirable than prescription of a single agent or a minimal number of drugs (oligopharmacy).

Some axioms of drug therapy are:

1) If dosage and duration have been sufficient, failure to respond to treatment may be evidence of an inaccurate diagnosis. However, no drug is always effective in every case for the condition it is meant to treat; sometimes another drug from the same category will be effective. Drug choice depends primarily on diagnosis and secondarily on specific signs or symptoms.

2) The categories of drugs are fairly specific for the conditions they are intended to treat. Multiple use of drugs within the same category is to be discouraged because most studies have shown that no

combination is better than an adequate dose of just one drug. Further, if drugs are combined, the patient may experience the undesirable side effects of both.

3) Simultaneous use of drugs belonging to two or more categories is rarely advisable because most studies have shown that, at best, such combinations are no better than administration of a single agent. In most cases they are worse, sometimes even dangerous. In a sense, the hypothesized mechanisms of action of the two types of drugs are often mutually opposite. Many drugs potentiate the unwanted effects of another drug.

QUIZ, Section I.

1. From the following select three steps in drug therapy. Circle the correct answers.

   a. Arrive at a diagnosis.
   b. Choose a psychotomimetic agent.
   c. Choose a psychotherapeutic agent.
   d. Administer the agent chosen in adequate dose and duration.
   e. Use doses which will promptly cure the condition in a couple of days.

TRUE or FALSE: Circle the correct letter.

T F 2. One very important reason for taking a detailed drug history is to avoid the occurrence of adverse drug interactions.

T F 3. Oligopharmacy is generally preferable to using multiple drugs.

T F 4. Simultaneous use of drugs belonging to two or more categories is frequently advisable because most studies show that combinations are better than administration of a single agent.

T F 5. Use of multiple drugs will decrease the number and types of side effects.

T F 6. The choice of drug to be used depends primarily on diagnosis and secondarily on specific signs and symptoms.

II. ANTIPSYCHOTIC DRUGS

The terms antipsychotic, antischizophrenic, and neuroleptic agents are often used interchangeably in the literature. All three are equally appropriate. Neuroleptic is a term more frequently used in Europe, and it means that the agent has the capacity to mimic neurological disease. Antipsychotic and antischizophrenic are more pragmatic terms as befit American philosophy. Antipsychotic is an appropriate term because all neuroleptics influence favorably some of the signs or symptoms of most psychoses, whether they are the result of CNS derangement (Huntington's chorea), toxic insult (amphetamine poisoning), or more purely functional (Schizophrenia). The schizophrenias are the most frequent types of psychoses, hence the appropriateness of the term antischizophrenic agents. This group of psychotherapeutic agents consists of six chemically different types of drugs: rauwolfia alkaloids, phenothiazines, thioxanthines, butyrophenones, indoleamines, and tricyclic dibenzoxazepines. Their main use is usually the treatment of psychoses other than affective psychosis.

A.   RAUWOLFIA ALKALOIDS

The chemical structure of these alkaloids and reserpine is given below:

Figure 16-1

CONFIGURATION OF RAUWOLFIA ALKALOIDS

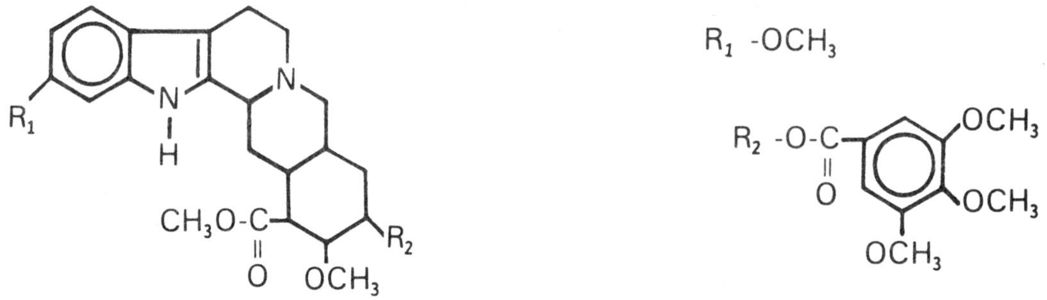

Rauwolfia derivatives, of which reserpine is the principal agent, were among the first drugs noted to have an antipsychotic action, but are rarely used today in the USA because their antipsychotic potential is weaker compared with more modern neuroleptics. They also have more unwanted effects than other drugs now used to treat Schizophrenia or other psychoses. These unwanted effects include hypotension, gastrointestinal signs and symptoms (nausea, vomiting, diarrhea), lethargy, impotence, and depression. Reserpine-induced arterial hypotension is very well known in medical practice since some clinicians still use it as an antihypertensive. For this reason, when taking a drug history one should remember that the psychiatric complication of depression may occur with reserpine use. It has been estimated that 5-15% of patients receiving reserpine may develop depression. This is sometimes sufficiently severe to lead to suicide or to require antidepressant medication or electroconvulsive therapy (ECT). Reserpine is frequently used in experimental animal studies to accomplish a massive depletion of stored

ANSWERS, Section I.

1. a, c, d
2. T
3. T
4. F
5. F
6. T

CNS monoamines (dopamine, noradrenaline, and serotonin). It is important to remember reserpine primarily as an experimental tool because the above amines are thought to play vital roles as neurotransmitters at synaptic (receptor) sites of the CNS. For such reason, these putative neurotransmitters are also called biogenic amines (see Table 16-4, p. 821). Although unpopular in American psychiatry, reserpine may be a rational alternative to the use of other antipsychotic agents in some selected cases. One such reasonable alternative is presented by some chronic schizophrenics with controlled but observable symptoms who would relapse upon drug withdrawal, but who have a strong propensity to develop tardive dyskinesia, a serious complication caused by most antipsychotics (see p. 823).

Reserpine is an antipsychotic with minimal risk of tardive dyskinesia. This may be due to another rather unique pharmacological property of reserpine, namely its central and peripheral cholinergic activity. It will be seen later that most other antipsychotics have from mild to very strong anticholinergic potential. It will also be seen that anticholinergics usually aggravate tardive dyskinesia.

B. PHENOTHIAZINES

It is important to recognize the phenothiazine nucleus. This is given below:

Figure 16-2

COMMON NUCLEUS TO ALL PHENOTHIAZINE DERIVATIVES

PHENOTHIAZINE NUCLEUS

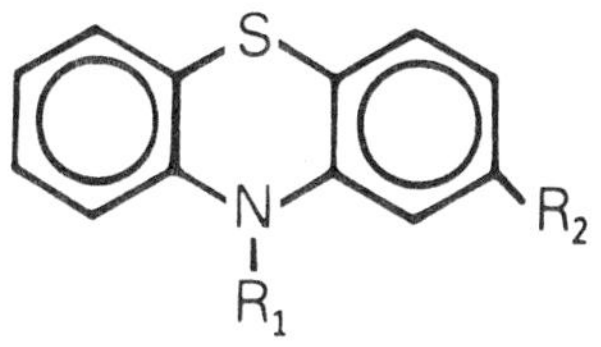

On the above moiety are based the various phenothiazine derivatives used as antipsychotic agents. Based on whether a chlorine, fluorine atom(s), or other radicals are attached at position X, neuroleptics with widely differing potencies and side effects can be synthesized. Also depending on whether an aliphatic (aminoalkyl, straight carbon-chain), a piperidine (one amino nitrogen atom incorporated into a cyclic structure), or a piperazine (two amino nitrogen atoms into cyclic structure) radical is bound at position R, other phenothiazine derivatives are obtained which differ markedly in their potency and specific side effects.

Phenothiazines with one or three fluorine atoms at position X and a piperazine radical at position R are particularly potent antipsychotic agents. Some
of these features are illustrated in the figure below.

Figure 16-3

CHANGES AT X AND R PRODUCE A VARIETY OF
PHENOTHIAZINE NEUROLEPTICS

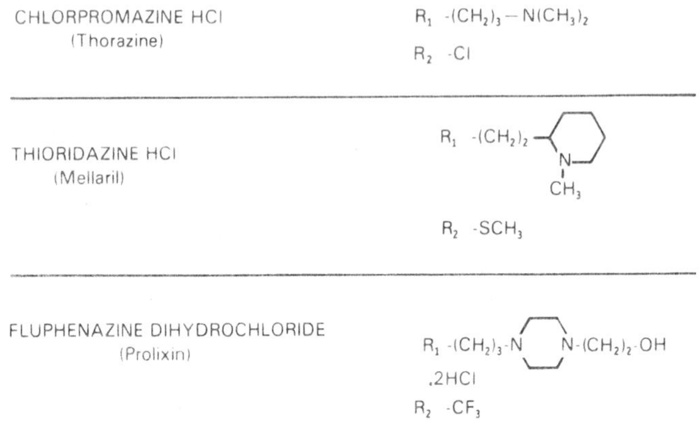

CHLORPROMAZINE HCl
(Thorazine)

R_1 $-(CH_2)_3-N(CH_3)_2$

R_2 $-Cl$

THIORIDAZINE HCl
(Mellaril)

R_1 $-(CH_2)_2$ ⬠ N-CH$_3$

R_2 $-SCH_3$

FLUPHENAZINE DIHYDROCHLORIDE
(Prolixin)

R_1 $-(CH_2)_3-N$ ⬠ $N-(CH_2)_2-OH$

$.2HCl$

R_2 $-CF_3$

Phenothiazines are drugs of choice for Schizophrenia. They are also effective in treating the early stage of mania, the psychotic phenomena induced
by LSD ingestion, amphetamine psychosis, and the agitation or psychosis of
some Organic Brain Syndromes.

Phenothiazines have sometimes been promoted as useful in treating anxiety,
but they have more unwanted and potentially dangerous or irreversible
side effects than other drugs used to treat anxiety. Therefore, the
nonpsychiatric practitioner should never use phenothiazines to treat
anxiety states. Psychiatrists must be prepared to provide compelling
reasons for selecting phenothiazines in the treatment of anxiety without
psychotic phenomenology.

Many drugs in this category have been synthesized by substituting on the
phenothiazine nucleus (see Fig. 16-2). The nature of the substitution has
much to do with dosage and unwanted effects. Nearly 20 such agents are
clinically available. The most popular phenothiazines are listed with their
commercial names and approximate daily dose in Table 16-2. We shall learn
to use one drug from each of the three general categories. Other
phenothiazines will resemble in their dosage, properties, and side effects
one of these three. The therapeutic effect of the phenothiazines is their
antipsychotic effect. Psychotic signs and symptoms are the specific
targets of phenothiazine administration. The sedating and hypnotic side
effects of phenothiazines are frequently used for therapeutic purposes,
rather than as untoward side effects, in the agitated or insomniac patient.

The three phenothiazines that we will consider are: chlorpromazine (Thorazine), thioridazine (Mellaril), and fluphenazine (Prolixin). They are represented in Fig. 16-3. The therapeutic or antipsychotic effect of these drugs
is similar. They differ mainly in dosage and unwanted effects. Chlorpromazine and thioridazine have predominantly a complex of side effects consisting

of hypotension, sedation, and anticholinergic signs, while fluphenazine has predominantly extrapyramidal side effects. A typical daily dose of chlorpromazine and thioridazine is 500 mg, while 10-20 mg daily may be an average dose for fluphenazine. The mechanism of action for the phenothiazines' therapeutic or antipsychotic effect is not clearly understood but it is thought to be related to the dopamine blocking action that these drugs exert at central receptor sites. It has become general consensus that blockade of dopaminergic receptors at sites in the neostriatum (caudate nucleus, putamen) is responsible for the so-called extrapyramidal side effects induced by administration of neuroleptics, including phenothiazine derivatives. Extrapyramidal side effects will be described later (see pp. 818-820). The therapeutic or antipsychotic effects are also thought to be dependent on the blockade of dopaminergic receptors or autoreceptors, but not necessarily of those confined to the neostriatum.

The location in the CNS of those dopaminergic receptors whose blockade by neuroleptics improves the signs and symptoms of psychosis is not clear. Limbic structures, or perhaps better, mesolimbic regions are popular candidates. Mesolimbic regions refer to medial structures of the limbic system. The limbic system is an assortment of phylogenetically old anatomical regions heavily and complexly interconnected. Phylogenetically old means that its presence in the brain can be traced to very early species (reptiles) in the phyletic scale. The limbic system is thought to mediate and modulate the sphere of emotions. The limbic brain is also called the visceral or emotional brain. Of these limbic structures one has attracted much attention in recent years. This is the nucleus accumbens which in the human brain is to be found rostroventrally to the head of the caudate nucleus at about the level of the anterior commissure. The nucleus accumbens also receives heavy dopaminergic innervation.

Figure 16-4

DIAGRAMMATIC REPRESENTATION OF NEUROTRANSMITTER PATHWAYS WITHIN THE BRAIN AND BRAINSTEM

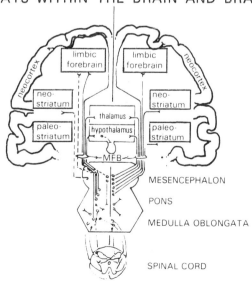

From: Fuxe, K. and Andén, N. Studies on central monoamine neurons with special reference to the nigro-neostriatal dopamine neuron system. In E. Costa, L.J. Côté, and M.D. Yahr (Eds.), Biochemistry and pharmacology of the basal ganglia. New York: Raven Press, 1966, p. 127 (figure 3). Reprinted by permission.

Figure 16-4 is a classical diagram of main monoamine pathways. For simplicity, catecholaminergic pathways have been drawn on the left side (norepinephinre as solid lines and dopamine as dashed lines) and indoleamine pathways on the right.

If the student desires to become more enlightened about the accumbens and the limbic system in general, he is encouraged at this point to turn to textbooks of neuroanatomy and neurophysiology.

The phenothiazines' widespread influence on the central and autonomic nervous systems may produce remarkable effects. Tolerance to some of the side effects does develop. One should start a patient on small doses of a phenothiazine and allow tolerance to some of the unwanted side effects to develop. Psychiatrists select a particular phenothiazine on the basis of the side effects they want or will accept. For example, chlorpromazine's side effect of sedation is sometimes desirable during the early course of treatment of agitated Schizophreniform or other psychoses.

Some of the major side effects of phenothiazine administration are listed in Table 16-1 (see next page) with their mechanism of occurrence.

TABLE 16-1

MECHANISM OF ACTION OF ANTIPSYCHOTIC DRUG SIDE EFFECTS

Side Effect	DA	NE	ACh	Unknown	Allergic	Idiosyn-cratic	Toxic Impurity
Hypotension		B					
Sleepiness		B					
Sedation		B					
Dizziness		B					
Fainting		B					
Dry mouth			B				
Blurred vision			B				
Constipation			B				
Urine retention			B				
Tachycardia			B				
Gynecomastia	B						
Prolactinemia	B						
Dystonia	B		A				
Parkinson-ism-like	B		A				
Tardive dyskinesia	A						
Jaundice						✓	or ✓
Agranulo-cytosis						✓	
Skin rash					✓		
Akathisia				✓			
Seizure				✓			

DA, NE, ACh are dopamine, norepinephrine, and acetylcholine receptors respectively; B = blockade; A = activation.

Table 16-2 provides a more complete list of the usual phenothiazines employed as antipsychotic agents.

TABLE 16-2

TYPICAL PHENOTHIAZINES IN CLINICAL PRACTICE

Generic Name	Trade Name	Usual Oral Dose (mg/day)
Phenothiazines		
Aliphatic		
Chlorpromazine	Thorazine	100-700
Triflupromazine	Vesprin	30-200
Piperidine		
Mesoridazine	Serentil	50-400
Piperacetazine	Quide	20-160
Thioridazine	Mellaril	100-700
Piperazine		
Acetophenazine	Tindal	20-160
Butaperazine	Repoise	5-110
Carphenazine	Proketazine	25-400
Fluphenazine	Prolixin, Permitil	2-60
Perphenazine	Trilafon	8-64
Trifluoperazine	Stelazine	5-40

Keep in mind the general rules given below, namely:

1) Phenothiazines with lower therapeutic dose are more likely to induce parkinsonian-like side effects.
2) Aliphatic and piperidine compounds are less powerful inducers of parkinsonian-like side effects.
3) Sedating, hypotensive, and anticholinergic side effects are usually inversely related to parkinsonian-like symptomatology.
4) Thioridazine is the most anticholinergic of the phenothiazines.
5) Nonphenothiazine anticholinergic agents are usually employed to treat phenothiazine-induced parkinsonian-like symptomatology.

C. THIOXANTHENES

As a group, thioxanthenes resemble the phenothiazines in structure and action. Indeed, thioxanthenes became the first nonphenothiazine antipsychotic agents derived by alteration of the tricyclic core of the phenothiazine nucleus. The thioxanthenes are also divided into aliphatic types such as chlorprothixene (Taractan) and piperazine types (thiothixene, Navane), which resemble the aliphatic and piperazine phenothiazine derivatives respectively. The resemblance also applies to the dose range and side effects. The same general rules outlined above for phenothiazines apply to the thioxanthenes. These drugs are illustrated in the figure found on the next page.

Figure 16-5

TYPICAL THIOXANTHENES

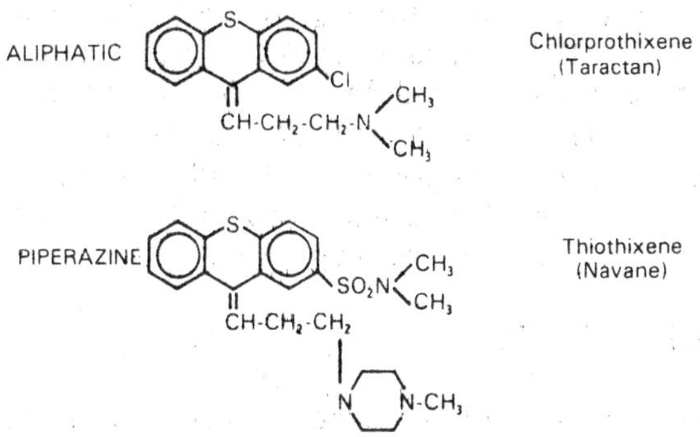
ALIPHATIC
S
Cl
CH-CH2-CH2-N
CH3
CH3
Chlorprothixene
(Taractan)
PIPERAZINE
S
SO2N
CH3
CH3
CH-CH2-CH2
N
N-CH3
Thiothixene
(Navane)

Because individuals are sometimes resistant to, or intolerant of, one or more of the phenothiazines, it is important to have other antipsychotic drugs from which to choose. Studies involving large numbers of patients have revealed no significant difference in the therapeutic or antipsychotic effect between thioxanthenes and phenothiazines.

D. BUTYROPHENONES

The fourth group of antipsychotic drugs is the butyrophenones, which are not structurally related to the phenothiazines, thioxanthenes, or rauwolfia alkaloids. They are phenylbutylpiperidines. Haloperidol (Haldol) is the only important example of this group marketed in the U.S. Its chemical configuration is shown below.

Figure 16-6

CHEMICAL CONFIGURATION OF HALOPERIDOL

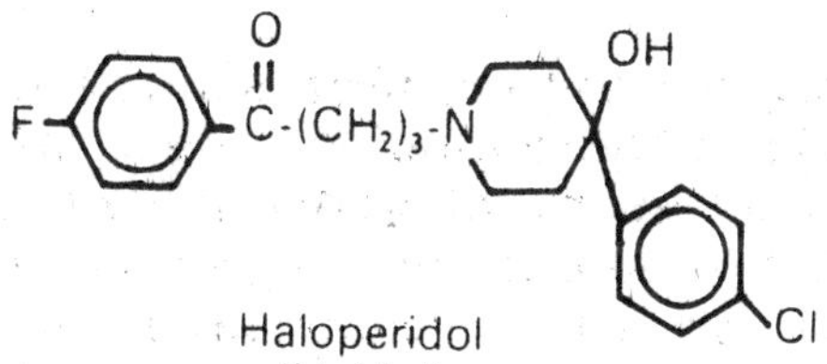
O
OH
F
C-(CH2)3-N
Cl

Haloperidol
(Haldol)

Haloperidol has little anticholinergic and sedative effect, and liver toxicity and convulsions are rarely reported with its use. However, there is a high incidence of Haldol-induced extrapyramidal side effects.

The usual daily dose range of haloperidol is 1-16 mg. This drug is very popular for the treatment of schizophrenic manifestations in apathetic patients, Organic Brain Syndromes with psychosis of the elderly, and, initially, in the treatment of manic or hypomanic episodes. Haloperidol has also become the drug of choice for the treatment of a colorful but bizarre and distressing condition afflicting children up to the early teens. It is called Gilles de la Tourette syndrome and consists of behavior deterioration, grimaces, motor tics, groaning or barking sounds, and compulsive utterance of obscenities, typically four letter words.

These symptoms may get worse under stress or fatigue. Although for a long time of obscure etiology (since 1885), current evidence suggests that Gilles de la Tourette disease may be caused by a genetic and metabolic defect resulting in hyperactivity of the dopaminergic system similar to that of tardive dyskinesia, levodopa-induced dyskinesia, or Huntington's chorea. The dose of haloperidol for the effective treatment of Tourette's syndrome may need to be raised far above the usual range of 1-16 mg daily. It has been recommended that gradual and careful increase to 150-200 daily may be necessary before treatment with haloperidol is abandoned.

E. INDOLEAMINE DERIVATIVES

These neuroleptics are unrelated to the phenothiazines, thioxanthenes, or butyrophenones. The basic nucleus of the indoleamine derivatives resembles instead that of reserpine and serotonin. This moiety is shown below to be shared by all three compounds: reserpine, serotonin, and molindone.

Figure 16-7
INDOLEAMINE COMPOUNDS

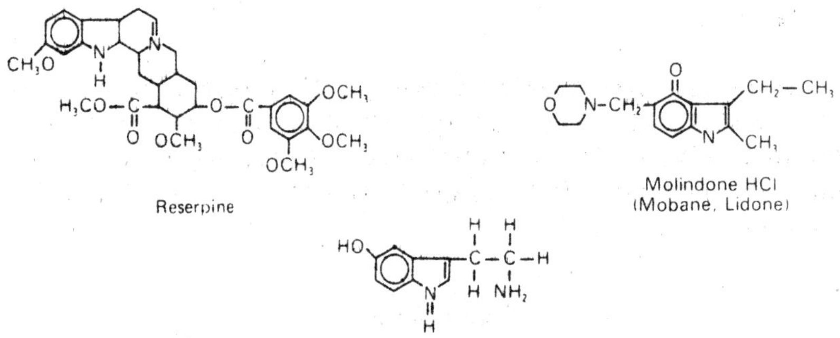

Reserpine

Molindone HCl
(Mobane, Lidone)

5-Hydroxytryptamine
[5-HT]
(Serotonin)

Molindone (Moban) is the only derivative of this nucleus recently marketed in the U.S. It is a synthetic dihydroindolone derivative. Serotonin is an indole alkylamine. There is a theory of causation of Schizophrenia ("indole theory"), contending that an unknown but abnormal metabolite of serotonin (or 5-hydroxytryptamine, or 5-HT) is responsible for this condition. This hypothesis was partly responsible for stimulating some research which eventually led to the synthesis of molindone. Serotonin is found in the brain, particularly in the limbic system. The indole nucleus is shared by all the following compounds: serotonin (a central biogenic amine), reserpine (an older neuroleptic, hardly used nowadays as an antipsychotic), LSD (a psychotogenic compound), and molindone (a newer neuroleptic). The rationale behind the use of molindone as an antipsychotic agent is that, based on receptor theory, the similarity between all these indole-derivative substances renders conceivable that they are capable of occupying the same receptor sites (serotonergic) on nerve cell membranes. Occupation by serotonin would lead to normal function, occupation by an aberrant metabolite of serotonin would cause Schizophrenia (indole theory), occupation by LSD, a compound foreign to the brain, would cause--indeed causes--toxic psychosis, and occupation by reserpine or molindone would prevent any abnormal serotonin metabolite or LSD from occupying those same serotonergic receptor sites at the same time and thus bring about a therapeutic effect.

Molindone, however, shares with other neuroleptics the one property which has been found to correlate best with antipsychotic efficacy or potency, and this is an ability to block central dopaminergic receptor sites. Thus, you have above an outline of the theory followed by a statement of the facts. Theory and fact may not necessarily match each other. But the drug works as an antipsychotic with a potency which is roughly comparable to that of trifluoperazine (Stelazine).

F. TRICYCLIC DIBENZOXAZEPINES

Loxapine succinate (Loxitane, Lederle) is the only important, recently released, agent in this category. The chemical structure of this neuroleptic is shown below:

Figure 16-8

STRUCTURE OF LOXITANE (RIGHT) AND ITS TRICYCLIC NUCLEUS (LEFT)

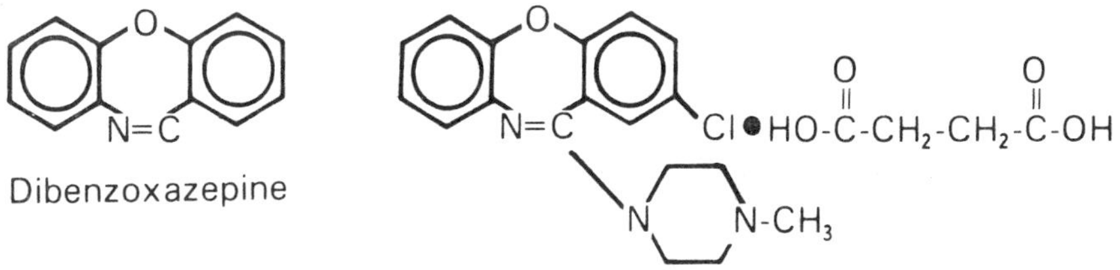

Dibenzoxazepine

Loxapine succinate
(Loxitane)

Note the lower three-ring part of this structure. It is reminiscent of the tricyclic (three rings) configuration of one of the classes of antidepressants, which will be described later (see p. 828). The pharmacological responses to loxapine are similar to those of other classes of antipsychotic agents discussed earlier (phenothiazines, thioxanthenes, butyrophenones, and indoleamines). The exact mode of action of loxapine has not been established yet. It appears to reduce the firing threshold of CNS neurons mediating polysynaptic circuits. Particularly sensitive are such neurons located in the reticular formation of the brain stem. Loxapine has also been found to have potent anti-emetic effect in animals, a property which is also general to most phenothiazines. Following oral administration, peak serum levels usually occur within two hours. About 50% of a single oral dose is excreted within the first 24 hours. These pharmacokinetic data are important in guiding a rational schedule of administration. The therapeutic dose range for loxapine is 50-200 mg. An average starting dosage is 10 mg tid or qid. The approximate relative mg equivalence of loxapine is half that of trifluoperazine and thiothixene in potency and ten times that of chlorpromazine. These conversion estimates are important when one is considering switching a patient from one neuroleptic to another.

G. RULES OF ANTIPSYCHOTIC DRUG USE

1. Administration of Antipsychotic Agents.

   a. Begin at relatively low doses and swiftly increase the dose until a therapeutic response is achieved or deleterious side effects intervene.
   b. It is wiser in the long run to settle momentarily for a moderate therapeutic response than to push impatiently for a maximal therapeutic effect which may be missed because the patient has reached the toxic range.
   c. Neuroleptics usually improve the status of patients with chronic Schizophrenia, but they are hardly ever curative in this population. Therefore, maintenance therapy is often required for many months or years.
   d. Interpolation of drug holidays is advisable. These can be short-term (weekends without medications) or long-term (one month each year without medication). Drug holidays are useful because they provide a basis for: (1) reassessment of the need for, and amount of, chemotherapy, (2) home weekend trials without medication and the reassurance that perhaps the patient is ready to manage without drugs, (3) freeing nurses' time for engaging in other modalities of interaction or therapy with inpatients, (4) reducing drug expenses, and (5) decreasing serious complications (i.e., dyskinesia, see p. 821) or unmasking their existence.

2. Relative Potencies of Antipsychotic Agents.
   Table 16-3 below provides an approximate equivalence of the usually prescribed neuroleptic agents. This table is a useful guideline for switching patients from one antipsychotic to another. For example, the antipsychotic potency of 100 mg of chlorpromazine is approximately equal to that of 2 mg of haloperidol. These equivalencies do not apply to the capacity to induce specific side effects. Also they are more accurate for acute management and the lower dosage ranges than for chronic maintenance and the higher dosage requirements.

TABLE 16-3
USUAL ORAL DOSE AND EQUIVALENCE

Neuroleptic	Oral mg
Chlorpromazine	100
Thioridazine	100
Triflupromazine	40
Mesoridazine	40
Loxapine	15
Molindone	12
Perphenazine	10
Trifluoperazine	7
Thiothixene	6
Fluphenazine	2
Haloperidol	2

3.   Long-acting or Depot Neuroleptic Agents.
     There are about seven available depot neuroleptic forms. Only two
     will be considered here. These are the enanthate and decanoate
     esters of fluphenazine. The hydrochloride salt of fluphenazine
     listed in Table 16-3 is not a depot form but a short-acting prepar-
     ation. The enanthate is usually effective for 1-2 weeks and the
     decanoate for 2-3 weeks. They are currently available for intra-
     muscular injection. They are specially indicated for patients with
     chronic Schizophrenia who are unreliable drug takers. They are
     frequently prescribed for outpatient populations. It is recommended
     that therapy be initiated with a relatively small dose (2.5 mg) which
     is usually well-tolerated. Otherwise, the risk of acute EPS is mark-
     edly increased. If the initial 2.5 mg dose is well tolerated, it is
     repeated on the 3rd, 5th, and 8th day. Then the dose is doubled
     (5 mg) on day 12 and increased to 12.5 mg (0.5 ml) on day 19. A
     week later (26th day) a 25 mg dose is injected. Thereafter, 25 mg
     or more is given every 14 days or more for several months. Chronic
     patients being switched from oral neuroleptics to depot fluphenazine
     should be first given a wash out period or drug holiday for at least
     one week before instituting depot fluphenazine according to an em-
     pirical conversion formula, or better yet, initiation with a small
     dose (2.5 mg) as described above.

QUIZ, Section II.

Circle the correct answer(s). One or more than one answer may be correct.

1.   In the schematic representation shown in Figure 16-4, three distinct
     structures are indicated as receiving dopaminergic innervation. These
     are (select three):

     a.   MFB
     b.   limbic forebrain
     c.   thalamus
     d.   neocortex
     e.   neostriatum
     f.   paleostriatum
     g.   pituitary

2.   Some of the most common side effects of phenothiazines include

     a.   sedation.
     b.   respiratory distress.
     c.   orthostatic hypotension.
     d.   EPS.
     e.   diarrhea.
     f.   anticholinergic or atropine-like effects.

3. Choose the correct statements.

   a. Thiothixene is more sedating than chlorprothixene.
   b. Thiothixene is less sedating than chlorprothixene.
   c. Average dose of chlorprothixene is half that of fluphenazine.
   d. Chlorpromazine is more sedating than thiothixene.

4. On the basis of the information provided above, rank the following doses of various agents from the most (lst) to the least (4th) antipsychotic potency.

   ____ a. chlorpromazine 50 mg   ____ b. loxapine 30 mg
   ____ c. thiothixene 5 mg   ____ d. trifluoperazine 10 mg

5. Arrange in sequence the three fluphenazine compounds below from the longest to the shortest acting.

   ____ a. enanthate
   ____ b. hydrochloride
   ____ c. decanoate

6. Which of the following types of psychoses can be treated by phenothiazines?

   a. Schizophrenia
   b. mania
   c. toxic psychosis
   d. organic psychosis
   e. retarded depression
   f. all of the above

7. The side effects of reserpine include

   a. hypotension.   e. impotence.
   b. nausea and vomiting.   f. lethargy.
   c. diarrhea.   g. none of the above.
   d. depression.

8. Sequence the following phenothiazines from most to least parkinsonian-like potential.

   ____ a. chlorpromazine
   ____ b. fluphenazine
   ____ c. triflupromazine
   ____ d. thioridazine
   ____ e. trifluoperazine

Circle the letter corresponding to the <u>one</u> correct response.

9. The order in which you have them now (if quiz 8 is done correctly) should represent the order from

   a. most to least sedating effect.
   b. least to most sedating effect.

10. Thioridazine should be at the

    a. top of the list.
    b. mid-range of the list.
    c. bottom of the list.

11. Fluphenazine should be at the

    a. bottom.
    b. top.
    c. mid-range.

12. Now, draw below that portion of the molecule which is common to the three substances shown in Figure 16-7.

13. The compound that you have drawn above is most closely related to

    a. indoleamine.
    b. chlorpromazine.
    c. norepinephrine.

14. The side effects of reserpine are caused by

    a. increased cholinergic and decreased noradrenergic central activity.
    b. increased cholinergic and decreased noradrenergic peripheral activity.
    c. increased cholinergic and decreased noradrenergic central and peripheral activity.
    d. decreased noradrenergic activity alone.
    e. decreased cholinergic activity alone.

Use the following case study to answer questions 15-18. Circle the letter corresponding to the one correct response.

A 58-year-old female with a protracted history of chronic Schizophrenia and no manifestations of depression presents at the clinic. Her delusions and other signs of a thought disorder are marginally controlled by haloperidol (a butyrophenone), 10 mg qid, but she decompensates upon drug withdrawal. She knows (correctly) that haloperidol may cause tardive dyskinesia and wishes to stop this medication (adapted from Janowsky et al., 1978).

15. If the patient stops her medication, it is likely that she will

    a. remain in good psychologic control.
    b. improve.
    c. relapse.

16. A rational alternative to stopping her medication completely is

    a. to switch her to a phenothiazine and tell her it is safe.
    b. to discontinue her medications completely every other year.
    c. to send her to a hypnotist.
    d. none of the above.

17. A more rational alternative to stopping her medication completely is to

    a. switch to reserpine.
    b. switch to propranolol.
    c. switch to chlordiazepoxide (Librium).
    d. begin alphamethyldopa (Aldomet).

18. If the patient accepts the choice of being switched to reserpine, this is a rational choice because

    a. reserpine is a relatively good antipsychotic agent with less potential to cause tardive dyskinesia.
    b. reserpine does not cause too many side effects.
    c. reserpine is a derivative of a plant root, and thus is morally better than a chemical.

19. Haloperidol is pharmacologically most comparable to

    a. chlorpromazine.
    b. thioridazine.
    c. fluphenazine.

20. Which of the following sequences strikes you as being most rational?

    a. admission to the hospital with schizophreniform episode, immediate antipsychotic medication with good response and adjustment, home weekend pass without antipsychotic medication one week later
    b. same patient, antipsychotic medication, weekend drug holiday while in the hospital with continued good response and adjustment, medication again, home weekend without medication
    c. same patient, no medication during first week following admission with good adjustment to the ward, home weekend pass with antipsychotic medication for the first time

21. Your patient has been started on 200 mg of chlorpromazine tid, for treatment of an acute episode of agitation, delusions, and threatening gestures. These appear to be responding well to chlorpromazine, but within a few days he develops a severe skin rash thought to be an allergic reaction to the phenothiazine. Select your best alternative among those offered below.

   a. Increase the dose of thorazine since it is antihistaminic.
   b. Reduce thorazine by half.
   c. Switch to haloperidol 4 mg tid.
   d. Combine an anticholinergic agent with the phenothiazine.
   e. Leave chlorpromazine as is and recommend suntanning.
   f. Switch to fluphenazine 10 mg tid.

Use the following Case Study to answer question 22.

A 19-year-old student is admitted to the hospital because he hears accusatory voices telling him that he is a faggot and that he is to die soon. Speech is incoherent, rushed, and inappropriate. He appears very anxious, fearful, and suspicious. Prior to admission he had not been eating, sleeping, or going to class for several days. Physical and neurological examinations were within normal limits.

22. At this point the best approach would be

   a. discharge with a prescription for sleeping pills.
   b. fluphenazine 2 mg daily.
   c. immediate electroconvulsive therapy.
   d. chlorpromazine and thioridazine combined, 100 mg of each daily.
   e. Chlorpromazine 50 mg orally, followed by 100 mg every hour until relaxation or drowsiness occurs.

Use the following Case Study to answer question 23.

The patient is a 24-year-old male, brought to the hospital by his family, who complains that he has become increasingly agitated and threatening during the past few days, not sleeping at night, and talking to himself. The patient appears hostile and agitated, and admits that he has had difficulty sleeping because the radiator in his room is giving off poisonous gases.

23. Of the two phenothiazines below, which would be the best choice?

   a. chlorpromazine
   b. fluphenazine

Use the following Case Study to answer question 24.

A 30-year-old white, moderately overweight female is brought to the hospital by her family, who states that she has become increasingly withdrawn and seclusive over the past several months. She was hospitalized for treatment of Schizophrenia a year ago. She was on medication for six months. Mental status examination reveals an apathetic woman who gives no information spontaneously, but responds to questions with one or two words. There is marked flatness of affect. She admits to auditory hallucinations and states that the Chinese have gained control of her thoughts through acupuncture.

24. She should receive a phenothiazine which is

    a. sedating.
    b. nonsedating.

Use the following Case Study to answer question 25.

An 8-year-old boy is diagnosed as having a Gilles de la Tourette syndrome, mainly on the basis of muscle jerks, facial twitches, bizarre throaty noises, and utterance of obscenities.

25. The first drug of choice to be entertained is

    a. thioridazine.
    b. molindone.
    c. haloperidal.
    d. dilantin.

26. On a mg per mg basis, molindone as an antipsychotic is prescribed in doses most closely resembling those of

    a. thioridazine.
    b. chlorprothixene.
    c. chlorpromazine.
    d. trifluoperazine.

TRUE or FALSE: Circle the correct letter.

T   F   27. It is not feasible to improve the manifestations of psychosis by means of more than one chemical variety of compounds.

T   F   28. Phenothiazines are drugs of choice for treating anxiety.

T   F   29. Side effects of phenothiazine, such as sedative or hypnotic effects, are often considered therapeutic effects in treating agitated and insomniac patients.

T   F   30. The main therapeutic effect of phenothiazines is the antipsychotic effect.

On the basis of the information provided in Figure 16-2, match the following drugs on the left with the entries on the right.

_____31. chlorpromazine   a.   most potent antipsychotic
_____32. thioridazine   b.   aminoalkyl derivative
_____33. fluphenazine   c.   piperidine derivative

Match the following CNS regions with the side effects or therapeutic effect.

_____34. neostriatum   a.   hormonal alterations
_____35. retina   b.   extrapyramidal effects
_____36. hypothalamus   c.   antipsychotic effects
_____37. limbic forebrain   d.   pigmentary retinopathy

Match the following drugs with the items on the right. Each letter may be used once, more than once, or not at all.

_____38. chlorpromazine   a.   more sedating, hypotensive, and
_____39. thioridazine   anticholinergic
_____40. fluphenazine   b.   dopamine receptor blocker
                                c.   most extrapyramidal potential

Match the following numbered items with the entries on the right. Each letter may be used once, more than once, or not at all.

_____41. serotonin   a.   antipsychotic
_____42. reserpine   b.   putative neurotransmitter
_____43. molindone   c.   enzyme

Match the following numbered items with the entries on the right.

_____44. obscenities   a.   presumed etiological factor
_____45. dopaminergic hyperactivity   in Tourette's syndrome
_____46. dopamine receptor blockade b.   coprolalia
                                c.   haloperidol

Match the daily dose range which should go with each of the following thio-xanthenes.

_____47. thiothixene   a.   2 - 60 mg.
_____48. chlorprothixene   b.   40 - 600 mg.

Match items 49 and 50 with the appropriate EPS.

_____49. chlorpromazine   a.   more EPS
_____50. fluphenazine   b.   less EPS

Complete the following.

51.   Blockade of dopamine receptor sites in the _____ is
      thought to be responsible for the antipsychotic effects of phenothiazines.

52. Blockade of dopamine receptors in the _____ is thought to be responsible for the extrapyramidal effects of phenothiazines.

53. Low dose phenothiazines correlate best with _____ side effects and high dose phenothiazines with _____ effects.

54. We have described five classes of antipsychotics. These are the _____, the _____, the _____, the _____, and the _____.

55. Indicate the recommended therapeutic schedule for depot fluphenazine (fill in blank spaces).

Depot fluphenazine	mg IM	Day
Initial dose	_____	_____
2nd "	_____	_____
3rd "	_____	_____
4th "	_____	_____
5th "	_____	_____
6th "	_____	_____
7th "	_____	_____
Next "	_____	_____
Next "	_____	_____

III. ANTICHOLINERGIC DRUGS

Anticholinergic (AC) drugs are not, strictly speaking, psychotherapeutic agents because, when they are prescribed for psychiatric patients, they are not aimed at the amelioration of any psychiatric signs or symptoms. Rather they are used exclusively for the reduction of one type of side effects caused by neuroleptic agents. It is useful to remember in this context that the term neuroleptic means "mimicking neurological disease." For these reasons, anticholinergic agents are presented in this chapter following the neuroleptic agents. Therefore, in this discussion we will review first those neurological signs and symptoms that neuroleptic agents usually produce during the course of antipsychotic therapy. These manifestations are frequently referred to as extrapyramidal symptomatology (EPS). It is called EPS because there is little doubt that these phenomena largely represent disruption of neural circuits outside the classical pyramidal or voluntary motor system. The structures primarily involved are the neostriatum or caudate and putamen. These two nuclei receive heavy dopaminergic innervation from the substantia nigra. It will be recalled that most neuroleptic agents are characterized by their ability to block central dopaminergic receptors. The usual EPS will now be described.

  1. Dystonia.
      Involuntary tonic contraction of skeletal muscles. Usually induced early and abruptly by neuroleptics with the most potent dopamine

blocking action (i.e. haloperidol, depot fluphenazines). Any striated muscle group may be involved. Spasms of the musculature may cause oculogyric crises, blepharospasm, blinking, tongue protrusion or twisting, facial grimaces, tics, trismus, torticollis, retrocollis, dysphagia, respiratory distress, frozen unilateral shoulder shrugging, tortipelvis, scoliosis, truncal flexion to one side (Pisa Tower syndrome), carpo-pedal spasms, bizarre writhing motions of limbs, toe dorsiflexion, dystonic gait, urinary bladder spasms, and even grand mal seizures. Most of these disorders yield promptly to anticholinergic medications. It is thought that dystonic disturbances induced early during neuroleptic medication represent hyperactivity of dopaminergic neurons caused by the initial increase in turnover and synthesis of dopamine which occurs transiently at the initiation of neuroleptic therapy along with dopamine receptor blockade.

2. Acute Dyskinesia.
Dystonic variant in which muscles contract in a clonic rather than tonic pattern. It closely resembles tardive dyskinesia (p. 823), from which it must be distinguished. Acute dyskinesia usually has an early onset and responds promptly to parenteral AC medication. Tardive dyskinesia, on the contrary, usually has a more delayed onset and is often aggravated by AC drugs (see pp. 821, 823). As in dystonia, it is thought that acute dyskinesia is an early manifestation of dopaminergic predominance triggered by the neuroleptic.

3. The Rabbit Syndrome.
This phenomenon closely resembles the chewing movements of rabbits. It is seen more often in middle age or in the edentulous elderly. Because tardive dyskinesia has a predilection for the orofacial musculature, the rabbit syndrome may be taken to represent incipient late dyskinesia. It appears to be, however, a Parkinsonian form of EPS since it occurs early in neuroleptic therapy, disappears with neuroleptic withdrawal, and also responds to AC therapy.

4. Akathisia.
It means an inability to sit still. It is subjectively experienced as motor restlessness or "jitters." The patients are always in motion, as if having a restless legs syndrome. These patients, if commanded to sit, will tap their feet or shift their legs continuously. If standing, they keep on shifting their body weight from one leg to the other which imparts a sidewise rocking to their trunk. At other times the rocking is to and fro as if doing and undoing their steps. This compulsion for continual motion may prevent sleep at night. Akathisia is sometimes mistaken for agitation. This phenomenon responds poorly to AC medication; indeed it is the least responsive of all EPS except for tardive dyskinesia. For this reason it is felt that akathisia may occur outside of the central extrapyramidal circuits. Diazepam, methylphenidate, and Na valproate have been claimed to improve akathisia.

5. Parkinsonian-like Symptomatology.
   It is thus called because it resembles the naturally occurring Parkinson's disease which consists primarily of hypokinesia, tremor, and rigidity. This triad in its totality is the most frequent neurological side effect induced by neuroleptics. Other signs of Parkinson's disease may also occur. Hypokinesia means reduced motor activity, which decreases in amount and rate. Thus patients appear slow, anergic, and expressionless (amimia). Some patients may look depressed and the diagnosis of akinesia may be overlooked. Some patients complain of the experience of not being themselves which may lead them to reject neuroleptic medication. Their appearance may be zombie-like. Complete akinesia may appear as akinetic mutism or as catatonia. At this stage, the development of hyperthermia, sweating, drooling, tachycardia, dyspnea, seizures, and unstable BP (hypothalamic crisis) must be expected and dealt with by discontinuation of the neuroleptic because it may otherwise cause death. Tremor may be localized to the upper extremities or, in more severe cases, it may be generalized to include neck muscles, tongue, jaw, and lower extremities. The rigidity of Parkinson's disease as induced by neuroleptics is to be distinguished from the spasticity of more focal pyramidal and/or extrapyramidal syndromes. While the resistance to passive limb manipulation in spasticity gives way at a given point of muscle stretch (clasp-knife effect), rigidity does not melt away at any point within the range of stretch, but rather gives a cogwheel or ratchet-like effect. The discontinuous resistance is thought to implicate the superimposed tremor usually present in these patients.

It will be appreciated from the above descriptions that any of the neuroleptic-induced neurological side effects can mimic many neurological disorders or psychiatric manifestations including schizophrenic stereotypies, catatonia, and hysterical behavior. It is beyond the scope of this chapter to discuss a detailed differential diagnosis. Table 16-4 summarizes some important features of these neuroleptic-induced extrapyramidal side effects .

The student should bear in mind that tardive dyskinesia has been inserted at the bottom of the following table only to emphasize its contrasting features as compared to the other EPS. It is important to think of tardive dyskinesia as a serious complication and of all the other EPS as side effects, most of which can readily be corrected usually with AC agents, with other drugs, or by withdrawal or reduction of the neuroleptic. Tardive dyskinesia is not reliably amenable to any of these measures. For this reason the usual AC agents will now be briefly described. Tardive dyskinesia will then be reviewed with the implication that AC drugs are contraindicated in its treatment.

ANSWERS, Section II.

1. b,e,g	16. d	34. b	51. limbic forebrain
2. a,c,d,f	17. a	35. d	52. Neostriatum
3. b,d	18. a	36. a	53. EPS, sedating
4. b,d,c,a	19. c	37. c	54. Rauwolfia alkaloids
5. c,a,b	20. b	38. a,b	Phenothiazines
6. a,b,c,d	21. c	39. a,b	Thioxanthenes
7. a,b,c,d,e,f	22. e	40. b,c	Butyrophenones
8. b,e,c,a,d	23. a	41. b	Indoleamine derivatives
9. b	24. b	42. a	55. 2.5 1
10. c	25. c	43. a	2.5 3
11. b	26. d	44. b	2.5 5
12. (indole structure, N–H)	27. F	45. a	2.5 8
	28. F	46. c	5 12
	29. T	47. a	12.5 19
	30. T	48. b	25 26
13. a	31. b	49. b	25 or more 14 or more days later
14. c	32. c	50. a	25 or more 14 or more days later
15. c	33. a		

TABLE 16-4

FEATURES OF NEUROLEPTIC-INDUCED EXTRAPYRAMIDAL SIDE-EFFECTS

	Inci-dence	On-set	NT Predom.	NT Deficit	AC	Other R_x
Dystonia	2-10%	Early, abrupt	DA		Effective	
Dyskinesia		Acute	DA		''	
Rabbit syndrome			DA		''	
Akathisia	21-45%	Early-middle	?	?	Poor	Switch neuroleptic drug, diazepam, methylphenidate, Na valproate
Parkinsonism	2-56%	Early	ACh	DA	Effective	
Akinesia			''	DA	''	Na valproate
Tremor	35%		''	DA	''	
Rigidity			''		''	Na valproate
			5-HT			
Tardive dyskinesia	5-50%	Late, insidious	DA	ACh GABA	Contraindicated	Na valproate, Baclofen

Abbreviations: NT neurotransmitter PREDOM predominance
AC anticholinergic agent DA dopamine ACh acetylcholine
5-HT 5-hydroxy tryptamine GABA gamma aminobutyric acid

Not all the anti-parkinsonian agents are indicated for the treatment of neuroleptic-induced side effects. Only the primarily anticholinergic and/or antihistaminic (AH) anti-parkinsonian drugs are indicated against the neuroleptic-induced side effects as presented in Table 16-4. The dosages of AC and AH are summarized in Table 16-5.

TABLE 16-5

USE OF ANTICHOLINERGIC AND ANTIHISTAMINIC AGENTS
IN NEUROLEPTIC-INDUCED PARKINSONIAN-LIKE SIDE EFFECTS

	Initial Oral Dose (mg)	Daily Dose Range	IM or IV
Anticholinergic			
Trihexyphenidyl	1-2	5-15	2
Biperiden (Akineton)	1-2	2-6	
Procyclidine (Kemadrin)	2-2.5	6-20	
Cycrimine (Pagitane)	1.25-5	5-20	
Anticholinergic-Antihistaminic			
Benztropine (Cogentin)	0.5-1	1-6	2
Antihistaminic			
Diphenhydramine (Benadryl)	25-50	25-50	25-50
Orphenadrine (Disipal)	50	300	

The following are guidelines for use of agents in Table 16-5.

1) They should not be combined routinely with neuroleptics at the initiation of antipsychotic therapy.
2) They are to be used to treat EPS but not to prevent it.
3) If concomitant administration with neuroleptics is required, they should be gradually discontinued after a few days.
4) It is usually preferable to decrease the dose of the neuroleptic than to add an anticholinergic.
5) The anticholinergics of long duration of action (trihexyphenidyl, benztropine) are used to mitigate the more enduring EPS (hypokinesia, rigidity, tremor).
6) The anticholinergics of shorter duration of action (biperiden, procyclidine) or the milder antihistamine agents (diphenhydramine, orphenadrine) are used to relieve the acute and more transient EPS (dystonia).

7) Parenteral administration should be reserved for the prompt elimination of acute dystonic reactions or severely handicapping EPS.

8) Anticholinergic agents can cause side effects of their own which
add to the powerful anticholinergic action of some neuroleptics;
this is a good reason for avoiding concomitant administration.

9) Elderly patients are particularly sensitive to anticholinergic effects;
they should be treated with lower doses of neuroleptics and the
milder antihistamines should be preferred over the anticholinergics.

10) Large doses of anticholinergics cause peripheral side effects (dry
mouth, blurred vision, cycloplegia, constipation, tachycardia, urinary retention); they also cause a central anticholinergic syndrome
characterized by cognitive disruption, delirium, ataxia, and hallucinations.

Tardive dyskinesia is a neuroleptic-induced neurological disorder which
stands apart from all other neuroleptic-induced EPS because: a) it usually,
if not always, emerges late (tardive), after a protracted period of antipsychotic use, b) there is no effective therapy for this potentially serious
complication, and c) in some patients it behaves as an irreversible process,
despite total withdrawal of the neuroleptic. It is characterized by stereotyped involuntary movements with special predilection for the mouth, face,
and shoulder muscles, although any part of the body may be affected. Sucking, smacking, groaning, jaw movements, tongue darting (as if chameleon's
fly-catching), oculogyric crisis, winking of eyelids, twisting and pulling of
the commissure of the lips and jerks of shoulder muscles may all be observed. The upper extremities may exhibit abrupt unpredictable and purposeless choreiform movements of the proximal musculature or slower and
writhing (snaking) motions (athetosis) of the more distal muscles. Thus,
the syndrome mimics Huntington's chorea which is an ominous heredo-degen-
erative neurological disease.

It is thought that the earliest sign of tardive dyskinesia may be a subtle
vermicular (worm-like) motion of the tongue, presumably at rest on the floor
of the mouth, but this sign is difficult to assess. It is important to suspect
and diagnose tardive dyskinesia early because the best prospect for recovery
is complete discontinuation of the neuroleptic. It is also important to remember that tardive dyskinesia may coexist with the more benign EPS. Therefore, it is not always a matter of diagnosing either one or the other. Thus,
EPS must be evaluated and identified early in its emergence instead of mask-
ing it with anticholinergic agents. A dose increase of the neuroleptic may
also mitigate or completely but temporarily suppress dyskinetic movements,
but this is only a stop-gap measure which is to be discouraged. Table 16-4
gave two GABA agonists (Na valproate and baclofen) as alternative treatment
approaches to tardive dyskinesia but they are still at an experimental stage.
There is as yet no reliable and established treatment of tardive dyskinesia.
The best approach is neuroleptic withdrawal and hope that it is reversible.

QUIZ, Section III.

Circle the letter corresponding to the one correct response.

1.   From a scrutiny of Table 16-4 it should be apparent that a theory underlies the pathophysiology of neuroleptic-induced EPS, including tardive dyskinesia. After studying Table 16-4 again, see if you can guess which of the statements proposed below is the correct one.

    a.   Excess norepinephrine at central receptor sites is exclusively responsible for EPS.
    b.   Neuroleptics block primarily central serotonin receptors, which in turn causes tardive dyskinesia.
    c.   Dopaminergic-cholinergic balance is important for absence of EPS, including tardive dyskinesia.
    d.   For as long as anticholinergic agents are administered jointly with neuroleptics, no EPS problems will emerge, including tardive dyskinesia.
    e.   Dopaminergic mesolimbic structures are the neural substrate of EPS, including tardive dyskinesia.

Use the following case study to answer questions 2-4

Your patient has developed auditory hallucinations, ideas of reference, a belief that her thoughts are being broadcast, and flat affect. You elect to treat her with fluphenazine 16 mg at bedtime. After the first three daily doses (4th day) she appears stiff, has finger tremors, exhibits drooling of saliva, and facial expression is hypomimic. You do nothing at this juncture but continue her on the same daily dose of fluphenazine. She blandly accepts your lack of response. The following (or 5th) day she emerges from bed with severe torticollis (neck bent to one side) and spasms of the same shoulder. This, she says, hurts and frightens her.

2.   What is the cause of the additional signs on the fourth and fifth days?

    a.   aggravation of the psychosis
    b.   extrapyramidal reaction
    c.   hysteria
    d.   fluphenazine
    e.   d causing b

3.   What was the sequence in the emergence of additional signs?

    a.   akathisia, pseudoparkinsonism
    b.   pseudoparkinsonism, akathisia, dystonia
    c.   pseudoparkinsonism alone
    d.   pseudoparkinsonism, dystonia
    e.   dystonia, aggravation of psychosis

4.   Indefinite treatment of this patient with benztropine 2 mg daily may cause a central anticholinergic syndrome characterized by

    a.   visual hallucinations.
    b.   disorientation.
    c.   confusion.
    d.   shifting levels of consciousness.
    e.   ataxia.
    f.   all of the above.
    g.   none of the above.

Use the following case study to answer questions 5-7.

A 60-year-old female comes to your office complaining that she has lost control of her tongue which keeps darting inside and outside of her mouth. Inspection further reveals that she also exhibits facial grimaces, winking, and sudden jerks of the head and the shoulder to one side. She further volunteers that she was discharged from the state hospital two months ago with a diagnosis of Schizophrenia and a prescription of Stelazine (trifluoperazine) and Haldol (haloperidol) which she had been taking for the last 20 years, until about 3 weeks ago when she ran out of medication. She exhibits no signs of psychosis at this time.

5.   The most likely diagnosis for the above signs is

    a.   Huntington's chorea.
    b.   Gilles de la Tourette syndrome.
    c.   hysteria.
    d.   levodopa-induced tardive dyskinesia.
    e.   neuroleptic-induced tardive dyskinesia.
    f.   Schizophrenia.

6.   What is the likely cause of the syndrome at this time?

    a.   discharge from the hospital
    b.   the anxieties of being on her own
    c.   a return to the stresses at home
    d.   abrupt cessation of antipsychotic use
    e.   none of the above

7.   What option is available to you at this time?

    a.   place her back on Stelazine and Haldol
    b.   administer anticholinergics
    c.   explain that at this juncture it is better to wait and see whether signs will worsen or improve and whether her mental condition will require medication

Case study continued: She returns a week later. The manifestations of the first visit remain the same, but her mental status has deteriorated. Exam elicits paranoid ideas and auditory hallucinations. She also appears to have less control over her emotions.

8.   The course to follow now is to

    a. place her on reserpine alone.
    b. resume Stelazine and Haldol.
    c. b plus anticholinergics.
    d. avoid all medications.

9.   Reserpine is

    a. antihypertensive with antipsychotic action.
    b. antihypertensive without antipsychotic action.
    c. an antipsychotic with great potential to cause, mask, or aggravate tardive dyskinesia.

10.   The abnormal movements in this patient may

    a. kill her eventually.
    b. intensify over time.
    c. respond many years later to levodopa.
    d. cause lower motor neuron disease and muscle flaccidity.

Circle the correct answer. One or more than one answer may be correct.

11.   Resumption of Stelazine and Haldol in this same patient is likely to lead to

    a. temporary decrease of abnormal movements.
    b. further intensification of the problem later.
    c. permanent cure of both abnormal movements and psychosis.

12.   Anticholinergic agents

    a. may intensify dyskinesia.
    b. are always effective in the treatment of dyskinesia.
    c. are usually effective in the treatment of most signs of neuroleptic-induced pseudoparkinsonism.

Match the following disorders with the appropriate descriptions

_____13.   pseudoparkinsonism   a.   mechanism not clear
_____14.   akathisia   b.   hyperactivity of dopaminergic neurons
_____15.   dystonia   c.   dopamine blockade plus acetylcholine activation

IV. ANTIDEPRESSANT DRUGS

Consistent with the classification of drugs by desired effect, the antidepressant drugs are used to treat depressions. There are three types of antidepressants:

1) Monoamine oxidase inhibitors (MAOI)
2) Tricyclic antidepressant drugs
3) CNS stimulants: Amphetamines

A. MONOAMINE OXIDASE INHIBITORS (MAOI)

MAOI describes the inhibition of an enzymatic reaction whereby an amine radical of brain monoamines (dopamine, norepinephrine, serotonin) is oxidized away into ammonium. Somehow it has tacitly been assumed that clinical response to MAOI, that is relief from depression, is dependent on that deamination. But there is no evidence that this is how or why MAOI work. There is much controversy as to their efficacy in the treatment of depression. There is even controversy as to whether they should be used or removed from the market. Indeed, in the U.S., the MAOI Marsilid was withdrawn from the market in 1960 because it was reported in association with instances of severe and even fatal liver damage. Then came the dread of hypertensive crises with intracranial hemorrhage which was attributed to potentiating interactions between the MAOI agent and tyramine-containing foodstuffs or sympathomimetic agents. Tranylcypromine, another MAOI, was also briefly withdrawn from the U.S. market as a result of the complications caused by hypertensive crises attributed to it alone or in combination with tyramine-containing ingestibles. The introduction of newer and seemingly safer antidepressants - the tricyclics, to be discussed later - finally made MAOI fall into disfavor. They are coming back, however, because, in the view of some researchers there are some types of tricyclic-resistant depressions which respond more favorably to MAOI. Meticulous care and caution have also reassured us that it is all right and rewarding to use them again judiciously. The important insight to be gained from all this is that nonpsychiatric practitioners should never use MAOI for the treatment of depression. The responsibility of selecting MAOI treatment should be placed on the psychiatrist. The student should bear in mind that MAOI potentiate the effects of tyramine which is contained in some foodstuffs and alcoholic beverages. They also potentiate the effects of sympathomimetic agents frequently present in over-the-counter drugs. Severe hypertensive crises and intracranial hemorrhage have resulted from these combinations. Further, MAOI prolong the effects of barbiturates, alcohol, meperidine, anti-parkinson drugs, and tricyclic antidepressants. If a patient has been receiving MAOI, it is necessary to wait at least three weeks before beginning treatment with tricyclic antidepressants. The careless combination of MAOI with some other drug may be exceedingly dangerous.

The dangers of combining MAOI with tricyclic drugs emphasize the importance of taking a drug history before instituting drug treatment for depression. The main MAOI used in psychiatry as antidepressants are those shown on the following page.

Figure 16-9

MONOAMINE OXIDASE INHIBITORS

HYDRAZINE

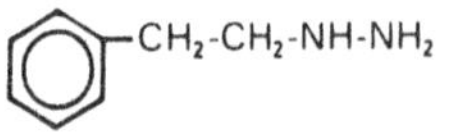

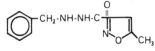

Phenelzine (Nardil)

NON-HYDRAZINE

Isocarboxazid (Marplan)

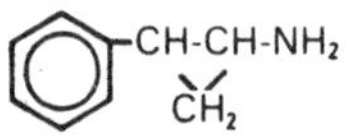

Tranylcypromine (Parnate)

B.   TRICYCLIC ANTIDEPRESSANTS

This group of antidepressant drugs, the tricyclics, is the one currently most used to treat depression. Mild or neurotic depressions usually do not warrant drug therapy and are generally unresponsive to drugs. Tricyclics are useful in the treatment of the more severe depressions. More discriminating guidelines will be given later.

The tricyclics are structurally rather similar to the phenothiazines and the thioxanthenes. Hence many of the side effects caused by these neuroleptics are also shared by the tricyclics. These striking structural similarities are shown below:

Figure 16-10

STRUCTURAL SIMILARITIES BETWEEN TRICYCLIC
ANTIDEPRESSANTS, PHENOTHIAZINES, AND THIOXANTHENES

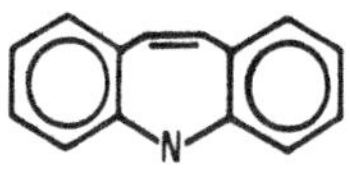

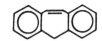

DIBENZAZEPINE   DIBENZOCYCLOHEPTADIENE

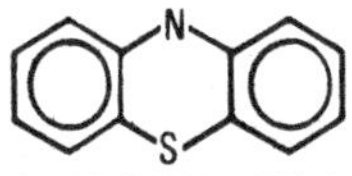

PHENOTHIAZINE 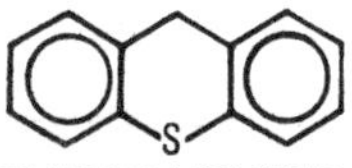   THIOXANTHENE

But their therapeutic or desired effects differ. Tricyclics may aggravate or precipitate Schizophrenia or mania, and chlorpromazine may aggravate or precipitate depression. Therefore, the first principle in drug therapy is to make as accurate as possible a diagnosis in order to avoid such developments.

Any of the unwanted effects of the phenothiazines may occur with the tricyclics, but their most common side effects are:

1) Sedation (often desirable)
2) Anticholinergic action
3) Hypotension

As with the phenothiazines, tolerance to the therapeutic effect of tricyclics does not usually develop, but some tolerance to the unwanted or side effects usually does develop, which is often a good outcome.

As we have stated, combining MAOI with tricyclic drugs can be dangerous. Tricyclics also interact with other drugs, such as phenothiazines and CNS depressants, including alcohol and narcotics. Polypharmacy is usually poor practice and must be avoided.

Tricyclics should not be used in the presence of closed-angle glaucoma. They should be used cautiously and in lower doses in elderly men, in whom bladder paralysis is a common complication. Some tricyclics have marked anticholinergic action. Amitriptyline has the greatest anticholinergic potency. Less anticholinergic potential is attributed to doxepin, primarily because it is usually prescribed in lower dosage than the other tricyclics and for milder depressions. Least anticholinergic effect is produced by desmethylimipramine and protriptyline. The unwanted effects of hypotension and cardiotoxicity should make one seriously consider alternative methods to drug therapy in treating depression in the presence of heart disease or in the elderly. The powerful anticholinergic action of amitriptyline is particularly to be avoided in such cases.

The tricyclics' mechanism of action in relieving symptoms of depression is thought to be the blockade of reuptake of some neurotransmitter amines. There are six main tricyclics in common usage; their trade names and dosage ranges are given in the table below.

TABLE 16-6

COMMONLY USED TRICYCLIC ANTIDEPRESSANTS

	mg/day	
a. Imipramine (Tofranil)	150-300	Dibenzazepine
b. Desmethylimipramine (Norpramin)	75-200	derivatives
c. Amitriptyline (Elavil)	150-300	
d. Nortriptyline (Aventyl)	40-100	Dibenzocycloheptadiene
e. Protriptyline (Vivactil)	30-60	derivatives
f. Doxepin (Sinequan)	200-300	

These drugs are structurally related and similar in effect, except that amitriptyline and doxepin have greater sedative and anticholinergic effects than the other tricyclics. The structural configuration of the six tricyclics listed in the preceding table is shown in Figure 16-11, below.

Figure 16-11

CHEMICAL CONFIGURATION OF TRICYCLIC ANTIDEPRESSANTS

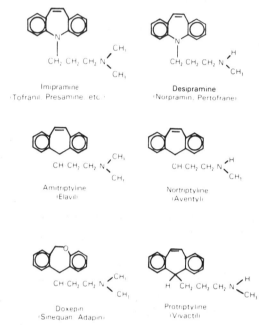

1. Guidelines for use of tricyclics.

    a. One generally chooses a particular tricyclic agent on the basis of whether or not a sedative effect is desired. For example, in an agitated depression one might prefer amitriptyline or doxepin.

    b. The onset of the tricyclics' therapeutic or antidepressant effect is slow, often being delayed for one or two weeks. However, if a tricyclic compound is administered in adequate dosage for four weeks without improvement, continued administration of the drug will probably not produce improvement.

    c. One should start the medication at a low dose, 25 mg tid or qid, to allow tolerance to sedative and autonomic effects to develop. If unwanted effects are troublesome, one should temporarily decrease the dosage.

Studies of large numbers of patients have shown that if one tricyclic is not effective with a particular patient, another may be tried and will sometimes be effective. But drugs should not be switched without a trial of three to four weeks because onset of the antidepressant action is slow.

2. Responders and Nonresponders to Tricyclics.
    There has been in recent years much writing focused on the pref-
    erential responsiveness of various types of depression to one or
    another of the available tricyclic antidepressants. A summary of
    this research should be profitable, even if at this stage it may still
    be a bit premature to draw conclusions. There is a general belief
    that practitioners can enhance their resourcefulness in the effective
    psychopharmacotherapy of the various depressive disorders by
    keeping in mind a few guidelines, some of which are fairly obvious.
    For example, the first is that if optimal doses of one compound for
    a sufficient period of time fail to improve the depression it is time
    to switch to another compound. This requires no ancillary informa-
    tion besides the clinical evolution of the disorder. A second guide-
    line is that those compounds that have been effective during past
    episodes, or, in their absence, in the treatment of similar episodes
    in blood relatives, should have priority in the selection. This
    empirical insight is based on the closer affinity of the chemistries
    of blood relatives and by implication on possible genetic similarity
    of the disorder. Are there biological tests that can be conducted
    to help decide on the choice of a particular antidepressant? Yes,
    various lines of evidence have suggested that methoxy-hydroxy-
    phenyl-glycol (MHPG) is the major metabolite of central norepineph-
    rine metabolism. Some laboratories, but not all, have found that in
    bipolar (BP) patients, manic and hypomanic episodes have relatively
    higher than normal urinary levels of MHPG while depressions corre-
    late with lower levels. Some depressed patients also respond to
    ECT with increase in urinary levels of MHPG, along with improve-
    ment of the condition. Other studies have found that depressed
    patients who respond favorably to imipramine or its demethylated
    derivative also exhibit increased urinary MHPG following treatment.
    Imipramine nonresponders show a decrease in MHPG excretion. An
    even smaller number of patients has yielded results suggesting that
    relatively high levels of MHPG can serve as predictors of favorable
    response to amitriptyline. Thus, MHPG excretion may become a
    biochemical criterion for choosing amitriptyline or imipramine in the
    treatment of patients with depression. Laboratories equipped to
    make MHPG determinations in urine are quickly emerging in various
    parts of the country. Are there other pharmacological predictors of
    drug response if MHPG determinations cannot be conducted? Yes,
    this involves the use of one pharmacological agent to predict re-
    sponse to another. A good example is dextroamphetamine. A tran-
    sient mood elevation in response to acute amphetamine administration
    may predict subsequent response to imipramine, but failure of
    response to amitriptyline. This is explained as follows: amitripty-
    line preferentially blocks reuptake of serotonin by nerve terminals
    with little or no effect on norepinephrine reuptake, while imipramine
    is less selective and blocks the reuptake of both norepinephrine and
    serotonin. Neither tricyclic seems to block the reuptake of DA.
    Amphetamines cause a massive extrusion of catecholamines, both NE
    and DA, from nerve terminals. Therefore, amphetamine and imi-
    pramine share one feature; they both facilitate the presence of

norepinephrine at noradrenergic receptor sites, although by different mechanisms. On the other hand, amphetamine and amitriptyline do not have anything in common in this regard. What we have just said about imipramine applies even more neatly to desipramine because this compound very selectively blocks NE reuptake without affecting the serotonin system. Thus, desipramine is the very opposite of amitriptyline. At the concentrations likely to be found in vivo, say in therapeutic regimes, most researchers have found all the usual tricyclic antidepressants to be ineffective in causing any significant changes on dopaminergic systems.

It may be useful to summarize at this point what each one of the usual tricyclic antidepressants does to the various putative neurotransmitters. The consensus is that desmethylimipramine is a very potent blocker of norepinephrine reuptake. It is indeed very selectively so, and as such it may be considered the very opposite of amitriptyline which blocks very powerfully and exclusively the reuptake of serotonin. Therefore, if one is thinking in terms of a deficiency of either serotonin or norepinephrine, one way to save on time and expense is to choose either desmethylimipramine or amitriptyline and switch to the other if no improvement occurs with adequate doses and duration of treatment.

Usually, the first choice is decided on the basis of convenience or not of sedation. If sedation is deemed desirable, amitriptyline is usually chosen. Other tricyclic antidepressants, interestingly, seem to ride in between the two extremes represented by desmethylimipramine, an exclusive blocker of norepinephrine reuptake, and amitriptyline, an exclusive blocker of serotonin reuptake. That is to say, imipramine, and even the secondary amine derivative of amitriptyline (which is nortriptyline), both have less selective action, in the sense that they block both monoamines under discussion - serotonin and norepinephrine. The differences between these two tricyclics (imipramine and nortriptyline) are very slight in terms of their preferential capacity to block monoamine reuptake.

Imipramine seems to have a mild preference for blockade of serotonin reuptake, while nortriptyline appears to have slight preference for norepinephrine blockade. Choosing imipramine blindly would not lead to insurmountable complications of rationale. This is so because imipramine is converted in vivo to desmethylimipramine, its secondary amine. Indeed the rate of conversion to the secondary amine is such that the ratio of desmethylimipramine to imipramine in plasma is somewhat greater than unity. This means that ingestion of imipramine yields in plasma more desmethylimipramine than imipramine. Hence, a greater blocking of norepinephrine reuptake will result. Since there is good agreement that imipramine effectively blocks serotonin reuptake, the blind choice of imipramine has a pretty good chance of being a wise one. Table 16-7 below summarizes the preferential blockade of neurotransmitter reuptake by the various tricyclic antidepressants.

TABLE 16-7

TRICYCLIC BLOCKADE OF NEUROTRANSMITTER UPTAKE

Tricyclic	NE	5-HT	DA
1. Amitriptyline	−	++++	−
2. Nortriptyline	+++	++	−
3. Imipramine	++	+++	−
4. Desmethyl-imipramine	++++	−	−

Recent reviews indicate that the tricyclics in general are more effective in unipolar depressives who also have vegetative symptoms. Identifying features include an insidious onset, anorexia, weight loss, middle-of-the-night or late insomnia, and psychomotor disturbance. Usually a psychomotorically agitated patient will receive amitriptyline, while a retarded patient is more likely to be given imipramine. This retarded group of patients is usually referred to as endogenously depressed. Endogenous symptoms can be observed however in so-called reactive depressions with a clear cut precipitating environmental change. Unfavorable response to tricyclics is predicted in the bipolar illness, or at least not as favorable as it would be to lithium therapy. Unfavorable response is also predicted by the presence of delusions or neurotic, hypochondriacal, and hysterical personality traits along with a chronic characterological depression. For this last group psychotherapy is perhaps the best approach. In any event, the drug which has been chosen should not be withdrawn when improvement occurs. Tricyclics should be continued for at least two to four months after complete remission of signs and symptoms of depression, otherwise depression often recurs.

A judgment about the indications and contraindications of tricyclic antidepressants must also consider a discernment of the pharmacological possibilities in the bipolar-unipolar spectrum. This is of prime importance to the clinician. Some types of pharmacological treatments appear to be differentially effective in bipolar (BP) and unipolar (UP) illness. Most studies, for example, have shown that lithium is somewhat more effective an antidepressant in BP than in UP patients. When lithium is used as a prophylactic, however, the difference in response between BP and UP patients seems to fade away. Also, rebound hypomania in depressed patients treated with tricyclic compounds occurs more frequently, as would be expected, in BP than in UP patients. Thus, as a prophylactic measure, tricyclics should perhaps be used only in UP depressed patients. But general rules at this stage in our understanding must be applied with caution, and the treatment approach must be individualized.

One must remember that the onset of antidepressant action is slow, usually one to two weeks. If improvement does not occur within four weeks, the tricyclic drug should be discontinued. Another tricyclic drug should be tried, or electroconvulsive therapy (ECT) may be used alone or concomitantly with a tricyclic drug.

Antidepressant drugs have not been as effective as ECT in the relief of depression, but drugs are more pleasant to administer than ECT and offer the rudiment of a rational framework for therapy, whereas the mode of action of ECT remains largely unknown.

3. Tricyclic Plasma Levels.
   When tricyclic antidepressants are administered orally on a chronic basis, the steady-state plasma levels vary markedly from individual to individual. Steady-state occurs when the output of the drug equals its input. It is, therefore, appropriate to wonder what the impact of this variability is on the treatment outcome since it appears that it is the plasma level of the drug, rather than the actual oral dose, that is most directly related to the therapeutic effect. It is precisely because of this inter-individual variability that the actual oral dose may be irrelevant to treatment results and plasma level determinations may one day become a prerequisite for valid, accurate, reliable, and, therefore, meaningful assessment of these pharmacokinetically and pharmacodynamically complex agents. Several groups have been investigating this problem since Asberg and collaborators found a curvilinear relationship for nortriptyline in 1971. Since then, more than 100 works have been published on tricyclic plasma levels in the world literature. Asberg described poor response at both low (below 50 ng/ml) and high levels (above 175 ng/ml), hence a curvilinear (U shape) profile. The mid-range delimited by lower and upper plasma levels is called the "therapeutic window." Asberg speculated that at a middle range, reuptake of monoamines is blocked and this leads to improvement of depression, while at higher plasma levels nortriptyline might cause a neuroleptic-like blockade of receptor sites which would preclude improvement of depressive symptomatology. Asberg's results have since been largely confirmed by technically adequate studies. It is interesting that nortriptyline was initially selected, and indeed the number of studies of plasma levels of this tricyclic far exceeds that of other tricyclics. The reasons are that: a) reliable methodology was available for nortriptyline but not for imipramine or amitriptyline, and b) both imipramine and amitriptyline are parent compounds which are converted in the body into desmethylated compounds with antidepressant properties of their own and, therefore, determination of these metabolites is also required.

There are indications that genetic factors play a role in the disposition of psychotherapeutic agents. It has been shown for example that monozygotic twins, on a standard dose of nortriptyline, maintain similar plasma levels, while dizygotics do not.

What about imipramine? Strangely enough, there is not much work available on the pharmacokinetic vicissitudes of this very effective tricyclic. This is a strange situation only on the surface. There are not many investigations of imipramine plasma levels. This is only because until recently it has been technically more difficult to simultaneously measure plasma levels of imipramine and desmethylimipramine, which is the therapeutically active secondary amine derivative of imipramine by desmethylation.

There is much less information on plasma levels-clinical outcome correlations for amitriptyline, protriptyline, desipramine and doxepin. Yet amitriptyline is the most profusely used antidepressant in the U.S.A. A linear relationship has been proposed for amitriptyline, but this claim requires more and better designed studies. A therapeutic window has been proposed for protriptyline but an upper limit has not yet been demonstrated. Much less can be said of desmethylimipramine and doxepin. A therapeutic window may also apply to doxepin.

Thus, the idea that most patients handle drugs in much the same way must be discarded in favor of the more rational concept that there is a correlation between plasma levels and therapeutic or toxic effect. The studies of correlations with this focus in mind have taught us much about inter-individual differences in absorption, metabolism, and interactions between drugs in individual patients. This trend in medicine began with the anticonvulsant agents in 1968, followed by digoxin in 1971. It has had a great impact in psychiatry with lithium plasma levels, and the problem is now beginning to be elucidated for the tricyclic antidepressants and neuroleptic agents. The fact that patients taking the same dosage have exhibited a 10- to 20-fold variation in their plasma levels has clouded the significance of this research effort, but it appears that the wide variation rather has at its basis factors which have not been controlled or are unknown at the present stage of technical development. Any or all of these factors together may account for the fact that two patients on the same tricyclic dose may differ in the amount of drug available to the target (receptor site) by a factor of 800. It would appear that tricyclic plasma levels depend on a variety of factors besides dose, such as genetic makeup, intake of other drugs, and perhaps smoking and drinking habits.

Unfortunately plasma level determinations are still expensive and not widely available as yet. For the time being, therefore, most clinicians have to satisfy themselves with clinical guidelines for gauging drug response, such as the presence or absence of autonomic side effects. Thus, if these side effects do not become apparent along with a failure to improve, they may suggest that increasing the dosage of the tricyclic will be appropriate. Conversely, side effects which are not severely handicapping or do not suggest signs of toxicity may be an indication that the dosage should not be decreased. Since it is estimated that about 20-40% of the patients on a schedule of tricyclic therapy fail to obtain any improvement, it would be very instructive to determine the percentage of such patients falling outside the therapeutic range of drug plasma levels.

Table 16-8 summarizes the range of therapeutic plasma levels in nanograms/ml (ng/ml). These have been averaged from the most reliable studies and are only tentative. An important consideration in this selection has been that these studies have measured not only the parent drug, but also the active metabolite. It also provides the estimated toxic plasma levels.

TABLE 16-8

PLASMA LEVELS OF TRICYCLIC ANTIDEPRESSANTS

	Therapeutic Range (ng/ml)	Toxic (ng/ml)
Amitriptyline + Nortriptyline	138-210	$\geq$400
Nortriptyline	43-167	$\geq$500
Protriptyline	100-200	?
Imipramine + D-imipramine	157-250	$\geq$700
Doxepin + D-doxepin	110-150	$\geq$500

It is obvious from the preceding discussion that future studies of neurotransmitter metabolites in body fluids and investigations of the correlation between plasma levels of tricyclic and therapeutic response will have to be integrated.

4. Treatment of Tricyclic Toxicity.
    The treatment of tricyclic toxicity should begin with an accurate diagnosis. Tricyclic antidepressants have built-in anticholinergic action which will give the first and most reliable cues as to diagnosis. It is useful to keep in mind that desmethylimipramine is the least anticholinergic of the usual tricyclics, and that amitriptyline has the highest anticholinergic potency. Amitriptyline is one of the most frequently overdosed drugs with suicidal intent, and this risk is particularly aggravated by the availability of large dose capsules. If a standard therapeutic daily dose of desmethylimipramine is given an anticholinergic value of unity, equivalent doses of imipramine, nortriptyline, and amitriptyline will have 2.3, 3.3, and 18 times the anticholinergic potency of desmethylimipramine. The elderly depressed patient on a regimen of tricyclics is particularly prone to chronic toxicity. Acute toxicity is most frequently

due to ingestion of an overdose. In both, there will be signs and symptoms of peripheral muscarinic receptor blockade. The usual sequence is tachycardia, warm dry skin and mucosae, mydriasis, urinary retention and gastrointestinal hypomotility. Central nervous system muscarinic receptors are also hyporesponsive. This "central anticholinergic syndrome" is first signaled by impaired cognitive function and restlessness. As the syndrome aggravates, consciousness and perception become impaired and confusional states (delirium) dominate the picture. If in doubt about the diagnosis, a "test" of 2 mg of physostigmine injected slowly intravenously will produce a dramatic reversal of the central anticholinergic syndrome in five minutes. A single dose has diagnostic value but will hardly suffice as therapy because physostigmine has a very short half-life. Repeated intravenous injections are not advisable, however, because they may induce extreme shifts in the level of consciousness. It is desirable to start an intravenous continuous infusion of physostigmine following a positive "test dose." It has been recommended that the rate of infusion be at about 4 mg of physostigmine per hour. Infusion can then be interrupted every six hours for about 30 minutes to reassess the patient's mental status. Physostigmine-induced peripheral cholinergic crisis can be prevented by intravenous injection of 30 mg of propantheline every six hours. Tricyclic-induced cardiac arrhythmias and other heart conduction problems have also been found to be very effectively controlled by alkalinization with sodium bicarbonate or lactate. It is important to remember that neostigmine cannot substitute for physostigmine because, while it will counteract the peripheral cholinergic blockade caused by the tricyclic, it will not improve the central anticholinergic syndrome. This is because physostigmine readily passes the blood-brain barrier, while neostigmine does not appear to exhibit such passage. Of course, all the other lifesaving measures against tricyclic overdose are mandatory. These should be carried out by the specialized physician in the intensive care unit. It is interesting that physostigmine's efficacy as an antidote against anticholinergic blockade has been known for over a century, but only within the last decade has been disinterred from near oblivion in view of the escalating tricyclic antidepressant overdose problem. It still remains to be determined, however, whether physostigmine can reduce the mortality rate caused by massive overdoses of the tricyclic.

C. CNS STIMULANTS: AMPHETAMINES

Amphetamines are not really used to treat depression because they have short action and are ineffective in the long run. They also pose high risks of dependence, tolerance, and eventually toxic amphetamine psychosis, or rebound depression when the drug is withdrawn. As stated earlier, dextroamphetamine may be used for a short period of several days, only to predict pharmacologically what type of tricyclic drug response your patient may exhibit. A transient mood elevation in response to small doses of dextroamphetamine is thought to augur a therapeutic response to imipramine and desmethylimipramine, but not to amitriptyline. The idea, therefore, is to switch from the amphetamine to imipramine or its congener if there was an amphetamine-induced improvement or to amitriptyline if there was no improvement after a short period of amphetamine administration.

QUIZ, Section IV.

Circle the letter corresponding to the one correct response.

1. You see a 35-year-old female who appears markedly depressed and with psychomotor retardation but no suicidal intent. You come to the conclusion that she may respond to a tricyclic antidepressant. Your inquiry into past drug history elicits that she has been taking Parnate (MAOI), 20 mg tid, for the last three months without improvement of her depression. She has never been on any other antidepressant drug, nor has she received electroconvulsive therapy. To carry out your plan of initiating therapy with a tricyclic antidepressant requires

    a. ascertainment that she is not consuming tyramine-containing foodstuffs or beverages.
    b. three-week wash out period before a tricyclic is initiated.
    c. a call to the physician who had treated her before to tell him that his approach was wrong and dangerous.

2. In treatment of a retarded depression you might prefer to select

    a. amitriptyline.
    b. doxepin.
    c. desmethylimipramine.

3. In using tricyclics to treat depression the drug should be continued for _____ before deciding that it is ineffective.

    a. 3 days
    b. 7 - 15 days
    c. 4 weeks
    d. 2 months

4. Tricyclics are more useful in treating

    a. unipolar depression.
    b. bipolar depression.

5. Amitriptyline is more useful in treating

    a. agitated depression.
    b. retarded depression.

6. Therapeutic effect of drugs correlates best with

    a. dose.
    b. plasma levels.

7. You decide to treat her with

    a.   haloperidol 5 mg qid.
    b.   amitriptyline 150 mg daily.
    c.   thyroid medication.
    d.   vitamins.

8. A week later she reports having taken 150 mg daily of amitriptyline and feeling worse. Now she appears confused, disoriented, and is hallucinating visually. You decide to

    a.   change her diagnosis from depression to Schizophrenia.
    b.   decrease amitriptyline to 75 mg daily.
    c.   switch her to imipramine.
    d.   discontinue amitriptyline and observe closely every 2 days.

9. Two days later thinking is clear and there are no hallucinations or disorientation, but depression remains as on the first visit. You decide that the patient has been suffering from

    a.   depression with added central anticholinergic delirium during the last few days.
    b.   Multi-infarct Dementia for the last three months.
    c.   plain depression with exacerbation lately.

10. Your best choice at this point is to start her on

    a.   a MAOI (tranylcypromine).
    b.   intensive psychotherapy.
    c.   desmethylimipramine 75 mg daily initially.

Circle the correct answer(s). <u>One</u> or <u>more</u> <u>than</u> <u>one</u> answer may be correct.

11. Choose the most appropriate statement(s) below.

    a.   Amitriptyline preferentially blocks reuptake of serotonin.
    b.   Serotonin reuptake is not blocked by amitriptyline.
    c.   Amphetamines cause release of catecholamines from nerve terminals.
    d.   Serotonin is the only biogenic amine released from nerve terminals by amphetamines.
    e.   Amphetamine and imipramine have in common the facilitation of presence of norepinephrine at noradrenergic receptor sites.
    f.   Tricyclic antidepressants cause significant changes on dopaminergic systems.

12. Frequent causes of atropinic psychosis are

    a.   fluphenazine.
    b.   haloperidol.
    c.   thioridazine plus artane.
    d.   amitriptyline.

TRUE or FALSE: Circle the correct letter.

T   F   13. Amitriptyline is a dibenzazepine derivative.

T   F   14. The only structural difference between amitriptyline and doxepin is that the latter has an oxygen in the middle ring.

T   F   15. Desipramine and nortriptyline are demethylated derivatives of imipramine and amitriptyline respectively.

T   F   16. The only difference between the parent drugs imipramine and amitriptyline is an N-C and a C=C ring, respectively connected to the side-chain.

T   F   17. Dopamine uptake is markedly blocked by most tricyclic antidepressants.

T   F   18. The capacity to block serotonin and norepinephrine uptake is the same for all tricyclic antidepressants.

Match the following lettered items with the numbered entries:

____19. phenothiazine   a. neuroleptic
____20. dibenzocycloheptadiene   b. tricyclic antidepressant
____21. thioxanthene   c. monoamine oxidase inhibitor
____22. dibenzazepine   d. barbiturate

Match the following:

____23. 6, 6, 6 ring   a. tricyclic antidepressant
____24. 6, 7, 6 ring   b. neuroleptic

25. Sequence the four tricyclics in Table 16-7 from the most to the least potent blocker of serotonin reuptake on the left below, and from the most to the least potent blocker of norepinephrine reuptake on the right.

_____   _____

_____   _____

_____   _____

_____   _____

V. ANTIMANIC DRUGS

The symptoms and signs of mania and hypomania can be controlled by the administration of lithium carbonate. Lithium is considered by most authorities the drug of choice for treating hypomania and mania. The first trials of lithium for the treatment of Affective Disorders were made by Cade (1949) in Australia. His observations led him to conclude that: 1) the onset of action was relatively long (7-10 days); 2) normalization of manic behavior occurred at 1-3 weeks; 3) if normalization is regained, the patient does not feel under the effects of sedation which is often associated with other psychotherapeutic agents; 4) manic episodes tend to recur on lithium withdrawal more often than on lithium maintenance (thus a prophylactic effect was foreshadowed); 5) higher doses are required initially; later lower maintenance doses are sufficient to sustain improvement; 6) toxicity affects primarily the gastrointestinal and central nervous systems. Since Cade's 1949 four-page publication, a great deal of work has been conducted on lithium, and these original observations have been confirmed in the essentials. In some important ways lithium therapy for mania has provided very desirable guidelines for psychopharmacology in general. Lithium carbonate is such a simple molecule compared with every other psychopharmacological agent. The lithium ion cannot undergo further metabolism in the body. Lithium is easily quantified in plasma, and indeed very accurate methods for measuring its plasma levels were soon developed.

Then the concept of a therapeutic range or "window" began to develop by comparing plasma levels with degrees of clinical improvement. As with tricyclics, therapeutic window means the upper and lower limits of lithium plasma levels within which optimal improvement occurs. Not too long ago therapeutic windows between I and 2.5 mEq/L were considered on an average as desirable, but in more recent years the results of more refined research suggest that it is best to settle for therapeutic windows between 0.6 and I.2. There are patients, however, who require relatively large or small doses of lithium to reach levels within the therapeutic range.

A useful and relatively quick way of determining the dosages required to achieve a plasma level within the more currently entertained therapeutic window is to give an initial 600 mg dose of lithium carbonate and obtain a single level determination 24 hours later. The plasma level obtained correlates very highly with the steady-state level, or that stabilized level usually 5 to 8 days after the patient has been receiving a fixed dosage. At this point lithium input equals output. Upon receiving the report of blood level 24 hours following the 600 mg single dose of lithium carbonate, check in the table below the dosage required for a therapeutic window inferred from your report.

TABLE 16-9

MANAGEMENT OF LITHIUM THERAPY

Your 24 hour plasma level after single oral dose of 600 mg (mEq/L)	Total daily dosage predicted to achieve a therapeutic window between 0.6 and 1.2 mEq/L	Recommended schedule
<0.05	3,600 mg	900 mg QID
0.05-0.09	2,700 mg	900 mg TID
0.10-0.14	1,800 mg	600 mg TID
0.15-0.19	1,200 mg	600 mg BID
0.20-0.23	900 mg	300 mg TID
0.24-0.30	600 mg	300 mg BID
>0.30	300 mg	300 mg IXD *

You do not have to memorize this table, but it will be extremely helpful to carry it in your pocket when you make your rounds in the early morning. Patients who fall within the last population (*) in the table (24 hours plasma level > 0.30) are brittle and difficult to regulate. They eliminate lithium very slowly and readily become toxic. With such patients extreme caution must be exercised. Plasma level determinations at more frequent intervals (daily initially) are appropriate in these cases. If the therapeutic range is not reached on the schedule recommended in the table (300 mg once daily), the dosage may be doubled. If the patient still fails to reach the level in the therapeutic range, there is little to be gained by a further increase because the likelihood of toxicity in this type of patient is very great. It is better to think of him as a poor candidate for lithium therapy.

As with most other drugs, including the psychotherapeutic agents, the elderly are more prone to experience side effects or develop toxicity under lithium therapy. But with caution and within the guidelines provided above, elderly patients can be treated successfully with lithium. Side effects may occur even within the therapeutic range or in the absence of toxicity. Side effects, therefore, do not necessarily suggest that the total daily dosage should be lowered or that the lithium regimen ought to be discontinued altogether.

There are some ancillary measures which may help the clinician in his effort to distinguish tolerable side effects from lithium-induced toxicity.

You probably remember that at the beginning of the section we summarized Cade's observations which included the systems chiefly affected by lithium toxicity.

One way to evaluate lithium-induced neurotoxicity is to obtain an electro-encephalogram (EEG). It has been shown that this neurotoxicity is highly correlated with the induction of EEG changes. The value of an EEG may encompass more than the determination of lithium toxicity because various reports have pointed out the emergence of neurological deterioration in patients suspected of having progressive brain damage following a lithium regimen alone or in combination with other psychopharmacological agents. Some of these suspected neurological patients had lithium plasma levels within the customarily accepted therapeutic range. Therefore an EEG, thorough neurological examination, mental status, and perhaps other neurodiagnostic evaluations, should be conducted in lithium candidates before therapy is instituted.

Lithium has definite therapeutic potential in the great majority of manic and hypomanic patients. The overall improvement rates of mania treated with lithium is 60 to 100%. There is also a clear-cut evidence for prophylactic efficacy against recurrence of mania. The evidence of therapeutic efficacy of lithium in depressive episodes is less strong for bipolar depressed patients and least for unipolar depression. Somewhat more impressive is the evidence for the prophylactic efficacy of lithium in both unipolar and bipolar depressed patients. But there are no reliable or easy methods of identifying lithium responders within the wide spectrum of the affectively ill population. Dramatic response to lithium is often observed to run in families among first

ANSWERS, Section IV._____

1.	b	15.	T	
2.	c	16.	T	
3.	c	17.	F	
4.	a	18.	F	
5.	a	19.	a	
6.	b	20.	b	
7.	b	21.	a	
8.	d	22.	b	
9.	a	23.	b	
10.	c	24.	a	
11.	a,c,e	25.	1	4
12.	c,d		3	2
13.	F		2	3
14.	T		4	1

---

degree relatives. This is consistent with what we know of the genetics of Affective Disorders (see Chapter 8). This illustrates the worth of taking thorough family histories of mental illnesses and their responsiveness to psychopharmacological agents before proceeding to institute pharmacotherapy.

The onset of effect of lithium therapy is relatively slow (7 to 10 days). This is a longer lag period than for the sedating effects of neuroleptics. For this reason, neuroleptics are the drugs of choice for the initial management of severely active hypomanics or dangerously agitated manics.

The comparative efficacy of lithium and the neuroleptics in mania bears more discussion. There are claims of complete normalization of manic patients on lithium versus partial improvement on neuroleptics. There are other claims that neuroleptics make manic patients look quiet while remaining underneath deceivingly manic. Lithium, on the other hand, is claimed to exert a more complete and specific effect on the entire manic picture without inducing sedation as neuroleptics often do. Despite these claims, a group of authoritative reviewers has recently concluded that "after over 25 years of study and clinical use of lithium. . . .its comparative efficacy with neuroleptics is still not fully resolved." (Gerbino et al., 1978, p. 1264).

We feel that the most important consideration in favor of lithium over neuroleptics in the long-term treatment of mania and hypomania is that these conditions usually represent one facet of a bipolar illness. Therefore, depressive episodes in these patients are more likely to be precipitated or aggravated by neuroleptics than by lithium. As discussed earlier, there are some claims that lithium may also be prophylactic against recurrence of depressive episodes.

The mechanism of action of this simple compound in Affective Disorders is still not clearly elucidated. Several potential aspects of its effects have been demonstrated. Because this ion can substitute for Na^+, K^+, Mg^{2+}, and Ca^{2+} at various cellular sites and can alter or diminish neurophysiological regulation or the responsiveness to neural or neuromuscular stimulation, most of the attention and effort have focused on the effects of lithium on electrolyte balance across membranes, including those of muscle fibers and neurons. It has been suggested that in severe mania there may be an abnormal tendency for intracellular sodium concentration to increase, and that lithium may be therapeutic by correcting this abnormality. But the basic concept of abnormally increased intracellular sodium is not solidly established, and the specific mechanism by which lithium might correct this abnormal distribution of sodium is not clear. A second strategy vigorously pursued in the last decade has been to study the short- and long-term effects of lithium administration on neurotransmitter systems. Thus, considerable evidence has been accumulated to support the view that lithium in therapeutic concentrations exerts antagonistic actions at brain synapses mediated by biogenic monoamines.

Indeed, lithium-induced actions which have been demonstrated at presynaptic nerve terminals include all of the following:

1) Enhancement of NE synthesis.
2) Inhibition of NE release.
3) Inhibition of DA release.
4) Inhibition of DA turnover.
5) Enhancement of NE reuptake.
6) Enhancement of DA reuptake.
7) Inhibition of NE retention.
8) Inhibition of DA retention.
9) Enhancement of 5-HTP reuptake.
10) Enhancement of 5-HTP conversion to 5-HT.
11) Conversion to 5-HT turnover rate.
12) Increase of 5-HIAA accumulation in forebrain regions upon electrical stimulation of raphe (serotonergic) cell bodies.

(The student need not memorize all or any of these effects, but he should read them once or twice just to have a grasp of the effort expended in elucidating the mode of action of lithium.)

It is too early to venture a comprehensive hypothesis as to how some or all of these effects may induce improvement in mania, and particularly the mood-normalizing and prophylactic action in recurrent depressions of Bipolar Affective Disorders.

The medical evaluation of a candidate for lithium therapy should include a physical examination, laboratory tests of renal function, electrolytes, thyroid profile, fasting blood sugar, complete blood count, EKG, and, as stated earlier, EEG plus mental status and neurological examination.

The most frequent initial problem associated with lithium therapy is gastrointestinal distress and intolerance (nausea, vomiting, diarrhea). This can be minimized or eliminated by increasing the dose gradually and by prescribing the total daily dosage on a tid or qid schedule with or just after each meal.

Central nervous system side effects such as light-headedness and fine resting tremor are frequent and need not alter the lithium regimen. Only a clear increase in tremor or deterioration of handwriting should be suspected as a clue to incipient intoxication. Neurotoxicity will then often be accompanied by drowsiness, giddiness, ataxia, weakness, slurred speech, blurred vision, and tinnitus. In the face of these signs, lithium intake should be decreased without delay and without waiting for a plasma lithium level determination. If this is not done, more severe signs of neurotoxicity will emerge in the form of neuromuscular irritability as verified by increased deep tendon reflexes, nystagmus, progressive deterioration of sensorium (lethargy, stupor, coma, and death), and convulsions, or less frequently choreoathetosis. Even before this stage is reached, the EEG may reveal generalized slowing (4-6 Hz). Serious toxicity can be expected at plasma levels of 2 mEq/L or more. For this reason, it has recently been felt that attempting to reach such levels for therapeutic purposes is unnecessarily risky.

In the elderly patient on a protracted lithium regimen, subtle forms of organic mental derangement (delirium) must be guarded against. Pre-existing severe renal insufficiency is a contraindication against lithium therapy. Lithium-induced nephrogenic diabetes insipidus may become a serious concern. In this syndrome, lithium is thought to interfere with the normal action of antidiuretic hormone (ADH) on the renal tubule. The result is similar to that of diabetes insipidus of post-pituitary disease: inordinate polydipsia and polyuria of very dilute urine. This complication requires reduction or discontinuation of lithium intake. If that cannot be afforded, thiazide diuretics may help correct this complication.

Recently there has been a flurry of reports indicating that lithium therapy may cause another related complication called lithium-induced nephrotoxicity. The contention so far is that lithium causes glomerular and tubular damage which are verifiable upon kidney biopsy. Functionally, renal concentrating capacity and creatinine clearance are also thought to be reduced. The implications of these findings, even if preliminary, are that lithium is not a totally innocuous therapy and that it should not be instituted lightly for less clearly defined clinical conditions than mania and hypomania.

Protracted lithium therapy may induce goiter of a benign, diffuse, nontoxic type and a slightly hypothyroid profile at most. Whether lithium should be discontinued or thyroxin instituted jointly with, or in place of, lithium should be decided in consultation with an endocrinologist.

The use of lithium during pregnancy and lactation ought to be avoided. If there is an urgent indication for lithium therapy, two guidelines must be kept in mind:

1) At the beginning of pregnancy lithium clearance increases and anti-manic efficacy decreases.
2) Post-delivery diuresis and natriuria may cause compensatory lithium retention and toxicity.

QUIZ, Section V.

Circle the correct answer(s). <u>One</u> or <u>more</u> <u>than</u> <u>one</u> answer may be correct.

1.   Which of the following systems is/are most affected by lithium toxicity?

   a. respiratory
   b. visual
   c. gastrointestinal
   d. blood and lymphatics
   e   central nervous
   f. genital

2.   Check three amines which lithium may antagonize at brain synapses.

   a. tyrosine hydroxylase
   b. serotonin
   c. tyramine
   d. choline acetylase
   e. dopamine
   f. angiotensin
   g. butazolidine
   h. norepinephrine
   i. pitocin

3.   Three complications of concern in lithium therapy are

   a. nephrotoxicity.
   b. neurotoxicity.
   c. interference with ADH function.
   d. respiratory insufficiency.

4.   Lithium is of use in

   a. treatment of mania and hypomania.
   b. prophylaxis against recurrence of mania.
   c. prophylaxis in bipolar depressed patients.

5.   From the following, select the therapeutic lithium plasma level.

   a. 1.0 mEq/L
   b. 2.0 mEq/L
   c. 0.1 mEq/L
   d. 2.5 mEq/L

Match the following headings with the lettered items. Indicate the initial management for each of these manic-hypomanic patients.

___6.   lithium alone
___7.   chlorpromazine
         plus lithium

a. patient appears verbally exuberant, mildly anxious, manageable, and motivated for pharmacotherapy
b. patient brought to emergency room in the wee hours after spending half of the night running wild around the house of his former girlfriend, stark-naked, hollering "but I love you, sweet-heart"

VI. ANTIANXIETY DRUGS

The terms antianxiety, anxiolytic, and minor tranquilizer are more or less interchangeable and euphemistically connote that these drugs fight anxiety or melt it away, or tranquilize in a lesser way than the neuroleptics or major tranquilizers. Many drugs over the years have been used for that purpose. The latest since the beginning of the 20th century have been bromides, alcohol, paraldehyde, chloral hydrate, barbiturates, meprobamate, benzodiazepines, and beta-adrenergic blockers. This discussion will be confined to phenobarbital and the benzodiazepines because they are superior to all the other anxiolytic agents. Important parameters for these two drugs are compared in summary form in the table below.

TABLE 16-10

COMPARISON BETWEEN PHENOBARBITAL AND BENZODIAZEPINES

Features	Phenobarbital	Benzodiazepines
1. Cost ($)	Cheap	Expensive
2. Safety margin	Narrow	Comfortable
3. Overdose lethality	Great	Small
4. Withdrawal	Life-threatening	Mild
	Infrequent	Infrequent
5. Addictive risk	Low	Even lower
6. Fetal effects	Substantial	Mild
7. CNS effects	Depresses excitation	No excitatory effect
	Enhances GABA	Enhances GABA
	Inhibition	Inhibition
8. CNS locus of action	Diffuse	More selective (limbic)
9. Adverse drug interactions	Many, strong	Few, mild

It can be seen from the table above that the benzodiazepines are more desirable and safer, and that the only advantage of phenobarbital over the benzodiazepines is that it is far less expensive.

But since anxiolytics are more often used in general medicine than in psychiatry, it is important to know that in drug comparisons phenobarbital appears as effective an antianxiety agent as any of the more modern anxiolytics. Thus, phenobarbital is often used for the reduction of neurotic anxiety and dysphoric states.

Phenobarbital is a long-acting barbiturate with a prolonged half-life. These features distinguish phenobarbital from the shorter-acting barbiturates in that it infrequently causes physical dependence or a withdrawal syndrome; however, these very features complicate the management of acute overdose. Its limited capacity to produce euphoria (feeling of well being) also decreases its potential for abuse.

Phenobarbital stimulates the synthesis and activity of the liver microsomal enzyme systems which may lead to serious metabolic alterations of other drugs administered concomitantly.

Phenobarbital also increases the production of porphyrins. For this reason, phenobarbital or any other shorter-acting barbiturates are always contraindicated in patients known to suffer from porphyria.

Of the benzodiazepines, we will discuss only chlordiazepoxide (Librium), diazepam (Valium), flurazepam (Dalmane), and oxazepam (Serax). These newer anxiolytics were developed in search for safer agents than the older anxiolytics. Benzodiazepines have become the most popularly used, and perhaps abused, drugs in the entire pharmacological paraphernalia. It will be useful to think of these four benzodiazepines from the beginning in terms of their most frequent indications. These are given in Table 16-11.

TABLE 16-11

FEATURES AND INDICATIONS OF BENZODIAZEPINES

Benzodiazepine	Pharmacology	Indications and Dose (mg)
Chlordiazepoxide (Librium)	Rapid oral absorption Half-life 6-30 hr	Alcoholic withdrawal 5-25 QID
Diazepam (Valium)	Rapid absorption Euphoriant → abuse, acute intoxication Lipophilic Prolonged elimination	Alcoholic withdrawal Anxiety control Seizure control 2-10 TID
Flurazepam (Dalmane)	More sedative Less anxiolytic Less tolerance	Hypnotic Nighttime sedation 15-30 H S
Oxazepam (Serax)	Most rapid metabolism and clearance No active metabolites No tissue accumulation Most potent anti-convulsant	Convulsion control DT control Hepatic insufficiency in elderly 10-30 QID

ANSWERS, Section V. _____

1. c,e
2. b,e,h
3. a,b,c
4. a,b,c
5. a
6. a
7. b

_____

The chemical configurations of these agents are shown in Fig. 16-12.

Figure 16-12

CHEMICAL STRUCTURE OF BENZODIAZEPINES

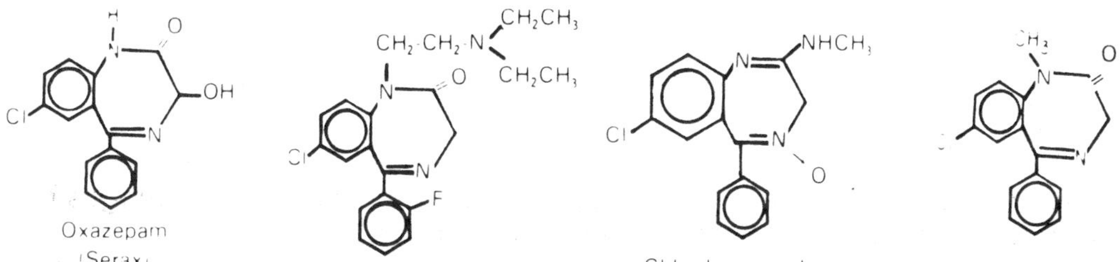

Oxazepam
(Serax)

Flurazepam
(Dalmane)

Chlordiazepoxide
(Librium)

Diazepam
(Valium)

Pharmacologically the benzodiazepines, as well as older anxiolytics, depress CNS function in a concentration-dependent fashion. They all have anticonvulsant and muscle-relaxant actions. Doses which produce mild CNS depression and muscle relaxation are presumably also anxiolytic. Larger doses cause a toxic brain syndrome which may eventually result in respiratory depression, coma, and death. Upon chronic administration, most sedative tranquilizers, including the benzodiazepines, will cause the user to develop tolerance; that is, a gradually greater dose will be required to achieve the same effect. All the anxiolytics herein discussed also exhibit "cross-tolerance," or the ability of one agent to produce tolerance to the effects of others in the group. This phenomenon can be used to advantage in the treatment of withdrawal from other barbiturates. Anxiolytics, including the benzodiazepines, have negligible potential to cause either autonomic nervous system disruption, which is typical of neuroleptics and tricyclic antidepressants, or extrapyramidal symptomatology which, as you have seen (pp. 818-820), is a frequent side effect of most neuroleptics.

The indications for anxiolytics are: short-term treatment of relatively transient acute and disruptive behavioral expressions of anxiety, tension, and fear. They are not indicated as the primary approach to severe psychosis or depression. They are widely used in general medicine and surgery

for the control of short-lived painful syndromes and as preoperative sedation. They are used by psychiatrists for the control of moderately severe
anxiety in neurotic and depressed patients. They may also be useful in the
more severely depressed patients during the delayed onset of antidepressant
effects of tricyclic compounds. Whichever the target symptoms, it is advisable to use anxiolytics only for brief periods because tolerance may lead to
decreased effectiveness, increase in dose, dependency, abuse and addiction.
Long-term psychotherapy should be the treatment of choice for the more verbal, introspective, and psychologically oriented patient. A combination of
physician optimism and conviction about the efficacy of these agents plus low
socioeconomic class, and poor verbal and psychological ability on the part of
the patient appear to warrant a favorable response to anxiolytic medication.

QUIZ, Section VI.

Circle the letter corresponding to the <u>one</u> correct response.

1. Compared with modern antianxiety agents, phenobarbital is

    a. as effective.
    b. less effective.
    c. more effective.

Match the following lettered items with the appropriate numbered heading(s).
Each lettered item may be chosen once or more than once.

___2.	muscle dystonias	a.	amitriptyline
___3.	arterial hypotension	b.	haloperidol
___4.	most anticholinergic antidepressant	c.	thioridazine
___5.	hypnotic non-antidepressant	d.	flurazepam

ANSWERS, Section VI._____

1.   a
2.   b
3.   a,c
4.   a
5.   d

_____

POST-TEST

For the following questions, circle the letter corresponding to the <u>one</u> correct answer.

Use the following case study to answer questions 1-4.

A 70-year-old female comes to your office with complaints of decreased appetite and energy, loss of interest in activities, and cessation of involvement with friends and neighbors. These have gradually become worse for the last three months. Another doctor has treated her with amitriptyline 75 mg daily for the past two months without much improvement. There have been no previous similar episodes or other past psychiatric disturbances. Mental Status: Thinking logical, no delusions or hallucinations.

1. You decide to treat her with

   a. haloperidol 5 mg qid.
   b. amitriptyline 150 mg daily.
   c. thyroid 30 mg daily.
   d. multivitamins.
   e. lithium carbonate 300 mg tid.

2. A week later she reports, stating that she feels much worse. She now appears confused, disoriented, and has visual hallucinations. You decide to

   a. increase haloperidol to 10 mg qid.
   b. increase amitriptyline to 250 mg daily.
   c. switch her to imipramine.
   d. discontinue amitriptyline and observe closely every two days.
   e. increase lithium to 600 mg daily.

3. Two days later thinking is clear and there are no hallucinations or disorientation but presenting symptoms remain as on the first visit. You decide the patient has been suffering from

   a. depression with added central anticholinergic delirium during the last few days.
   b. Multi-infarct Dementia for the last three months.
   c. plain depression with exacerbation lately.
   d. hysterical neurosis.
   e. Schizophrenia.

4. From the following, select the therapeutic lithium level to treat mania.

   a. 1.0 mEq/L
   b. 2.0 mEq/L
   c. 0.1 mEq/L
   d. 2.5 mEq/L
   e. 3.0 mEq/L

Use the following case study to answer questions 5-6.

An elderly man with severe arterial hypertension has been maintained with fair success on the antihypertensive guanethidine for a long period. Recently he became so psychotic as to pose the need for specific medication.

5.   Your choice for the treatment of this psychosis is

    a.   imipramine.
    b.   chlorpromazine.
    c.   amitriptyline.
    d.   reserpine.
    e.   none of the above.

6.   Imipramine, amitriptyline, and chlorpromazine have in common which of the following?

    a.   release all norepinephrine, dopamine and serotonin from neurons
    b.   blockade of guanethidine uptake into noradrenergic neurons
    c.   hypotensive; therefore, more effective in combination with guanethidine
    d.   decrease blood volume through diuresis
    e.   none of the above

Use the following case study to answer questions 7-9.

A 60-year-old female comes to your office complaining that she has lost control of her tongue which keeps darting inside and outside of her mouth. Inspection further reveals that she also exhibits facial grimaces, winking, and sudden jerks of the head and shoulder to one side. She further volunteers that she was discharged from the state hospital two months ago with a diagnosis of Schizophrenia and a prescription for Stelazine (trifluoperazine) and Haldol (haloperidol) which she has been taking for the last 20 years until about three weeks ago when she ran out of medication. She exhibits no evidence of psychosis at this time.

7.   The most likely diagnosis for the above signs is

    a.   Gilles de la Tourette syndrome.
    b.   hysteria.
    c.   levodopa-induced tardive dyskinesia.
    d.   neuroleptic-induced tardive dyskinesia.
    e.   Schizophrenia.

8.   What is the likely trigger of this syndrome at this point?

    a.   discharge from the hospital
    b.   the anxieties of being on her own
    c.   a return to the stresses at home
    d.   abrupt cessation of antipsychotic medication
    e.   none of the above

9. Which of the following options will you choose at this time?

    a. Place her back on Stelazine and Haldol.
    b. Administer anticholinergics.
    c. Explain that at this juncture it is better to wait without medication and see whether signs will worsen or improve and whether her mental condition will require medication later.
    d. Advise immediate return to the state hospital.

10. A 19-year-old student is admitted to the hospital because he hears accusatory voices telling him he is a faggot and that he is to die soon. Speech is incoherent, rushed, and inappropriate. He appears very anxious, fearful, and suspicious. Prior to admission he had not been eating, sleeping, or going to class for several days. At this point the best approach would be

    a. Valium, 5 mg tid.
    b. fluphenazine, 2 mg daily.
    c. electroconvulsive therapy.
    d. chlorpromazine and thioridazine combined, 100 mg of each daily.
    e. chlorpromazine, 50 mg orally, followed by 100 mg every hour until relaxation or drowsiness occurs.

11. If specific treatment of phenothiazine-induced hypotension is required, use

    a. norepinephrine.
    b. epinephrine.
    c. isoproterenol.
    d. reserpine.
    e. levodopa.

12. In regard to drug therapy of psychoses, which of the following statements is (are) true?

    a. Only one variety of chemical compounds is useful in improving the manifestations of psychoses.
    b. Simultaneous use of drugs belonging to two or more categories is frequently advisable because most studies show that combinations are better than a single agent.
    c. Use of multiple drugs will decrease the number and types of side effects.
    d. Oligopharmacy is generally preferable to using multiple drugs.
    e. Adverse drug interactions are rare.

13. Your patient has been started on 200 mg of chlorpromazine tid for treatment of an acute episode of agitation, delusions and threatening gestures. These appear to be responding well to chlorpromazine but within a few days he develops a severe skin rash thought to be an allergic reaction to the phenothiazine. Select the one best alternative from the following.

    a. Increase the dose of chlorpromazine since it is antihistiminic.
    b. Reduce chlorpromazine by half.
    c. Switch to haloperidol 4 mg tid.
    d. Leave chlorpromazine as is and add an anticholinergic agent.
    e. Leave chlorpromazine as is and recommend suntanning.

14. Some phenothiazines have effects similar to

    a. nicotine.
    b. muscarine.
    c. physostigmine.
    d. atropine.

15. Tricyclic drugs used to treat depression vary most in

    a. effectiveness.
    b. dose.
    c. unwanted reactions.
    d. degree of sedative effect

For the following questions, <u>one</u> or <u>more</u> <u>than</u> <u>one</u> answer may be correct. Circle the correct answer(s).

16. Drug choice primarily depends on

    a. diagnosis.
    b. dynamic formulation.
    c. specific signs or symptoms.
    d. an understanding of the doctor-patient relationship.

17. Which of the following produce <u>severe</u> physiological addiction?

    a. benzodiazepines
    b. phenothiazines
    c. amphetamines
    d. barbiturates

18. Side effects of reserpine include

    a. hypotension.
    b. depression.
    c. nausea and vomiting.
    d. impotence.

19. The "central anticholinergic syndrome" occurring with concomitant signs of peripheral muscarinic receptor blockade is characterized by

   a. impaired cognitive functioning.
   b. restlessness.
   c. impaired consciousness.
   d. impaired perception.

20. Complications of concern in lithium therapy include

   a. nephrotoxicity.
   b. neurotoxicity.
   c. interference with antidiuretic hormone function.
   d. respiratory insufficiency

21. Which of the following statements is (are) correct?

   a. Antipsychotics are additive with each other.
   b. Chlorpromazine in larger doses counteracts amphetamine intoxication or psychosis.
   c. MAOI-phenothiazine combinations may produce arterial hypotension and severe extrapyramidal symptoms.
   d. Phenothiazines combined with other phenothiazines cause enhanced sedation and respiratory depression.

22. Which of the following statements regarding Phenothiazines is (are) correct?

   a. Phenothiazines are drugs of choice for treating anxiety.
   b. Side effects of phenothiazines such as sedative or hypnotic effects are often considered therapeutic effects in treating agitated patients.
   c. Increasing doses of phenothiazines are required with increasing age of the patient to obtain a therapeutic response.
   d. The main therapeutic effect of phenothiazines is the antipsychotic effect.

23. Which of the following statements is (are) true?

   a. Phenothiazines used at lower doses (1-10 mg) are more likely to induce parkinsonian-like side effects than those used at higher doses (100-500 mg).
   b. Sedating, hypotensive and anticholinergic side effects are usually inversely related to parkinsonian-like symptomatology.
   c. Thioridazine is the most anticholinergic of the phenothiazines.
   d. Nonphenothiazine anticholinergic agents are usually employed to treat phenothiazine-induced parkinsonian-like symptomatology.

24. Phenothiazines are <u>not</u> a good first choice to treat anxiety because

   a. they are ineffective.
   b. withdrawal reactions are more serious than with other drugs.
   c. dependency and addiction occur more readily than with other drugs.
   d. they have more serious side effects than antianxiety drugs.

25. The anticholinergic effects of tricyclics suggest caution in their use with patients who have

   a. prostatic hypertrophy.
   b. spastic colon.
   c. certain types of glaucoma.
   d. complaints of chronic pain.

26. If most tricyclic drugs are ineffective at the upper limit of their dosage range,

   a. dosage should be increased.
   b. another tricyclic should be added.
   c. an MAOI inhibitor should be added.
   d. electroconvulsive therapy may be indicated.

27. Tardive dyskinesia

   a. usually emerges late after a protracted period of antipsychotic use.
   b. is characterized by stereotyped involuntary movements, especially of the mouth, face, and shoulder muscles.
   c. has no effective treatment.
   d. in some patients behaves as an irreversible process despite total withdrawal of the neuroleptic.

28. Phenothiazines vary in

   a. dosage.
   b. sedative effect.
   c. anticholinergic effect.
   d. capacity for extrapyramidal reactions.

29. Haloperidol is useful in the treatment of
   a. Schizophrenia.
   b. mania.
   c. Organic Brain Syndromes with psychosis of the elderly.
   d. Gilles de la Tourette syndrome.

30. Which of the following may be useful in treating mania?

   a. barbiturates
   b. phenothiazines
   c. benzodiazepines
   d. lithium carbonate

31. Amphetamines are <u>not</u> used for serious depressions because of

    a. significant incidence of toxic reactions.
    b. toxic reactions with other drugs.
    c. paradoxical sedation.
    d. ineffectiveness.

32. Pigmentary retinopathy may result from overdose of

    a. thioxanthenes.
    b. trifluoperazine (Stelazine).
    c. chlorpromazine (Thorazine).
    d. thioridazine (Mellaril).

33. The "central anticholinergic syndrome" is dramatically reversed by

    a. physostigmine, 2 mg I.V.
    b. chlorpromazine, 100 mg po.
    c. Valium, 10 mg I.V.
    d. imipramine, 50 mg po.

Match the following disorders with the lettered items. Lettered items may be used once, more than once or not at all.

___34. akathisia
___35. pseudoparkinsonism

a. norepinephrine blockade
b. mechanism not clear
c. dopamine blockade plus acetylcholine activation

PRE-TEST ANSWERS

1. b,d	13. a,c	25. b
2. a,b,c,d	14. a,b,c	26. d
3. a,b,c,d	15. d	27. a
4. d	16. a,b,c,d	28. a
5. d	17. a,b,c,d	29. d
6. a,b,c,d	18. a,b,c,d	30. e
7. a,b,c,d	19. a	31. a
8. a,c	20. a,b,c,d	32. d
9. d	21. c	33. b
10. d	22. d	34. c
11. b,d	23. d	35. a
12. d	24. c	36. c

POST-TEST ANSWERS

1. b	14. d	26. d
2. d	15. d	27. a,b,c,d
3. a	16. a,c	28. a,b,c,d
4. a	17. d	29. a,b,c,d
5. d	18. a,b,c,d	30. b,d
6. b	19. a,b,c,d	31. a,b,c,d
7. d	20. a,b,c	32. d
8. d	21. a,b,c,d	33. a
9. c	22. b,d	34. b
10. e	23. a,b,c,d	35. c
11. a	24. d	
12. d	25. a,c	
13. c		

REFERENCES

Baldessarini, R. J. Chemotherapy. In A. M. Nicholi (Ed.), The Harvard guide to modern psychiatry. Cambridge, Mass.: The Belknap Press of Harvard University Press, 1978.

Cade, J. F. Lithium salts in the treatment of psychotic excitement. Medical Journal of Australia, 1949, 2, 349-352.

Clark, W. G., & Del Guidice, J. (Eds.) Principles of psychopharmacology, (2nd Ed.) New York: Academic Press, 1978.

Freedman, A. M., Kaplan, H. I., & Sadock, B. (Eds.) Comprehensive textbook of psychiatry, Vol. II. Baltimore: The Williams & Wilkins Co., 1975.

Gerbino, L., Oleshansky, M., & Gershon, S. Clinical use and mode of action of lithium. In M. Lipton, A. DiMascio, & K. Killam (Eds.), Psychopharmacology: A generation of progress. New York: Raven Press, 1978.

Glick, R. A., Meyerson, A. T., Robbins, E., & Talbot, J. A. (Eds.) Psychiatric emergencies. New York: Grune & Stratton, 1976.

Greenblatt, D. J., & Shader, R. I. Treatment of the alcohol withdrawal syndrome. In R. I. Shader (Ed.), Manual of psychiatry therapeutics. Boston: Little, Brown and Co., 1975.

Janowsky, D. S., Addario, D., & Schuckit, M. A. Psychopharmacology - Case studies. New York: Medical Examination Publishing Co., Inc., 1978.

Seiden, L. S., & Dykstra, L. A. Psychopharmacology - A biochemical and behavioral approach. New York: Van Nostrand Reinhold Co., 1977.

Slaby, S. E., Lieb, J., & Tancredi, L. R. Handbook of psychiatric emergencies. New York: Medical Examination Publishing Co., Inc., 1975.

CHAPTER 17
Psychosocial Treatments
Thomas E. Steele, M.D.

CHAPTER OUTLINE

Learning Objectives

Pre-Test

Post-Test

Pre-Test/Post-Test Answers

References

LEARNING OBJECTIVES

After reading this chapter, the student will be able to:

1. Define psychotherapy

2. Distinguish psychosocial therapy from somatic therapy.

3. List factors common to various forms of psychotherapy.

4. Distinguish psychotherapeutic context from psychotherapeutic technique.

5. Describe four psychotherapeutic contexts, and cite possible indications for each.

6. Define transference and countertransference.

7. Describe the major factors responsible for improvement in interactional group psychotherapy.

8. Distinguish psychoanalysis from psychoanalytic psychotherapy.

9. Define essential features of psychoanalytic technique.

10. Describe six "lessons" that are learned, according to Strupp, in dynamic psychotherapies.

11. List four attributes of the "reactive environment" in milieu therapy, as described by Maxmen, Tucker, & LeBow.

12. Describe four factors in the illness situation that foster the existence of societal guidelines for healer and patient behavior.

PRE-TEST

For the following questions, <u>one</u> or <u>more</u> <u>than</u> <u>one</u> answer may be correct. Circle the correct answer(s).

1. According to Maxmen, Tucker, & LeBow, which of the following is/are characteristic(s) of the "reactive environment"?

   a. primary emphasis on intrapsychic difficulties, with a secondary focus on behavior
   b. utilization of knowledge of the antecedents and consequences of a patient's behavior in order to alter it
   c. subordination of other treatment modalities to the goals of individual psychotherapy
   d. less emphasis upon confidentiality between patient and staff member, and more emphasis upon interchange of information among staff
   e. similarity of specific behavioral goals (such as increased expression of feelings) for most patients
   f. general agreement on specific patient goals among staff, despite staff's coming from different disciplinary backgrounds
   g. interchangeable treatment personnel, despite different disciplinary backgrounds, with regard to implementing specific diagnostic and therapeutic measures

2. Choose the correct statement(s) concerning interactional group psychotherapy, as described by Yalom.

   a. Overt expression of painful feeling states is discouraged.
   b. Catharsis and inspiration are major therapeutic factors.
   c. Group cohesiveness and imparting of information are major therapeutic factors.
   d. Interpersonal learning and universality are major therapeutic factors.
   e. The primary task of the leader is to foster communication among group members.

3. Choose the correct statement(s) about brief psychotherapy.

   a. Time is the principal dimension that distinguishes brief psychotherapy from other approaches.
   b. Use of a specific technique (direct interpretation) is the principal dimension that distinguishes brief psychotherapy from other approaches.
   c. Brief (or short-term) psychotherapy is an example of a specific treatment context.

4. According to Parsons, which of the following statements is/are correct?

    a. Societal factors influence doctors' and patients' behavior.
    b. Individual factors do not influence doctors' and patients' behavior.
    c. The healer's role is functionally diffuse.
    d. The uncertainty of medical knowledge contributes to the need for socially-sanctioned behavioral guidelines.

5. Choose the correct statement(s) about family therapy.

    a. Because an individual's distress may be symptomatic of a less-obvious problem in the family system, the family therapist should not give psychotropic medication to the "identified patient."
    b. Treatment of a married couple may affect the behavior of their children.
    c. Family therapy might be indicated when the presenting problem is a 9-year-old child with a well-documented learning disability resulting from perinatal hypoxia.
    d. Fluid generational boundaries are generally a sign of a well-functioning family system.

6. Choose the correct statement(s) about psychoanalysis.

    a. Interpretation of transference is an essential element of psychoanalysis.
    b. Other therapeutic approaches may share common therapeutic factors with psychoanalysis.
    c. Meeting five times a week is an essential element of psychoanalysis.
    d. Resistance can be both an impediment to the progress of treatment and a useful source of information.

TRUE or FALSE. Indicate which of the following statements are true (T) and which are false (F) by circling the appropriate letters.

T   F   7. Transference is an inappropriate, unconscious reaction based upon previous experience.

T   F   8. Transference occurs in individual psychotherapy, but not in multiple-person therapy contexts.

T   F   9. Psychotropic drugs should <u>not</u> be combined with psychodynamic psychotherapy.

T   F   10. Psychotropic drugs should <u>not</u> be given to patients with unconscious conflicts.

T   F   11. Psychoanalysis represents both a therapeutic technique and a specific therapeutic context.

T   F   12. Psychosocial therapy should <u>not</u> be used when organic factors play a significant role in a patient's dysfunction.

T   F   13. Psychotropic drugs may be indicated when experiential factors play a significant role in a patient's dysfunction.

T   F   14. Biochemical/neurophysiologic factors play a major role in the content of hallucinations.

T   F   15. Success of a therapeutic technique based upon a given theory of personality implies that that theory is correct.

T   F   16. The DSM-III diagnosis may be of little help in choosing a treatment strategy in psychodynamic psychotherapy.

T   F   17. Resistance in psychoanalysis does _not_ occur when transference is properly interpreted.

T   F   18. Strupp considers imitation of the therapist to be a major therapeutic factor in dynamic psychotherapy.

I.   INTRODUCTION

The psychosocial therapies encompass an extremely broad range of practices. In contrast to somatic therapies (such as drugs, psychosurgery, or electro-convulsive therapy), which involve direct introduction of a physical or chemical agent into the body of the patient, psychosocial therapies are symbolic interventions primarily involving communication (both verbal and nonverbal) between therapist and patient. The term "psychosocial" recognizes the importance of interpersonal as well as intrapsychic processes in the genesis and treatment of disorders.

Although no universal agreement exists concerning the indications for somatic or psychosocial treatments, authorities generally concur that somatic therapy is an important aspect of the treatment of disorders--such as Schizophrenia or the major Affective Disorders--in which a neurochemical abnormality is presumed to play a primary or major role. Psychosocial therapies, by contrast, are aimed more at disorders in which learning, broadly defined, plays a significant role. Thus, if a patient suffers chronic low self-esteem because his parents were critical and aloof--i.e., he did not learn at an early age that he was a lovable person and that people could be expected to give warmth and affection--then a psychosocial therapy would be appropriate. However, if a patient's low self-esteem reflects an episodic Affective Disorder rather than an enduring, learned pattern, then somatic treatment (in this case, antidepressants) would be more appropriate. For many patients, some combination of somatic and psychosocial therapies may be more useful than either alone. It is important to note that while it is possible to administer a psychosocial therapy alone, a "pure" somatic therapy does not exist since the patient's response is influenced by symbolic factors (such as the placebo response, the quality of the doctor-patient relationship, the meaning of the illness to the patient, and the culturally-sanctioned role of the healer), as well as by the intrinsic properties of the somatic agent.

QUIZ, Section I.

Classify the following as somatic (S) or psychosocial (P) therapy by circling the appropriate letter.

S   P   1.   Marital couple group therapy.

S   P   2.   ECT

S   P   3.   Prolixin decanoate 25 mg IM q 2 weeks.

S   P   4.   Hypnosis

S   P   5.   Systematic desensitization for fear of flying

S   P   6.   Psychodrama

II.   TREATMENT CHOICE

Some of the confusion surrounding indications for and efficacy of the various psychosocial therapies arises from a failure to distinguish <u>context</u> from <u>technique</u> (Abroms, 1969).   Individual psychotherapy is not a specific technique, but rather a relationship context (one therapist and one patient) in which a technique is applied.   Similarly, group therapy, marital couple therapy, and family therapy are contexts rather than techniques.   Within a given context, various techniques may be utilized, depending upon the nature of the patient's problem and goals and the therapist's areas of expertise.   Examples of techniques, which will be discussed more fully in this and other chapters, include procedures such as free association, systematic desensitization, operant conditioning, role-playing, interpretation of dreams, giving advice, or hypnosis.   The relevant question in choosing a therapeutic approach is not, "Does individual psychotherapy 'work'?," but rather, "Does technique A, applied in context B, exert a salutary effect on specified target behaviors, symptoms, or feelings?"

Given the plethora of psychotherapeutic schools, theories, techniques, and practitioners, it is probably impossible to offer a definition of psychotherapy that would encompass the activities of all those who consider themselves "psychotherapists."   However, if we restrict our attention only to those therapies that have a reasonably systematic theoretical basis and that have stood the test of time, we could define psychotherapy as:

1)   a procedure whereby a trained and socially-sanctioned therapist
2)   tries, via symbolic interventions,
3)   to modify or remove behaviors, thoughts, or feelings
4)   that are a source of distress to the patient (or, in some instances, to others) and/or that interfere with the patient's psychosocial functioning.

Item 1) in this definition excludes advice or support from well-meaning friends or relatives; while such interventions may well be helpful, they are not psychotherapy.   Similarly, while effective care for physical illness by a physician or forgiveness of sin by a priest may make people feel better, such efforts do not constitute formal psychotherapy.

Regarding the social sanctioning of the therapist, Parsons (1950) has presented a penetrating analysis of the relationships between social structure and general medical practice, and has discussed how social as opposed to individual factors influence how doctors and patients behave toward one another.   These factors are social rather than individual in that they reflect well-defined (if seldom articulated openly) institutionalized expectations rather than individual personality traits of doctors or patients.   Several characteristics of the illness situation call forth these expectations: being sick is distressing and anxiety-provoking; the patient is relatively helpless and "at the mercy of" the doctor; the physician has unusual liberties to probe the patient--both physically and emotionally--in intimate ways, to cut him, and to drug him; and medical knowledge is incomplete, and clinical decisions are fraught with uncertainty. Given such stresses, it is obvious that socially-sanctioned guidelines, rather than the whims of individuals, are needed if doctors and patients are to carry out their respective responsibilities.

One example of Parsons' way of classifying interactions is the dichotomy of functional specificity vs. functional diffuseness. The healer's role is functionally specific: the physician's specific task is to help increase the well-being and adaptive behavior of the patient, and the physician's and patient's obligations to one another are restricted to those which further the goals of treatment. The doctor is not a universal wise person who is expected to advise the patient on his investments or how he should vote--just as the banker is not expected to inquire into a loan-seeker's dietary habits or sex life. In contrast, the relationship of a patient to a friend or relative is functionally diffuse and carries a different set of expectations and responsibilities. While a friend may be expected to listen sympathetically to one's troubles, he is not expected to "do something" definitive about them; nor is the doctor expected to go to the movies with the patient if the patient desires companionship.

A second way in which social sanction affects therapy is through what is generally accepted by the culture as a reasonable modus operandi. A therapy based upon exorcism of demons is unlikely to gain wide currency in a technologically-oriented society that reveres the scientific method. Similarly, a therapy emphasizing the interplay within the individual of unconscious impulses and conflicts is not consonant with a society that views disordered behavior as divine punishment.

Item 2) in the definition of psychotherapy merely distinguishes the psychosocial therapies from the somatic therapies. It is well to remember that the particular symbols that may be efficacious are determined by both individual and societal factors. Even if placebos are effective via the release of endorphins, only certain symbolic forms will carry the meanings that are transduced by the brain into endorphin release.

Item 3) in the definition distinguishes the goals of psychotherapy--change in behavior, thought, or feeling--from other medical goals.

Item 4) sets further limits upon the goals of therapy. Improvement in personal comfort and/or psychosocial functioning may seem modest goals compared to such aims as "mental health," "self-actualization," or "personality growth," but the former, being more specific, are more readily definable by both patient and therapist, and are more susceptible to clinical and experimental verification.

Given the complexity of human personality and the multitude of biological, psychological, and sociocultural factors that shape human development, proper choice of a treatment context and technique requires considerable

ANSWERS, Section I. _____

1.	P	5.	P
2.	S	6.	P
3.	S	7.	P
4.	P	8.	S

_____

skill. Indeed, even the identification of the problem(s) and the formulation of appropriate goals may prove difficult. Patients may consciously or unconsciously conceal the "real" reason for their distress, and the presenting problem may be only a "ticket of admission" that allows the patient to enter into a healer-patient relationship that will provide the context for the later unfolding of more fundamental distresses. Furthermore, goals and strategies of treatment may remain unclear until much more is known about the patient's premorbid functioning. For example, a patient who is severely depressed may be quite withdrawn and reclusive; follow-up treatment for a patient who has never acquired adequate interpersonal skills will differ markedly from treatment of a person whose previously-adequate skills are temporarily impaired by acute illness.

What are the sorts of problems that bring a patient to psychotherapy? At one level, as mentioned above, problems consist of various sorts of personal discomfort and impaired psychosocial functioning. Personal discomfort may include such distresses as: decreased self-esteem; excessive shyness; inordinate sadness; anxiety in its many guises; various circumscribed phobias; unhappiness with the choice of mate or occupation; obsessional thoughts; dissatisfaction with one's sexual performance or sexual object choice; and so on. Examples of psychosocial dysfunction include: impaired performance as a student, parent, or spouse; inability to form close and satisfying relationships with peers; difficulty sustaining employment in an occupation commensurate with one's abilities and interests; and so on.

It should be obvious that difficulties in the personal and psychosocial spheres interpenetrate: a junior executive who unconsciously harbors resentment against his father (because of his father's aloof and overly critical manner of relating during the executive's childhood) may behave irritably with his superiors and stubbornly refuse to perform in accordance with the demands of his position; thus, his occupational performance will suffer. His anger may instead be displaced onto seemingly less-threatening targets such as his wife, and this--plus the financial difficulties resulting from his failure to advance occupationally--may contribute to marital discord. Or, a young woman's lack of skill in peer relationships may lead her to become overly attached to and dependent upon her parents. This may not only interfere with her further contact with peers (which might facilitate her learning more effective ways of relating to them), but also may lead to discord within the family as the parents' extrafamilial interests give way to their daughter's demands.

Choice of appropriate treatment demands a careful teasing-out of primary and secondary sources of distress. In the above example of the junior executive, treatment of marital discord might be necessary--yet would be clearly inadequate as the sole therapeutic intervention. In the example of the homebound woman, therapy focusing upon the family's difficulties might seem a logical choice--but would be inadequate unless supplemented by a therapy that would increase the patient's skill and comfort in dealing with her peers outside the home.

Detre and Jarecki (1971) emphasize that specifying the area of dysfunction aids in the choice of treatment context. If a person's primary difficulty is in forming and maintaining intimate relationships or in relating to persons occupying a particular role (such as authority figures--e.g., teachers, or supervisors), then individual therapy would be a logical choice. If discomfort or lack of skill in transacting with peers is a major source of distress, then group therapy would be a suitable matrix. If a child's dysphoria or misbehavior is judged to be reactive to discord in the parents' marriage, then family therapy would be a logical treatment context. Perhaps this would be followed by marital couple therapy as the reactive nature of the youngster's problem becomes more apparent. If the child's difficulties continued even after marital harmony was restored, then a therapeutic context involving only the child would be appropriate, and intervention with the parents might be limited to measures that ensure their cooperation with their child's treatment.

A word about "short-term" treatment is in order. Short-term (or its synonyms "brief," or "time-limited") is not a specific context or technique; rather, it is a time dimension that reflects the belief that certain approaches encompassing various techniques in various contexts can accomplish certain goals in less time than one might think. The breadth of the concept is illustrated by a recent monograph that includes articles on brief group psychotherapy, brief family therapy, and short-term sexual counselling, as well as brief psychodynamic individual psychotherapy (Sloane & Staples, 1979).

As a means of illustrating initial context selection, consider the four cases below in terms of the following context alternatives:

1) Individual therapy.
2) Group therapy.
3) Couple therapy.
4) Family therapy.
5) Somatic therapy is indicated, regardless of specific treatment context.

Case 1. A middle-aged woman is intensely afraid of driving a car; this fear developed after her husband told her that he was having an extramarital affair. A major consequence of her driving phobia is that her husband spends much of his free time chauffeuring her about. Previous history of emotional problems is denied.

Case 2. A middle-aged woman is intensely afraid of driving a car; this fear developed when her oldest child, a son, reached the age at which he could get his learner's permit for driving. He had expected his mother to help teach him to drive. Past history reveals that the woman experienced considerable distress when she left her parental home and made several "false starts" with abortive attempts at independence. She was able to move away from home permanently only after her marriage at age 28. She has always been quite sensitive to separations--e.g., she has become quite distressed in the past when friends have moved away. She performs well in her job as an assistant manager of a department store.

Case 3. A middle-aged woman is intensely afraid of driving a car; this fear developed gradually over several weeks and reflects her increasing conviction that she is such an evil person that she would surely harm someone were she to drive. She is also afraid that enemy agents have tampered with her car. There is no previous history of emotional problems.

Case 4. A middle-aged woman is intensely afraid of driving a car; this fear developed after a move to a different state in connection with her husband's promotion. Throughout her married life she has been a "stay-at-home" because of her considerable discomfort (primarily, symptoms of anxiety) around other people. She dreads meeting new people--especially neighbors and her husband's business associates and their spouses. She remembers feeling shy and "out-of-it" throughout high school and college, although she has had two or three close friends over the years. She has never enjoyed driving a car, although previously she was able to drive on errands such as shopping or chauffeuring the children.

Symptoms per se may be relatively nonspecific in that a variety of psychosocial or neurochemical events may lead to similar constellations of behavior. In the preceding cases, the presenting symptom of a driving phobia is the final common pathway for the expression of several different sorts of difficulty. In Case 1, the phobia seems to serve as a way of occupying her husband's time in order to preclude his seeing his paramour; the phobia has interactional as well as intrapsychic consequences, although the wife may not be consciously aware of them. We do not know whether he told her of the affair to relieve his guilt or to punish her or for some other reason, but we do know that he told his wife rather than her discovering it herself, again suggesting that there is an interactional (between husband and wife) function of the affair. Thus, marital couple therapy would be a logical choice of therapeutic context.

In Case 2, the phobia seems to be serving to avoid separation from her son. Her problems with separation are long-standing; we have no evidence (at present) that either forming peer relationships or functioning at work represents a problem for the patient. Because the difficulties seem limited to extreme sensitivity to separation in one-to-one relationships, individual therapy would be a logical treatment context.

In Case 3, the driving phobia seems to be a symptom of a first episode of a major disorder--probably a depression (her belief that she is an evil, dangerous person) with associated paranoid ideation. Somatic therapy is indicated as a first approach; a more accurate assessment of her need for more extensive psychosocial therapy can be made when her acute psychosis is in remission.

In Case 4, the phobia seems related to the woman's marked difficulties in interacting comfortably with peers. Perhaps the phobia's unconscious purpose is to allow the patient to stay at home, thereby shielding her from the anxiety-provoking circumstance of dealing with others. She seems able to form one-to-one relationships--as evidenced by her having had close friends--on those rare occasions when she is able to surmount the initial period of intense distress. Group therapy would be an appropriate context for improving her transactional skills and comfort.

The preceding paragraphs posit that the appropriate therapeutic context is the one most closely matching the area of difficulty: interactional problems between husband and wife suggest marital couple therapy; social awkwardness or generalized interpersonal discomfort suggests group therapy; dysfunction or distress in both parent and child suggests family therapy; problems in intimate, one-to-one relationships suggest the individual therapy context. In practice, such matching is not always possible. Universal agreement about this schema does not exist. Some therapists, for example, might believe that problems in the mother-child dyad are at the root of most psychological distress and thus recommend individual therapy for most patients; others might suggest family or group therapy for most patients since most problems have presumably arisen in, and manifest themselves in, an interpersonal context. Furthermore, factors such as the availability of the desired context and clinicians' own preferences and therapeutic repertoire may, in practice, outweigh theoretical considerations.

That a spectrum of therapeutic approaches may be associated with beneficial changes in patients suggests that certain <u>common</u> <u>factors</u> may be present in effective therapies--factors that are partially independent of both therapeutic context and particular therapeutic technique. Before exploring these factors further, it will be useful to review the causes of disturbances in feelings, thoughts, and behaviors that lead a person to want or need psychosocial therapy.

Psychiatric disorders, to oversimplify at this time, may be divided into two broad classes: those that result from learning and experience; and those that are relatively autonomous or endogenous. Our knowledge of child development tells us that each infant is born with certain instincts, drives, and needs that are variously satisfied, channelled, or thwarted by others as the child grows. The response of the environment--represented especially by the parents--to these needs is determined by an amalgam of factors that reflect the parents' own upbringing, the vicissitudes of their lives, and the prevailing sociocultural milieu. While an infant has a certain minimum need for food and shelter in order to survive, infants (and indeed most primates) also have interpersonal and emotional needs that must be met if the infant is to grow into an adult who functions effectively and comfortably. A person's sense of self-esteem and self-worth originally develops, in large part, as a reflection of how others seem to view the person. The child who is cared for with consistent warmth or affection is likely to see the world as gratifying and see himself as a worthwhile human being; the child cared for by indifferent, hostile, or inadequate parents will see not only the world, but also himself, as flawed. As each succeeding task of psychosocial development is approached, the reservoir of past experience and present opportunities will contribute to structuring the individual's experiential world. Erikson, in Childhood and Society (1963), has presented a lucid and influential account of how the child's biological/psychological maturation and development interact with and are shaped by the psychological and cultural milieu of the environment. Because each developmental stage is influenced by those that have gone before it, the severity of learned impairments in psychosocial functioning is roughly proportional to the age at which development first begins to miscarry. Thus, the person who experienced severe psychological trauma (e.g., parental brutality or abandonment) from infancy onward is likely to experience great difficulty in numerous spheres--e.g., in experiencing a sense of comfort or security in human relationships; in loving and being loved by others; and in trusting the intentions and goodwill of others and one's self. If certain basic tasks (such as developing a sense of trust, beginning to achieve personal autonomy, and developing initiative) are accomplished with relative comfort, then problems arising from impaired learning at later ages--such as excessive shyness in adolescence resulting from inadequate earlier experience with peers--may be more amenable to the process of relearning that is a part of most psychosocial therapies.

That "problems in learning" are involved in the genesis of various psychosocial dysfunctions does not, of course, mean that therapy is simply the replacement of ignorance with facts. Experience with the fundamental issues of human existence--love and hate, sexuality, aggression, attachment and loss, dominance and submission, dependence and independence, and so on--occurs in situations characterized by high emotional arousal, and much of our present-day view of ourselves and others reflects unconscious as well as conscious processes (Chapter Two describes the functioning of the unconscious realm of mental existence, including the mechanisms of defense that are involved in channelling conflict-laden wishes, impulses, and ideas).

For example, a man's erectile impotence could reflect his equating, unconsciously, his wife with his mother. His anxiety upon approaching his wife sexually might then be understood as representing a signal that it is dangerous to approach a forbidden sexual object. A psychotherapeutic treatment that intended to change his perception of sex with his wife (which would involve a detailed exploration of his earlier relationships with his mother and father) should then alleviate the sexual dysfunction.

On the other hand, sexual dysfunction need not result from such antecedent conflict. For example, another man might develop impotence with his wife because his lack of knowledge of female sexuality renders him a clumsy and hasty lover, which results, over time, in his wife's becoming angry and withdrawn when he approaches her sexually. This in turn makes the possibility of a sexual encounter with her sufficiently aversive that his arousal is impaired. In this instance anxiety is a major contributor (via adrenergic discharge) to the impotence, as well as a result of it (via the threat to his self-esteem implied by his erectile difficulty).

In the first case the anxiety was one manifestation of an unconscious conflict and the impotence was another. In the second instance a behavioral approach (see Chapter 18) aimed at increasing the man's knowledge of sexual technique and at extinguishing the connection between sexual arousal and the various aversive feelings might be the preferred treatment. (Things may not be as simple as they seem: why has the man failed to develop adequate sexual knowledge? What interferes with the couple's working this out on their own, rather than withdrawing from one another?) Such problems may persist or emerge even after the focal symptom has been relieved, in which case additional therapeutic approaches may be needed. On the other hand the problem may vanish once the primary symptom is successfully treated. Again, it should be evident that choosing an appropriate therapy depends upon a detailed understanding of the nature and the genesis of the dysfunction.

While some disorders result primarily from learning and experience, others seem to be relatively autonomous. To illustrate, consider the symptoms of the Schizophrenias and the Major Affective Disorders: although life experiences may sensitize a person to particular sorts of stresses or may predispose to particular patterns of reacting to stresses, occurrence of such symptoms as insomnia, hallucinations, or delusions may reflect biologic/physiologic factors rather than learning per se. The particular content of an hallucination tends to be experientially determined, reflecting psychological factors. For example, one depressed man may hear a woman's voice accusing him of sexual perversions, while another may hear a man's voice castigating him for his laziness. However, the presence of the symptom of hallucinations, regardless of the content, represents an altered neurophysiologic state, and this state can be influenced far more by somatic treatment than by psychosocial treatment.

Thus, while psychosocial treatments may play a crucial therapeutic role in the major disorders (i.e., those presumed to have strong biologic determinants), this role generally is not in the treatment of symptoms per se. For example, a patient with Schizophrenia might engage in group therapy in order to acquire or maintain the interactional skills that could reduce the tendency to become more isolated and withdrawn. A depressed woman might be involved in marital couple therapy so that she and her husband could better understand the illness and each partner's reaction to it. Her husband might learn that her decreased libido is a symptom of illness rather than a personal rejection, and she might learn that her husband's withdrawal from her stems from his sense of helplessness in coping with her illness, rather than lack of concern for her.

A common error in thinking about psychosocial and somatic therapies is the failure to consider carefully which sorts of disturbances in the patient are amenable to which particular approach. It should be obvious from the examples in preceding sections that the need for somatic treatment does not preclude a need for psychosocial treatment; each can be effective in dealing with certain sorts of dysfunction and quite ineffective when used inappropriately. If an acutely depressed patient with low self-esteem has a history of excellent premorbid functioning with a benign and undistorted self-concept, then that patient's self-esteem is likely to return to normal when the depression remits; somatic treatment, rather than psychotherapy designed to improve self-esteem, would be appropriate. On the other hand, a patient with a life-long overly-critical view of himself--that has arisen from his internalization of his parent's seeming coldness and indifference--will profit far more from a psychosocial approach than from a drug. Similarly, the schizophrenic's delusions will respond more to an antipsychotic drug than to psychotherapy--but the fear of intimacy and social awkwardness that predispose to social isolation (which in turn fuels the patient's sense of alienation and heightens his tendency to idiosyncratic or bizarre thinking) can best be ameliorated psychosocially. Even the presence of unequivocal organic illness does <u>not</u> preclude a need for psychosocial intervention, as the following vignette indicates:

Allen was a 17-year-old boy whose 11th grade academic performance was declining. He experienced difficulty concentrating, had little interest in his studies, and felt increasingly distressed (sad, worried, angry) as the school year progressed. His grades in previous years had been average in most subjects and above-average in art and music. His father hoped that Allen would study mechanical engineering in college and, eventually, join the family's engineering firm. Although Allen was seen as a generally bright and pleasant person who made friends easily, he had been regarded as an "underachiever" throughout secondary school by both his teachers and by his college-educated parents.

There was no family history of psychiatric illness. Until this year, Allen had had minimal exposure to illicit drugs. However, as his grades and his self-confidence fell (and as pressure from teachers and parents mounted), he began to smoke marijuana several times per week in an effort to relieve his dysphoria. Although occasionally relaxing, the marijuana frequently led to frightening perceptual distortions and he stopped using it. A counsellor found him to be mildly depressed and moderately anxious and felt that his underachievement at school represented a rebellion against authority in general and his parents (especially his father) in particular; his interest in art and music was interpreted as a subtle defiance of his "he-man" father. A period of individual psychotherapy, focusing on Allen's ambivalence about pleasing his parents and about achieving success resulted in some diminution of his anxiety and self-blame, but did not affect his school performance or his worry about his future educational plans.

A more detailed review of his past history revealed the following:

   1) He had had a febrile illness and a seizure at age three years which were followed by a persistent but very minimal facial asymmetry and a transient set-back in the pace of developmental milestones.

2) Following the above-mentioned illness he had seemed mildly awkward motorically to his mother; this lasted for several months, then
seemed to disappear.

3) Allen had considerable trouble learning to read when he first went
to school. This was thought possibly to represent a refractive error, but visual acuity was normal when tested. Over the next few
years his ability to read gradually improved somewhat, but reading
remained a struggle and he never read for pleasure.

4) Allen's grades in elementary school were very poor in arithmetic
and history, average in English, "Science" (primarily human health
and descriptive biology), and Social Studies, and excellent in art
and mechanical drawing. His teachers liked him, although they
felt he did not apply himself sufficiently to his work and thus was
not "living up to his potential." He was not required to repeat any
grades.

On formal mental status testing, Allen gave the impression (via his good
vocabulary and grammar) of above-average intelligence. However, his performance on tasks requiring quantitative knowledge and abilities was sur-
prisingly poor: he experienced considerable difficulty and became increasingly anxious and tearful at one point while attempting serial subtractions.
He did not know the boiling point of water and thought it might be 500 miles
from New York to Paris and 5000 miles from the Earth to the Moon. His
fund of information in nonquantitative areas, however, was quite good. He
expressed considerable guilt over "letting my parents down," and felt hopeless about school since he seemed unable to master some things, no matter
how hard he tried. He dreaded the idea of college, feeling sure that he
would flunk out.

Because of the suggestion of brain dysfunction--the history consistent with
a mild encephalitis at age three, the history of dyslexia, and the marked
difficulty in areas requiring quantitative reasoning and knowledge--more extensive neuropsychological tests were obtained. These revealed that Allen
had a chronic, nonprogressive cerebral dysfunction that interfered significantly with the recognition, retention, and processing of quantitative data.
There was also a much less severe interference with letter recognition and
word processing. Allen's visuospatial abilities--including copying geometric
figures from memory, imaginary rotation in space of three-dimensional forms,
and recognizing embedded figures--were well above average.

In addition, Allen's vocational interests and aptitudes were formally assessed.
As might be expected from the neuropsychological tests (and from his history), his aptitude for work requiring quantitative mastery--such as accounting, engineering, or physics--was quite low. By contrast, his aptitude
for and interest in work that drew upon his visuospatial skills--such as
drafting, interior design, and commercial art--were quite high.

How can we interpret what we know about Allen? What role might psycho-social interventions play? Although Allen's fundamental problem is disordered brain function which is presumably a sequella of a mild encephalitic episode at age three, much of his current distress results from his and his environment's <u>reactions</u> <u>to</u> his dysfunction. His school problems have been viewed, erroneously, as "underachievement"--i.e., a failure of motivation or willpower--rather than as symptoms of a subtle neurologic illness or perceptual dysfunction. To be sure, Allen's problems with areas that are intrinsically difficult for him have led to discouragement and demoralization that have in turn impaired his performance in areas where he is not neurologically handicapped--yet these secondary difficulties could probably have been avoided if the primary problem had been recognized. The areas of psychosocial intervention for Allen included:

1) Redefinition of the problem as a perceptual dysfunction rather than "underachievement;" this was discussed in detail with Allen and was also explained to his parents and to his school advisor.

2) Allen's feelings about having a handicap needed to be explored in some detail. To him, perceptual dysfunction meant "brain damage" or "mentally retarded," terms which held distressing connotations for him and led, temporarily, to a further lowering of his self-esteem. As he gained a better perspective on the meaning of his dysfunction and on the impact it might have upon his future, his guilt over his school work and over disappointing his parents began to abate.

3) It was apparent that he had neither the interest nor the aptitude to pursue a career in engineering. It is quite possible that some of his lack of interest could indeed represent a rejection of or rebellion against his father, but it is equally plausible that the deficit in aptitude preceded the lack of interest. In working with Allen, it seemed more productive to focus on areas to which he brought both talent and interest. He began to consider the possibility of attending a school for design or for commercial art, rather than a traditional college. Given his average overall I.Q., it might have been possible, if he were highly motivated, to struggle through a four-year liberal arts curriculum. However, since he had little interest in a conventional college program, it would have been futile to pursue one. An engineering major was completely out of the question.

4) His parents needed help in understanding why it made little sense for him to try to attend college, and they also needed to understand that his not pursuing engineering was not simply his way of rejecting them. His father, a hard-driving businessman as well as a fiercely competitive amateur athlete, was especially upset at Allen's interest in the arts; this smacked of homosexuality to him.

In summary, a variety of psychosocial approaches were used--individual meetings with Allen, family meetings involving Allen and his parents, a meeting with his parents alone, and consultation with his school--even though "the problem" was fundamentally a neurologic disorder.

QUIZ, Section II.

Classify the following as therapeutic technique (T) or therapeutic context (C) by circling the appropriate letter.

T   C   1.   Male and female co-therapists meet weekly for 90 minutes with seven patients who suffer varying degrees of social awkwardness.

T   C   2.   A patient is helped to lose a phobia of snakes by watching the therapist handle a snake.

T   C   3.   A therapist instructs a couple with sexual dysfunction to abstain from intercourse for two weeks.

T   C   4.   A therapist and a patient with poor academic performance meet twice a week.

T   C   5.   A therapist encourages the patient to report whatever thoughts enter his mind, even if they seem trivial or embarrassing.

T   C   6.   A husband and wife, their delinquent 15-year-old son, and their apparently problem-free 10-year-old daughter meet weekly with a clinical psychologist.

Circle the correct answer(s). One or more than one answer may be correct.

7.   Psychotherapy, as defined earlier, would include which of the following?

   a.   A minister with training in pastoral counseling suggests different ways of communicating for a married couple who complain of excessive arguments.
   b.   A group of mothers discuss among themselves the nuances of breast feeding in order to help new mothers nurse their infants successfully.
   c.   A depressed parishioner experiences some relief upon receiving absolution for his sins during his confessional.
   d.   A psychologist suggests to a student that his difficulties with his teacher may be related to previous difficulties with his mother.
   e.   A shaman tried to relieve a headhunter's erectile impotence by having him draw a picture of a bull.
   f.   A surgeon informs a frightened woman that the breast biopsy revealed the lesion to be benign.

8. According to Parsons, functional specificity of the healer's role implies that

   a. a generalist should not perform a procedure if a specialist is available.
   b. a psychotherapist should try to meet all of a patient's emotional needs.
   c. the major difference between a psychotherapist and a friend is that you don't have to pay a friend.
   d. a therapist should have a doctoral degree.
   e. a therapist's expertise is not expected to extend beyond certain areas.

9. Which of the following reflect societal, rather than individual, factors in the choice of a psychotherapist?

   a. A young professional woman prefers to discuss her problems with a female rather than a male therapist.
   b. An Australian aborigine, failing to understand how the missionary physician could help him with his prolonged grief, prefers to be treated by a shaman.
   c. A construction worker refuses to see a psychiatrist, but will discuss his sexual difficulties with his family physician.

TRUE or FALSE: Circle the correct letter.

T F 10. Experiential factors play no role in the symptom patterns of psychotic disorders.

T F 11. Psychological factors exert relatively minor influence upon the presence or absence of delusions.

T F 12. Biochemical/neurophysiologic factors play a major role in determining the specific content of hallucinations.

T F 13. Psychosocial treatment should rarely be combined with psychopharmacologic treatment.

T F 14. Antidepressant drugs should not be used in treating a depressed middle-aged man if severe marital conflict is present.

T F 15. Patients with unconscious conflicts should not receive psychotropic drugs.

T F 16. Combined drug-psychosocial therapy can readily reverse the effects of deficient parenting in the first two to three years of life.

T   F   17. Psychosocial treatments are more likely to be effective when
            learning (broadly defined) is a major source of the patient's
            problems.

III.   THERAPEUTIC FACTORS

The scheme described earlier for selecting a therapeutic context is reasonably straightforward. By contrast, the choice of therapeutic technique within a given context is considerably more problematic: a technique of treatment is intimately related to a theory of normal and abnormal personality development, yet no truly comprehensive theory of human personality exists (Coleman, 1968). The therapy conducted by a clinician with major allegiance to a psychoanalytic view, wherein unconscious conflict and the mechanisms of defense are major determinants of symptom formation, will bear little obvious resemblance to therapy conducted by a behaviorist who finds that conditioning paradigms provide more cogent explanations of behavior .

That clinicians with widely divergent theories can obtain equally impressive results suggests several possibilities: common factors may underlie superficially different therapeutic techniques; the success or failure of a therapeutic technique bears little relation to the truth or falsity of the theory upon which it is based; what clinicians say or believe that they are doing does not correspond completely with their actual behavior; and certain symptoms may remit with the passage of time alone. Probably all these statements have some validity. In the following paragraphs we will consider factors that may be common to effective therapeutic techniques.

Hope, trust, the placebo response--these are present in medicine in general as well as in psychotherapy. One does not wish to do away with these elements as "unscientific"; they are meliorative in themselves, and they also help sustain the relationship between patient and therapist through periods of difficulty. Hope and trust are not necessarily fostered by the therapist's saying, "Cheer up! I will help you," but rather by the therapist's conveying a consistent interest in and respect for the patient.

Another effective element in therapies is the clinician's empathy for the patient--that is, the clinician's ability accurately to identify, via experiencing in attenuated form, the patient's feeling states. Empathy seems to be conveyed by nonverbal as well as verbal channels; saying "I understand" or "I know how you feel" to a patient rings hollow unless true. If patients feel persistently misunderstood--and understanding a patient is not the same as agreeing with or sharing all of the patient's perceptions--they are unlikely to become sufficiently engaged in treatment to allow other, more specific factors to operate.

Warmth, positive regard, and caring represent a third group of relatively nonspecific therapeutic factors. Although the therapist may not like or approve of, or may even be repelled by, certain aspects of the patient, the therapist needs to feel--and the patient needs to perceive--a certain concern for the person of the patient that goes beyond the therapist's feelings about any particular symptoms or behavior. As with empathy, this humane concern cannot be created or conveyed on demand.

Although a distinction is sometimes drawn between "supportive" therapies and those with ambitious goals of extensive behavioral change, it should be evident that the above-mentioned factors are supportive indeed. Many patients whose difficulties are amenable to a psychosocial approach will feel varying degrees of demoralization, shame, or alienation simply as a result of having a problem that affects their social function, in addition to the specific distresses that represent the problem per se. That someone will listen, try to understand, accept rather than judge, and try to be helpful is supportive and gratifying in itself; that that someone is a trained, socially-sanctioned, and respected healer creates a powerful field within which more specific techniques of therapy can be employed.

QUIZ, Section III.

TRUE or FALSE: Circle the correct letter.

T   F   1.   Failure of a therapeutic technique based upon a given theory of personality implies that that theory is incorrect.

T   F   2.   Success of a therapeutic technique based upon a given theory of personality implies that that theory is correct.

T   F   3.   Successful treatment of phobias by psychoanalytic psychotherapy would indicate that conditioning has no role in the genesis or maintenance of phobic symptoms and/or that behavior therapy should not be used to treat phobias.

T   F   4.   Unconscious factors may be involved in creating or maintaining a symptom that can be successfully treated with behavior therapy.

Classify the following therapeutic techniques as specific (S) or nonspecific (N) by circling the correct answer.

S   N   5.   Free association

S   N   6.   Catharsis and abreaction

S.   N   7.   Conveying a sense of understanding

S   N   8.   Conveying insight

S   N   9.   Role-playing

S   N   10.   Faith in the therapist

S   N   11.   Systematic desensitization

IV. PSYCHODYNAMIC PSYCHOTHERAPIES

One of the most influential and enduring psychosocial techniques is that of psychoanalytic or psychodynamic psychotherapy; psychoanalysis stands at the more formal end of this spectrum. In psychoanalysis, the patient re-experiences, through the relationship with the analyst, significant events and relationships from the past--especially childhood--that have contributed to the formation of the patient's personality and problems. Conflicts from early years influence and distort the patient's perception of the present, but because these early experiences have been rendered unconscious by repression, they are unavailable to conscious scrutiny and modification. The primary goal of psychoanalysis is to promote insight--i.e., to bring these experiences from unconsciousness to consciousness--so that the patient can perceive and act in the present with a freedom of choice that is not possible when one is burdened with the excess baggage of unresolved conflict. Implied in the therapeutic process of psychoanalysis are both cognitive factors and "economic" (referring to psychic energy) factors . The patient cognitively understands the past and the present in a new and less distorted light, and the psychic energy that was consumed by intrapsychic conflict becomes available for consciously chosen uses.

A major technique in psychoanalysis is the use of free association. "Free association" means that the patient should, in the analytic session, say whatever comes to mind, no matter how odd, trivial, or embarrassing these thoughts might be, without consciously selecting or censoring what is said. This partially frees the patient's associations from the logic and obligations of ordinary conversation; this will gradually reveal certain themes that are not readily available to the patient's consciousness.

Yet, despite the admonition to speak with complete candor, both conscious and unconscious processes will interfere with the patient's verbal productions; the patient no longer associates freely. The patient may consciously avoid speaking of something that is a source of shame, or the patient may fear that he will evoke the analyst's disapproval. In addition, as potentially anxiety-provoking material is approached, mechanisms of defense may shield conflict-laden material from conscious awareness.

This process of avoidance that interferes with the basic task of the analysis is termed resistance. Paradoxically, although resistance serves as a block to the progress of the analysis, it also provides invaluable clues to the nature of the patient's conflicts. Resistance may take many forms: anxious silence; stubborn silence; talking about the weather; forgetting an appointment; or flattering the analyst, to name but a few. These and other forms of resistance may occur in a variety of contexts: when the patient experiences sexual thoughts, angry thoughts, or affectionate thoughts; or when the patient thinks of reporting signs of progress in therapy; or when the analyst is about to go on vacation; or many others. The particular form and particular context of the resistance often illuminate conflicts that otherwise would not be apparent. As resistances are identified, understood, and then removed by interpretation (see below), the work of the analysis proceeds.

1. C (group therapy)
2. T (modeling, or imitation)
3. T (giving advice)
4. C (individual therapy)
5. T (free association)
6. C (family therapy)
7. a,d,e
8. e
9. b

10. F
11. T
12. F
13. F
14. F
15. F
16. F
17. T

The use of <u>transference</u> is another hallmark of psychoanalysis. Transference is an unconscious process whereby thoughts or feelings arising in a significant past relationship (such as with a parent) are displaced onto another person (in this case the analyst) in a manner that is inaccurate or inappropriate to the current situation. For example, a woman whose father was cold and distant will at various times tend to see the analyst (whether the analyst is male or female) as cold and distant, even if the analyst is in fact attentive and sympathetic. At another time the same woman may react to the analyst as if he or she were the patient's doting and indulgent grandmother--even though the analyst's behavior has not changed. A man may fear that the analyst will retaliate harshly if he (the patient) dares to express the slightest annoyance; this fear is based not upon an accurate assessment of the analyst's character, but rather results from the patient's displacing early memories and experiences with his mother onto the analyst. Note that transference does <u>not</u> encompass all feelings toward the therapist--just those that are unconscious, based on previous relationships and inappropriate to the present situation. Thus, if the analyst falls asleep during the patient's therapy hour or forgets the patient's name, the patient's anger is an appropriate response to the current situation rather than a transference response. In this instance one would suspect that the therapist was experiencing <u>countertransference</u> toward the patient (which is exactly the same process as transference except that the direction of feeling is reversed--i.e., from therapist to patient rather than patient to therapist). To foster the development of transference, the analyst is relatively inactive and nondirective; thus, to the degree that the analyst is a "blank screen," the patient's perceptions of the analyst tend to represent fantasies and projected memories--which are invaluable aids to understanding the patient--rather than reactions to the real person of the analyst. When the transference to the analyst has developed sufficiently a "transference neurosis" exists, and core conflicts from the patient's earlier life are re-experienced with great intensity.

Transference is an extraordinarily useful process in therapy. Through it, past relationships become alive in the present and thus far more accessible to understanding. By experiencing first-hand the patient's ways of relating, the therapist gains a far more vivid and accurate understanding than is provided by the patient's second-hand accounts of significant outside relationships. Transference is a general phenomenon in human relationships (especially in those fraught with emotion, such as doctor-patient relationships), but it receives specific attention only in psychotherapeutic settings and, especially, in psychoanalysis.

The major specific technique of the analyst is interpretation. At the more superficial levels, interpretation consists simply of calling attention to the patient's behavior ("You're unusually quiet today." "It seems difficult for you to talk about your husband." "You were fifteen minutes late today."). More complex interpretations might try to link the patient's transference manifestations with elements of the patient's history ("You seem afraid to express any anger at me, even when it might be justified. It's as if you're afraid something bad will happen--like your feeling that you caused your mother's stroke."). The cinema psychoanalyst dazzles the patient by identifying deeply-buried complexes in the first therapy hour; in fact, an interpretation must be based upon data available to both the patient and the analyst if it is to be useful and comprehensible. Consequently, material that is thoroughly repressed will become available only when layer after layer of defense has been carefully and painstakingly eliminated through interpretation. Interpretations that accurately link the patient's current thoughts and feelings in the transference situation with their historical antecedents are especially efficacious in bringing important material into consciousness in a way that promotes change in the patient.

Certain technical procedures are commonly used in psychoanalysis. The patient reclines on a couch, which encourages the patient's associative reverie. The analyst sits out of the patient's view so that the developing transference will be influenced as little as possible by the actual person of the analyst (although Freud's initial rationale for this was, apparently, his dislike of being looked at all day by his patients). Sessions are held frequently (four or five times a week) in order to foster the development of the transference relationship and to attenuate the influence of the patient's day-to-day life upon the material discussed in the analytic hours. One should not, however, view these technical trappings as the essence of a psychoanalysis. The essentials of the psychoanalytic process are the use of free association and interpretation and the formation and resolution of the transference neurosis in order to resolve unconscious conflict and produce insight.

DSM-III diagnostic categories, based as they are upon readily observable phenomena rather than inferences about underlying psychic mechanisms, are of little help in identifying patients suitable for psychoanalysis. Such difficult-to-operationalize constructs as ego strength, capacity to relate, and motivation are far more useful, in the hands of experienced clinicians, than formal diagnoses. In general, patients who have benefitted from psychoanalysis include those whose problems are characterized by anxiety; mild depression without marked vegetative symptoms; obsessional or phobic complaints; various personality disorders (with the exception of antisocial personality); psychosomatic problems; and sexual difficulties.

Although the analyst's attention and commitment to the patient are supportive and gratifying factors, the relative nonresponsiveness and anonymity of the analyst may be experienced by some patients as an unbearable deprivation. Impulsive patients who are unable or unwilling to interpose thought between impulse and action are not suitable for classical psychoanalysis, nor are patients whose current situation contains so many realistic stresses that they are unable to spare the requisite emotional energy for the work of the analysis. Patients who are psychotic, who lack the capacity to enter into an intense therapeutic relationship, or who would regress severely in the analytic situation are also unsuitable, as are patients in crisis who need quick, focused help. Because the time (years) and emotional effort required are so great, psychoanalysis is obviously not the treatment of choice for self-limited or mildly annoying problems that cause little or no psychic suffering.

While there is agreement that psychoanalytic treatment can be effective--sometimes stunningly so--there is no consensus on whether its results are sufficiently better or more enduring than those obtained from therapies that are considerably less arduous. Both therapists and patients, especially in years past, sometimes held exaggerated views on what psychoanalysis might reasonably be expected to accomplish--as if a malfunctioning Chevrolet could, with sufficiently devoted repair and tuning, be turned into a Porsche.

Psychodynamic individual psychotherapy, which utilizes many psychoanalytic concepts and techniques, is probably the most widely-employed combination of therapeutic context and technique; it is useful in treating a far broader spectrum of patients than is appropriate for psychoanalysis per se. As in psychoanalysis, the transference relationship provides both a source of information and a vehicle for change as do clarification and interpretation of resistance. However, psychoanalytic psychotherapy is less intense than psychoanalysis: sessions are generally less frequent (once or twice per week); the therapist does not strive to maintain the anonymity that fosters the fully-developed transference neurosis; and the goals of treatment are likely to be more focal or limited than the psychoanalytic ideal of thoroughly resolving all infantile childhood neurotic conflicts. The therapist in psychoanalytically oriented psychotherapy is generally more active or directive than the psychoanalyst; the psychotherapist may pursue particular lines of inquiry that seem especially relevant at the moment, while the psychoanalyst--less burdened by time constraints and the need to deal with external crises in the patient's life--lets the material unfold as it will in order to minimize his influence upon it. The psychoanalytically oriented psychotherapist may use medication, may meet from time to time with others in the patient's life such as a spouse, or may depart in other ways from the constraints of classical psychoanalytic technique.

There is, in fact, no unitary technique of psychodynamic or psychoanalytic-ally oriented psychotherapy; rather, there are therapists whose understand-ing of the patient is enhanced to varying degrees by a knowledge of psy-choanalytic theory and whose therapeutic technique and interventions are influenced to varying degrees by a knowledge of psychoanalytic technique. At the nonanalytic end of the therapeutic spectrum, psychoanalytic theory might contribute much to an understanding of the patient, even though non-specific factors or medication is responsible for maintaining or improving the patient's adjustment.

Psychodynamic psychotherapy has been employed in treating a broad range of dysfunctions. As with psychoanalysis, a formal DSM-III diagnosis is less useful in suggesting a treatment strategy than is a precise description of the particular difficulties and of the situations in which they occur. Patients not suitable for formal psychoanalysis--such as those unable to tolerate its deprivational aspects, or unable to "let go" sufficiently to form an intense transference neurosis, or unable for whatever other reason to invest the requisite time and psychic energy--may be treated successfully with psycho-dynamic psychotherapy.

This chapter began by emphasizing the role of psychosocial treatment in dis-orders where learning plays a major role; it is appropriate to consider in more detail the nature of re-learning or un-learning that occurs in dynamic psychotherapies. Strupp (1969) describes several "lessons" that successfully treated patients learn, among which are:

1) You are fully responsible for your own actions. Your biological heritage and earlier experiences are influential, and the past is irreversible, but you have more latitude in shaping the present and future than you may have been willing to admit. Blaming others (parents, society, etc.) for your troubles is self-defeating and ineffectual.

2) You reach goals through realistic action, rather than through sit-ting and wishing. In general, the greater the effort expended, the more satisfying the results. Some things are, realistically, unattainable; the wish for such things must be abandoned or modified. Further, you must often delay gratification--you can't always get what you want when you want it.

3) Your own satisfaction--rather than the praise and applause of others --will have to be sufficient reward for your achievements. This does not mean that it is wrong or immoral to be praised or to enjoy praise, but rather that you will become progressively more disap-pointed and resentful if you seek affirmation of your worth from others rather than from your own internal standards (which must be realistic).

4) Certain interpersonal maneuvers are ineffective and self-defeating--although they may not be as dangerous as previously supposed. For example, angry feelings are not lethal; feelings must not be con-

fused with acts. Ingratiation and negativism are not useful ways to influence others. Nurturing grudges and always trying to "get even" is generally a waste of time and energy. By contrast, co-operation with others is more likely to get you what you want.

5) You have rights, and should stand up for them. On the other hand, there are also higher authorities whom you need to respect and accept. If a particular situation is uncongenial to you, it is more productive to seek out another; staying in the situation and engaging in efforts to compete with or rebel against persons in higher positions is usually futile. Accepting authority does not mean abandoning your freedom; rather, the acceptance frees you from nonproductive struggles that inhibit your freedom of choice and action.

6) You should be honest with yourself about your feelings and motives. This does not mean that you promiscuously confess all of your less desirable tendencies (although they are universal), nor that you castigate yourself because you are not perfect. Recognizing your impulses is not justification for acting upon them--you will be judged by your actions, not your fantasies--but an increased knowledge of your feelings and motivations may help you to take more appropriate action.

Strupp considers identification to be the major process responsible for the learning that takes place in psychodynamic psychotherapy. For this process to occur, the patient must be open to the therapist's influence, which in turn requires strong emotional ties between patient and therapist. The mobilization of feelings, especially those about the therapist and the patient-therapist interaction, heightens the effectiveness of the cognitive learning that occurs in therapy. Despite the desire to be helped the patient will erect obstacles to a more open, close relationship with the therapist; the removal (via interpretation) of these resistances is thus a major prerequisite to the patient's identification with the therapist. As resistances are removed, the transference can intensify so that the patient is emotionally aroused and highly receptive to the therapist's corrective influence.

It is essential to realize that identification does not refer to a superficial aping of the therapist's mannerisms or an uncritical adoption of the therapist's particular foibles and prejudices. Rather, what is identified with includes the therapist's tolerance and acceptance (which contrast with the patient's excessive self-criticism); the therapist's calm (in the face of the patient's anxiety); and the therapist's refusal to be drawn into the patient's various self-defeating maneuvers (such as excessive passivity, guilt-inducement, exploitation, coercion, etc.) as they are repeated in the transference.

Inasmuch as the human psyche is not organized upon disciplinary lines, it may be presumptuous to attribute the relief of all sorts of distress entirely to one's favorite therapeutic factor, to the exclusion of all others. Processes occurring in widely divergent types of therapies must have, in common, the ability to create and nurture the patient's openness to change. All humans possess an unconscious, whose workings are reasonably well-described by psychoanalytic theory--yet this does not preclude the therapist's intentional or unintentional shaping of behavior via subtle reinforcement of particular themes throughout the therapeutic hour. Similarly, the effectiveness of desensitization in treating certain phobias does not imply that the patient's transferential wish to please the therapist plays no role. While considerable advances have been made in assessing the success or failure of various psychosocial techniques, the actual conduct of treatment remains more an art than a science. Fortunately, a growing body of data confirms the efficacy of this art (Andrews & Harvey, 1981).

QUIZ, Section IV.

Circle the correct answer(s). <u>One</u> or <u>more</u> <u>than</u> <u>one</u> answer may be correct.

1. Transference

    a. is an appropriate but unconscious reaction based upon previous experience.
    b. may involve thoughts as well as feelings.
    c. includes all the patient's feelings about the therapist.
    d. may occur in supportive therapies as well as in psychoanalysis.

2. Essentials of the psychoanalytic process include

    a. attention to transference phenomena.
    b. interpretation as the therapist's primary activity.
    c. efforts to bring unconscious material into consciousness.
    d. the use of the couch.

3. Resistance in psychoanalysis

    a. will not occur with well-motivated patients.
    b. is primarily a conscious process.
    c. will not occur if interpretations are well-timed and appropriate.
    d. may be a source of useful information as well as an impediment to progress.

4. Choose the correct statements about psychoanalysis.

    a. Nonspecific factors may contribute to patient improvement.
    b. The analyst's interpretations address unconscious material only.
    c. A female therapist might be reacted to as if she were the patient's father.
    d. Countertransference includes all the analyst's unconscious feelings about the patient.

5. Psychodynamic psychotherapy

    a. may be used in conjunction with psychotropic medication.
    b. may be useful in treating patients with anxiety disorders but not with personality disorders.
    c. is not used in treating patients with Affective Disorders.
    d. may utilize transference and interpretation of resistance.

6. Compared to psychoanalysis, psychodynamic psychotherapy

    a. usually involves more ambitious goals.
    b. may involve greater overt activity by the therapist.
    c. places greater emphasis on the transference neurosis.
    d. encompasses a broader range of therapeutic techniques.

7. Which of the following phrases about individual psychodynamic psychotherapy is(are) correct?

    a. may be employed with other therapeutic contexts (e.g., marital couple or group)
    b. psychoanalytic theory plays a greater role than psychoanalytic technique
    c. less-restrictive criteria for patient selection
    d. description of patient's dysfunctional behavior less useful than DSM-III diagnosis

8. Which of the following is(are) considered by Strupp to be major factors in the success of dynamic psychotherapy?

    a. identification with the therapist
    b. re-experiencing early childhood traumas
    c. interpretation of resistance
    d. role-playing
    e. transference

TRUE or FALSE: Circle the correct letter.

T   F   9. Certain therapist-patient behaviors in psychoanalytic psychotherapy may be understood via an operant conditioning (behavioral) paradigm.

T   F   10. Formal psychoanalysis discourages the processes of identification that Strupp describes in dynamic psychotherapy.

T   F   11. Cognitive learning in psychotherapy is enhanced by emotional arousal.

T   F   12. The patient's desire to please the therapist is a major obstacle to the patient's progress in dynamic psychotherapy.

Among the lessons learned in psychotherapy are, according to Strupp:

T F 13. that one needs to stand up for one's rights while respecting the rights of others

T F 14. that one must persist in the struggle against authority figures when those figures are arbitrary or unreasonable

T F 15. that one must develop strategies for "one-upping" one's colleagues and competitors

T F 16. that one's parents (or other significant early caretakers) are to blame for one's present or future problems

T F 17. that if you wish for something with sufficient intensity, you are likely to get it

T F 18. that people are judged more by their actions than by their unconscious fantasies or feelings

Classify the following patients as possibly suitable for psychoanalysis (S), or probably unsuitable for psychoanalysis (U) by circling the correct letter.

S U 19. A 24-year-old woman, married with one child, who feels considerable guilt over her thoughts of having an extramarital affair.

S U 20. A 43-year-old business executive finds himself increasingly inefficient at work because he feels compelled to count the holes in the acoustical tile ceiling. He has had occasional periods of ritualistic behavior since his mid-teens, but these have not previously interfered significantly with his ability to function.

S U 21. A 38-year-old politician who has been involved in many "shady" business deals throughout his adult life becomes depressed when his wife leaves him following his arrest for embezzling campaign funds; he feels that, because his alcoholism had interfered with his judgment, she is judging him too harshly.

S U 22. A 29-year-old woman loses her zest for work following her promotion to vice-president of a medium-sized firm. She feels uncertain whether she wishes to pursue a promising career in business, or "give up the rat race and get married."

S U 23. A 58-year-old man with mild but longstanding problems in relating to authority becomes quite anxious upon learning that he has lung cancer.

V. MULTIPLE-PERSON CONTEXTS

A. GROUP THERAPY

Although psychodynamic theory can contribute to understanding the behavior of individuals seen in group or family therapy contexts, these contexts provide, by their very nature, additional therapeutic factors that are not present in the individual context. The type of group described here will be the Interactional Group (Yalom, 1975); there are many other types of therapy groups with widely differing theories and practices, and it must be emphasized that the following comments may not apply to groups other than the Interactional Group. The Interactional Group is intended to produce significant and lasting changes in patients, and must be distinguished from short-term groups dealing with crisis situations, from groups (such as groups of parents in prenatal clinic) where imparting information is a major method and goal, and from groups (such as Alcoholics Anonymous) in which catharsis and inspiration are major therapeutic factors. While inspiration, catharsis, and imparting information may be helpful in the Interactional Group, the following factors seem to make especially important contributions to successful therapy: interpersonal learning; universality; and group cohesiveness. The therapist's (or therapists'--groups are often led by co-therapist pairs) major function in an Interactional Group is not to be the purveyor of wisdom or the answer man, but rather to create a climate in which patients will gradually reveal themselves to one another, become more aware of and honest about themselves, and be willing over time to risk giving up old but familiar maladaptive patterns.

Interpersonal learning assumes particular importance in the group context. The patient in a therapy group learns how he or she affects others; it can be less painful for one's "blind spots" or self-defeating interpersonal maneuvers to be pointed out by a fellow patient than by the therapist. One can also become aware of one's own reactions to a variety of others--which is one argument favoring a degree of heterogeneity in group composition. Including both males and females of various ages and with varying sorts of difficulties expands the opportunities for interpersonal learning; the group serves as a social microcosm and as a laboratory where new ways of experiencing and relating to others may be tried. Thus, a 35 year old man may learn in the group that he tends to deal with women in a seductive fashion, with most men in a combative fashion, but with older men in a self-effacing manner. Some of this information could be gleaned over time in individual psychotherapy--via the patient's transference reactions to the therapist as well as his direct (but inevitably somewhat distorted) reports of his interactions with others--yet in the group these patterns are particularly vivid, and may emerge more rapidly than in individual psychotherapy. A related aspect of interpersonal learning in groups is the opportunity for patients to identify with various aspects of other group members--to "try on," as it were, different ways of experiencing and reacting to other group members and to the therapist. Initially this may seem more imitation than identification, but with the passage of time certain changed ways of feeling and behaving can become natural aspects of the patient's repertoire. As noted earlier, identification is a critical process in individual dynamic psychotherapy as well as in interactional group psychotherapy.

A second major therapeutic factor in the Interactional Group is universality: an individual's sense that one is not totally alone, that other human beings harbor aggressive and sexual fantasies, and that one's "darkest secrets" are not unique, nor quite as terrible, when they are finally shared with the group. Many patients lack the social/transactional skills that foster enduring and gratifying relationships with others, and the resulting isolation tends to heighten an individual's sense of unique undesirability. The sense of universality engendered by the group is gratifying in itself, and also fosters further sharing and risk-taking within the group.

A third factor, group cohesion, is defined as the attractiveness that the group has for its members--how important, how valued is the group to each member? Yalom (1975) views group cohesion as analogous to "relationship" in individual psychotherapy: a certain quality and intensity of relationship (or group cohesion) must exist for the patient to become involved in and committed to therapy, yet the relationship itself--or the cohesiveness of the group--serves also as a vehicle for effecting change. Thus, group cohesion is both a necessary pre-condition for change and a means to accomplish it.

The empathy and life experiences that help the clinician function as an effective individual psychotherapist are valuable to the group psycho-therapist as well. However, if the group becomes merely a forum where individuals await their turn for individual counselling from the leader, the distinctive and powerful advantages of the interactional group will have been squandered.

B. FAMILY THERAPY

A major tenet of most family therapists is that the individual is but one component of an interacting system. Therefore, an individual's "problem" can be seen as an effort to restore, albeit in a less optimal way, homeostasis or balance to a system that has been stressed from within or without. A consequence of this view is that an individual's problems cannot be understood or treated unless that person's "significant others"--typically, the family--participate in treatment. A common example would be an early adolescent who begins to get into fights at school, can't concentrate on homework, and becomes involved in petty theft. The clinician learns upon interviewing the parents that these problems began following the onset of covert but intense marital discord; thus, the child's difficulties seem to be in some way related to the parents' distress. While it can be argued that successful treatment of the parents (for example, by marital couple psycho-therapy) would lead automatically to improvement in the child, a family ther-apist might point out that the child's behavior now also causes problems for the parents and that the parents' distress has "spilled over" onto the child in a particularly maladaptive way. Consequently, treating the child only, or the parents only, would be unlikely to ameliorate whatever factors have led this particular family unit to be dysfunctional in these particular ways. As in this example, the "identified patient"--that is, the most overtly-symp-tomatic person--may not be the most severely disturbed member of the fam-ily: the child whose parents' marriage is rife with discord may believe (perhaps unconsciously) that his misbehavior will provide the rallying point for his quarrelling parents.

ANSWERS, Section IV.

1.	b,d	9.	T	17.	F
2.	a,b,c	10.	F	18.	T
3.	d	11.	T	19.	S
4.	a,c	12.	F	20.	S
5.	a,d	13.	T	21.	U
6.	b,d	14.	F	22.	S
7.	a,b,c	15.	F	23.	U
8.	a	16.	F		

Failure to observe generational boundaries represents another form of family dysfunction. The parent who overidentifies with his or her adolescent child --perhaps in response to dissatisfaction in marriage or career, or concern over aging--not only appears foolish but also fails to provide an appropriate future role model for the child and an appropriate companion for the spouse. Or a child may, because of inadequacy, passivity, or lack of interest, be thrust prematurely into assuming responsibilities that are more appropriately parental. Discord between the parents may lead to their vying for the allegiance of their children, rather than toward effort to solve their problems. The resulting parent-child coalitions are unstable, a source of distress to the child and to the excluded parent, and inimical to the integrity and functioning of the family. Incest represents an extreme example of an inappropriate coalition that violates generational boundaries; viewing the phenomenon in a systems context often reveals that the problem is not confined to the sexual partners, but is also being covertly or even overtly encouraged by the "nonparticipant" spouse.

A number of techniques may be employed in treating families. Members are encouraged to communicate honestly and directly with one another, rather than via family intermediaries or via destructive behaviors. Efforts are made to understand the sources of various angers, disappointments, or resentments within the family, and to clarify each family member's misconceptions about the motives and feelings of others. When generational boundaries are blurred, if dysfunctional coalitions have formed, or if a family member is being "scapegoated," the family therapist tries to understand why such things are occurring and endeavors to help the family find less destructive and more rewarding means of solving its problems.

It is impossible in this chapter to begin to do justice to the many theoretical and practical aspects of the various schools of family therapy; the goal of this section must be limited to suggesting the flavor of a systems approach to treating psychopathology. Reviews such as Whiteside's (1979) provide a guide to more detailed accounts of family assessment and treatment.

C. MILIEU THERAPY

Any hospitalization--whether for medical, surgical, or psychiatric treatment-- involves the patient with a health care team. In nonpsychiatric settings, however, the function of the team is to administer a more-or-less technolog- ically sophisticated treatment to a patient who is unable to take more than a passive role in his care. The functions of the various team members are subordinate to implementing the diagnostic and treatment recommendations of the physician, and other hospitalized patients are certainly not expected to contribute to each other's care. Although psychiatric inpatient treatment in some settings may also follow this model--i.e., the hospital serves in essence as a specialized hotel in which the major treatment event is the patient's daily session with the psychiatrist--those services that utilize milieu therapy are able to extend the treatment potential of inpatient care well beyond the limits of round-the-clock supervision, room, and board.

While universal agreement on the definition of milieu treatment does not exist, Maxmen, Tucker, & LeBow's description (1974, p. 33) of the "reactive en- vironment" encompasses the overall philosophy of a therapeutic milieu: "the unit's overall structure maximally utilizes and coordinates the entire staff's efforts towards the rehabilitation of the patient's particular behavior problems ...In such an environment the entire staff is primarily concerned with the patient's specific activities and responds to them in an integrated and con- sistent manner." (emphasis added).

Several concepts are implicit in this definition. Observation of patient be- havior in a variety of settings--in one-to-one relationships with various professionals, in transactions with other patients, when dealing with family members, etc.--greatly increases the opportunity for a comprehensive assess- ment of the patient's problems, and provides a variety of contexts for ther- apeutic interventions. Since psychosocial dysfunction is, as discussed in Section II of this chapter, manifest by various observable behaviors, doc- tors, nurses, social workers, activities therapists, and indeed other patients are in a position to identify and help modify various maladaptive symptoms and interactional patterns. Open communication among various staff members reduces the likelihood of staff working at cross purposes with one another, and promotes continual updating and integration of information about the patient. Because the patient is immersed in the hospital environment around the clock, staff and other patients are able to observe and control the ante- cedents and consequences of various behaviors to a greater degree than is possible in an outpatient setting. Provided that treatment goals are chosen with great care--that is, provided they are appropriate for and acceptable to the patient and the setting which he will enter upon leaving the hospital --this "leverage" offered by a reactive environment can be extremely bene- ficial.

Also implicit in the concept of a reactive milieu is the need for treatment plans to be individualized. Most patients may participate in individual and group psychotherapeutic sessions, but this should be done with a specific rationale in each case rather than "because it's available" or in order to fill the day. Similarly, goals for different patients will differ greatly: a shy, depressed young man may need considerable encouragement and prodding to communicate with others and to learn to practice social skills, while a loud and boisterous hypomanic woman may need considerable encouragement to sit quietly, keep her more flamboyant thoughts to herself, and listen to others. Principles of individual, group, and family therapies described earlier in this chapter are applicable to inpatient as well as outpatient settings.

Staff must share a commitment to individualized treatment programs and must not be overly wedded to any single approach: if Patient A needs intensive psychosocial intervention, patient B needs large doses of imipramine, Doctor C thinks drugs are a "crutch," and Nurse D thinks "just talking" is a waste of time--a cohesive therapeutic milieu cannot flourish.

This section has provided only the briefest overview of milieu treatment. Maxmen, Tucker, & LeBow (1974) offer a lucid and far more detailed discussion of theoretical and practical aspects of inpatient psychiatric treatments.

QUIZ, Section V.

In the following questions, one or more than one answer may be correct. Circle the correct answer(s).

1. According to Yalom, which of the following is/are major therapeutic factor(s) in Interactional Groups?

    a. interpersonal learning
    b. catharsis/ventilation
    c. group cohesiveness
    d. working-through the transference relationship
    e. universality
    f. advice-giving
    g. imparting information

2. Major function(s) for the therapist in the Interactional Group include(s)

    a. fostering communication among members.
    b. interpreting the group members' dreams.
    c. recommending individual psychotherapy for more severe problems.
    d. encouraging group members to be direct with one another.

3. Which of the following statements is/are true concerning a systems approach to the family?

    a. The most overtly disturbed member--the "identified patient"--may be responding to distress in other family members.
    b. Psychotropic medication should not be given to the "identified patient."
    c. Incest represents pathologically rigid generational boundaries.
    d. A strong husband-wife bond represents a dysfunctional coalition.
    e. Marital couple therapy is contraindicated if a childhood behavioral disorder is present in the couple's child.

4. Which of the following statements is/are consistent with Maxmen and associates' view of effective milieu treatment?

    a. Staff physicians, but not staff social workers, need some familiarity with psychotropic medication as well as with psychosocial modalities.
    b. An "activities therapy" such as crocheting might be appropriate in helping assess whether an elderly woman taking lithium is experiencing significant tremor.
    c. The primary function of the inpatient milieu is to provide systematic support for intensive individual psychotherapy when outpatient care is no longer feasible.
    d. A comprehensive milieu program provides family psychotherapy for all patients.
    e. A major function of around-the-clock hospitalization is weaning most patients from psychotropic medication.
    f. An "activities therapy" such as crocheting might be appropriate in helping assess whether a 40-year-old truck driver taking lithium is experiencing significant tremor.
    g. In order to protect patient confidentiality, it is important that doctors and nurses carefully monitor what they tell each other about their unit's inpatients.
    h. Open expression of feelings might be strongly encouraged for some patients, but strongly discouraged for other patients.

ANSWERS, Section V. _____

1. a,c,e
2. a,d
3. a
4. b,h

POST-TEST

For the following questions, <u>one</u> or <u>more</u> <u>than</u> <u>one</u> answer may be correct. Circle the correct answer(s).

1.   According to Maxmen, Tucker, & LeBow, which of the following is/are characteristic(s) of the "reactive environment"?

      a. primary emphasis on intrapsychic difficulties, with a secondary focus on behavior
      b. utilization of knowledge of the antecedents and consequences of a patient's behavior in order to alter it
      c. subordination of other treatment modalities to the goals of individual psychotherapy
      d. less emphasis upon confidentiality between patient and staff member and more emphasis upon interchange of information among staff
      e. similarity of specific behavioral goals (such as increased expression of feelings) for most patients
      f. general agreement on specific patient goals among staff, despite staff's coming from different disciplinary backgrounds
      g. interchangeable treatment personnel, despite different disciplinary backgrounds, with regard to implementing specific diagnostic and therapeutic measures

2.   Choose the correct statement(s) concerning Interactional Group psychotherapy, as described by Yalom.

      a. Overt expression of painful feeling states is discouraged.
      b. Catharsis and inspiration are major therapeutic factors.
      c. Group cohesiveness and imparting of information are major therapeutic factors.
      d. Interpersonal learning and universality are major therapeutic factors.
      e. The primary task of the leader is to foster communication among group members.

3.   Choose the correct statement(s) about brief psychotherapy.

      a. Time is the principal dimension that distinguishes brief psychotherapy from other approaches.
      b. Use of a specific technique (direct interpretation) is the principal dimension that distinguishes brief psychotherapy from other approaches.
      c. Brief (or short-term) psychotherapy is an example of a specific treatment context.

4.   Choose the correct statement(s) about family therapy.

a.   Because an individual's distress may be symptomatic of a less-obvious problem in the family system, the family therapist should not give psychotropic medication to the "identified patient."
b.   Treatment of a married couple may affect the behavior of their children.
c.   Family therapy might be indicated when the presenting problem is a 9-year-old child with a well-documented learning disability resulting from perinatal hypoxia.
d.   Fluid generational boundaries are generally a sign of a well-functioning family system.

5.   Choose the correct statement(s) about psychoanalysis.

a.   Interpretation of transference is an essential element of psychoanalysis.
b.   Other therapeutic approaches may share common therapeutic factors with psychoanalysis.
c.   Meeting five times a week is an essential element of psychoanalysis.
d.   Resistance can be both an impediment to the progress of treatment and a useful source of information.

6.   According to Strupp, which of the following statements is/are correct?

a.   A patient should be held responsible for his present and future behavior, even if he has experienced an unhappy childhood.
b.   Becoming more effective at eliciting praise from others is a significant source of self-esteem.
c.   Successfully treated patients learn to ignore the distinctions between feelings and behavior.
d.   Successfully treated patients learn to maintain their goals, no matter how unattainable they seem.

7.   According to Parsons, which of the following statements is/are correct?

a.   Societal factors influence doctors' and patients' behavior.
b.   Individual factors do not influence doctors' and patients' behavior.
c.   The healer's role is functionally diffuse.
d.   The uncertainty of medical knowledge contributes to the need for socially-sanctioned behavioral guidelines.

TRUE or FALSE: Circle the correct letter.

T   F   8. Transference is an inappropriate, unconscious reaction based upon previous experience.

T   F   9. Transference occurs in individual psychotherapy, but not in multiple-person therapy contexts.

T   F   10. Psychotropic drugs should not be combined with psychodynamic psychotherapy.

T   F   11. Interpretation is used in psychoanalysis, but rarely in less-intensive psychotherapies.

T   F   12. Societally-determined expectations may serve to reduce certain strains inherent in the clinician-patient situation.

T   F   13. Psychotropic drugs may be appropriate for patients with unconscious conflicts.

T   F   14. A depressed patient whose premorbid social functioning was impaired will not benefit from psychotropic drugs.

T   F   15. Psychoanalysis represents both a therapeutic technique and a specific therapeutic context.

T   F   16. Psychosocial therapy may be appropriate when organic factors play a significant role in a patient's dysfunction.

T   F   17. Psychotropic drugs may be indicated when experiential factors play a significant role in a patient's dysfunction.

T   F   18. Experiential factors play little or no role in the symptom patterns of psychotic disorders.

T   F   19. Biochemical/neurophysiologic factors play a major role in the specific content of hallucinations.

T   F   20. Psychosocial treatments are more likely to be effective when learning (broadly defined) is a major source of the patient's problems.

T   F   21. Success of a therapeutic technique based upon a given theory of personality implies that that theory is correct.

T   F   22. Unconscious factors may be involved in creating or maintaining a symptom that can be successfully treated with behavior therapy.

T   F   23. The DSM-III diagnosis is usually very helpful in choosing a treatment strategy in psychodynamic psychotherapy.

T   F   24. Resistance in psychoanalysis does not occur when transference is properly interpreted.

T   F   25. Strupp considers imitation of the therapist to be a major therapeutic factor in dynamic psychotherapy.

PRE-TEST ANSWERS

1.	b,d,f		10.	F
2.	d,e		11.	T
3.	a		12.	F
4.	a,d		13.	T
5.	b,c		14.	F
6.	a,b,d		15.	F
7.	T		16.	T
8.	F		17.	F
9.	F		18.	F

POST-TEST ANSWERS

1.	b,d,f		13.	T
2.	d,e		14.	F
3.	a		15.	T
4.	b,c		16.	T
5.	a,b,d		17.	T
6.	a		18.	F
7.	a,d		19.	F
8.	T		20.	T
9.	F		21.	F
10.	F		22.	T
11.	F		23.	F
12.	T		24.	F
			25.	F

REFERENCES

Abroms, G. M. The new eclecticism. Archives of General Psychiatry, 1969, 20, 514-523.

Andrews, G., & Harvey, R. Does psychotherapy benefit neurotic patients? Archives of General Psychiatry, 1981, 38, 1203-1208.

Coleman, J. V. Aims and conduct of psychotherapy. Archives of General Psychiatry, 1968, 18, 1-6.

Detre, T. P., & Jarecki, H. G. Modern psychiatric treatment. Philadelphia: J.B. Lippincott, 1971.

Erikson, E. H. Childhood and society (2nd ed.). New York: W.W. Norton, 1963.

Maxmen, J. S., Tucker, G. J., & LeBow, M. Rational hospital psychiatry. New York: Brunner/Mazel, 1974.

Parsons, T. Social structure and dynamic process: The case of modern medical practice. In T. Parsons, The social system. New York: The Free Press, 1951.

Sloane, R. B., & Staples, F. R. (Eds.) Symposium on brief psychotherapy. In Psychiatric clinics of North America, Vol. 2, No. 1. Philadelphia: W.B. Saunders, 1979.

Strupp, H. H. Toward a specification of teaching and learning in psychotherapy. Archives of General Psychiatry, 1969, 21, 203-212.

Whiteside, M. F. Family therapy. In S. I. Harrison (Ed.), Basic handbook of child psychiatry, Vol. III. New York: Basic Books, 1979.

Yalom, I. D. The theory and practice of group psychotherapy (2nd ed.) New York: Basic Books, 1975.

CHAPTER 18

Behavioral Treatment
Alberto B. Santos, M.D.
John C. Roitzsch, Ph.D.

CHAPTER OUTLINE

LEARNING OBJECTIVES

After completing this chapter you will be able to:

1. Contrast the principles of psychoanalytic and behavioral theory.

2. Contrast the nature of the psychotherapeutic process in psychoanalytic and behavioral therapy.

3. Name and describe three basic models of behavioral learning.

4. Describe the concept of contingency learning or operant conditioning.

5. Distinguish between negative reinforcement and punishment.

6. Discuss the concept of extinction as it applies to behavioral treatment techniques.

7. Contrast various reinforcement schedules used in operant conditioning.

8. Distinguish between primary and secondary reinforcers.

9. Discuss the process of shaping by successive approximation.

10. Define "Reciprocal Inhibition" in the contexts of behavior therapy.

11. Name and describe the commonly used behavioral treatment techniques.

12. State what clinical conditions would indicate a particular behavioral treatment modality.

13. Cite the theoretical principles on which the therapeutic strategy of cognitive therapy is based.

PRE-TEST

For the following questions, <u>one</u> or <u>more</u> <u>than</u> <u>one</u> answer may be **correct**. Circle the correct answer(s).

1. Behavioral theories of psychopathology

    a. emphasize intrapsychic conflict.
    b. reject the effect on individuals of biogenetic and sociocultural influences.
    c. are firmly rooted in the psychoanalytic model.
    d. developed from learning theory.

2. Behavioral models of learning include

    a. classical conditioning.
    b. modeling.
    c. operant conditioning.
    d. reaction formation.

3. The efficacy of behavior modification is, to a large extent, **attributed to**

    a. the regressive transference phenomenon.
    b. genetic analysis.
    c. the "drift" hypothesis.
    d. operant or classical conditioning.

4. Behavioral principles include which of the following?

    a. Behavior is maintained because it is reinforced.
    b. Maladaptive behavior is a result of fixations.
    c. What can be learned can be unlearned.
    d. Reinforcement diminishes the occurrence of new behaviors.

5. In order to relieve symptoms through behavioral **techniques the** therapist must delineate

    a. the frequency of the symptom under differing circumstances.
    b. possible social cues.
    c. possible environmental and physiological reinforcers.
    d. possible factors which may act as punishers of **more adaptive** behavior.

6. Behavioral techniques

    a. are concerned with symptom removal.
    b. require a directive, active approach from the therapist.
    c. are based on experimentally derived concepts.
    d. develop the patient's understanding about the psychodynamic origins of the symptom.

7. Progressive relaxation is used in

    a. token economy systems.
    b. implosive therapy.
    c. aversive conditioning.
    d. classical systematic desensitization.

8. Response prevention is a useful technique in the treatment of any behavior where the prevention of escape and/or avoidance behavior is important, but is used most effectively in

    a. Simple Phobias.
    b. Avoidant Personality Disorders.
    c. Agoraphobia.
    d. obsessive compulsive rituals.

9. Assertiveness training

    a. can be used to help people who fail to stand up for their own rights in a firm, effective, and appropriate manner.
    b. can be performed in a group setting.
    c. involves the principle of behavioral shaping.
    d. is the treatment of choice in Tourette's syndrome.

10. The token economy system

    a. can be easily applied to any general hospital unit regardless of length of stay.
    b. employs behavioral shaping techniques.
    c. originated in criminal institutions.
    d. has been used to aid in the treatment of Schizophrenia and mental retardation.

11. Aversive conditioning

    a. is a useful adjunct to the treatment of Bipolar Affective Disorders.
    b. involves the use of a noxious stimulus.
    c. must be done subtly without the patient's conscious consent.
    d. may be useful in treating patients with Buerger's disease who smoke.

12. With biofeedback

    a. an individual can learn to control physiological activities such as heart rate, vasodilatation, and gastric acid secretion.
    b. good results are obtained in the treatment of tension and neuro-vascular migraine headaches.
    c. skin temperature can be raised.
    d. an individual with Raynaud's Disease may have a better prognosis.

13. Cognitive therapy is based on the theoretical assumption(s) that

    a. feelings and behaviors are preceded by patterns of thinking.
    b. feelings and behaviors are products of an individual's way of interpreting information.
    c. patterns of cognitive processing are changeable.
    d. changing the way one feels will be followed by cognitive changes.

I. INTRODUCTION

The historical development of general medical therapeutics is, in part, characterized by scientists claiming supremacy over each other's regimens. This phenomenon is especially evident in the development of the psychotherapies. The psychoanalytic movement in the psychotherapies was triggered by the work of Jean-Martin Charcot, a French neurologist, who in the late 1800's studied hysterical symptomatology through the use of hypnosis. Charcot's contributions were expanded into a widely accepted exploratory clinical technique by Sigmund Freud. Within this movement various "schools of thought" emerged, each debating for differing theoretical principles. These "schools," however, are similar in that they all emphasize the degree to which individuals are driven by unconscious forces. It follows then that the central goal in psychoanalytically based psychotherapy is the achievement of conscious awareness of these unconscious forces by means of analytic insight (see chapter 17 on the analytic model).

During the late 1950's the behavioral movement in psychotherapy emerged. The behaviorists based their approach on the growing body of knowledge about the process of learning, spearheaded by the contributions of Ivan Pavlov and B. F. Skinner, and derived primarily from animal laboratory experiments. The behavioral "school" asserts that much behavior, including symptoms in psychopathology, is learned, and if learned, can be unlearned. This approach does not deny the existence of biological or cultural influences. Most behaviorists are aware of the interaction of different influences on behavior. They do, however, focus on the scientific method, i.e., the forming and testing of hypotheses modifying them as needed. The major therapeutic goal is on the removal of disturbing symptoms through techniques which are firmly based on objective, observable data. The concept of the unconscious and the subjective focus of psychoanalytic therapy were discarded. Understandably, this led to much debate between the dynamic-analytic therapists and the behavior therapists. In recent years, however, many behaviorally trained and psychodynamically trained psychotherapists have begun to learn and apply clinically therapeutic principles from both camps as dictated by the patient's specific problem. Regardless of their differences, both of these models of practice are well-established in the professional community.

This chapter will provide an introductory overview of the nature of behavioral approaches to health care. It should be noted that the question of what mode of psychotherapy is most useful, for what type of patient, is an area of much current collaborative research, and will not be addressed here in depth.

II. BASIC PRINCIPLES OF BEHAVIORAL LEARNING THEORY

There are three basic types of learning paradigms on which behavioral treatment techniques are based. These are: A. Classical conditioning; B. operant conditioning; and C. modeling.

A. CLASSICAL CONDITIONING

The principles of classical conditioning were clearly elucidated by Ivan Pavlov, a physiologist, during the late 1920's and the 1930's. Pavlov cannulated the salivary glands of dogs in order to measure salivation. Meat powder, when presented to the dogs, elicited salivation. He then paired (presented simultaneously) another stimulus such as a bell or a particular tone with the meat powder. He found that after several pairings of the tone with the meat powder, the presentation of the tone alone produced salivation. In this particular case, the meat powder is called the unconditioned stimulus (since it normally elicits salivation), and the salivation is the unconditioned response (since it naturally occurs in the presence of meat powder). When the bell or tone is presented alone, i.e., not paired with the meat powder, it will not produce salivation. It is then called a neutral stimulus. After several pairings of the tone with the meat powder, the tone alone results in salivation. When this occurs, the tone is called the conditioned stimulus. Since the salivation is now occurring as a response to the conditioned stimulus (tone), it is referred to as the conditioned response.

A conditioned response can be elicited not only by the conditioned stimulus but also by stimuli similar to the original conditioned stimulus. For example, tones of different frequencies from the original tone (conditioned stimulus) can also elicit the conditioned response, although the response will be weaker than with the original tone. The more similar a stimulus is to the original conditioned stimulus, the more likely the response will approach the magnitude of strength of the original conditioned response. This phenomenon is called stimulus generalization. A well-known experiment by Watson and Rayner (1920) involving an 11-month old boy, Albert, illustrates the development of a learned fear ("phobia") through classical conditioning and stimulus generalization.

In the beginning of the experiment Albert played with a rat, exhibiting no fear of the animal. After a time, the presentation of the rat (neutral stimulus) was paired several times with a loud noise (unconditioned stimulus) which startled and frightened (unconditioned response) Albert. Consequently, just the presentation of the rat (conditioned stimulus) frightened Albert (conditioned response). Through stimulus generalization, Albert responded with fear to other stimuli which were furry (other animals, stuffed animals, fur coats), although in a progressively weaker manner, depending upon the degree of similarity to the original stimulus.

If the conditioned stimulus is continually presented without occasional pairing with the unconditioned stimulus, the conditioned response will eventually fail to occur. This is called extinction. There are different definitions of extinction for classical and operant conditioning. Both result in a cessation of responding. It needs to be noted, however, that phobias are maintained on an operant paradigm. Avoidance or escape results in negative reinforcement through anxiety reduction. More about this later.

Classical conditioning occurs, therefore, when a stimulus which does not normally elicit a given response acquires the power to do so by being paired with a stimulus that does normally elicit the given response. This is a reflexive, involuntary type of behavioral learning.

B. OPERANT CONDITIONING

Along with classical conditioning, operant conditioning is the basis for what is called behavior modification. B.F. Skinner studied this type of learning extensively. According to Skinner, the consequences of behavior actually control the behavior. Over a period of time, we learn that certain behaviors (operants) result in certain consequences from our environment. The connection between the behavior and the events from the environment which influence the behavior is called a contingency.

Operant conditioning consists of strengthening a desired response, which is already part of the organism's repertoire. This may be done through the presentation of a positive reinforcer or a negative reinforcer following the response. Diagramatically operant conditioning may be represented:

$$S \to R+ \text{ Reinforcement}$$

while classical (respondent) conditioning may be represented:

$$US \to UR$$
$$US + CS \to UR$$
$$CS \to CR$$

A reinforcer is anything which strengthens a response and prevents its extinction. Receiving something pleasant would be a positive reinforcer, while removing or losing something unpleasant would be a negative reinforcer. Reinforcers have the effect of increasing the occurrence of a behavior.

Punishment is usually perceived as receiving something unpleasant although it may also include losing something pleasant. In either event the result is the reduction in the occurrence of a behavior. Punishment is not the same as negative reinforcement. Punishment is unpleasant while negative reinforcement is pleasant since it results in the loss of something unpleasant. An example of a negative reinforcer would be performing a compulsive ritual resulting in the loss of anxiety, which is unpleasant. Punishment has the effect of suppressing the reinforced response, but does not generally result in permanent extinction. Nonreinforcement is necessary for extinction to occur. Experiencing the anxiety without performing the compulsive ritual would be an example of nonreinforcement.

Whether or not something is a reinforcer or a punishment depends on how it is perceived by the recipient. One man's meat is another man's poison. Keeping a child after school may seem to be a punishment, but if the child likes the teacher's attention (even though it is negative attention) it would be a reinforcer.

Reinforcers may also be divided into primary and secondary, as well as positive and negative. Primary reinforcers have the power to strengthen a response because they reduce a physiological drive such as hunger, sexual desire, pain, or thirst. Most of the reinforcers we receive are secondary reinforcers acquiring reinforcing strength by being associated or paired with primary or previously established reinforcers. For example, money has positive reinforcing properties because of its association with the acquisition of desired goods or services.

New behaviors may be too complex to be learned all at once; thus some behaviors must be shaped gradually. This is done by initially reinforcing any behavior which approximates the goal behavior. It is then necessary for successive behaviors to be more and more like the goal behavior before reinforcement is given. This process is called shaping behavior by the use of successive approximations. Teaching animals complex tricks or babies to talk is done using this process.

The manner in which reinforcement is given in behavior therapy is called a reinforcement schedule. The schedule of reinforcement indicates under what circumstances reinforcement will occur. The reinforcement may occur after every response (a 100% schedule), or less than every response (a partial schedule). Partial reinforcement schedules may be further subdivided into ratio and internal and fixed and variable schedules. If the schedule depends on the number of responses made before reinforcement is given, it is called a ratio schedule. If the schedule depends on the passage of time before reinforcement is given, it is called an interval schedule. When a reinforcement is given after a specific number of responses or time intervals, the subject is on a fixed schedule. When reinforcement is given after a random number of responses or unspecified time intervals, the subject is on a variable schedule. In summary, partial reinforcement schedules can be fixed ratio, variable ratio, fixed interval, or variable interval. The reinforcement schedule is important because a 100% schedule produces faster learning than a partial schedule, but a partial schedule produces learning which is more resistant to extinction. In fact, the schedule most resistant to extinction is a variable interval schedule, and this is the one which occurs most naturally in our daily lives. Usually, a continuous reinforcement schedule is used to initiate new behaviors with a gradual change to a partial schedule. This has the effect of rapid establishment of the behavior, as well as greater resistance to extinction.

Seldom is anyone reinforced every time a "desirable" response is made. For example, a mother may not be around to see the child be nice to a younger sibling or may not smile or praise him if she is present. Thus, the behavior is reinforced, not because of the number of responses, but because mother is there and decides to reinforce the behavior - a variable interval schedule.

C. MODELING

Observational learning or modeling occurs when we learn something by watching someone else do it. Modeling is roughly analogous to the concept of identification in psychoanalytic theory. Children may learn much of what they know by imitating (modeling) their parents, peers, or other important figures in their lives, such as "superheroes." They may also learn fears by observing others respond to a feared object or situation. It may be that we model some behaviors and not others, depending on an internal or external reinforcement. The reinforcers may not always be apparent however; therefore modeling appears to be a unique learning paradigm with properties not found in classical or operant conditioning.

Albert Bandura has extensively studied modeling behavior in children. The following outline was developed by Hilgard and Bower (1975, p. 601) to illustrate some of the factors studied by Bandura:

A. Stimulus properties of the model

    1. The model's age, sex, and status relative to that of the subject are paired. High-status models are more imitated.

    2. The model's similarity to the subject: The model may be either another child in the same room, or a child in a movie, or an animal character in a movie cartoon, etc. Imitation induced in the subject decreases as the model is made more dissimilar to a real person.

B. Type of behavior exemplified by the model

    1. Novel skills are compared to novel sequences of known responses. The more complex the skills, the poorer the degree of imitation after one observation trial.

    2. Hostile or aggressive responses. These are imitated to a high degree.

    3. Standards of self-reward for good versus bad performances. The subject will adopt self-reward standards similar to those of the model. Also, the subject will imitate the type of moral standards exhibited by an adult model. Techniques of self-control can be transmitted in this manner.

C. Consequences of model's behavior

    Whether the model's behavior is rewarded, punished, or "ignored" (neither reinforced nor punished) by other agents in the drama is varied. Rewarded behaviors of the model are more likely to be imitated.

D. Motivational set given to the subject

    1. Instructions given to the subject before he observes

the model provide him with high or low motivation to pay attention to and learn the model's behavior. High motivations might be produced by telling the subject that he will be rewarded commensurate with how much of the model's behavior he can reproduce on a later test. Under minimal instructions, learning is classified mainly as "incidental."

2. Motivating instructions may be given after the subject views the model and before he is tested. This aids in distinguishing learning from performance of imitative responses (p. 601).

READING NOTE: For further information about the principles of Learning Theory, the interested student is referred to Hilgard & Bower, Theories of learning. Englewood Cliffs, NJ: Prentice-Hall, Inc., 1975.

QUIZ, Section II.

Match the following terms with their corresponding descriptions.

In Pavlov's experiment

____ 1.	unconditioned stimulus	a.	salivation to meat powder
____ 2.	unconditioned response	b.	tone not paired with meat powder
____ 3.	conditioned stimulus		
____ 4.	conditioned response	c.	tone, previously paired with meat powder, now alone yields salivation
____ 5.	neutral stimulus		
		d.	meat powder
		e.	salivation to tone after pairings with meat powder

Match the following types of reinforcement with their corresponding descriptions.

____ 6.	negative reinforcement	a.	receiving something unpleasant
____ 7.	primary reinforcement	b.	reinforcement occurs after a random number of responses.
____ 8.	fixed schedules of reinforcement		
		c.	reduction of a physical drive
____ 9.	punishment	d.	removal of something unpleasant
____ 10.	secondary reinforcers	e.	reinforcement is given after a specific number of responses
____ 11.	variable schedules of reinforcement		
		f.	associated with previously established reinforcers

TRUE or FALSE: Indicate which of the following statements are true (T) and which are false (F) by circling the appropriate letters.

T   F   12. Stimulus generalization describes a phenomenon by which a conditioned response can be elicited by not only the conditioned stimulus, but also by stimuli similar to the original conditioned stimulus, although in a progressively weaker manner (depending on the degree of similarity).

T   F   13. Extinction results if a conditioned response stimulus is not reinforced.

III. DISTINGUISHING FEATURES OF BEHAVIOR THERAPY

There are features of behavior therapy which can be seen as unique from psychoanalytically based therapy in many respects.

A. CONCEPT OF PATHOLOGY

Behavioral theory focuses on types of behavior, normal and abnormal, that are products of how an individual has learned (or not learned) to respond to situations that life presents. The influences of biological and sociocultural factors on an individual's behavior are recognized. Maladaptive behavior or psychopathology, therefore, is not viewed as unconscious manifestations of repressed intrapsychic conflicts. Instead, maladaptive behavior is often thought to be learned and maintained according to the principles of learning theory outlined above, i.e., neither quantitatively nor qualitatively different in development and maintenance from other learned behaviors. For example, one may have learned to fear dark places directly because of being frightened in the dark as a child or through modeling a parent's fear of entering a dark place.

B. MODE OF CHANGE

Since the behaviorist views abnormal behavior problems as learned, change is achieved through a process of direct teaching and learning of new behavioral associations. The therapist must reinforce the new or desired behavior, and the patient must repeat and practice it both with and without the therapist. The goal of behavior therapy is the removal of a symptom through an overt, well-structured, directive procedure without emphasis on developing a patient's insight into the dynamic origins of the behavior.

Since the behavioral approach is focused on the removal of a "symptom" (complaint or problem as reported by the patient with help of the therapist in its delineation), it is imperative to investigate a variety of factors which may relate to the symptom: 1) the frequency and duration of the symptom under differing situations, 2) cues which might elicit and maintain the symptom, 3) possible environmental and physiological reinforcers, and 4) possible factors which may act as punishers of more adaptive behavior.

This information is studied in the context of the individual's life history, but without a focus on that individual's subjective, detailed, historical account of developmental conflicts if these conflicts are not related to the problem situation. A treatment program is then designed to reduce the frequency, duration, and severity of the problem. Periodic reassessment is important to insure that the program designed is successful.

C. NATURE OF THE THERAPEUTIC RELATIONSHIP

The therapist's task is to program, model, reinforce, inhibit, or shape specific behavioral responses. Although the role of the therapist varies according to the nature of the problem, in general, the therapeutic relationship, because of its directive nature, is similar to that of teacher and pupil. In contrast to the importance placed on the concept of transference in the psychodynamic model, in behavior therapy relatively little time is spent on direct exploration of the vicissitudes of the patient-therapist relationship. The behaviorist may use warmth, acceptance, and other means of relating to secure the patient's cooperation in the treatment plan and to strengthen the therapist's role as a social reinforcer (or nonreinforcer). The therapeutic alliance, however, is deliberately structured in such a way that attention is drawn to the patient's constructive and "healthy" behaviors and attitudes.

QUIZ, Section III.

TRUE or FALSE: Circle the correct letter.

T   F   1.   The behaviorist's concept of psychopathology focuses on repressed intrapsychic conflicts.

T   F   2.   Behavioral theory presumes that most behavior is a product of learning.

T   F   3.   Behavior therapy does not emphasize the need for the development of the patient's psychodynamic insight into the problem.

T   F   4.   The nature of the therapist-patient relationship in behavior therapy forces an inquiry into transferential phenomena.

IV.　TREATMENT TECHNIQUES AND THEIR INDICATIONS

Behavior therapy offers a large variety of conditioning, training, and other directive techniques. The behaviorist first identifies a specific target behavior or response to be modified. A behavioral formulation is then constructed focusing on environmental cues and other possible factors of influence as mentioned above which maintain the behavior (this is the behaviorist's analog to a dynamic formulation). Having completed the behavioral formulation, one can then choose a particular treatment technique and set specific treatment goals. A formal behavioral contract describing the treatment goals agreed upon by the therapist and the patient may be drawn up. Compliance with the desired behavior leads to reinforcement, while noncompliance may lead to punishment. For example, in a residential treatment center a teenager who observes a ten o'clock curfew will be permitted to continue going out at night, while violation of the curfew will lead to removal of the privilege.

A.　CLASSICAL SYSTEMATIC DESENSITIZATION

It has been suggested that a process of accidental pairing of a noxious stimulus with a normally benign stimulus is the basis of most simple phobias. When an individual experiences an unpleasant emotion such as anxiety or fear in response to a particular object or situation, extinction does not occur because the object or situation is avoided where possible. In fact the individual will avoid even thinking about the object or situation, since the thought alone might evoke the unpleasant response. Avoidance acts as a negative reinforcer since it prevents the individual from experiencing anxiety. If placed in the phobic situation, the individual leaves or escapes. This action reduces the anxiety, thus serving as a negative reinforcer and strengthening the avoidance behavior.

Joseph Wolpe (1958) developed a technique for treating conditioned fears such as that induced in the case of Albert, by Watson and Rayner. The basis for his technique was the general physiological principle that sympathetic and parasympathetic responses are mutually exclusive. Put another way, one cannot feel tense and relaxed at the same time. This phenomenon is called reciprocal inhibition: the pairing of an unpleasant experience (anxiety, fear) with a competitive pleasant one (eating, relaxation, or sexual arousal) will result in the inhibition of the unpleasant experience. Systematic Desensitization evolved from this principle.

Traditionally, the anxiety or fear response is paired with relaxation. The patient must first, however, learn to relax. A modification of Jacobson's (1938) progressive relaxation technique is used. This involves first tensing, then relaxing all the major muscle groups of the body in an orderly fashion (e.g., hands, arms, head, chest, abdomen, legs, feet). Learning of this technique is augmented by the therapist's modeling. The patient practices relaxation exercises as frequently as necessary until the muscle groups can be relaxed at will without having to employ a preceding increase in muscle tension. The procedure can be learned in a few weeks. The main goals are to have the patient first be aware of the difference between muscle relaxation and muscle extension and then be able to relax when desired.

The patient is also asked to construct a <u>hierarchy</u> of stimuli which depicts increasingly anxious situations. At the top of the hierarchy should be the maximally feared situation.

Once the hierarchy has been constructed and relaxation has been learned, the patient is asked to imagine vividly each scene in the hierarchy and then to relax so that the feared stimulus will be <u>paired</u> with the relaxation response. If a particular scene produces anxiety which overwhelms the relaxation response, the patient signals (e.g., lifts a finger) and may be asked to imagine an already practiced scene and work up the hierarchy again until all scenes are mastered. Relaxation at every step of the hierarchy should be accomplished before proceeding on to the next higher step. The patient is encouraged to expose himself outside the office to real-life stimuli which have already been mastered in the imagined situation.

In more recent years, it has been thought that the active induction of relaxation is not absolutely necessary in systematic desensitization. Nevertheless, the traditional mode of systematic desensitization has been used extensively and effectively in the treatment of <u>simple phobias</u>. Outcome studies done as long as four years after treatment have shown that patients remained symptom free.

****

GO TO VIDEOTAPE

****

B.　FLOODING

<u>Flooding</u>, unlike systematic desensitization where the situations are followed by relaxation, maximally raises the patient's anxiety with strong affect-laden imagery <u>from the beginning</u>. Relaxation is not emphasized and the patient is encouraged to encounter and master the feared stimulus as quickly as possible. The theoretical basis is that the nervous system cannot function indefinitely at maximum capacity; therefore, if a stimulus that elicits an anxiety response is continually presented, the response should wear out and so extinguish. This is different from pairing relaxation with a stimulus in order to reduce anxiety as is the case in systematic desensitization. This technique may be used to reduce or extinguish the anxiety to particular stimuli. It has also been used in cases of Dysthymic Disorders by having patients imagine the most helpless, hopeless situation possible and to maintain that image as long as possible. Continuation of this should wear out the anxiety or fear associated with the image.

Flooding, as well as systematic desensitization, can occur in the office through imagery (in vitro) or in real life (in vivo).

C. IN VIVO DESENSITIZATION AND FLOODING

It is now generally accepted that in vivo (real life) methods of desensitization and flooding are superior to in vitro (imagined) ones in terms of achieving extinction. Of course, in some cases it may be impractical or impossible to go directly to the real-life situation. In others the anxiety may be so debilitating or dangerous (as in patients with angina or asthma), that the traditional relaxation/imagery approach would be indicated.

In cases of Agoraphobia, (fear of crowded places), in vivo techniques of treatment appear to be superior over the in vitro approach. Flooding for Agoraphobia is widely done in groups. The therapist accompanies the patients and provides emotional support as the threatening situation is faced in vivo. Individuals in these groups appear to drop out of treatment less frequently than when treated alone with flooding. The group pressure may serve as a motivator, and the group process may be socially reinforcing. Agoraphobia may also be treated in vivo by gradually exposing a patient to feared situations in hierarchical order with support to help reduce anxiety in the situation.

D. EXTINCTION THROUGH RESPONSE PREVENTION

Thus far you have read about two techniques: systematic desensitization and flooding, in which the concept of extinction is of primary importance. A third technique which highlights this principle is response prevention, which can be used effectively for the treatment of obsessive compulsive rituals.

In a patient with a ritual, like handwashing, anxiety results from touching a possible contaminant and persists until the individual performs the ritual. To relieve the anxiety the patient engages in excessive hand-washing. Performing the ritual is negatively reinforcing since it relieves the anxiety. Even though the patient will say that the behavior is irrational, he continues to do it since it relieves the anxiety. The patient, if hospitalized, can be prevented from handwashing by either verbally declining a request to use the lavatory or possibly by periodically taking the handles off the water faucets. The patient is forced to experience high degrees of anxiety. As in flooding, the anxiety gradually subsides. Extinction takes place through nonreinforcement; that is, the relief of anxiety through handwashing is not allowed to occur. For the treatment of obsessive compulsive rituals other therapists have used modeling (the therapist touches the object and encourages the patient to do the same) or direct stimulus flooding (the patient is asked to contaminate himself as much as possible and remain in the feared situation until the anxiety subsides). The two techniques, response prevention and flooding, are often used together.

E. ASSERTIVENESS AND SOCIAL SKILLS TRAINING

Many people behave maladaptively in different social situations. They may either display a lack of assertion or behave in social situations in an inappropriate or ineffective manner. The goal of this technique is to increase the social effectiveness of the individual. Assertiveness training can be used to help people who generally (or in specific situations) fail to stand up for their own rights or needs in a firm, effective, and appropriate manner. Many people suffer significantly because of their inability to express their disappointments and anger in a productive way. For example, some individuals report that they "hold anger in until [they] explode." The "explosion" is usually nonproductive and self-defeating since the factors causing the anger continue to exist.

It is maintained that individuals who are inhibited from asserting themselves when appropriate are either afraid of making others angry at them or of their own anger becoming unmanageable. Consequently, they are usually passive in their interactions with others, even though they may be angry at themselves later for not being more assertive. As with many other maladaptive behaviors, the person experiences the short-term gain of a temporary relief of anxiety through avoidance, but there is a long-term loss as the behavior does not deal with the problem. Being assertive may cause more immediate anxiety, but should result in anxiety reduction over time as a person gains reinforcements for such assertive action.

The technique is as follows: the individual is instructed in the principles of being assertive and encouraged to be alert to situations where frustration has been experienced because of lack of assertion. As the situations are reported, alternative ways of responding are explored by the patient with the therapist. This process may be done individually or in groups and may involve <u>modeling</u> by the therapist. It may also involve <u>role playing</u> (acting) with the therapist, including <u>role reversal</u> (the patient takes the role of the object of his actions and the therapist acts the role of the patient). Role playing affords further opportunity for modeling. When done in a group, other patients may participate in the role playing or role reversal. In other social situations the problem may not be a lack of assertiveness but instead, inappropriate behavior. For example, teenagers may be ineffective in getting dates due to failure to use approaches which will be well-received. The approach to this problem would be similar to assertiveness training.

****

GO TO VIDEOTAPE

****

F. TOKEN ECONOMY SYSTEMS

Token economy systems evolved in the early 1960's as a means of motivating institutionalized chronic Schizophrenia patients who were apathetic and inactive. The approach is an attempt to apply the principles of operant conditioning to a large hospital-based, patient population. The behaviors to be reinforced and the reinforcers selected are often determined in collaboration with the patients. The behaviors selected should be health engendering, not primarily to achieve conformity to hospital rules. The reinforcers may include patient desired privileges as long as they are not contraindicated for therapy (e.g., not having to go to group). Points, token coins, or other means of keeping track of desirable behaviors are given, which in turn can be exchanged for reinforcers. Tokens minimize the delay between response and reinforcement. It has been shown that the tokens themselves become reinforcing in that patients will work for them, whether or not they can exchange them for things they want. It is necessary with this technique that the desired behaviors are well-defined, understood by the patient, and rewarded when they occur.

Token economy systems have been used mostly in long-term care facilities with good results. They are rarely used in general hospital units because of the relatively short stay of the patients or because of difficulty controlling reinforcers. Token economy systems have been used effectively in classroom settings for children with emotional, behavioral, and learning disturbances. It is also of value in improving self-help skills in individuals who are mentally retarded.

As previously noted, the token economy systems are an example of the clinical application of learning or behavioral change through operant conditioning. Similar operant techniques, but without the use of tokens, have been used effectively in the treatment of a variety of the common clinical conditions. These include: the training of speech in childhood autism, motivating the physically handicapped towards active participation in rehabilitation and physical therapy, the achievement of weight gain in anorexia nervosa, and motivating individuals towards diet control in the treatment of obesity.

In some of these cases the desired response to be reinforced (within the operant treatment paradigm) is not present at all in the individual's behavioral repertoire; thus it cannot be directly reinforced. In such cases, it is necessary to shape behaviors gradually until the desired response appears. This approach is formally called Behavioral Shaping. The patient is first reinforced for any response which resembles the desired target behavior. With time, the criterion for reinforcement is gradually narrowed towards the target behavior until only the desired behavior is reinforced.

G. AVERSIVE CONDITIONING

Aversive conditioning is a type of behavior therapy in which noxious stimulation or punishment is used to decrease the frequency of undesirable behavior. The noxious stimulus, typically a mild electric shock delivered immediately after the unwanted behavior, acts as a punisher. The treatment involves voluntary collaboration between the patient and therapist. As stated earlier, learning theory holds that punishment can suppress the frequency of occurrence of a learned response but does not usually extinguish it. Therefore, aversive conditioning is generally combined with other therapies. The noxious stimulus paired with the undesirable behavior produces fear or anxiety which results in inhibitory behavior.

Aversive conditioning is useful in treating behaviors which are dangerous, socially embarrassing, or unlawful. These include: alcoholism; sexual deviations such as pedophilia, fetishism, and exhibitionism; overeating; self-mutilation or head banging in autistic children; and smoking (as in cases of severe respiratory illnesses or vascular disease such as Buerger's where there is reduced blood flow to the periphery). For aversive conditioning to work best, alternative desirable behaviors should be reinforced.

H.   BIOFEEDBACK

Biofeedback is a relatively new but well established treatment for a variety of medical problems. It provides a technology by which an individual can learn to control voluntarily certain physiological activities by providing "feedback" information to the patient about those functions. A person may, for instance, receive feedback about his heart rate, skin temperature, or muscle tension. The feedback may consist of an actual numerical reading or an auditory or visual stimulus when the physiologic function falls above or below a set range. To illustrate its role in clinical medicine, consider the syndrome of tension headaches. We commonly see chronic muscular tension headaches in association with life stresses in individuals who, for one reason or another, are likely to be unaware of tension within themselves. Psychotherapeutic techniques can offer these individuals improved coping skills to defend against stress, as well as greater productive mastery over aggressive drives. Biofeedback can be extremely helpful in directly relieving the symptom (headache) and can be used alone or in conjunction with other therapeutic techniques aimed at increasing the patient's ability to cope effectively with stress.

Through the use of electrical monitoring devices (electromyograph) the individual is made aware of the precise level of tension in the occipitalis and frontalis muscles. The equipment monitors the information, amplifies it, and feeds it back through visual or auditory means reflecting the amount of muscular tension. Through this process of presenting previously unavailable physiological information, an individual can learn to bring under control certain bodily functions traditionally thought to be "involuntary." Successful performance in the treatment task may hopefully by itself be sufficient reinforcement for the patient so there will be a reduction of the symptoms which brought him for treatment. If the relationship between success at biofeedback and symptom reduction is not clear to the patient, then success at biofeedback will not provide adequate reinforcement to sustain an adequate level of practice. In these cases, other reinforcers (i.e., praise, money) may be used to increase the motivation to practice.

The precise role of psychological "mediational" factors (images, thoughts, feelings) in the achievement of voluntary control over physiological functions is not clear. To illustrate this issue, Olton and Noonberg (1980) present the following case examples:

> Several people, in attempting to decrease their heart rate through biofeedback, are simply told that when a light turns on it represents a slowed rate, and are asked to turn the light on (which they are able to do). When asked how they accomplished this goal, "one person replied that she imagined a peaceful, relaxing scene . . . Another person replied that he just concentrated on the feedback light and tried to turn it on; he had had no images

and he focused his thoughts on making his heart beat slower and turning the light on. A third person says that he felt a particular emotion, but the emotion was not associated with any visual image. He developed a feeling of being relaxed, peaceful, at ease with the world, satisfied with his role in life" (p.21).

The precise role, if any, of these cognitive processes for successful control in biofeedback is presently unknown.

One common use of biofeedback is in the treatment of headache syndromes (tension and migraines). For neurovascular migraine headaches, the patient is fed back information about the dilation and constriction of the temporal artery. This is done through a photosensor measuring the diameter of the artery. Measuring head and hand temperature is also used as a measurement of blood flow which would affect the dilation or constriction of the artery. The sensor gives direct feedback to the patient and he learns to control the dilation and constriction of the temporal artery. Giving feedback about the temperature of the head and hand allows the patient to decrease the blood flow (temperature) to the head and increase it to the extremities. The same technique can also be helpful to patients with Raynaud's disease. Biofeedback techniques are also being used and further developed for the treatment of asthma, peptic ulcers, tachycardia, hypertension, and epilepsy. They have also been used in other physical conditions such as cardiac arrhythmias (PVC's and the Wolff-Parkinson-White Syndrome) and for neuromuscular reeducation following injury (fecal incontinence from nerve damage; paralysis and paresis from cerebral strokes or nerve damage). In most situations, relaxation training increases the effectiveness of biofeedback.

****

GO TO VIDEOTAPE

****

QUIZ, SECTION IV.

Circle the letter corresponding to the one correct answer.

1. Classical systematic desensitization is a useful technique in an individual who experiences irrational anxiety or fear in the presence of a particular object or situation, and when _____ does not occur because the object or situation is avoided.

    a. positive reinforcement
    b. punishment
    c. extinction
    d. satiation
    e. negative reinforcement

2. In response prevention, extinction takes place through

   a. positive reinforcement.
   b. nonreinforcement.
   c. negative reinforcement.
   d. punishment.
   e. intermittent reinforcement.

3. Aversive conditioning is usually combined with other therapies because it is a form of

   a. positive reinforcement.
   b. negative reinforcement.
   c. punishment.
   d. delayed reinforcement.
   e. permanent reinforcement.

4. Biofeedback has been used successfully to treat all of the following except

   a. tension.
   b. migraine headaches.
   c. Raynaud's disease.
   d. myopia.
   e. paralysis from cerebral strokes.

TRUE or FALSE: Circle the correct letter.

T   F   5. Flooding is a more effective treatment for Agoraphobia than classical systematic desensitization.

T   F   6. Classical systematic desensitization is more frequently used for the treatment of simple phobias rather than Agoraphobia.

V. COGNITIVE THERAPY

Most of the early behaviorists considered cognitions (or thoughts) to be irrelevant in explaining behavior. Techniques of behavior modification were based on principles of either classical or operant conditioning. Remember that conditioning uses essentially a stimulus-response model (S-R) and not a model which includes the organism (S-O-R). The notion that thought or what has been called "inner speech" might play a role in learning was not pursued.

The cognitive-semantic therapists, beginning with Kelley (1955) and followed by Frank (1961), Ellis (1962), Beck (1970), and Singer (1974), wrote about the value of cognition in learning. Meichenbaum (1969), in the first of a series of studies, reported the effects of giving instructions and reinforcements on thinking and language. He maintained that an individual may give instructions to himself to perform a certain behavior, perhaps in imitation of instructions given by a parent or authority figure. Subsequently the individual may actually give himself praise for emitting the behavior.

Luria (1961, 1969) suggests a three step process in a child's acquisition of socialized behavior: 1) adults give overt instructions and control; 2) the child gives himself overt instructions; and 3) the child gives himself inner or covert instructions. Logically it seems to follow that a similar process would hold true for reinforcement, i.e., an adult gives verbal reinforcement, the child gives himself overt verbal reinforcement, and finally the child gives himself covert verbal reinforcement.

The concept of "self-instruction" may play an important role in a variety of behavioral therapy techniques, e.g., in systematic desensitization. In short, the "self-instruction" may become a form of negative reinforcement (removal of a noxious stimulus). For example, a person may covertly instruct himself to "calm down" in the face of an anxiety-producing situation. After some training, the pairing of self-instruction to "calm down" with the onset of an aversive stimulus may well produce the conditioned response of relaxing. Furthermore, this process may even generalize to situations similar to the original one.

The degree to which cognitions influence an individual's behaviors and moods is an area of current research and debate. Nevertheless, research into cognitive processes suggests that some psychopathology, in particular depressed mood and anxiety, may be influenced by cognitive errors in information processing or by firmly held irrational beliefs.

Present day cognitive therapy is one of the newly developed "talking" therapies which is assuming an important place within the realm of available psychological treatments. The basic assumption is that negative feeling states are not just a result of events in a person's life, but more specifically a result of the way that events are interpreted. As Beck, Rush, Shaw, & Emery (1979) point out:

> His cognitions (verbal or pictorial 'events' in his stream of consciousness) are based on attitudes or assumptions (schemas) developed from previous experiences. For example, if a person interprets all his experiences in terms of whether he is competent and adequate, his thinking may be dominated by the schema, 'Unless I do everything perfectly, I'm a failure.' Consequently, he reacts to situations in terms of adequacy even when they are unrelated to whether or not he is personally competent (p.3).

Ellis (1962) proposed that a major core of emotional disturbance is the faulty belief that self-worth is determined by what other people think of you. He noted that faulty or irrational styles of processing information were prevalent in individuals with emotional problems. Ellis (1962) described eleven commonly held irrational beliefs. They are irrational in that they don't realistically reflect the individual's past experiences:

1. The idea that it is a dire necessity for an adult human being to be loved or approved by virtually every significant other person in his community (p.61).

2. The idea that one should be thoroughly competent, adequate, and achieving in all possible respects, if one is to consider oneself worthwhile (p.63).

3. The idea that certain people are bad, wicked, or villainous and that they should be severely blamed and punished for their villainy (p.65).

4. The idea that it is awful and catastrophic when things are not the way one would very much like them to be (p.69).

5. The idea that human unhappiness is externally caused and that people have little or no ability to control their sorrows and disturbances (p.72).

6. The idea that if something is or may be dangerous or fearsome one should be terribly concerned about it and should keep dwelling on the possibility of its occurring (p.75).

7. The idea that it is easier to avoid than to face certain life difficulties and self-responsibilities (p.78).

8. The idea that one should be dependent on others and needs someone stronger than oneself on whom to rely (p.80).

9. The idea that one's past history is an all-important determinant of one's present behavior and that because something once strongly affected one's life, it should indefinitely have a similar effect (p.82).

10. The idea that one should become quite upset over other people's problems and disturbances (p. 85).

11. The idea that there is invariably a right, precise, and perfect solution to human problems and that it is catastrophic if this correct solution is not found (p.87).

In addition to such firmly held irrational beliefs, other forms of cognitive distortions can occur which may lead to maladaptive patterns of interpreting information. Such errors in information processing include for example: selective abstraction, the faulty process of differentially attending to and personally emphasizing negative detail in life experiences while discounting positive aspects, resulting in an overall negative evaluation of the experience; arbitrary inference, the faulty process of formulating a negative interpretation of an experience without a logical examination of the data base or from an insufficient data base ("jumping to conclusions" or "misreading others"); and overgeneralization, seeing a negative event as a continuous pattern of negative experiences. The task of the cognitive therapist is to identify both irrational beliefs and errors in information processing which lead to emotional unrest. Then, these cognitive distortions are attached and modified. For example, in depression-prone individuals, self-devaluating ways of interpreting information are challenged. As Kovacs and Beck (1978) point out:

> The depressed person's thinking and preoccupation represent erroneous and exaggerated ways of viewing oneself and events. The depressed person is overtly sensitive to obstacles to goal-directed activity, interprets trivial impediments as substantial, reads disparagement into innocuous statements by others, and, at the same time devalues himself or herself. The characteristic depressive preoccupations are stereotypical and are evident in self-report, fantasy, and dream content. Moreover, the cognitions are frequently irrelevant and inappropriate to the reality of the situation, and mirror a consistent negative bias against oneself (p.526).

The goal of this mode of therapy is to extinguish maladaptive cognitive processes and to substitute and reinforce more adaptive cognitive styles. Therapy consists of an active treatment in which the therapist challenges the patient's cognitions through verbal interaction or behavioral assignments designed to invalidate the maladaptive thoughts. In this manner maladaptive cognitions are addressed and modified. Sometimes the patient will keep daily records to help examine evidence against and in support of a particular maladaptive cognition. This work leads to the substitution of more reality-based interpretations of life events. As therapy progresses, patients begin to question their assumptions on their own without the help of the therapist. The capacity to conduct this process successfully alone is self-rewarding and is a key factor related to therapeutic efficacy.

****

GO TO VIDEOTAPE

****

POST-TEST

Circle the correct answer(s). <u>One</u> or <u>more</u> <u>than</u> <u>one</u> answer may be correct.

1. The behavioral orientation to therapeutics emphasizes

    a. the concept of the unconscious.
    b. the concept of regression.
    c. defense mechanisms.
    d. a focus on objective observable events.

2. When a stimulus which does not normally elicit a given response acquires the power to do so by pairing with a stimulus that normally elicits the given response, this is called

    a. shaping.
    b. operant conditioning.
    c. modeling.
    d. classical conditioning.

3. Operant Conditioning

    a. consists of strengthening a response which is already part of the organism's repertoire through the presentation of a reinforcer following the response.
    b. is based on the principles of contingency learning.
    c. employs the principle of shaping by successive approximation for the learning of more complex behaviors.
    d. achieves learning which is most resistant to extinction when a variable interval schedule is used.

4. According to the work of Bandura on modeling,

    a. high status models are more imitated.
    b. hostile or aggressive responses tend to be imitated to a high degree.
    c. rewarded behaviors of the model are more likely to be performed.
    d. techniques of self-control can be learned through the modeling paradigm

5. The behaviorist's task includes

    a. programming behavioral response.
    b. rewarding certain behaviors.
    c. punishing certain behaviors.
    d. shaping behaviors.

6. In behavior therapy

   a. the relationship between the therapist and the patient is like that of a teacher and a student.
   b. transference is carefully explored.
   c. the patient's "healthier" behaviors are actually reinforced.
   d. the therapist mostly follows the patient's flow of thought.

7. Classical systematic desensitization

   a. is based on the principle of reciprocal inhibition.
   b. is used in the treatment of Simple Phobias.
   c. can be described as the pairing of an unpleasant experience with a competitive pleasant one, with subsequent inhibition of the unpleasant experience.
   d. usually involves progressive relaxation techniques.

8. Flooding

   a. is more efficacious for the treatment of Agoraphobia than is classical systematic desensitization.
   b. involves the use of mental imagery and progressive relaxation techniques.
   c. is a form of in vivo desensitization.
   d. is based primarily on the concept of vicarious learning.

9. With response prevention,

   a. some Anxiety Disorders can be treated.
   b. extinction takes place through nonreinforcement.
   c. obsessive compulsive rituals can be successfully treated.
   d. the patient is forced to experience high degrees of anxiety.

10. Assertiveness training may involve

    a. role playing.
    b. role reversal.
    c. modeling.
    d. free association.

11. Aversive conditioning

    a. is usually combined with other therapies.
    b. is a modification of progressive relaxation.
    c. is used in treating behaviors which are dangerous, socially embarrassing, or unlawful.
    d. is a form of negative reinforcement.

12. Biofeedback has been used effectively in the treatment of

    a. diabetes mellitus.
    b. peptic ulcer disease.
    c. obesity.
    d. asthma.

13. Cognitive therapy is based on the theoretical assumption(s) that

    a. feelings and behaviors are preceded by patterns of thinking.
    b. feelings and behaviors are products of an individual's way of interpreting information.
    c. patterns of cognitive processing are changeable.
    d. changing the way one feels will be followed by cognitive changes.

PRE-TEST ANSWERS

1. d
2. a,b,c
3. d
4. a,c
5. a,b,c,d
6. a,b,c
7. d

8. d
9. a,b,c
10. b,d
11. b,d
12. a,b,c,d
13. a,b,c

POST-TEST ANSWERS

1. d
2. d
3. a,b,c,d
4. a,b,c,d
5. a,b,c,d
6. a,c
7. a,b,c,d

8. a,c
9. a,b,c,d
10. a,b,c
11. a,c
12. b,d
13. a,b,c

REFERENCES

Beck, A. Cognitive therapy: Nature and relation to behavior therapy. Behavior Therapy, 1970, 1, 184-200.

Beck, A. T., Rush, A. J., Shaw, B. F., & Emery, G. Cognitive therapy of depression. New York: The Guilford Press, 1980.

Ellis, A. Reason and emotion in psychotherapy. New York: Lyle Stuart Press, 1962.

Frank, J. Persuasion and healing. Baltimore: Johns Hopkins Press, 1961.

Hilgard, E. R., & Bower, G. H. Theories of learning. Englewood Cliffs, N.J.: Prentice Hall, Inc., 1975.

Jacobson, E. Progressive relaxation. Chicago: University of Chicago Press, 1938.

Kelley, G. The psychology of personal constructs (2 vols). New York: Norton, 1955.

Kovacs, M., & Beck, A. T. Maladaptive cognitive structures in depression. The American Journal of Psychiatry, 1978, 135 (5), 525-533.

Luria, A. The role of speech in the regulation of normal and abnormal behaviors. New York: Lineright, 1961.

Luria, A. Speech and formation of mental processes. In M. Cole & I. Maltzman (Eds.), A handbook of contemporary Soviet psychology. New York: Basic Books, 1969.

Meichenbaum, D. The effects of instructions and reinforcement on thinking and language behaviors of schizophrenics. Behavior Research and Therapy, 1969, 7, 101-114.

Olton, D. S., & Noonberg, A.R. Biofeedback: Clinical applications in behavioral medicine. Englewood Cliffs, New Jersey: Prentice-Hall, Inc., 1980.

Singer, J. Imagery and daydream methods in psychotherapy. New York: Academic Press, 1974.

Watson, J. B., & Rayner, R. Conditioned emotional reactions. Journal of Experimental Psychology, 1920, 3, 1-14.

Wolpe, J. Psychotherapy by reciprocal inhibition. Stanford: Stanford University Press, 1958.

SUGGESTED READING

Ayllon, T. & Azrin, N. H. The token economy: A motivational system for therapy and rehabilitation. New York: Appleton-Dentury-Crofts, 1969.

Bandura, A. Principles of behavior modification. New York: Holt, Rinehart and Winston, 1969.

Benjamin, S., Marks, I. M., & Hudson, J. Active muscular relaxation in desensitization of phobic patients. Psychological Medicine, 1972, 2, 381-390.

Celder, M. G., & Marks, I. M. Severe agoraphobia: A controlled prospective trial of behavior therapy. British Journal of Psychiatry, 1966, 112, 309-319.

Hodgson, R., Rachman, S., & Marks, I. M. The treatment of obsessive-compulsive behavior: Follow-up and further findings. Behavior Research and Therapy, 1972, 10, 181-189.

Karasu, T. B. Psychotherapies: An overview. American Journal of Psychiatry, 1977, 134, 851-863.

Lovaas, O. A program for the establishment of speech in psychotic children. In J.K. Wing (Ed.), Early childhood autism. Oxford: Pergamon Press, 1966.

Manning, D. E., & Whipple, S. H. Anorexia nervosa: Commitment to a multi-faceted treatment program. Psychosomatics and Psychotherapy, 1978, 30, 161-169.

Marks, I. M. Phobic disorders four years after treatment: A prospective follow-up. British Journal of Psychiatry, 1971, 118, 683-688.

Marks, I. M. Behavioral treatments of phobic and obsessive-compulsive disorders: A critical appraisal. In M. Hersen, M. Eisler, & P. M. Miller (Eds.), Progress in behavior modification (Vol. 1). New York: Academic Press, 1975.

Mills, H. L., Agras, W. S., Barlow, D. H., & Mills, J. R. Compulsive rituals treated by response prevention. Archives of General Psychiatry, 1973, 28, 524-529.

Rachman, S., Hodgson, R., & Marks, I. M. Treatment of chronic obsessive-compulsive neurosis. Behavior Research and Therapy, 1971, 9, 237-247.

Stunkard, A. New therapies for the eating disorders: Behavior modification of obesity and anorexia nervosa. Archives of General Psychiatry, 1972, 26, 391-395.

CHAPTER 19

Other Treatment Modalities

Philip T. Ninan, M.D.
Alberto B. Santos, M.D.

CHAPTER OUTLINE

LEARNING OBJECTIVES

After completing this chapter, you will be able to:

1. Cite the indications for electroconvulsive therapy.

2. Explain the method of administering ECT.

3. Discuss the effects of ECT and its possible complications.

4. Discuss the legal and ethical issues involved in ECT.

5. Explain the role of psychosurgery in psychiatry.

6. Explain the indications for, complications involved in and mode of using narcotherapy.

7. Discuss the use of hypnosis as an adjunct to psychotherapy.

8. Cite the theoretical principles on which the therapeutic strategy of cognitive therapy is based.

PRE-TEST

For the following questions, <u>one</u> or <u>more</u> <u>than</u> <u>one</u> answer may be correct. Circle the correct answer(s).

1. The indication(s) for ECT include

    a. Anorexia Nervosa.
    b. Schizophrenia, catatonic type.
    c. borderline personality organization.
    d. Major Depressive Disorder.

2. Atropine or Scopolamine is given prior to ECT to

    a. prevent bradycardia and dysrhythmias.
    b. reduce the pharyngeal secretions.
    c. prevent the parasympathetic (cholinergic) inhibition of the SA node caused by the seizure.
    d. potentiate the therapeutic effect of ECT.

3. The effect(s) of ECT include

    a. anterograde and retrograde amnesia which do not persist on objective testing.
    b. sympathetic effects like hypertension and tachycardia resulting from the release of catecholamines from the adrenal medulla.
    c. cerebral anoxia unless the patient is adequately ventilated with oxygen rich mixtures.
    d. increased turnover of central norepinephrine and increased tyrosine hydroxylase activity.

4. A "modified" ECT consists of

    a. cholinergic blockade prior to ECT.
    b. the use of short-acting general anesthetic.
    c. artificial, assisted breathing with oxygen rich mixtures.
    d. the use of succinylcholine to attenuate the skeletal muscular contractions of the seizure.

5. ECT should be given

    a. to violent obnoxious patients who refuse other forms of treatment.
    b. to patients committed to involuntary psychiatric treatment without their consent.
    c. when family members insist on its use even though the patient disagrees.
    d. none of the above.

6. Psychosurgery is

   a. not different from neurosurgery.
   b. a standardized form of psychiatric treatment.
   c. a first line of treatment for Schizophrenia.
   d. useful as a last resort in the treatment of some severe psychiatric disorders.

7. Narcotherapy

   a. uses narcotic drugs alone.
   b. can facilitate abreaction.
   c. is a form of truth serum.
   d. can result in psychotic episodes.

8. Hypnotherapy is

   a. a form of treatment which prominently uses suggestion.
   b. useful only for hysterical patients.
   c. an adjunct to psychotherapy.
   d. useful in patients with minimal brain dysfunction who have problems with sustained attention.

9. All of the following symptoms and signs of depressive illness respond well to ECT except

   a. psychomotor retardation.
   b. anorexia.
   c. pre-morbid maladaptive character traits.
   d. insomnia.
   e. middle of the night awakening.

10. A contraindication for ECT would be

   a. angina pectoris.
   b. brain tumor with raised CSF pressure.
   c. psychosis.
   d. the presence of degenerative dementia.
   e. ulcerative colitis.

11. The patient who might benefit most from ECT would be

   a. a violent patient with a psychotic agitated depression.
   b. a patient with Schizophrenia manifesting delusions of control.
   c. a patient with a stress-related psychosis that is a manifestation or part of a personality disorder.
   d. a patient with a dissociation disorder who is dysfunctional socially and vocationally.
   e. a patient with bulimia and anorexia nervosa.

12. With ECT, which of the following substances is (are) used to prevent bradycardia?

    a. short-acting barbiturates
    b. succinylcholine
    c. sodium pentothal
    d. atropine
    e. norepinephrine agonistic

I. SOMATIC THERAPIES

A. ELECTROCONVULSIVE THERAPY (ECT)

  1. History.
      As early as in the first century bioelectric discharges from the
      electric torpedo fish were used to cure headaches. In the 18th
      century electric shocks and the epileptogenic agent camphor began
      to be used as treatments for mental illness. However, the use of
      convulsive therapy, as a coherent therapeutic agent, began only in
      the early 20th century. Its use was based on the clinical observa-
      tion that patients suffering from mental illness and epilepsy often
      showed an improvement of their mental illness after an epileptic
      seizure. The prevalent theory was that mental illness and epilepsy
      could not coexist. Thus, insulin and other seizure-inducing sub-
      stances such as Metrazol were popularized as effective in producing
      convulsive treatments. Ugo Cerletti, a psychiatric research worker
      studying the effects of seizures on brain tissue in animals, sug-
      gested that electrical methods of inducing seizures were more
      reliable and technically more feasible. In 1938, Cerletti and Bini
      introduced the first electrically induced convulsion to a catatonic
      patient in Rome. Over the next 20 years ECT developed as a major
      tool of psychiatric treatment. With time, ECT became "modified"
      with the introduction of muscle relaxants, short-acting general
      anesthetics, atropine, and artificial, assisted ventilation.
      Initially, ECT was used fairly indiscriminately due to the lack of
      other effective treatment modalities. However, with the coming of
      age of psychopharmacology in the late 1950's and early 1960's, the
      indications for the use of ECT were refined. There are still
      situations where ECT is preferred over psychopharmacology - for
      example in patients suffering from a major depression who also have
      myocardial damage.

  2. Indications.

      a. Major Depressive Disorders.

          (1) Major Depressive Episode.
              Severe depression is the primary indication for ECT.
              Depressions labeled prior to DSM-III as endogenous,
              post-partum and involutional melancholia are particularly
              responsive to ECT. Both the unipolar and bipolar depres-
              sions respond well to ECT. Symptoms which predict a good
              response to ECT (Clare 1979) include early morning awak-
              ening, anorexia with weight loss, a decrease in libido,
              diurnal variation (so called "hypothalamic symptoms"),
              low self-esteem, feelings of worthlessness and hopelessness,
              preoccupation with guilt and suicide, somatic and other
              delusions, and pronounced psychomotor retardation.
              Sudden onset of symptoms, good insight, a pre-morbid
              obsessional personality, self-reproach, and a duration of

illness of less than one year are also favorable features. Hypochondriasis, hysterical features, anxiety, self-pity, and depersonalization are indicators of a poor response to ECT. Depressions of a mild nature (especially those of a reactive kind), dysphoria, and those forms of depression seen in borderline personality organizations are not indications for ECT.

Studies show that 70-85% of patients with severe depression show some response to ECT (versus 60-70% for tricyclic antidepressants and 30% for placebo). Delusional, endogenously depressed patients often fail to respond to an adequate trial of tricyclic antidepressants. Thus, there might exist a specific category of depressed patients who respond primarily to ECT, but no study has yet been able to consistently delineate this population. ECT is especially useful in depressed patients where rapid response is needed (for example, in dangerously suicidal patients). Such response is sometimes seen after one or two ECT procedures. It is also useful in patients with certain cardiac problems which contraindicate tricyclic antidepressants.

(2) Manic Episode.
Though lithium and phenothiazines have largely supplanted the use of ECT in mania, ECT is still useful, especially in severe mania where exhaustion can lead to death.

b. Schizophrenia.
The efficacy of ECT varies with the subgroups of Schizophrenia. In acute Schizophrenia, especially the catatonic variety, and with Schizophrenia with a strong affective component, ECT is particularly useful. Both ECT and neuroleptics are significantly less effective with chronic schizophrenics. Though the concurrent use of major tranquilizers and ECT is widespread, they potentiate each other, both in their therapeutic effects and side effects (especially when strongly anticholinergic neuroleptics are used). Following a course of ECT, neuroleptics may be used effectively to decrease the frequency of relapses. The number of ECT treatments necessary for Schizophrenia is significantly more than those needed for depression.

c. Other Psychiatric Disorders.
ECT has been used in a wide variety of psychiatric conditions including Anorexia Nervosa, severe obsessive compulsive disorders, toxic psychoses, chronic brain syndromes, and in organic brain syndromes. However, in the absence of reliable, valid studies, such treatments are not encouraged. Conditions which clearly do not respond to ECT include personality disorders, addictions, and sexual deviations.

3. Contraindications.
    Since ECT results in a transient rise in cerebrospinal fluid (CSF) pressure, any space-occupying lesion or pre-existing elevation of intracranial pressure is an absolute contraindication for ECT.

    A recent myocardial infarction raises the danger of arrythmias during a seizure.

    Particular care to prevent fractures and dislocations, especially of the spinal column, needs to be taken in patients prone to such effects during a seizure. This can be done by adequate muscle relaxation in patients with spinal pathology.

    Medical conditions which contraindicate general anesthesia can also be considered contraindicated for ECT.

4. Method of Administration.
    The following is a description of a model method of administering ECT suggested by the American Psychiatric Association (APA) by the Task Force on ECT (1978).

    (1) Preparation of the Patient: If the ECT is to be administered early in the morning, the patient is allowed nothing by mouth (NPO) from midnight. If the ECT is scheduled for the afternoon, a light nonsolid breakfast may be allowed. The bladder should be emptied before treatment.

    (2) The patient is placed on a bed adequately insulated to prevent grounding of the current through the patient. Dental appliances are removed if possible.

    (3) A scalp-vein needle is inserted into an accessible vein and taped to the skin. Increments of 0.25 mg Methscopolamine, or 0.5 mg Atropine are injected intravenously until there is a 10% increase in the heart rate. Subcutaneous Atropine may be given 45 minutes prior to ECT instead, but this makes titration of the dose to produce adequate cardiac cholinergic blockade difficult.

    (4) In patients with cardiopulmonary problems, two to three minutes of breathing 100% oxygen may be encouraged prior to the general anesthesia. The anesthetic agent is given intravenously. The dose of the anesthetic agent should be individualized to produce an adequate depth of anesthesia. Ventilation with 100% oxygen is initiated.

    (5) Succinylcholine is now injected in doses of 0.5 to 1.5 mg per kg, until adequate muscle paralysis is obtained.

(6) A mouth gag is put in place. The electrodes are placed on the head for bilateral ECT. Each electrode is placed 1½ inches perpendicularly above the midpoint of the line joining the external auditory meatus and the angle of the eye. For unilateral ECT, both electrodes are placed on the nondominant side of the head. The individual holding the electrodes is protected by suitable insulation and/or rubber or plastic gloves. The electrical stimulus is then administered.

(7) If a therapeutically adequate seizure is not evoked, a greater stimulus may be reapplied after an interval of 60 to 90 seconds.

(8) The mouth gag is removed and the teeth are checked. Secretions in the hypopharynx are removed, and artificial, assisted ventilation is applied until spontaneous respiratory activity occurs. The return of protective pharyngeal reflexes is monitored.

(9) Observation and monitoring of vital signs with attention to adequacy of ventilation during immediate post-treatment is important. Reassurance and reorienting on awakening are helpful. Some patients complain of post-ECT headache which responds to aspirin.

For depression, a course of 6 to 10 ECTs is usually adequate. These can be given three times per week. Response is most often seen after the first few treatments, with initial response seen in somatic symptoms, followed by an improvement in the mood and social behavior.

5. Effects of ECT.

    a. Neuropsychiatric or Central Effects.

        (1) EEG Changes.
            The immediate effect of ECT is a change in the EEG from the desynchronized resting pattern to a high amplitude synchronized pattern. Seizures are initiated in the central part of the brain and spread toward the cortices and the periphery. Following ECT, there are slow wave changes in the EEG pattern, though this varies with individuals and with the number and frequency of ECT procedures. The post-ECT EEG patterns have not been consistently correlated with therapeutic effects.

        (2) Cerebral Metabolic Changes.
            Following ECT, there is a rapid increase in cerebral blood flow, chiefly the result of a transient systemic hypertension. Metabolic changes in the brain correlate with the presence or absence of hypoxia. If hypoxia is present,

there is a marked reduction in brain ATP and phospho-creatine with an accumulation of lactate, signifying a shift to anaerobic metabolism. Such changes are not observed with ECT when adequate ventilation, especially with oxygen-rich mixtures, is provided. Since hypoxia could possibly aggravate amnesia and confusion and could potentially cause cardiac arrhythmias, proper ventilation during ECT is crucial.

Other changes which take place include a transient raising of intracranial pressure and increase in the permeability of the blood-brain barrier. No neuropathological changes have been systematically documented as a result of modified ECT.

(3) Effects on Neurotransmitters.
ECT results in an increased turnover of brain norepineph-rine and increase in tyrosine hydroxylase activity. There is longer-lasting increase in brain monoamine oxidase activity lasting for several weeks.

(4) Memory.
There is an acute amnestic state following ECT which is in some ways similar to that seen following a grand mal seizure, Korsakoff's syndrome, and with pathology in the hippocampal and diencephalic areas. There are two components to the amnesia - an impairment in new learning capacity, or anterograde amnesia, and an impairment in recalling events prior to the ECT, or retrograde amnesia.

Following a course of ECT (up to 15 ECTs), the antero-grade amnesia generally recovers within 4 to 6 weeks. Anterograde amnesia, for both verbal and nonverbal memory, appears to be less with unilateral than with bilateral ECT.

On objective testing, the retrograde amnesia following a course of ECT varies. Events which happened within a day or two of the ECT may be permanently forgotten. Memory for some events within the past one or two years may be lost, though this does not seem permanent. Loss of memory for events which happened a number of years prior to ECT seems to recover spontaneously.

Going by the subjective reports of long-lasting amnesia, there is a greater incidence of such amnesia reported following bilateral ECT than unilateral ECT. That these reports are not substantiated on objective testing might be due to the sensitivity of the tests used or due to the subjective sensitization to memory functioning as a result of ECT such that awareness of normal forgetting is increased.

(5) Psychological Reactions.
Undoubtedly, a number of patients experience the ECT treatment procedure as stressful. It is crucial that empathic support be provided and every effort be made to explicitly deal with both the realistic and unrealistic fears of the patient regarding the procedure.

b. Peripheral Effects of ECT.

(1) Parasympathetic Effects.
The peripheral spread of the seizure across the parasympathetic system can cause bradycardia and occasional asystole, unless this effect is blocked by the prior administration of atropine or scopolamine. Vagal inhibition of the S.A. node can lead to the pacemaker activity being usurped by the A.V. node or other ectopic foci which are not under parasympathetic inhibition.

(2) Effects on the Sympathetic System and the Adrenal Medulla.
The peripheral effects of the seizure on the sympathetic nerves result in release of norepinephrine in the heart and catecholamines from the adrenal medulla. These neurotransmitters cause hypertension (average increase of 50 to 100 mm of mercury) and tachycardia (average increase of 20 to 50 beats per minute). These effects rapidly return to normal within 5 minutes. These effects can be blocked by adrenergic blocking agents and with ganglionic blockers.

(3) Hypothalamic-Pituitary and Adrenal Cortical Effects.
There is increase in prolactin, growth hormone, ACTH, and cortical steroid levels following seizures.

c. Possible Adverse Reactions to ECT.

(1) Cardiac arrhythmias and arrest are possible complications of ECT. Death as the result of ECT happens to 1 in 10,000 patients, mostly due to cardiac compromise.

(2) Significant complications are possible with any of the drugs used during ECT. Atropine can cause a toxic delirium because of its ability to cross the blood-brain barrier. This condition is observed most frequently in elderly patients and those already on drugs with strong anticholinergic activity. Scopolamine, a quarternary anticholinergic, does not cross the blood-brain barrier and, therefore, is safer.

(3) Anaphylactic reactions to thiopental (Pentothal) and methohexital (Brevital) have been documented. The danger of pharyngeal spasm exists with the light level of anesthesia used in ECT.

(4) Succinylcholine is hydrolized by pseudocholinesterase in the plasma, thus limiting its action to around 5 minutes. But, pseudocholinesterase activity is affected by drugs used for myasthenia gravis, insecticides, and by genetic factors. Lithium might prolong the activity of succinylcholine. Pseudocholinesterase hydrolyzing activity can be measured in the laboratory prior to ECT if necessary.

(5) The development of epileptic seizures following "modified" ECT has been rarely reported in the literature. However, their incidence is no greater than that of the development of idiopathic epilepsy.

6. Theories on Mechanism of Action.
An explanation of how ECT works has been limited by the knowledge of the etiology of the disorder it treats. Thus, in the early days of ECT, theories stressed psychological and interpersonal mechanisms alone. More recently, the theories have moved to encompass the biological arena, as well as the psychological and social. Thus, therapeutic response may be related to alteration of the permeability of the blood-brain barrier, neuroendocrine changes, neurotransmitter-receptor alterations, and electrophysiologic mechanisms of the centrencephalic structures. It is known that the actual seizure is necessary for therapeutic effects. Sham ECTs and subthreshold shocks have failed to bring response in patients. Further, since a greater number of treatments is necessary in Schizophrenia than in depression and their efficacy is less in Schizophrenia, the mode of action of ECT probably differs in the two. Maintenance ECT (roughly once a month) is often found to be useful by some clinicians. Any theory of action of ECT must be able to explain this clinical observation.

7. Ethical and Legal Issues.
There are complex social, ethical, and legal issues surrounding the use of ECT. Increasing medical knowledge, politics, attitudes towards mental illness, and economic factors are often uncomfortably intertwined and do not automatically lead to the provision of optimum treatment for the patient. At the outset of this discussion, certain points need to made clear.

(1) ECT is an effective, acceptable though controversial, safe, and at times life-saving form of treatment.

(2) The provision of unmodified ECT today should be considered poor medical practice and should invite little toleration among both professionals and laymen.

(3) Since there are no proper studies looking at the effects of ECT on the developing brain, there are almost no situations when its use in children and adolescents is justified.

(4) To put things in perspective, the vast majority of patients who are treated with ECT receive it on a voluntary basis with informed consent and do not have any concomitant problems.

The major issue involved in a legal sense is the patient's <u>right to treatment</u> and his <u>right to refuse treatment</u>. There is also the question of whether the patient is <u>competent</u> to make the decision about his treatment, and this is often complicated in situations where the hospitalization or psychiatric treatment is on an involuntary basis.

The issue of the right to refuse treatment is dealt with within the framework of informed consent. Informed consent is the procedure whereby the treatment is adequately explained with its indications, procedure, possible side effects, and alternatives to the patient by an appropriate member of the treatment team. Adequate opportunity should be provided for questions to be raised, fears to be discussed and anxieties to be allayed. However, a number of issues revolve around the concept of informed consent. There are no adequate studies looking at the amount of factual information about ECT which is picked up by the patient through this procedure. There is the question of the statistical level of incidence of a particular side effect which must be present before it is included within the information provided. Does the information about possible side effects have a suggestive value and increase the incidence of side effects? How realistic is the expectation that any patient would consent to the procedure in view of the barrage of information about possible side effects, especially those related to memory deficits? How can a consent form valid for today cater to the changing social values of tomorrow? To what extent is the authoritative figure of the physician felt as a form of pressure by the patient to agree with the treatment procedure? Does the patient fear some fantasized negative reaction from the physician should he reject ECT? What guidelines should be provided to the physician to withdraw from the care of his patient if he feels that his therapeutic capacity has been neutralized by the patient's refusal for ECT? Obviously, many of these questions can be asked in reference to other forms of medical treatment.

From the point of view of the right to treatment, an interesting question can be raised. Since ECT is a safe and effective treatment modality, is it appropriate for the doctor to withhold the treatment when the patient's refusal to consent is more related to his primary pathology than to an objective evaluation?

Competence in psychiatry is an issue which is further complicated where ECT is concerned. Who makes the decision that the patient should be labeled incompetent? If the patient is incompetent, who makes the decision about whether he should or should not receive

ECT? If this should be members of his family, what is their investment in the patient? How often do their emotions, especially anger towards the patient, prevent them from making a valid decision? How practical is it to involve lengthy legal procedures when time is the essence of the issue?

A number of authors have pointed out the dangerous trend of legalistic and civil rights issues encroaching on the doctor-patient relationships. This changing of the doctor-patient role from supportive to oppositional is conducive to good legal care, but poor medical practice. In different states, legal procedures and legislative statutes have been used to restrict or make it difficult to practice ECT. This is an unfortunate state of affairs, especially since court rulings have usually been under emotionally laden climates related to the negligent use of ECT, rather than the objective evaluation of "modified" ECT by itself.

The APA Task Force on Electroconvulsive Therapy (1978) has noted, "Neither the complex nature of mental illnesses itself nor the attitudes of society permit simple and rapid remedies. In attempting to dissolve mental illness in behavioral and sociocultural theories, the modern critic has paid little attention to the pervasive and stubborn nature of severe interpersonal psychopathology and the suggestive evidence that at least some aspects of mental disorders spring from biological factors as yet poorly understood." (p. 135). Following are the recommendations of the APA Task Force on ECT with regards to ethical and legal matters.

(1) In situations where the patient is competent and consents to ECT, procedures should allow the patient to have the treatment within the context of the doctor-patient relationship, and without interference from others.

(2) Competent patients who refuse consent should not be treated. The psychiatrist should have the option of withdrawing from the case and the patient be transferred to the care of another psychiatrist.

(3) In the case of incompetent patients who are not capable of providing informed consent or do not protest the use of ECT, the psychiatrist should consult family members who in the best interest of the patient should make the decision. Informed consent from such relatives should be considered within the spirit of the doctrine of informed consent.

(4) In incompetent or involuntary patients who protest the use of ECT, legal representation and the court should be used to decide whether ECT is to be used or not.

```
******************************************************************

                        GO TO VIDEOTAPE

******************************************************************
```

B. PSYCHOSURGERY

1. Definition.
    The U.S. National Commission for the Protection of Human Subjects of Biomedical and Behavioral Research (1977) has defined psychosurgery as brain surgery on (a) normal brain tissue of an individual who does not suffer from any physical disease for the purpose of changing or controlling the behavior or emotions of such individual, or (b) diseased brain tissue of an individual if the primary object of the performance of such surgery is to control, change, or affect any behavioral or emotional disturbance of such individual.

    The results of psychosurgery have been disappointing on the whole, though some patients have responded dramatically. Adequate studies looking at patient selection, exact surgical lesion, and their effects are scarce. A variety of opinions exists among the leaders in the field of psychosurgery as to its indications. Therefore, it is most appropriate to look upon psychosurgery presently as (1) an alternative in some severe intractible conditions where all efforts at treatment and rehabilitation have failed, and (2) an experimental procedure.

2. Indications.
    The indications for psychosurgery are not absolute. Decisions need to be made on an individual basis. Psychosurgery should never be attempted as a first line of treatment. If psychotherapy, psychopharmacology, and if indicated, ECT, have all failed to achieve their goal, then psychosurgery may be considered in patients suffering from severe disturbances of mood. The greater the intensity and the more persistent the symptoms, the more appropriate it is to consider psychosurgery as an alternative. Phobias, chronic anxiety states, obsessive compulsive behavior all of a crippling nature, and marked, intractible depressions are possible indications for psychosurgery. Psychosurgery is considered much more controversial for Schizophrenia, obesity, aggressiveness, and assaultive behavior. It is not useful in psychopaths, alcoholics, drug addicts, and patients with diffuse brain damage or sexual deviants.

3. Method.
    Surgery involving the frontal lobes was initially the most popular, but with improved techniques other areas are being studied. Precise stereotactic instruments, using among other things, radio waves, freezing, electrocautery, radioisotopes, proton beams, ultrasound and thermocoagulation, have moved psychosurgery to a more exact science from the blind days of the leucotome. It has been found that lesioning of the amygdala is at times useful for

patients with unprovoked assaultive behavior. Lesioning of the medial limbic circuit is useful in psychic hyperactivity states and severe obsessive compulsive behavior. Lesioning of the lateral limbic circuit is useful in depression, perceptual, and hallucinatory disturbances.

C. NARCOTHERAPY

Cole and Davis defined narcotherapy as the "use of an intravenous injection of a drug, that may facilitate the uncovering of emotionally laden material in psychotherapy" (Cole & Davis, 1975, p. 1968).

Narcotherapy can be used to facilitate abreaction. The only therapeutic effect such an experience has is related to ventilation and to the subsequent working through of the experience so that it can be integrated into the rest of the personality. Such an effect is not the psychotropic effect of the drug, per se. The drug is only a facilitator of the experience by allowing the patient to enter into a state of consciousness whereby defenses are diminished and such processes are available for expression.

Narcotherapy is useful in situations in which affectively loaded material is not available to conscious memory, in which the energy which is locked up in forgetting the affectively loaded material needs to be released. There are potential dangers inherent in such a rapid unlocking of emotionally painful memories which have been defensively and actively repressed.

Narcotherapy should be employed only in the presence of a comfortable alliance with and trust in the therapist, and with a good understanding of the ego structure and ego capacity of the patient.

The most widely used narcotherapeutic agent is sodium pentothal which is given as a slow intravenous injection, the dosage varying with each individual (usually 0.25-0.5 gm). The patient is asked to count backwards from 100, and at the point where the patient is fading off into a drowsy state the injection is stopped and the patient is asked very direct questions in an authoritarian, but empathic manner. Some clinicians advocate the use of psychostimulants, like methylphenidate (25-40 mg), either alone or in addition to sodium pentothal. Narcotherapy is not the equivalent of a truth serum, though such fantasies in the patient might be associated with greater successes.

Sodium pentothal injections can also be used as: 1) a diagnostic tool in differentiating a catatonic state from a depression with severe psychomotor retardation (the depressed patient would tend to fall asleep while the catatonic patient would go through a phase when he might be able to communicate), 2) a method of facilitating speech with mute psychotic patients, and 3) an aid in differentiating organic from functional conditions (Santos et al., 1980). Essentially, in organic conditions where only subtle symptoms are present, small doses of sodium pentothal would tend to release grosser symptoms, whereas in functional conditions there may be elaboration of historical material and improvement in cognitive testing. The dangers of narcotherapy include its use in paranoid or pre-psychotic patients where the involuntary breakdown of defenses can result in a psychotic episode. Intravenous use of sodium pentothal can also lead to laryngeal spasm and death. Therefore, appropriate prophylaxis and availability of emergency measures are crucial.

QUIZ, Section I.

Circle the correct answer(s). One or more than one answer may be correct.

1. Which of the following statements is (are) true concerning ECT?

   a. With pre-existing raised CSF pressure, there is likelihood of cerebral herniation with ECT.
   b. ECT should not be given in patients with a potential for skeletal fractures.
   c. ECT is less safe than tricyclic antidepressants in patients with myocardial damage.

2. Which of the following is (are) not an effect(s) of ECT?

   a. The post-ECT changes in the EEG fall into a definite pattern and are valuable predictors of therapeutic outcome.
   b. Adequate assisted ventilation during ECT procedure prevents the danger of hypoxia in the brain.
   c. There is a short-term increase in the turnover of brain norepinephrine following ECT.
   d. A transient retrograde and anterograde amnesia is often seen on objective testing with ECT.

3. The theories on the mechanism of action of ECT

   a. include psychological, interpersonal and biological theories which attempt to explain the therapeutic effects of ECT.
   b. hypothesize that a seizure is not essential for the therapeutic effect of ECT as sham ECTs are as effective.
   c. claim that depression requires a lesser number of ECTs than Schizophrenia.

4. Psychosurgery is

   a. brain surgery on normal or diseased brain tissue when emotional, cognitive, or behavioral disturbance of a marked and intractable nature exists.
   b. a last alternative in severe psychopathology when other treatments have failed.
   c. a form of treatment in psychopaths and sexual deviants.

TRUE or FALSE: Circle the correct letter.

T F 5. Electrical currents in one form or another have been used in medical practice for nearly two thousand years.

T   F   6.   Initially, convulsive therapies were used under the belief that epilepsy and mental illness could not co-exist.

T   F   7.   The use of ECT declined with the availability of psychotropic medications.

T   F   8.   Therapeutic convulsions are induced today by electrical shocks under general anesthesia and muscle relaxants.

T   F   9.   The indications for ECT include Major Affective Disorders and Schizophrenia.

T   F   10.   Anorexia, insomnia, diurnal variation, and pronounced psychomotor retardation are symptoms which respond well to ECT.

T   F   11.   Schizophrenia usually requires a lesser number of ECTs than major depression for a therapeutic response.

T   F   12.   Sociopathic personality, sexual deviations, and borderline personality organization are indications for ECT.

T   F   13.   The concurrent use of psychotropic medications with ECT often accentuates neuropsychological side effects.

T   F   14.   Scopolamine is a quarternary compound which does not cross the blood-brain barrier.

T   F   15.   Scopolamine is safer than atropine because it does not cause anticholinergic delirium.

T   F   16.   Succinylcholine's action is limited to 5-7 minutes because it is rapidly hydrolyzed by plasma pseudocholinesterase.

T   F   17.   Post-ECT headaches are remarkably unresponsive to treatment.

From legal and ethical points of view the following are true or false:

T   F   18.   Unmodified ECT is still an acceptable form of treatment.

T   F   19.   There is little justification in the provision of ECT for adolescents and children.

T   F   20.   The vast majority of patients who receive ECT are competent and consent to the treatment voluntarily.

T   F   21.   Incompetent patients should receive ECT if their physician believes it is in their best interests.

T   F   22.   The concept of informed consent is ultimately a relative issue to be looked at within the doctor-patient relationship and within the larger arena of social factors.

T   F   23.   Competent patients who refuse ECT should not be given ECT.

Concerning Narcotherapy:

T F 24. Narcotherapy is both a diagnostic and therapeutic tool.

T F 25. Sodium pentothal is the most commonly used narcotherapeutic agent.

T F 26. Narcotherapy is a useful facilitator of catharsis.

II. HYPNOSIS AND HYPNOTHERAPY

A. HISTORY

Hypnosis as it is known today had its roots with Mesmer (1734-1815) who related the phenomenon to "animal magnetism," a force which he felt radiated from his hands. James Braid (1795-1860) coined the term hypnosis from the Greek word "hypnos" meaning sleep, and pointed out the importance of suggestion. Jean Charcot (1825-1893), a prominent French neurologist, proposed that hypnosis was a pathological condition linked to hysteria. Charcot's practice of hypnosis attracted, among others, Freud and Janet. However, it was Liebeault (1823-1904) who advanced hypnosis from the field of mysticism to science and left it with the indelible mark of psychology. Hypnosis came to age with its usage in World War II to treat traumatic states, and the post-World War II years saw a burgeoning of scientific societies and journals on hypnosis the world over. Today, it attracts an impressive following, both in the clinical field and in laboratory research.

B. DEFINITION AND CHARACTERISTICS

Speigel (1975) defined hypnosis as "an altered state of intense and sensitive interpersonal relatedness between hypnotist and patient, characterized by the patient's nonrational submission and relative abandonment of executive control to a more or less regressed, disassociated state" (p. 1843).

Some of the important characteristics of hypnosis as noted by Hilgard (1965) are:

1) Subsidence of the planning function in which the patient has the capacity for voluntary action, but finds little desire to take an action.

2) Redistribution of attention whereby the patient appears to concentrate selectively on limited stimuli or selectively disregards certain stimuli.

3) Availability of visual memories from the past and heightened ability of fantasy production. This capacity allows age regression, dream-like states, and hallucinations.

4) Reduction in reality testing and a tolerance for persistent reality distortion. This is analogous to the psychoanalytic concept of primary-process thinking.

5) Increased suggestibility is a core element of hypnosis and some authors declare all states of increased suggestibility are hypnotic in nature.

6) Role behavior is the capacity of the hypnotized subject to adopt a suggested role and play out complex activities within that role.

7) Amnesia for what transpired within the hypnotic state, though not an essential ingredient of hypnosis, is characteristic of deep hypnotic states and is often termed "somnambulistic." Amnesia can be actively removed by suggestion while under hypnosis. Subjects who reach this depth of hypnosis show an interesting phenomenon termed post-hypnotic compliance wherein, due to hypnotic suggestion, the subject at a pre-arranged signal feels compelled to carry out an act which he rationalizes.

C. CAPACITY FOR HYPNOSIS

The capacity for hypnosis is accepted as a relatively stable characteristic of the personality. It is either biologically determined or developed at an early age. The quickest way to test the hypnotic ability of a subject is to ask him to gaze upwards while holding his head straight, and slowly close his eyelids (Speigel, 1975). The greater the amount of sclera seen below the cornea, the greater the hypnotic ability. This is graded from 0 to 4, with 4 being the highest level of hypnotizability. However, this test has a 25% false-positive rate. Roughly 50% of the rest fall in grades 2 and 3. The capacity for hypnosis does not vary with gender--men are as hypnotizable as women. Children are more susceptible to hypnotism than adults, the peak years being between 8 and 12. There is possibly some mild decline in hypnotic ability with age. The hypnotic ability of patients with different psychiatric diagnoses is still debated. No diagnosis precludes hypnosis, nor is hypnotic ability a criteria for any diagnostic label. It would be expected that problems with sustained concentration would effect the hypnotic susceptibility.

D. MODE OF HYPNOTIC INDUCTION

Hypnotic induction is the transition from the normal state of consciousness to the hypnotic state. This can be achieved through various techniques under conditions conducive to relaxation. The subject can be asked to stare at an object, a metronome, gaze upwards, sway back and forth, hold his arm up, and any number of such procedures which require concentrated attention. With selective attention screening out other stimuli, there develops a disassociated state with blurring of ego-boundaries. The hypnotist merges with the subject's perception of the self. The depth of the state from a light trance to a deep somnambulistic state varies in the same subject from time to time and even within the same hypnotic episode.

1. a,b	10. T	19. T	
2. a	11. F	20. T	
3. a,c	12. F	21. F	
4. a,b	13. T	22. T	
5. T	14. T	23. T	
6. T	15. T	24. T	
7. T	16. T	25. T	
8. T	17. F	26. T	
9. T	18. F		

E. HYPNOSIS IN PSYCHOTHERAPY

Hypnosis has a specific place in psychotherapy. It is not a form of therapy by itself, but an adjunct to it. It must be used only by a therapist trained both in psychotherapy and hypnosis and within the context of the therapist-patient relationship.

Hypnosis used in psychotherapy has the capacity to reduce the length of the therapeutic intervention. Like dreams and free association, hypnosis can be another means of exploring the unconscious. It is often the most dramatic nonpharmacological tranquilizer available in the therapist's repertoire. It has the capacity to relax, directly relieve some symptoms and moderate the effects of others, and thus facilitate their investigation. Hypnosis is useful in the interpretation of symbolic material. It can have a hyperamnesic effect, especially with affectively loaded material.

Hypnosis is an altered state of consciousness which is very closely related to the personality and the intrapsychic processes of the person being hypnotized. The hypnotist is a facilitator and a means to get to these processes. However, because of the blurring of ego-boundaries and the hypersuggestibility of the state, subtle innuendoes by and expectations of the hypnotist can be incorporated into the experience of the patient. The transference relationship is intensified and contracted over time and can easily be dealt with inappropriately by the lesser-trained and inexperienced therapist. The hypnotist should perceive himself as an inducer, a guide, a facilitator, and an objective observer who should have the capacity to creatively innovate as novel situations arise.

It is important to recognize the nature of the transference relationship that develops within hypnosis. Since the roots of hypnotism lie in mysticism, and it has been only in the last century or so that it has entered the realms of science, this is often reflected within the transference feelings. The therapist is given the power, more of a wizard than that of a healer. Such fantasies of omnipotence can easily be incorporated into the fantasies of the hypnotist himself, thus possibly restricting the amplitude of clinical judgment.

F.   STRATEGIES OF HYPNOTHERAPY

Projection is an important mechanism in hypnotherapy. By placing the patient in a projective or hypothetical situation, the patient is encouraged to allow or magnify feeling states and mental imagery which are to some extent suppressed by cognition and social expectations. Age regression, whereby the patient regresses to an earlier stage of development, has always been a core therapeutic element in analytic and experiential forms of psychotherapy. Hypnosis is a useful tool to augment and intensify this regression. It helps focus on the actual surroundings of the critical period or traumatic experience and intensifies the affect associated with the experience. A useful way of doing this is to look back on prominent memories of the patient or to use an affective bridge, whereby the patient is asked to picture or think of a previous occasion when he experienced the same emotions. This may have a ventilatory or cathartic effect, apart from giving him better cognitive understanding and relating the experiences of his past to his present and specifically to his problems. If the emotion is too threatening, the patient can be asked to picture the scene on a television set so that he is somewhat removed from the experience. This kind of a cathartic experience may free emotional energy tangled within the previous conflict. It also allows patients some feelings of control over situations which might have happened at a time when they lacked that control. The patient can also be asked to project into the future and paint a picture of the way he would like to perceive himself in the future as a way of experiencing what life would be like without the problems which presently preoccupy him.

Hypnosis is most prominently used by behavioral and cognitive therapists where the emphasis is on removal of symptoms. Since direct suggestion for the removal of symptoms is ineffective, indirect suggestions can be used to clear the symptoms gradually. One mechanism is by initially moving the symptom from one part of the body to another through hypnotic suggestion. This gives the patient a feeling that he is in control of the symptom and gives him the option of giving up the symptom once he is ready to do so. If the patient complains of pain, the nature of the pain can be altered initially through hypnosis.

Physiological measures thought to be "involuntary" can be altered under hypnosis. As in biofeedback, hypnosis has been used to show that the autonomic nervous system can at least partially come under voluntary control. Thus, blood pressure, pulse rate, and muscle spasms, among others, have been shown to be altered through conscious control. There are a number of reports of hypnosis having been dramatically helpful in psychosomatic illnesses. The exact physiological mechanism of how hypnosis works in such cases is not known.

In conclusion, hypnosis has had a checkered career in psychiatry. Though at times it has promised much, it has often fallen short in delivery. However, a great deal of research is presently being done which might help illuminate the process by which hypnosis actually functions.

****

GO TO VIDEOTAPE

****

QUIZ, Section II.

Circle the correct answer(s). <u>One</u> or <u>more</u> <u>than</u> <u>one</u> answer may be correct.

1.   The characteristic(s) of hypnosis include

    a.   reduction in reality testing capacity.
    b.   selective concentration of attention on limited stimuli.
    c.   somnambulistic behavior with post-hypnotic compliance.
    d.   lack of a desire for voluntary action.
    e.   all of the above.

2.   Hypnosis is

    a.   a form of psychotherapy by itself.
    b.   a means of exploring the unconscious.
    c.   unrelated to the transference situation.
    d.   induced by the partial blurring of ego-boundaries.

3.   Hypnosis is

    a.   a useful tool in learning some control of the autonomic nervous system functions.
    b.   conducive to age-regression.
    c.   a prominent cathartic tool.

TRUE or FALSE: Circle the correct letter.

T   F   4.   Women are more hypnotizable than men.

T   F   5.   The capacity for hypnotizability is a relatively stable characteristic with some deterioration with age.

T   F   6.   Hysterical patients are more hypnotizable than patients with other diagnoses.

T   F   7.   Patients with attention disorders are less hypnotizable.

T   F   8.   The peak years of hypnotizability are between 8 and 12.

ANSWERS,   Section II._____

1.   e
2.   b, d
3.   a, b, c
4.   F
5.   T
6.   F
7.   T
8.   T

POST-TEST

For the following questions, <u>one</u> or <u>more</u> <u>than</u> <u>one</u> answer may be correct. Circle the correct answer(s).

1.   The indication(s) for ECT include

    a.   Anorexia Nervosa.
    b.   Schizophrenia, catatonic type.
    c.   borderline personality organization.
    d.   Major Depressive Disorder.

2.   The effect(s) of ECT include

    a.   anterograde and retrograde amnesia which does not persist on objective testing.
    b.   sympathetic effects like hypertension and tachycardia resulting from the release of catecholamines from the adrenal medulla.
    c.   cerebral anoxia unless the patient is adequately ventilated with oxygen rich mixtures.
    d.   increased turnover of central norepinephrine and increased tyrosine hydroxylase activity.

3.   ECT should be given

    a.   to violent obnoxious patients who refuse other forms of treatment.
    b.   to patients committed to involuntary psychiatric treatment without their consent.
    c.   when family members insist on its use even though the patient disagrees.
    d.   none of the above.

4.   All of the following symptoms and signs of depressive illness respond well to ECT <u>except</u>

    a.   psychomotor retardation.
    b.   anorexia.
    c.   pre-morbid maladaptive character traits.
    d.   insomnia.
    e.   middle of the night awakening.

5.   A "modified" ECT consists of

    a.   cholinergic blockade prior to ECT.
    b.   the use of short-acting general anesthetic.
    c.   artificial, assisted breathing with oxygen rich mixtures.
    d.   the use of succinylcholine to attenuate the skeletal muscular contractions of the seizure.

6.   Atropine or Scopolamine is given prior to ECT to

      a. prevent bradycardia and dysrhythmias.
      b. reduce the pharyngeal secretions.
      c. prevent the parasympathetic (cholinergic) inhibition of the SA node
          caused by the seizure.
      d. potentiate the therapeutic effect of ECT.

7.   A contraindication for ECT would be

      a. angina pectoris.
      b. brain tumor with raised CSF pressure.
      c. psychosis.
      d. the presence of degenerative dementia.
      e. ulcerative colitis.

8. . The patient who might benefit most from ECT would be

      a. a violent patient with a psychotic agitated depression.
      b. a patient with Schizophrenia manifesting delusions of control.
      c. a patient with a stress-related psychosis that is a manifestation or
          part of a personality disorder.
      d. a patient with a dissociation disorder who is dysfunctional socially
          and vocationally.
      e. a patient with bulimia and anorexia nervosa.

9.   With ECT, which of the following substances is (are) used to prevent
      bradycardia?

      a. short-acting barbiturates
      b. succinylcholine
      c. sodium pentothal
      d. atropine
      e. norepinephrine agonistic

10.   Psychosurgery is

      a. not different from neurosurgery.
      b. a standardized form of psychiatric treatment.
      c. a first line of treatment for Schizophrenia.
      d. useful as a last resort in the treatment of some severe psychiatric
          disorders.

11.   Narcotherapy

      a. uses narcotic drugs alone.
      b. can facilitate abreaction.
      c. is a form of truth serum.
      d. can result in psychotic episodes.

12. Hypnotherapy is

    a. a form of treatment which prominently uses suggestion.
    b. useful only for hysterical patients.
    c. an adjunct to psychotherapy.
    d. useful in patients with minimal brain dysfunction who have problems with sustained attention.

PRE-TEST ANSWERS

1. b,d
2. a,b,c
3. a,b,c,d
4. a,b,c,d
5. d
6. d

7. b,d
8. a,c
9. c
10. b
11. a
12. d

POST-TEST ANSWERS

1. b,d
2. a,b,c,d
3. d
4. c
5. a,b,c,d
6. a,b,c

7. b
8. a
9. d
10. d
11. b,d
12. a,c

REFERENCES

Clare, A. Psychosurgery and electroconvulsive therapy. In P. Hill, R. Murray, & A. Thorley (Eds.), Essentials of postgraduate psychiatry. New York: Grune and Stratton, Inc., 1979.

Cole, J. O., & Davis, J. M. Narcotherapy. In A. M. Freedman, H. I. Kaplan, & B.J. Sadock (Eds.), Comprehensive textbook of psychiatry (2nd ed.). Baltimore: Williams and Wilkins Co., 1975, 1968-1969.

Electroconvulsive therapy (Task Force Report No. 14). Washington, D.C.: American Psychiatric Association, September 1978.

Hilgard, E. R. The experience of hypnosis. New York: Harcourt, Brace, and World, Inc. 1965.

Santos, A., Manning, D., Waldrop W. Delirium or psychosis? Diagnostic use of the sodium amabarbital interview. Psychosomatics, 1980, Vol. 21, 863-864.

Speigel, H. Hypnosis: An adjunct to psychotherapy. In A. M. Freedman, H. I. Kaplan, & B. J. Sadock (Eds.), Comprehensive textbook of psychiatry (2nd ed.). Baltimore: Williams and Wilkins Co., 1975, 1843-1850.

U.S. National Commission for the Protection of Human Subjects of Biomedical and Behavioral Research, 1977. Report and Recommendations: Psychosurgery U.S. DHEW Publ. No. (OS) 77-0001.

APPENDIX A

ADJUSTMENT DISORDER

The DSM-III lists eight types of Adjustment Disorders. These disorders are related directly to psychosocial stressors in that a specific Adjustment Disorder is seen as a maladaptive response to the stressor.

The diagnostic criteria for Adjustment Disorder are:

A. A maladaptive reaction to an identifiable psychosocial stressor, that occurs within three months of the onset of the stressor

B. The maladaptive nature of the reaction is indicated by either of the following:

   (1) impairment in social or occupational functioning
   (2) symptoms that are in excess of a normal and expectable reaction to the stressor

C. The disturbance is not merely one instance of a pattern of overreaction to stress or an exacerbation of one of the mental disorders previously described.

D. It is assumed that the disturbance will eventually remit after the stressor ceases or, if the stressor persists, when a new level of adaptation is achieved.

E. The disturbance does not meet the criteria for any of the specific disorders listed previously or for Uncomplicated Bereavement.

   The eight types of Adjustment Disorder are:

   Adjustment Disorder with Depressed Mood (309.00)

   Adjustment Disorder with Anxious Mood (309.24)

   Adjustment Disorder with Mixed Emotional Features (309.28)

   Adjustment Disorder with Disturbance of Conduct (309.30)

   Adjustment Disorder with Mixed Disturbance of Emotions and Conduct (309.40)

   Adjustment Disorder with Work (or Academic) Inhibition (309.23)

   Adjustment Disorder with Withdrawal (309.83)

   Adjustment Disorder with Atypical Features (309.90)

For more detail regarding Adjustment Disorder, see pages 299-302 of the DSM-III.

APPENDIX B

V CODES

In some instances, persons seek and receive assistance for conditions which do not fit the criteria of a standard DSM-III diagnosis. The DSM-III (1980) lists "V Codes for Conditions Not Attributable to a Mental Disorder That Are a Focus of Attention or Treatment" (p. 331). These are adapted from the ICD-9-CM.

The V Codes may be used appropriately when no mental disorder is found; when evaluative information is not yet adequate to make a diagnosis; or when a mental disorder is present, but the focus of attention or treatment is on a condition which is not due to the disorder. In the DSM-III the following V Codes are listed:

V65.20	Malingering
V62.89	Borderline Intellectual Functioning
V71.01	Adult Antisocial Behavior
V71.02	Childhood or Adolescent Antisocial Behavior
V62.30	Academic Problem
V62.20	Occupational Problem
V62.82	Uncomplicated Bereavement
V15.81	Noncompliance with Medical Treatment
V62.89	Phase of Life Problem or Other Life Circumstances Problem
V61.10	Marital Problem
V61.80	Other Specified Family Circumstances
V62.81	Other Interpersonal Problems

For further information regarding the use of these categories, see pages 331-334 of the DSM-III.